HEALTH

THE BASICS

REBECCA J. DONATELLE

MOORPARK EDITION

Taken from:
Health: The Basics, Eighth Edition
by Rebecca J. Donatelle

Custom Publishing

New York   Boston   San Francisco
London   Toronto   Sydney   Tokyo   Singapore   Madrid
Mexico City   Munich   Paris   Cape Town   Hong Kong   Montreal

**Pearson
Custom Publishing**
is a division of

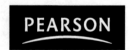

www.pearsonhighered.com   ISBN 10: 0-558-36453-5
                                 ISBN 13: 978-0-558-36453-3

BRIEF CONTENTS

CONTENTS

Part Four: Building Healthy Lifestyles

9 Nutrition: Eating for Optimum Health   250

10 Managing Your Weight: Finding a Healthy Balance   287

11 Personal Fitness: Improving Health Through Exercise   320

Part Five: Preventing and Fighting Disease

12 Cardiovascular Disease, Diabetes, and Cancer: Reducing Your Risk   346

13 Infectious and Noninfectious Conditions: Risks and Responsibilities   383

Health Education

The objective of the Health Education major is the development and education of students in preparation for professional careers in a variety of health fields. The curricula, based upon a foundation in the liberal arts and the natural and behavioral sciences, are directed to special preparation for the various activities in the specific health fields.

Dean

Lori Bennett, Phone (805) 378-1515

Full-time Faculty

James Bittner, Stephen Burkhart, Ronald Halleran, Traycie Kephart, Remy McCarthy, Delbert Parker

Counselors

Michael Johnson, Donna Proske Allyn

Health Education Transfer Information

Students planning to transfer need to consult with a counselor, prepare a Student Education Plan, and take advantage of support services available in the Career Transfer Center located in the Administration Building, (805) 378-1536. Transfer students interested in specializing in Health Education who wish to qualify for an Associate in Science Degree could explore Health Information Technology or Nursing Science as a possible major.

Health Education Courses

HED M01 – 2 Units
Health and Society

Prerequisites: None
Class Hours: 2 lecture
Focus is on the nature and function of health in our society. Overview of major health concepts designed to contribute to the students understanding of healthy living. Concepts included are: personal fitness; nutrition; mental health; personal relationships; harmful substances; environmental health; communicable diseases; chronic and degenerative disease; reproduction and contraception; and consumer health.
Applies to Associate Degree. Transfer credit: CSU; UC
(HED M01, M02 and M07 combined: maximum credit, one course)

HED M02 – 2 Units
Women's Health

Prerequisites: None
Class Hours: 2 lecture
Focuses on nature and function of women's health in our society. Introduces major female health problems, emphasizing both the individual's and the community's role in understanding medical advances and implementing their effects.
Applies to Associate Degree. Transfer credit: CSU; UC
(HED M02, M01, M07 combined: maximum credit, one course)

HED M03 – 3 Units
Nutrition, Fitness and Stress Management

Prerequisites: None
Class Hours: 3 lecture
Offers an integrated approach to good health and physical fitness through the study of basic principles of exercise, nutrition and human behavior. Applies specific topics of current concern such as maintaining healthy weight, prevention of heart disease and stress management. Stresses incorporating healthful habits and techniques into ones' daily life. Provider approved by the California Board of Registered Nursing. Provider number CEP2811 for 45 contact hours.
Applies to Associate Degree. Transfer credit: CSU

HED M05 – 3 Units
First Aid and CPR

Prerequisites: None
Class Hours: 3 lecture
Introduces procedures for rendering assistance in emergency first aid situations. Successful course completion qualifies student for the American Red Cross Standard First Aid certificate and the Adult Cardiopulmonary Resuscitation card (Adult CPR, AED card) and Child and Infant CPR Certifications.
Applies to Associate Degree. Transfer credit: CSU; UC

HED M06 – 3 Units
Prevention and Treatment of Athletic Injuries

Prerequisites: None
Class Hours: 2 lecture, 3 lab
Introduces basic concepts, skills and practices for the athletic trainer, including medical aspects of athletic training, athletic therapy, modalities, strength, conditioning, rehabilitation and diagnostic techniques. Provides hands-on experience responding to the athletically injured. Does NOT fulfill PE/Health requirement for Associate Degree.
Applies to Associate Degree. Transfer credit: CSU; UC

HED M07 – 3 Units
Personal Health

Prerequisites: None
Class Hours: 3 lecture
Introduces components and skills of health and wellness, reviewing positive behavioral changes and their effect on life. Emphasizes self-responsibility based on self-analysis and assessment.
Applies to Associate Degree. Transfer credit: CSU; UC
(HED M07, M01 and M02 combined: maximum credit, one course)

HED M10A – 0.5 Unit
Alcohol Awareness

Prerequisites: None
Class Hours: 0.5 lecture
Examines the physical, psychological and social effects of alcohol use and abuse including history, case studies, and treatment modes. Emphasizes local information and resources.
Applies to Associate Degree. Transfer credit: CSU

HED M10B – 0.5 Unit
AIDS Seminar
Prerequisites: None
Class Hours: 0.5 lecture
Introduces full range of information on AIDS, including prevention, testing, counseling, support groups, and medical care. Uses speakers and film to enhance discussion. Reviews local services.
Applies to Associate Degree. Transfer credit: CSU

HED M10C – 0.5 Unit
Women's Health Issues
Prerequisites: None
Class Hours: 0.5 lecture
Emphasizes importance of women's participation in own health care, since present decisions affect future health and wellness. Reviews specific health issues for discussion and application.
Applies to Associate Degree. Transfer credit: CSU

HED M10D – 0.5 Unit
Weight Management
Prerequisites: None
Class Hours: 0.5 lecture
Examines the fat cell and the functions of fat in the body. Reviews the effects of weight, including physiological, social, and cultural causes. Emphasizes nutrition, exercise, and lifestyle changes as means to weight management. Evaluates fad diets in order to formulate safe, realistic meal planning.
Applies to Associate Degree. Transfer credit: CSU

Health Education
HED M10E – 0.5 Unit
Athletic Injuries Seminar
Prerequisites: None
Class Hours: 0.5 lecture
Examines medical aspects of athletic injury management, including prevention, first-aid, treatment, evaluation and reconditioning.
Applies to Associate Degree. Transfer credit: CSU

HED M10F – 0.5 Unit
Stress Management
Prerequisites: None
Class Hours: 0.5 lecture
Examines physical, emotional, cognitive, and behavioral aspects of stress, including sources, symptoms, physiology of the stress response, burnout, and effective coping strategies such as induction of the relaxation response.
Applies to Associate Degree. Transfer credit: CSU

HED M10G – 0.5 Unit
Cardiopulmonary Resuscitation
Prerequisites: None
Class Hours: 0.5 lecture
Teaches proficiency in blocked airway management and basic cardiopulmonary resuscitation techniques in adult, child and infant situations. Procedures applicable to individuals with cardiovascular disease but also to those suffering from sudden death due to drowning, electrocution, sensitivity reaction, asphyxia, drug overdose, heart attack and anesthesia idiosyncrasy. Reviews early warning signs, risk factors and

prevention of heart disease. May be taken for a total of four (4) times for credit. (Only 0.5 unit total may be applied to health requirement).
Applies to Associate Degree. Transfer credit: CSU

HED M10H – 0.5 Unit
Domestic Violence/Issues and Information
Prerequisites: None
Class Hours: 0.5 lecture
Introduces definition of domestic violence and abuse, including review of behavioral characteristics of domestic violence, interplay of power and control in a relationship, cycle of violence, and social and legal resources available.
Applies to Associate Degree. Transfer credit: CSU

HED M10J – 0.5 Unit
Date Rape/Self Defense
Prerequisites: None
Class Hours: 0.5 lecture
The focus of this course is on recognizing the sexual, physical, and psychological abuse that may occur in dating relationships. Topics to be included are elements of a healthy relationship, appropriate communication strategies, risks and vulnerabilities in dating relationships, and self-defense tactics.
Applies to Associate Degree. Transfer credit: CSU

HED M10K – 0.5 Unit
Smoking and Your Health
Prerequisites: None
Class Hours: 0.5 lecture
Examines the primary and secondary effects of tobacco use (smoking and chewing) and reviews ways to stop its use. Applies to Associate Degree. Transfer credit: CSU

HED M10M – 0.5 Unit
Healthful Eating
Prerequisites: None
Class Hours: 0.5 lecture
Examines the foundation of nutrition science; nutrients, their individual requirements, nutrition guidelines, diets and fad diets, and nutritional standards. Discusses consumer issues, personal food choices, and the role of diet in the prevention of disease. (Same course as NTS M10M).
Applies to Associate Degree. Transfer credit: CSU

HED M10N – 0.5 Unit
Men's Health
Prerequisites: None
Class Hours: 0.5 lecture
Explores connections between the way men live their lives (exercise, nutrition, stress) and the quality of their health. Emphasizes need for men to participate in own health care, since present decisions affect future health and wellness.
Applies to Associate Degree. Transfer credit: CSU

HED M10P – 0.5 Unit
Fitness for Life
Prerequisites: None
Class Hours: 0.5 lecture
Introduces key concepts in physical fitness, developing practical tools to

assess personal levels of fitness and to create successful exercise programs in injury-free environments. Reviews consumer tips for health and fitness industry.
Applies to Associate Degree. Transfer credit: CSU

HED M10Q – 0.5 Unit
Health and Sexuality
Prerequisites: None
Class Hours: 0.5 lecture
Introduces health and human sexuality, including review of basic sexual anatomy, physiology of sexual response, sexually transmitted diseases, common impediments to healthy sexual functioning, sexual enhancement, and communication skills for achieving greater intimacy.
Applies to Associate Degree. Transfer credit: CSU

HED M10R – 0.5 Unit
Nutrition and Diabetes Management
Prerequisites: None
Class Hours: 0.5 lecture
Provides an overview of diabetes, with an emphasis on diabetes nutrition and the psychological and social impact on the individual. Includes step-by-step survival skills for dealing with the daily routine of diabetes care. Demonstrates the process of carbohydrate counting and exercise as the cornerstone of diabetes management. Provides strategies for preventing diabetes complications. (Same course as NTS M10R)
Applies to Associate Degree. Transfer credit: CSU

Health Education: Health Information Management
HED M10S – 0.5 Unit
Sports and Exercise Nutrition
Prerequisites: None
Class Hours: 0.5 lecture
Examines sports nutrition and exercise for athletes and non-athletes. Introduces social and behavioral aspects by examining the components of fitness, body composition and the diet for optimal performance. Evaluates the dangers of "making weight," the use of supplements, and fad diets. Provider approved by the California Board of Registered Nursing. Provider number CEP2811 for 7.5 contact hours. (Same course as NTS M10S).
Applies to Associate Degree. Transfer credit: CSU

HED M10T – 0.5 Unit
Nutrition and Cancer Prevention
Prerequisites: None
Class Hours: 0.5 lecture
Assesses the relationship of nutrition, exercise, and lifestyle choices in reducing the risks of cancer and examines the American Cancer Society's prevention guidelines. Includes psychological, social, physiological, medical, and nutritional aspects. (Same course as NTS M10T).
Applies to Associate Degree. Transfer credit: CSU

HED M22A/B – 1 to 3 Units
Independent Studies in Health Education
Prerequisites: A previous course in Health Education
Class Hours: 1 to 3 as arranged
Allows an independent project (approved by instructor and dean) to expand knowledge of health education through research, lab work or field

trips. Includes one-on-one work with instructor. May be taken for a maximum of six (6) units.
Applies to Associate Degree. Transfer credit: CSU

HED M60A-Z – 0.5 to 3 Units
Topics in Health Education
Prerequisites: To be determined
Class Hours: To be determined
Each course deals with a specific topic not covered in general offerings. When offered, each course is announced in the semester's Schedule of Classes.
Applies to Associate Degree. Transfer credit: determined by transfer institution.

HED M80 – 1 to 4 Units
Internship in Health Education
Prerequisites: Completion of or concurrent enrollment in one course in the discipline.
Class Hours: 3 to 33 work experience hours as arranged
Provides on-the-job learning to enhance coursework under the direct supervision of faculty and industry supervisors. Both supervisors provide feedback and written evaluations. Some meetings and workshops may be required as part of the course. To take this course, contact the Career Transfer Center, (805) 378-1536. May be taken for a total of four (4) times for credit. (Same course as WEXP M20.)
Applies to Associate Degree. Transfer credit: CSU

Physical Education

Physical Education classes offer students an opportunity to enrich their education with emphasis on improved individual physical well-being as well as professional career options.

Dean
Lori Bennett, Phone (805) 378-1515

Full-time Faculty
James Bittner, Stephen Burkhart, Howard Davis, Donald Green, Ronald Halleran, Traycie Kephart, Remy McCarthy, Delbert Parker, Sherry Ruter, Nancy Stewart, Willard Thurston

Athletic Counselor
Traci Franks

Counselors
Donna Proske Allyn, Michael Johnson

Degree Option in Physical Education
Associate Degree in Human Performance
To earn an Associate in Arts Degree with a major in Human Performance, students complete 32.5 specified units, plus General Education Degree Requirements. This pre-professional program is designed to prepare students for transfer to bachelor's degree programs in Physical Education, Physical Therapy, Athletic Training, Coaching and Fitness Management.

Physical Education

In addition to General Education Degree Requirements, complete the following:

Required Courses... Units

PE M90	Introduction to Human Performance	2.0
PE M91	Foundations of Fitness	3.0
HED M01	Health and Society	2.0
HED M05	Safety and First Aid	3.0
HED M06	Prevention and Treatment of Athletic Injuries	3.0
PSY M01A	Introduction to Psychology	3.0
ANAT M01	General Anatomy	4.0
PHSO M01	Human Physiology	5.0
NTS M01	Nutrition	3.0
Units from RECOMMENDED COURSES		4.5

TOTAL minimum units required in major area 32.5

Recommended Courses: Choose three 1.5-unit courses, one from each area: Team, Individual and Cardiovascular.

TEAM: PE M23C/D (Baseball); PE M24C/D (Basketball); PE M25C/D (Football); PE M27C/D (Soccer); PE M28C/D (Softball); PE M29C/D (Track); PE M30A/C/D (Volleyball) or any College Athletics activity (PE M62 to PE M79).

INDIVIDUAL: PE M02B (Free Weights); PE M06A/C/D (Golf); PE M08 (Power Lifting); PE M11A/C/D (Tennis); PE M38 (Wrestling) or any dance activity class (see DANC).

CARDIOVASCULAR: PE M01A (Walking); PE M03A (Running); PE M04 (Aerobics); PE M07 (Step-Aerobics); PE M12 (Extreme Aerobic Mix); or PE M15 (Cardio Kick Boxing)

See General Education Degree Requirements and Transfer Information.

A General Note on Transferability of Physical Education Courses*

An Associate Degree requires one or more PE/Dance activity classes for a minimum of 1.5 units total. Any combination of P.E. activity courses of a particular kind (e.g., body conditioning, golf, tennis, etc.) may be taken a total of four (4) times. Students planning to take more than 4 units of Physical Education activity courses should consult a counselor. The California State University (CSU) system accepts all P.E. courses for comparable semester credit, but the University of California (UC) system will only accept a total of four (4) units of credit. This UC transfer-status limitation is indicated below by the asterisk*.

Degree and Certificate Program in Exercise Science

The Exercise Science Program provides two tiers of opportunity for students seeking a career in fitness and health.

The Certificate of Achievement in Exercise Science: Fitness Specialist is an 18-unit core program that prepares students for an entry level career in the fitness and health industry. The program provides knowledge and leadership skills essential for students training to become Personal Trainers and/or Group Fitness Instructors.

The Associate of Science Degree in Exercise Science combines the 18 core units in the Certificate of Achievement for Exercise Science: Fitness Specialist and the General Education Degree Requirements. The degree prepares students for career entry into the fitness and health industry, and provides the academic foundation necessary for transfer to a 4-year institution in the field of Exercise Science and Kinesiology.

Associate of Science Degree in Exercise Science

To earn an Associate in Science Degree in Exercise Science, students complete 18 or more specified units and General Education Degree Requirements.

Required Courses... Units

PE M91	Foundations of Fitness	3.0
PE M95	Personal Training Principles	3.0
PE M96	Teaching Group Fitness	3.0
HED M05	First Aid and CPR	3.0
Program Electives (select a minimum of 6 units)		6.0

TOTAL... 18.0

Program Electives (select a minimum of 6 units)............... Units

*ANAT M01	Human Anatomy	4.0
*BIOL M01	Introduction to Biology	4.0
HED M03	Nutrition, Fitness and Stress Management	3.0
HED M06	Prevention and Treatment of Athletic Injuries	3.0
PE M80	Internship in Physical Education	1.0-4.0
*PHSO M01	Human Physiology	5.0

*Students planning on transferring to a university should select ANAT M01, BIOL M01, PHSO M01.

Certificate of Achievement in Exercise Science: Fitness Specialist

To earn a Certificate of Achievement in Exercise Science: Fitness Specialist, students complete 18 or more specified units.

Required Courses... Units

PE M91	Foundations of Fitness	3.0
PE M95	Personal Training Principles	3.0
PE M96	Teaching Group Fitness	3.0
HED M05	First Aid and CPR	3.0
Program Electives (select a minimum of 6 units)		6.0

TOTAL... 18.0

Program Electives (select a minimum of 6 units)...............Units

ANAT M01	Human Anatomy	4.0
BIOL M01	Introduction to Biology	4.0
HED M03	Nutrition, Fitness and Stress Management	3.0
HED M06	Prevention and Treatment of Athletic Injuries	3.0
PE M80	Internship in Physical Education	1.0-4.0
PHSO M01	Human Physiology	5.0

Physical Education Courses

PE M01A – 1 to 1.5 Units
Walking for Fitness

Prerequisites: None
Class Hours: 0.5 or 1 lecture, 1.5 or 2 lab
Provides exercise and fitness training, emphasizing cardiovascular conditioning to improve muscle tone.
Applies to Associate Degree. Transfer credit: CSU; UC*

PE M02A – 0.5 to 1.5 Units
Body Conditioning/Fitness Center

Prerequisites: None
Class Hours: 0.25 to 1 lecture, .75 to 2 lab
Designed to develop and encourage positive attitude and habits with regard to cardiovascular efficiency, muscular strength and endurance, flexibility and body composition. Allows individual scheduling of required lab hours.
Applies to Associate Degree. Transfer credit: CSU; UC*

PE M02B – 1 to 1.5 Units
Body Conditioning/Free Weights

Prerequisites: None
Class Hours: 0.5 or 1 lecture, 1.5 or 2 lab
Introduces overall body conditioning. Emphasizes improving the

cardiovascular system, enhancing flexibility, and increasing muscular strength. Includes jogging, stretching, and specific free weight exercises. Applies to Associate Degree.
Transfer credit: CSU; UC*

Physical Education

PE M03A – 1 to 1.5 Units
Running for Fitness and Conditioning
Prerequisites: None

Class Hours: 0.5 or 1 lecture, 1.5 or 2 lab

Emphasizes improved physical health and cardiovascular fitness through running and overall conditioning. Includes endurance training with a gradual increase in distance.

Applies to Associate Degree. Transfer credit: CSU; UC*

PE M03B – 1 to 1.5 Units
Sprinting for Fitness and Conditioning
Prerequisites: None

Class Hours: 0.5 or 1 lecture, 1.5 or 2 lab

Uses sprinting to improve physical fitness and general health. Emphasizes maximum speed performance and enhanced cardiovascular efficiency.

Applies to Associate Degree. Transfer credit: CSU; UC*

PE M04 – 1 to 1.5 Units
Body Conditioning through Rhythmics/Aerobics
Prerequisites: None

Class Hours: 0.5 or 1 lecture, 1.5 or 2 lab

Introduces series of simple but vigorous dances that improve circulation, respiration, digestion, agility, flexibility, coordination and rhythm as well as endurance and strength. Includes supervised practice.

Applies to Associate Degree. Transfer credit: CSU; UC*

PE M05 – 1.5 Units
Bowling
Prerequisites: None

Class Hours: 1 lecture, 2 lab

Introduces rules, etiquette, safety and techniques of bowling. Meets off campus.

Applies to Associate Degree. Transfer credit: CSU; UC*

PE M06A – 1 to 1.5 Units
Beginning Golf
Prerequisites: None

Class Hours: 0.5 or 1.0 lecture, 1.5 to 2.0 lab

Introduces basic rules and skills needed for playing golf. Includes development of skills and analysis of technique. May be taken for a total of four (4) times for credit.

Applies to Associate Degree.Transfer credit: CSU; UC*

PE M06C – 1.0 to 1.5 Units
Intermediate Golf
Prerequisites: PE M06A

Class Hours 0.5 or 1.0 lecture, 1.5 to 2.0 lab

Expands golfing skills through more extensive review of techniques and increased practice. May be taken for a total of four (4) times for credit.

Applies to Associate Degree. Transfer credit CSU, UC*.

PE M06D – 1.0 to 1.5 Units
Advanced Golf
Prerequisites: PE M06A

Class Hours: 0.5 or 1.0 lecture, 1.5 to 2.0 lab

Studies biomechanical principles of golf as preparation for golf competition. May be taken for a total of four (4) times for credit.

Applies to Associate Degree. Transfer credit: CSU, UC*

PE M07 – 1.0 to 1.5 Units
Cardio Sculpting
Prerequisites: None

Class Hours: 0.5 or 1 lecture, 1.5 to 2 lab

Guidance in using cardiovascular activity circuits, body sculpting with free weights, and core strength activities using STEP platforms. Works the major muscle group in the lower body and tones and strengthens the upper body and core. Focus on improving cardiovascular condition, core strength, muscle endurance, upper body strength, and weight management. May be taken for a total of four (4) times for credit.

Applies to Associate Degree. Transfer credit: CSU; UC*

PE M08 – 1 to 1.5 Units
Power Lifting/Free Weights
Prerequisites: None

Class Hours: 0.5 or 1 lecture, 1.5 or 2 lab

Introduces weight training and conditioning to build strength, power, and bulk. Focuses on the development of upper body strength, rehabilitation and strengthening of knee joints, and refinement of power lifting for the lower body. Emphasizes quickness, coordination, balance and speed through competitive drills and routines. May be taken for a total of four (4) times.

Applies to Associate Degree. Transfer credit: CSU; UC*

PE M10 – 1 to 1.5 Units
Shaping and Toning
Prerequisites: None

Class Hours: 0.5 or 1 lecture, 1.5 to 2 lab

Provides improvement of the cardiovascular system, enhanced flexibility and increased muscular strength. Includes cardiovascular/aerobic conditioning, stretching exercises and specific free weight exercises to strengthen the entire body. May be taken for a total of four (4) times.

Applies to Associate Degree. Transfer credit: CSU; UC*

PE M11A – 1 to 1.5 Units
Beginning Tennis I
Prerequisites: None

Class Hours: 0.5 or 1 lecture, 1.5 to 2 lab

Introduces beginning tennis skills, including etiquette, rules, and basic techniques. May be taken a total of four (4) times for credit.

Applies to Associate Degree. Transfer credit: CSU; UC*

PE M11C – 1 to 1.5 Units
Intermediate Tennis
Prerequisites: PE M11A

Class Hours: 0.5 or 1 lecture, 1.5 to 2 lab

Expands strategies, rules and techniques of tennis, emphasizing both singles and doubles play. May be taken for a total of four (4) times for credit.

Applies to Associate Degree. Transfer credit: CSU; UC*

PE M11D – 1 to 1.5 Units
Advanced Tennis

Prerequisites: PE M11C
Class Hours: 0.5 to 1 lecture, 1.5 to 2 lab
Expands experienced players individual techniques. Reviews rules and strategies for both singles and doubles play. Emphasizes tournament play.
Applies to Associate Degree. Transfer credit: CSU; UC*

Physical Education
PE M12 – 1 to 1.5 Units
Extreme Aerobic Mix

Prerequisites: None
Class Hours: 0.5 to 1 lecture, 1.5 to 2 lab
Develops a high level of cardiovascular efficiency. Promotes strength and flexibility through a variety of high-energy activities. Utilizes aerobic dance, funk, hip-hop, step, cardio kickboxing, and plyometrics to achieve a high level of conditioning and coordination. May be taken for a total of four (4) times.
Applies to Associate Degree. Transfer credit: CSU; UC*

PE M13 – 2 Units
Hiking and Backpacking

Prerequisites: None
Class Hours: 1 lecture, 2 lab
Uses lecture, field study and experience to Introduce sport of hiking and backpacking. Covers conditioning, skills, information and resources. Emphasizes safety procedures. Requires field trips.
Applies to Associate Degree. Transfer credit: CSU; UC*

PE M14 – 3 Units
Pep Squad

Prerequisites: None
Class Hours: 1 lecture, 6 lab
Provides training and practice techniques necessary to be a cheerleader. Requires field trips. May be taken for a total of three (3) times.
Applies to Associate Degree. Transfer credit: CSU; UC*

PE M15 – 1 to 1.5 Units
Cardio Kick Boxing

Prerequisites: None
Class Hours: 0.5 to 1 lecture, 1.5 to 2 lab
Offers a comprehensive and balanced program that develops proficiency in cardio kick boxing skills as well as physical and general health. Works every major muscle group in the upper and lower body, varying movements and speed to accommodate the fitness level of all students.
Applies to Associate Degree. Transfer credit: CSU; UC*

PE M16 – 1 to 1.5 Units
Flexible Strength/Pilate's Mat

Prerequisites: None
Class Hours: 0.5 to 1 lecture, 1.5 to 2 lab
A training technique designed to strengthen and tone muscles, improve posture, provide flexibility and balance, and create a more streamlined shape. Designed to emphasize the core muscles – the abdominal area, lower back, hips, and buttocks – thereby providing a strong foundation for any lab.
Applies to Associate Degree. Transfer credit: CSU; UC*

PE M17 – 1.5 Units
Conditioning for Athletic Competition

Prerequisites: None
Class Hours: 1 lecture, 2 lab
Designed to properly prepare and condition prospective athletes for competition. Athletics require an advanced degree of skill and preparation. Athletes engaged in competition need specific conditioning to insure optimal opportunity to perform at peak levels and have a more injury-free experience.
Applies to Associate Degree. Transfer credit: CSU; UC*

PE M18 – 1 to 1.5 Units
Core Stability and Stretch

Prerequisites: None
Class Hours: 0.5 to 1 lecture, 1.5 to 2 lab
Implements a variety of core (abdominal/trunk) training techniques including functional integrated resistance exercise, stability balls, yoga, and Pilate's, this class will focus on concepts and practices that develop core stability and overall flexibility for healthier living. May be taken for a total of four (4) times for credit.
Applies to Associate Degree. Transfer credit: CSU; UC*

PE M19A – 0.25 Unit
Golf Clinic

Prerequisites: None
Recommended Prep: Prior background and previous experience in the sport.
Class Hours: 0.2 lecture, 0.3 lab
Provides an intense skill-building clinic for those already familiar with the sport. May be taken for a total of four (4) times.
Applies to Associate Degree. Transfer credit: CSU; UC*

PE M19B – 0.25 Unit
Tennis Clinic

Prerequisites: None
Recommended Prep: Prior background and previous experience in the sport.
Class Hours: 0.2 lecture, 0.3 lab
Provides an intense skill-building clinic for those already familiar with the sport. May be taken for a total of four (4) times.
Applies to Associate Degree. Transfer credit: CSU; UC*

PE M19C – 0.25 Unit
Field Hockey Clinic

Prerequisites: None
Recommended Prep: Prior background and previous experience in the sport.
Class Hours: 0.2 lecture, 0.3 lab
Provides an intense skill-building clinic for those already familiar with the sport. May be taken for a total of four (4) times.
Applies to Associate Degree. Transfer credit: CSU; UC*

PE M19D – 0.25 Unit
Soccer Clinic

Prerequisites: None
Recommended Prep: Prior background and previous experience in the sport.
Class Hours: 0.2 lecture, 0.3 lab

Provides an intense skill-building clinic for those already familiar with the sport. May be taken for a total of four (4) times.
Applies to Associate Degree. Transfer credit: CSU; UC*

PE M19E – 0.25 Unit
Basketball Clinic
Prerequisites: None
Recommended Prep: Prior background and previous experience in the sport.
Class Hours: 0.2 lecture, 0.3 lab
Provides an intense skill-building clinic for those already familiar with the sport. May be taken for a total of four (4) times.
Applies to Associate Degree. Transfer credit: CSU; UC*

Physical Education
PE M19F – 0.25 Unit
Hiking Clinic
Prerequisites: None
Recommended Prep: Prior background and previous experience in the sport.
Class Hours: 0.2 lecture, 0.3 lab
Provides an intense skill-building clinic for those already familiar with the sport. May be taken for a total of four (4) times.
Applies to Associate Degree. Transfer credit: CSU; UC*

PE M19G – 0.25 Unit
Wrestling Clinic
Prerequisites: None
Recommended Prep: Prior background and previous experience in the sport.
Class Hours: 0.2 lecture, 0.3 lab
Provides an intense skill-building clinic for those already familiar with the sport. May be taken for a total of four (4) times.
Applies to Associate Degree. Transfer credit: CSU; UC*

PE M19H – 0.25 Unit
Volleyball Clinic
Prerequisites: None
Recommended Prep: Prior background and previous experience in the sport.
Class Hours: 0.2 lecture, 0.3 lab
Provides an intense skill-building clinic for those already familiar with the sport. May be taken for a total of four (4) times.
Applies to Associate Degree. Transfer credit: CSU; UC*

PE M19I – 0.25 Units
Self-Defense/Assault Clinic
Prerequisites: None
Recommended Prep: Prior background and previous experience in the sport.
Class Hours: 0.2 lecture, 0.3 lab
Provides an intense skill-building clinic for those already familiar with the sport. May be taken for a total of four (4) times.
Applies to Associate Degree. Transfer credit: CSU; UC*

PE M19J – 0.25 Unit
Stretching Clinic
Prerequisites: None
Class Hours: 0.2 lecture, 0.3 lab
Introduces stretching techniques. Develops each individuals stretching program to increase and maintain flexibility. May be taken for a total of four (4) times.
Applies to Associate Degree. Transfer credit: CSU; UC*

PE M19K – 0.25 Unit
Snowboarding Clinic
Prerequisites: None
Class Hours: 0.2 lecture, 0.3 lab
Designed as an intense skill-building clinic for snowboarders involving a trip to a ski resort. May be taken for a total of four (4) times for credit.
Applies to Associate Degree. Transfer credit: CSU; UC*

PE M20 – 1.5 Units
Adapted Physical Education
Prerequisites: None
Class Hours: 1 lecture, 2 lab
Meets special needs of students unable to participate in regular physical education activity classes. Provides individualized adapted fitness program. Requires evaluation by college physician to determine appropriate physical activity for each participant. May be taken for a total of four (4) times for credit.
Applies to Associate Degree. Transfer credit: CSU, UC*

PE M21 – 1 to 1.5 Units
Field Hockey
Prerequisites: None
Class Hours: 0.5 to 1 lecture, 1.5 to 2 lab
Introduces fundamentals of field hockey, including individual skills (passing, receiving and dribbling) as well as offensive and defensive tactics and team strategy.
Applies to Associate Degree. Transfer credit: CSU; UC*

PE M22A/B – 1 to 3 Units
Independent Studies in Physical Education
Prerequisites: A previous course in Physical Education
Class Hours: 1 to 3 as arranged
Allows an independent project (approved by instructor and dean) to expand knowledge of physical education through research, lab work or field trips. Includes one-on-one work with instructor. May be taken for a maximum of six (6) units.
Applies to Associate Degree. Transfer credit: CSU; UC (determined after admission)

TEAM ACTIVITIES
PE M23C – 1 to 1.5 Units
Intermediate Baseball
Prerequisites: None
Class Hours: 0.5 to 1 lecture, 1.5 to 2 lab
Develops intermediate techniques and strategies for baseball. Emphasizes skills levels for use in games. Applies to Associate Degree. Transfer credit: CSU; UC*

PE M23D – 1 to 1.5 Units
Advanced Baseball
Prerequisites: PE M23C
Class Hours: 0.5 to 1 lecture, 1.5 to 2 lab
Develops advanced skills in baseball, emphasizing methods and styles of play. Requires participation in fall baseball program.
Applies to Associate Degree. Transfer credit: CSU; UC*

PE M24C – 1 to 1.5 Units
Intermediate Basketball
Prerequisites: None
Class Hours: 0.5 to 1 lecture, 1.5 to 2 lab
Develops intermediate techniques and strategies in basketball. May be taken a total of four (4) times for credit.
Applies to Associate Degree. Transfer credit: CSU; UC*

Physical Education
PE M24D – 1 to 2 Units
Advanced Basketball
Prerequisites: PE M24C or varsity high school experience
Class Hours: 0.5 to 1.5 lecture, 1.5 to 2.5 lab
Introduces advanced skills and techniques in basketball. Uses game experience to develop different styles and formats of play. Develops cardiovascular fitness.
Applies to Associate Degree. Transfer credit: CSU; UC*

PE M25A – 1 to 1.5 Units
Beginning Football
Prerequisites: None
Class Hours: 0.5 to 1 lecture, 1.5 to 2 lab
Develops beginning skills in football and reviews the history of the sport.
Applies to Associate Degree. Transfer credit: CSU; UC*

PE M25C – 1 to 1.5 Units
Intermediate Football
Prerequisites: None
Class Hours: 0.5 to 1 lecture, 1.5 to 2 lab
Develops intermediate skills in football. Introduces theory behind different styles of play.
Applies to Associate Degree. Transfer credit: CSU; UC*

PE M25D – 1 to 1.5 Units
Advanced Football
Prerequisites: None
Class Hours: 0.5 to 1 lecture, 1.5 to 2 lab
Develops advanced skills in football. Introduces theory behind different styles of play.
Applies to Associate Degree. Transfer credit: CSU; UC*

PE M26 – 1 to 1.5 Units
Team Sports
Prerequisites: None
Class Hours: 0.5 to 1 lecture, 1.5 to 2 lab
Introduces basic rules, techniques and strategies of various seasonal team sports, including soccer, softball, football and basketball. Provides practice in each sport.
Applies to Associate Degree. Transfer credit: CSU; UC*

PE M27A – 1 to 1.5 Units
Beginning Soccer
Prerequisites: None
Class Hours: 0.5 to 1 lecture, 1.5 to 2 lab
Develops skills, rules, techniques and strategies of soccer. Requires participation. Co-educational.
Applies to Associate Degree. Transfer credit: CSU; UC*

PE M27C – 1 to 1.5 Units
Intermediate Soccer
Prerequisites: None
Class Hours: 0.5 to 1 lecture, 1.5 to 2 lab
Develops intermediate skills and strategies of soccer. Requires participation. Co-educational.
Applies to Associate Degree. Transfer credit: CSU; UC*

PE M27D – 1 to 1.5 Units
Advanced Soccer
Prerequisites: None
Class Hours: 0.5 to 1 lecture, 1.5 to 2 lab
Develops advanced skills and strategies. Requires participation. Co-educational.
Applies to Associate Degree. Transfer credit: CSU; UC*

PE M28A – 1 to 1.5 Units
Beginning Softball
Prerequisites: None
Class Hours: 0.5 to 1 lecture, 1.5 to 2 lab
Introduces the basic skills and strategies of fast-pitch softball. Requires participation. Co-educational.
Applies to Associate Degree. Transfer credit: CSU; UC*

PE M28C – 1 to 1.5 Units
Intermediate Softball
Prerequisites: None
Class Hours: 0.5 to 1 lecture, 1.5 to 2 lab
Develops intermediate skills and strategies of fast-pitch softball. Requires participation. Co-educational.
Applies to Associate Degree. Transfer credit: CSU; UC*

PE M28D – 1 to 1.5 Units
Advanced Softball
Prerequisites: None
Class Hours: 0.5 to 1 lecture, 1.5 to 2 lab
Develops advanced skills and strategies. Requires participation. Co-educational.
Applies to Associate Degree. Transfer credit: CSU; UC*

PE M29C – 1 to 1.5 Units
Intermediate Track
Prerequisites: None
Class Hours: 0.5 to 1 lecture, 1.5 to 2 lab
Introduces intermediate techniques and strategies in track and field. Prepares for a competitive season, emphasizing skills needed for proficiency. Required of varsity track candidates.
Applies to Associate Degree. Transfer credit: CSU; UC*

PE M29D – 1 to 1.5 Units
Advanced Track
Prerequisites: PE M29C
Class Hours: 0.5 to 1 lecture, 1.5 to 2 lab
Practices advanced skills and strategies of track and field for a competitive season. Required of all varsity track candidates.
Applies to Associate Degree. Transfer credit: CSU; UC*

PE M30A – 1 to 1.5 Units
Beginning Volleyball I
Prerequisites: None
Class Hours: 0.5 to 1 lecture, 1.5 to 2 lab
Introduces basic rules and techniques of power volleyball.
Applies to Associate Degree. Transfer credit: CSU; UC*

PE M30C – 1 to 1.5 Units
Intermediate Volleyball
Prerequisites: PE M30A
Class Hours: 0.5 to 1 lecture, 1.5 to 2 lab
Provides practice of the fundamental skills and strategies of volleyball, allowing two and three-player games. Requires participation.
Applies to Associate Degree. Transfer credit: CSU; UC*

Physical Education
PE M30D – 1 to 1.5 Units
Advanced Volleyball
Prerequisites: PE M30C
Class Hours: 0.5 to 1 lecture, 1.5 to 2 lab
Continues skills development for the advanced player, allowing two and threeplayer volleyball. Requires participation.
Applies to Associate Degree. Transfer credit: CSU; UC*

PE M35 – 1.5 Unit
T'ai Chi Ch'uan
Prerequisites: None
Class Hours: 1 lecture, 2 lab
Introduction to the history and philosophy of T'ai Chi Ch'uan and its relationship to exercise, health, self-awareness, relaxation, balance and harmony. The Yang Simplified Form of 24 movement patterns (known for improving body awareness, efficiency of daily activity and its relationship to self-defense techniques) will be taught. May be taken for a total of four (4) times for credit.
Applies to Associate Degree. Transfer credit: CSU; UC*

PE M36A – 2 Units
Analysis of Sexual Assault and Self-Defense
Prerequisites: None
Class Hours: 2 lecture, 1 lab
Reviews issues of personal assault and rape, reviewing readings and physical responses. Introduces self-defense techniques. May be taken a total of four (4) times for credit.
Applies to Associate Degree. Transfer credit: CSU; UC*

PE M37A – 1 to 1.5 Units
Beginning Martial Arts
Prerequisites: None
Class Hours: 0.5 to 1 lecture, 1.5 to 2 lab
Introduces the basic skills of martial arts, including punching, kicking, blocking, and grappling. Participation in the class will require the development of flexibility, endurance, strength, coordination, and concentration. May be taken for a total of four (4) times for credit. (Formerly PE M37)
Applies to Associate Degree. Transfer credit: CSU: UC*

PE M37C – 1 to 1.5 Units
Intermediate Martial Arts
Prerequisites: PE M37A
Class Hours: 0.5 to 1 lecture, 1.5 to 2 lab
Introduces the intermediate skills of martial arts, including punching, kicking, blocking, katas, sparring and grappling. Participation in the class will require the development of flexibility, endurance, strength, coordination and concentration. May be taken for a total of four (4) times for credit.
Applies to Associate Degree. Transfer credit: CSU; UC*

PE M38 – 1 to 1.5 Units
Wrestling
Prerequisites: None
Class Hours: 0.5 to 1 lecture, 1.5 to 2 lab
Introduces the basic skills of wrestling, including takedowns, rides, escapes and falls. May be taken a total of four (4) times for credit.
Applies to Associate Degree. Transfer credit: CSU; UC*

PE M39 – 1 to 1.5 Units
Nia Fusion Fitness
Prerequisites: None
Class Hours: 0.5 to 1 lecture, 1.5 to 2 lab
Nia is a whole-body conditioning practice that includes cardiovascular, strength, flexibility, and mind-body components. Combines concepts and movements from Jazz and Modern Dance, Tae Kwon Do, Tai Chi, Aikido, Yoga, and other movement forms, resulting in a creative and energizing workout. With a focus on non-impact movements, Nia is easy-to-learn, adaptable to all levels of ability, and performed to a variety of motivating music. Improves overall conditioning and enhances the mind-body connection. May be taken for a total of four (4) times for credit.
Applies to Associate Degree. Transfer credit: CSU; UC*

PE M40 – 1 to 1.5 Units
Core Fitness with Cardio Ball
Prerequisites: None
Class Hours: 0.5 to 1 lecture, 1.5 to 2 lab
Uses inflatable stability balls, medicine balls, and mini-inflatable balls, to improve both cardiovascular and core fitness. Includes ball drumming, seated low impact moves on the ball, plyometric leaps and resistance exercises for a high energy workout adaptable to most levels of fitness and ability. Combines cardiovascular and core exercises designed to burn calories and tone muscles while moving to the beat of a variety of music styles. May be taken for a total of four (4) times for credit.
Applies to Associate Degree. Transfer credit: CSU; UC*

INTERCOLLEGIATE ATHLETICS
(Passing a physical exam required for participation)
PE M62 – 3 Units
Golf - Women
Prerequisites: None
Class Hours: 1 lecture, 9 lab
Highly competitive. Requires advanced skills, travel, and competition against other institutions. Demands time beyond normal load. May be taken for a total of three (3) times for credit.
Applies to Associate Degree. Transfer credit: CSU; UC*

PE M63A – 3 Units
Volleyball - Men
Prerequisites: None
Recommended Prep: Understanding of volleyball skills, rules, and strategies.
Class Hours: 10 lab
Highly competitive. Requires advanced skills, travel, and competition against other institutions. Demands time beyond normal load. May be taken for a total of three (3) times for credit.
Applies to Associate Degree. Transfer credit: CSU; UC*

PE M63B – 1 Unit
Off Season Volleyball - Men
Prerequisites: None
Recommended Prep: Understanding of volleyball skills, rules and strategies and the ability to work with other students.
Class Hours: 3 lab
Highly competitive, requires advanced skills, for students who are interested in intercollegiate volleyball. May be taken for a total of four (4) times for credit.
Applies to Associate Degree. Transfer credit: CSU; UC*

Physical Education
PE M64A – 3 Units
Soccer - Men
Prerequisites: None
Recommended Prep: Understanding of soccer skills, rules, and strategies.
Class Hours: 10 lab
Highly competitive. Requires advanced skills, travel, and competition against other institutions. Demands time beyond normal load. May be taken for a total of three (3) times for credit.
Applies to Associate Degree. Transfer credit: CSU; UC*

PE M64B – 1 Unit
Off Season Soccer - Men
Prerequisites: None
Recommended Prep: Understanding of volleyball skills, rules and strategies and the ability to work with other students.
Class Hours: 3 lab
Highly competitive, requires advanced skills, for students who are interested in intercollegiate soccer. May be taken for a total of four (4) times for credit.
Applies to Associate Degree. Transfer credit: CSU; UC*

PE M65A – 3 Units
Soccer - Women
Prerequisites: None
Recommended Prep: Understanding of soccer skills, rules, and strategies.
Class Hours: 10 lab
Highly competitive. Requires advanced skills, travel, and competition against other institutions. Demands time beyond normal load. May be taken for a total of three (3) times for credit.
Applies to Associate Degree. Transfer credit: CSU; UC*

PE M65B – 1 Unit
Off Season Soccer - Women
Prerequisites: None
Recommended Prep: Understanding of volleyball skills, rules and strategies and the ability to work with other students.
Class Hours: 3 lab
Highly competitive, requires advanced skills, for students who are interested in intercollegiate soccer. May be taken for a total of four (4) times for credit.
Applies to Associate Degree. Transfer credit: CSU; UC*

PE M66 – 3 Units
Baseball - Men
Prerequisites: None
Recommended Prep: Understanding of baseball skills, rules, and strategies.
Class Hours: 1 lecture, 9 lab
Highly competitive. Requires advanced skills, travel, and competition against other institutions. Demands time beyond normal load. May be taken for a total of three (3) times for credit.
Applies to Associate Degree. Transfer credit: CSU; UC*

PE M67 – 3 Units
Basketball - Men
Prerequisites: None
Recommended Prep: Understanding of basketball skills, rules, and strategies.
Class Hours: 1 lecture, 9 lab
Highly competitive. Requires advanced skills, travel, and competition against other institutions. Demands time beyond normal load. May be taken for a total of three (3) times for credit.
Applies to Associate Degree. Transfer credit: CSU; UC*

PE M68 – 3 Units
Basketball - Women
Prerequisites: None
Recommended Prep: Understanding of basketball skills, rules, and strategies.
Class Hours: 1 lecture, 9 lab
Highly competitive. Requires advanced skills, travel, and competition against other institutions. Demands time beyond normal load. May be taken for a total of three (3) times for credit.
Applies to Associate Degree. Transfer credit: CSU; UC*

PE M69 – 3 Units
Cross Country - Men
Prerequisites: None
Recommended Prep: Understanding of cross country skills, rules, and strategies.

Class Hours: 1 lecture, 9 lab
Highly competitive. Requires advanced skills, travel, and competition against other institutions. Demands time beyond normal load. May be taken for a total of three (3) times for credit.
Applies to Associate Degree. Transfer credit: CSU; UC*

PE M70 – 3 Units
Cross Country - Women
Prerequisites: None
Recommended Prep: Understanding of cross country skills, rules, and strategies.
Class Hours: 1 lecture, 9 lab
Highly competitive. Requires advanced skills, travel, and competition against other institutions. Demands time beyond normal load. May be taken for a total of three (3) times for credit.
Applies to Associate Degree. Transfer credit: CSU; UC*

PE M71 – 3 Units
Football - Men
Prerequisites: None
Recommended Prep: Understanding of football skills, rules, and strategies.
Class Hours: 1 lecture, 9 lab
Highly competitive. Requires advanced skills, travel, and competition against other institutions. Demands time beyond normal load. May be taken for a total of three (3) times for credit.
Applies to Associate Degree. Transfer credit: CSU; UC*

PE M72 – 3 Units
Golf - Men
Prerequisites: None
Class Hours: 1 lecture, 9 lab
Varsity sports are highly competitive and require an advanced degree of skill. Students engaged in varsity sports should expect to compete against other institutions, travel, and put in additional hours beyond the normal activity load. May be taken for a total of three (3) times for credit.
Applies to Associate Degree. Transfer credit: CSU; UC*

PE M73 – 3 Units
Softball - Women
Prerequisites: None
Recommended Prep: Understanding of softball skills, rules, and strategies.
Class Hours: 1 lecture, 9 lab
Highly competitive. Requires advanced skills, travel, and competition against other institutions. Demands time beyond normal load. May be taken for a total of three (3) times for credit.
Applies to Associate Degree. Transfer credit: CSU; UC*

Physical Education
PE M74 – 3 Units
Tennis - Men
Prerequisites: None
Recommended Prep: Understanding of tennis skills, rules, and strategies.
Class Hours: 1 lecture, 9 lab
Highly competitive. Requires advanced skills, travel, and competition against other institutions. Demands time beyond normal load. May be taken for a total of three (3) times for credit.
Applies to Associate Degree. Transfer credit: CSU; UC*

PE M75A – 3 Units
Tennis - Women
Prerequisites: None
Recommended Prep: Understanding of tennis skills, rules, and strategies.
Class Hours: 10 lab
Highly competitive. Requires advanced skills, travel, and competition against other institutions. Demands time beyond normal load. May be taken for a total of three (3) times for credit.
Applies to Associate Degree. Transfer credit: CSU; UC*

PE M75B – 1 Unit
Off Season Tennis - Women
Prerequisites: None
Recommended Prep: Understanding of volleyball skills, rules and strategies and the ability to work with other students.
Class Hours: 3 lab
Highly competitive. Requires advanced skills, for students who are interested in intercollegiate tennis. May be taken for a total of four (4) times for credit.
Applies to Associate Degree. Transfer credit: CSU; UC*

PE M76 – 3 Units
Track - Men
Prerequisites: None
Recommended Prep: Understanding of track skills, rules, and strategies.
Class Hours: 1 lecture, 9 lab
Highly competitive. Requires advanced skills, travel, and competition against other institutions. Demands time beyond normal load. May be taken for a total of three (3) times for credit.
Applies to Associate Degree. Transfer credit: CSU; UC*

PE M77 – 3 Units
Track Women
Prerequisites: None
Recommended Prep: Understanding of track skills, rules, and strategies.
Class Hours: 1 lecture, 9 lab
Highly competitive. Requires advanced skills, travel, and competition against other institutions. Demands time beyond normal load. May be taken for a total of three (3) times for credit.
Applies to Associate Degree. Transfer credit: CSU; UC*

PE M78 – 3 Units
Volleyball Women
Prerequisites: None
Recommended Prep: Understanding of volleyball skills, rules, and strategies.
Class Hours: 1 lecture, 9 lab
Highly competitive. Requires advanced skills, travel, and competition against other institutions. Demands time beyond normal load. May be taken for a total of three (3) times for credit.
Applies to Associate Degree. Transfer credit: CSU; UC*

PE M79 – 3 Units
Wrestling Men
Prerequisites: None
Recommended Prep: Understanding of wrestling skills, rules, and strategies.
Class Hours: 1 lecture, 9 lab

Highly competitive. Requires advanced skills, travel, and competition against other institutions. Demands time beyond normal load. May be taken for a total of three (3) times for credit.

Applies to Associate Degree. Transfer credit: CSU; UC*

PE M80 – 1 to 4 Units
Internship in Physical Education

Prerequisites: Completion of or concurrent enrollment in one course in the discipline.

Class Hours: 3 to 33 work experience hours as arranged

Provides on-the-job learning to enhance coursework under the direct supervision of faculty and industry supervisors. Both supervisors provide feedback and written evaluations. Some meetings and workshops may be required as part of the course. To take this course, contact the Career Transfer Center, (805) 378-1536. May be taken for a total of four (4) times for credit. (Same course as WEXP M20)

Applies to Associate Degree. Transfer credit: CSU

PE M90 – 2 Units
Introduction to Human Performance

and Physical Education

Prerequisites: None

Class Hours: 2 lecture

Introduces aims, objectives and contemporary issues of Physical Education and Human Performance. Requires projects and fieldwork. Does NOT fulfill general education PE requirement.

Applies to Associate Degree. Transfer credit: CSU; UC

PE M91 – 3 Units
Foundations of Fitness

Prerequisites: None

Class Hours: 2 lecture, 3 lab

Provides a foundation for fitness enthusiasts and those interested in pursuing a career as a fitness professional. Emphasizes muscular, cardiorespiratory, and other physiological processes essential to understanding the effects and benefits of exercise. Includes basic muscle and bone anatomy in relationship to the study of movement, with the purpose of understanding safe and effective exercise program design. Does NOT fulfill general education PE requirement.

Applies to Associate Degree. Transfer credit: CSU; UC

PE M95 – 3 Units
Personal Training Principles

Prerequisites: None

Recommended Prep: PE M91

Class Hours: 2 lecture, 3 lab

Introduces leadership skills and the fundamentals of personal training to successfully prepare students for a national personal training certification. Offers
knowledge and practical experience in exercise and fitness testing, injury prevention, client assessment and counseling techniques. Examines fitness components and exercise science with an emphasis on conditioning and fitness program design.

Applies to Associate Degree. Transfer credit: CSU; UC (under review)

Physical Education Physics
PE M96 – 3 Units

Teaching Group Fitness

Prerequisites: None

Recommended Prep: PE M91

Class Hours: 2 lecture, 3 lab

Introduces the concepts and practice of teaching group fitness. Emphasizes teaching principles, techniques, and safety practices for a wide range of contemporary group fitness modalities. Attention will be placed on the learning process and learning strategies for the teaching of motor skills. Provides preparation for group fitness certification, and practical experience in group fitness leadership.

Applies to Associate Degree. Transfer credit: CSU; UC (under review)

Physical Science

Physical Science courses prepare students for a diversity of professions requiring an understanding of the fundamentals of the physical sciences. Such professions include teaching science at the secondary level, serving as a technical administrator in government and industry, or completing legal work with patents, scientific librarianship, and scientific journalism.

Dean

Kim Hoffmans, Phone (805) 378-1459

Full-time Faculty

Balazs Becht, Clinton Harper, Ron Wallingford

Counselors

Donna Proske Allyn, Edna Ingram, Danita Redd

Physical Science Courses
PHSC M01 – 3 Units
Principles of Physical Science

Prerequisites: MATH M03

Class Hours: 3 lecture

Introduces facts, principles and laws from physics, chemistry, and astronomy. Includes motion, force, energy, wave motion, electricity and magnetism, light, atomic and nuclear structure, chemical bonding and chemical reactions, solutions, organic chemistry, the solar system and planet Earth.

Applies to Associate Degree. Transfer credit: CSU; UC (no credit if taken after a college course in Astronomy, Chemistry, Geology or Physics)

PHSC M01L – 1 Unit
Principles of Physical Science Laboratory

Prerequisites: Completion of or concurrent enrollment in PHSC M01

Class Hours: 3 lab

Provides hands-on experience with fundamental concepts from physics and chemistry.

Applies to Associate Degree. Transfer credit: CSU; UC.

PHSC M22A/B – 0.5 to 3 Units
Independent Studies in Physical Science

Prerequisites: A previous course in Physical Science

Class Hours: 0.5 to 3 as arranged

Allows an independent project (approved by instructor and dean) to expand knowledge of physical science through research, lab work or field trips. Includes one-on-one work with instructor. May be taken for a maximum of six (6) units.

Applies to Associate Degree. Transfer credit: CSU; UC (determined after admission)

PHSC M80 – 1 to 4 Units
Internship in Physical Science

Prerequisites: Completion of or concurrent enrollment in one course in the discipline.

Class Hours: 3 to 33 work experience hours as arranged

Provides on-the-job learning to enhance coursework under the direct supervision of faculty and industry supervisors. Both supervisors provide feedback and written evaluations. Some meetings and workshops may be required as part of the course. To take this course, contact the Career Transfer Center, (805) 378-1536. May be taken for a total of four (4) times for credit. (Same course as WEXP M20)

Applies to Associate Degree. Transfer credit: CSU

PREFACE

At no time in our nation's history have so many people been tuned in to health. It's hard to have a conversation without hearing health come into the discussion and even more difficult to watch TV, surf the Internet, or read a newspaper or magazine without seeing health as headline news. The threat of pandemic flu, new strains of infectious diseases, sexually transmitted infections, polluted drinking water, global warming, catastrophic environmental events, and bioterrorism make us anxious about insidious risks to health. At the same time, looming threats of heart disease, cancer, and diabetes and epidemic increases in obesity-related illnesses cause us to worry about what we eat, whether we exercise, and how we care for our bodies. Adding to these concerns are worries over a health care system that is increasingly unable to provide high-quality care at a reasonable cost for all Americans. What will our futures look like? Who is going to protect us and keep us healthy? What can we do to ensure healthy years for ourselves and our loved ones?

These questions and countless others face us each and every day. We make decisions that may impact our own health or the health of others, based on a media blitz of information that is confusing to even the most savvy consumer. Are we obese because we were exposed to a virus, or is it lack of willpower, lack of exercise, or genetics—or a combination of all of the above? Is it a high-fat diet or inflammation that leads to artery clogging and heart disease, or is it something we don't yet fully understand? Is the tap water we drink safe, or is it necessary to buy bottled water? Can we trust our grocery stores and food suppliers to provide safe food? What changes can we make to reduce risk now? In the future? Where should we start? What sources of information are accurate? Although it may seem that the issues are overwhelming and that health troubles are mounting daily, there is good news. But to understand more clearly the infinite ways that our actions influence health, we first need to look back and see how far we've advanced.

The health challenges that we face today could not have been imagined by our ancestors. Although pandemic disease has always been part of the human experience, most of today's issues were unthinkable just a generation or two ago. Disease and illness were seen as phenomena people had little power over, and people who became sick from an infectious disease either weathered the illness and recovered or, in all too many cases, died. Few choices were available in foods, medicines, and services; consequently, health care decisions usually focused on cleanliness, avoiding known hazards, and staying away from others who were sick. Over the decades, our list of options for improved health has steadily grown. Improvements in vaccines and antibiotics, new treatments for a wide range of illnesses, and new scientific knowledge about risks and hazards have helped us sift through the information overload and begin to make some sense of things.

Juxtaposed against the threats to health are advances in medical research, recognition that we need to do more to remove barriers and reduce disparities for some groups, new attention to policies designed to preserve health and protect against harm, and improved strategies for promoting health and preventing premature disease and disability. Technologies continue to be developed, with concomitant improvements in diagnosis of disease and treatment. Newspapers and scientific journals report evidence that dietary choices, exercise behaviors, and improvements in interpersonal relationships really matter. At no time in history has it been more evident that by taking action, an individual can prevent illness and prolong a productive, fully functional life. The better individuals prepare themselves to make wise decisions, and the more community leaders and representatives of the health care system work together to help achieve and maintain excellent health, the more likely that everyone's quality of life will improve.

Each fall, a new class of students enters college with improved access to health information and a better understanding of the complex interactions of risk factors that may influence their health. They are demanding safer campuses, healthier foods in cafeterias, and improved opportunities for fitness and social interactions. They are working to reduce risks from unsafe sex, too many drugs, and campus cultures that support too much partying. At the same time, they are faced with an astounding, often contradictory and confusing, array of health information through the simple click of a mouse; the routine switching on of the television, cell phone, or other media device; or the casual perusal of a magazine. Because there is no one recipe for achieving health, it is important for students to have choices; to know where to turn for reliable, scientifically valid information and support when they encounter problems; and to consider carefully how their actions may affect them and those around them.

After more than 30 years of teaching public health students from a wide range of health and other disciplines and after working on several editions of this book, I continue to be excited about the tremendous opportunities that students today have to make a difference in their health, the health of their loved ones, and the health of others. Part of my goal in writing this book is to help students be better decision makers and agents of change as they view today's health controversies and those that will shape their future—not just in the arena of personal health behaviors, but also in the larger realm of public policy and community behaviors, which ultimately can help the global population live smarter, longer, and better. In short, this book is designed not just to teach health facts but to present health as a much broader concept, something that everyone desires and deserves. Recognizing that many of today's health problems know no international boundaries, we challenge students to think globally as they consider health risks and seek creative solutions to health problems. By reading, questioning, gaining greater understanding of the factors that contribute to individual and societal health, and contemplating possible actions that may reduce risk, *Health: The Basics* prepares students for their own development, as well as a possible future in a health-related field.

New to This Edition

Page by page, *Health: The Basics* packs maximum information into a smaller and moderately priced text that will move students from just thinking about health improvements to being actively involved in their own health behavior changes. It is designed to provide the latest information in an engaging manner, to guide students in accessing reliable health information and services, and to encourage them to make health decisions based on the best science, rather than on pop mythology. The most noteworthy changes to the text as a whole include the following:

- A brand-new design features new chapter openers, vibrant colors, redesigned boxes, and overall updating. The redesign of the text provides the same pedagogical standards as in previous editions of *Health: The Basics,* with a modern and bold look aimed at engaging the student.
- New photographs in every chapter enhance the visual appeal and pedagogical value of the text. These new photos include images of birth control methods discussed in the text, the effects of tobacco smoke on lung tissue, the Bod Pod® body composition measurement machine, stretching exercises, and common pathogens.
- Did You Know?, a new, eye-catching art feature, highlights interesting health facts and statistics, many of which relate directly to the American college student population.
- Updates on the status of our nation's health include new discussions of the concept of healthy life expectancy, improving overall quality of life, the existence of health disparities that affect specific U.S populations, and key information about risk reduction for major areas that are within individual control.
- Global health issues receive expanded coverage. In an era of constant travel and instant communication, we would be remiss in not addressing the interaction of individual, community, and global health. Updates include information on global warming, disease statistics for different countries, and discussion of health-related policies outside the United States.

Chapter-by-Chapter Updates

The Eighth Edition has been updated, chapter by chapter, line by line; whether using classic references, current research from professional journals, or reputable national data sources, we have tried to provide students with not only the most current information, but also sources for further exploration. Figures, tables, feature boxes, and photos have all been added to, improved on, and updated. The following is a chapter-by-chapter listing of some of the most noteworthy changes, updates, and additions.

Chapter 1: Promoting Healthy Behavior Change
The focus on healthy behavior change has been enhanced with new information on the six critical health behaviors identified by the CDC and with discussion of the concepts of self-efficacy and internal versus external locus of control. New information has been added about the causes and prevalence of health disparities among U.S. populations, as have new statistics about global health trends. New figures illustrate some of the key determinants of health, the health-related impediments to academic performance among college students, and tips for overcoming obstacles to behavior change.

Chapter 2: Psychosocial Health
Information on the role psychosocial health plays in overall wellness has been updated. New information covers the importance of adequate sleep to overall wellness, information on common sleep problems, the role of spirituality in psychosocial health, tips for building self-esteem, expanded coverage of obsessive-compulsive disorder and depression, and the prevalence of mental health issues on college campuses.

Chapter 3: Managing Stress
The chapter now includes new coverage of the unique stressors international students face. We also have expanded the coverage of the impact of finances on stress and added a feature box discussing the relationship between stress and accumulated body fat.

Chapter 4: Preventing Violence and Abuse
Expanded and updated coverage on violence includes the latest facts and figures on trends in crime, economic implications of crime, and the emotional and physical burden of violent crime among selected populations, particularly college students. New to this edition are several figures detailing crime rates on campus, coverage of how campuses have responded to incidents such as the Virginia Tech shootings, and expanded coverage of drug-facilitated "date" rape.

Chapter 5: Healthy Relationships and Sexuality
Changes include the latest statistics about marriage and family structure in the United States, discussion of sexual orientation as a continuum, and an exercise for examining personal feelings about sexual orientation; reports on student misperceptions of sexual activity among their peers; and two new figures detailing the phases and hormonal control of the menstrual cycle.

Chapter 6: Birth Control, Pregnancy, and Childbirth
This chapter provides the latest information on contraceptive methods available to students today, including their relative effectiveness and key issues regarding their use. New photos of the various methods have been added to better students' understanding of their contraceptive options. Lea's Shield, FemCap, Ortho Evra, NuvaRing, the sponge, Seasonale, and Mirena are among the products described and assessed. Information on emergency contraception and its safety, efficacy and availability has been expanded. The coverage of abortion has been updated with the latest on its legality, on the federal abortion ban and the surrounding controversy, and on the emotional aspects of abortion.

Chapter 7: Addictive Behaviors, Licit and Illicit Drugs
The chapter offers new coverage of addiction and addictive behaviors, including the increase of compulsive gambling among college students, along with updates on the dangers and prevalence of "club drugs," methamphetamine, OxyContin, and other widely publicized drugs. A new feature looks at the emerging trend of prescription drug misuse and abuse.

Chapter 8: Alcohol, Tobacco, and Caffeine
Information about the effects of alcohol on mood and the dangers of combining alcohol and other depressants has been added. A new self-assessment focuses on evaluating personal drinking habits. Coverage of tobacco use has been updated with a section discussing the phenomenon of "social smoking," especially among college students, and a feature on protecting oneself and others from secondhand smoke. New photographs include images comparing a healthy liver to a liver with cirrhosis, a photo of leukoplakia, and images comparing healthy lung tissue to a smoker's lung tissue.

Chapter 9: Nutrition
Updated coverage of nutrition offers the latest statistics on Americans' consumption patterns and discusses the USDA's new MyPyramid Plan, including its key goals and features, and the role of physical activity in the new plan. Other additions are a new figure giving serving size guidelines, information on portion distortion, review of popular dietary supplements, and feature box evaluating some of the latest "diet hype."

Chapter 10: Managing Your Weight
Discussion of the global epidemic of obesity and the relationship between obesity and other major health problems has been updated to include the latest information on risk factors for obesity, health problems related to obesity, and new methods for assessing body composition. In addition, we've added a feature box analyzing popular diets, new tips on sensible snacking, additional focus on weight and body image, and the latest statistics about eating disorders among college students.

Chapter 11: Personal Fitness
A greatly revised fitness chapter emphasizes the distinction between physical activity for overall health and wellness and exercise for weight management or for athletic performance. The chapter also includes new figures on the FITT principle and the health benefits of exercise, new photos of stretching exercises, new self-assessments for muscular endurance and flexibility, new information on evaluating fitness products and equipment, and suggestions for dealing with specific obstacles to creating and following a fitness program.

Chapter 12: Cardiovascular Disease, Diabetes, and Cancer
We have combined the chapters on cardiovascular disease and cancer and have added diabetes coverage to it. This combination emphasizes the behavioral changes students can undertake to reduce their risks for all three types of major disease. Statistics and research about CVD and diabetes risk and incidence have been updated throughout, along with new information about potential long-term complications of diabetes. The chapter includes the latest morbidity and mortality statistics from the American Cancer Society, focus on lifestyle risk factors contributing to specific cancers, and a new feature with tips for protecting your skin from the sun and the threat of skin cancer. We also added new figures on the prevalence of CVD, the warning signs of cancer, and the correlation between tobacco use and lung cancer mortality.

Chapter 13: Infectious and Noninfectious Conditions
New and updated coverage includes the latest research and statistics on such prominent threats as avian influenza, West Nile virus, meningitis, SARS, "mad cow disease," hepatitis, and tuberculosis. Coverage of sexually transmitted infections has been updated with the latest statistics and developments, including information about the new HPV vaccine. In addition, we have expanded our discussions of sleep apnea, other sleep disorders, and asthma and have added a new feature box looking at the problem of antibiotic resistance. New figures illustrate the human immune response, adult immunization recommendations, and methods of HIV infection. New photos of common pathogens and of herpes, HPV, and syphilis infections reinforce the reality of infectious disease threats to college students.

Chapter 14: Life's Transitions
Updates include the latest information on life expectancy, health care costs, and Alzheimer's disease. A new feature box presents strategies for helping a friend who is mourning a death, and a new

self-assessment looks at one's personal anxiety over death and ways to address it.

Chapter 15: Environmental Health

Expanded coverage includes discussions of our roles and responsibilities for promoting environmental health, conservation, and protection. We have updated information on overpopulation and its impact on our planet's resources, added new material on the role of carbon dioxide in air pollution and global warming, and presented the latest statistics on water and land pollution in the United States. New topics include the impact of environmental tobacco smoke, molds, and household cleaners on indoor air quality. New figures illustrate world population growth, world oil consumption, the enhanced greenhouse effect, rates of recycling and waste generation, and decibel levels of various activities.

Chapter 16: Consumerism

New and updated information on health care consumerism in the United States includes discussion of health insurance coverage among college students and other groups of young adults and the latest developments in Medicare. A new Assess Yourself box encourages students to become better health care consumers. Two new figures illustrate the extent of health care expenditures in the United States and the breakdown of those expenses.

Chapter 17: Complementary and Alternative Medicine

The updated CAM chapter contains expanded explanations of Ayurveda and homeopathy and new information on massage therapy, including discussion of different types of massage and a new feature box on the benefits of massage therapy for lower back pain. A new Assess Yourself box looks at students' supplement "savvy," and the text incorporates the latest research on popular supplements, such as gingko biloba, St. John's wort, echinacea, glucosamine, and SAMe. In addition, we have added discussion of USP verification procedures and the new FDA regulations for supplements. New figures illustrate the four domains of CAM, the reasons Americans use CAM, and evaluating the potential risks and benefits of CAM treatments.

Maintaining a Standard of Excellence

With every edition, the challenge has been to make the book better than before and to provide information and material that surpass the competition at every level. As such, we have painstakingly considered our reviewer feedback from the previous edition and strengthened and improved pedagogical standards.

We believe that optimum health changes will occur only in environments that are conducive to change, in which individuals can maximize resources to make long-term behavior changes.

In *Health: The Basics*, we have striven to establish both the individual and social context of health and disease and to promote the importance of health to society as a whole. This dual focus, in which we acknowledge the many factors that may influence health decision making, presents students with a more realistic approach to their own health. The roles that the community, health policies, and health services play in disease prevention and health promotion are integrated throughout the text, while individual decision making through critical thinking and awareness continues to form the cornerstone of each chapter.

Features and Learning Aids

Each chapter in *Health: The Basics* includes the following proven pedagogical features designed to help students learn the material, think about healthy behavior skills, and apply the concepts to their own lives:

- **Chapter objectives** summarize the main competencies students will gain from each chapter and alert students to the key concepts covered in upcoming material.
- **Chapter opener questions** capture students' attention and engage them in what they will be learning later in the chapter. Questions are repeated within the chapter, where answers can be found.
- **What Do You Think?** critical-thinking questions appear throughout the text, encouraging students to pause and reflect on material they have read.
- **Assess Yourself** boxes help students evaluate their health behaviors and consider possible changes, and the **Make It Happen!** section within each box provides students with the opportunity to use the results of the self-assessment to create a plan for healthy behavior change.
- **Skills for Behavior Change** boxes focus on practical strategies that students can use to improve health or reduce their risks from negative health behaviors.
- **Try It Now!** features, which appear throughout the chapter, describe simple actions a student can do immediately to improve overall health and encourage positive lifestyle changes.
- **Health Headlines** boxes highlight new discoveries and research, as well as interesting trends in the health field.
- **Spotlight on Your Health** boxes focus attention on specific health and wellness issues that relate to college-aged students. Statistical information and trends help students recognize risks as they relate to particular behaviors and outcomes.
- **Consumer Health** boxes promote critical-thinking skills and informed consumerism by increasing awareness of the health market and focusing on particular consumer issues.
- **Health in a Diverse World** boxes expand discussion of health topics to diverse groups within the United States and around the world.

- **A running glossary** defines words on the page where students first encounter them, emphasizing and supporting understanding of material.
- **Taking Charge** sections wrap up the chapter content with a focus on application by the student. The Summary, multiple-choice Chapter Review questions (with answers in the back of the book), Questions for Discussion and Reflection, Accessing Your Health on the Internet, and Further Reading sections offer more opportunities to explore areas of interest. References for the chapter are also provided.
- **Preventing Injuries and Providing Emergency Care.** This section, appearing at the end of the book, discusses unintentional injuries and describes procedures that may prevent injury and save lives.
- **Behavior Change Contract.** Blank copies are included at both the front and back of the book. A sample filled-in contract is also included in the back.

Supplementary Materials

Available with *Health: The Basics, Eighth Edition* is a comprehensive set of ancillary materials designed to enhance learning and facilitate teaching.

Student Supplements

- **MyHealthLab** (www.aw-bc.com/myhealthlab). This online resource lets students access a wide range of print and media supplements that make studying convenient and fun. New to this edition of MyHealthLab are self-assessments that allow students to respond completely anonymously while still allowing instructors to see that they've completed the assignment. Additional contents include an interactive e-book, *ABC News* Lecture Launcher video clips, and over 70 electronic self-assessments. Contents also include the Behavior Change Log Book and Wellness Journal, links to Research Navigator (three databases of credible and reliable source materials), and activities available on the text's Companion Website.
- **Companion Website** (www.aw-bc.com/donatelle). This easy-to-navigate site offers *New York Times* articles relevant to the text content and over 70 electronic self-assessments. The website also offers practice quizzes, open-ended critical-thinking questions, hypothetical case studies, and links for the websites described at the end of each chapter. The website includes the Flashcard program and Glossary, with the entire list of terms and their definitions from the textbook available for study.
- **Take Charge of Your Health! Worksheets.** This pad of 50 self-assessment activities allows students to further explore their health behaviors and make steps towards positive change.

- **Behavior Change Log Book and Wellness Journal.** This assessment tool helps students track daily exercise and nutritional intake and create a long-term nutrition and fitness prescription plan. It includes behavior change contracts and topics for journal-based activities.
- *Live Right! Beating Stress in College and Beyond.* *Live Right!* gives students useful tips for coping with stressful life challenges both during college and for the rest of their lives. Topics include sleep, managing finances, time management, coping with academic pressure, and relationships. This book also presents an objective overview of some of the health-oriented products on the market.
- *Eat Right! Healthy Eating in College and Beyond.* This handy, full-color 80-page booklet provides students with practical guidelines, tips, shopper's guides, and recipes that turn healthy eating principles into blueprints for action. Topics include healthy eating in the cafeteria, dorm room, and fast-food restaurants; planning meals on a budget; weight management; vegetarian alternatives; and effects of alcohol on health.
- **MyDietAnalysis.** Powered by ESHA Research, Inc., MyDietAnalysis features a database of nearly 20,000 foods and multiple reports. This easy-to-use program allows students to track their diet and activity for up to three profiles and to generate and submit reports electronically.
- **Tutor Center.** Students can visit www.aw-bc.com/tutorcenter for round-the-clock support from tutors that can help them get through some of the more difficult concepts they might encounter in their personal health course.

Instructor Supplements

A full resource package accompanies *Health: The Basics* to assist the instructor with classroom preparation and presentation, including an overhauled test bank now organized around Bloom's Taxonomy, and updated course management offering anonymous MyHealthLab self-assessments.

- **MyHealthLab** (www.aw-bc.com/myhealthlab). This online resource is loaded with valuable, free teaching resources that make giving assignments and tracking student progress easy. Powered by CourseCompass, the preloaded content in MyHealthLab includes *ABC News* Lecture Launcher video clips, PowerPoint slides, Test Bank questions, Instructor Resource Manual material, and more. The anonymous self-assessments (new to this edition) let students to answer completely anonymously while still allowing instructors to see that they've completed the assignment; the entire class's results are aggregated in the gradebook. Students are likely to be more open and honest about their experiences in an anonymous format, and instructors are able to get a more concrete idea of what to focus on in classroom lectures.

- *ABC News* **Lecture Launcher Videos.** Created in partnership with *ABC News*, these 24 clips, each 8 to 12 minutes in length, will enliven lectures, spark classroom discussion, and engage students. The videos are also integrated in the PowerPoint lectures and are available as separate full-screen videos on the Media Manager and through MyHealthLab.

- **Teaching Tool Box.** Developed to support adjunct and part-time faculty teaching the personal health course, and also to be invaluable to veteran instructors, this kit offers all the tools instructors need to guide students through the course. The box includes the Course-at-a-Glance Quick Reference Guide, Health Support Manual (with First-Time Teaching Tips), Instructor Resource Manual with Media Guide, Test Bank, Media Manager with *ABC News* Lecture Launcher videos and TestGen, MyHealthLab Instructor Access Kit, *Great Ideas: Active Ways to Teach Health and Wellness,* and Transparency Acetates. The Tool Box also includes the supplemental materials available for students, such as the Behavior Change Logbook and Wellness Journal, Take Charge of Your Health! worksheets, *Eat Right!*, and *Live Right!*.

- **Course-at-a-Glance Quick Reference Guide.** This valuable supplement acts as a roadmap to the Teaching Tool Box. The available resources are broken down by chapter, and further by page number, so instructors can easily see what resources are available for each chapter in the book. One side lists resources for instructors to use when preparing for a lecture or while in class. The other side outlines where to find the resources students can use in their homework or in-class activities.

- **Health Support Manual: First-Time Teaching Tips and Visual Lecture Outlines.** Organized by chapter, this key manual provides a step-by-step visual guide to the resources available to instructors. It includes information on available PowerPoint lectures with the accompanying figures and art, integrated Lecture Launcher video discussion questions, tips and strategies for managing large classrooms, suggestions for integrating MyHealthLab and MyDietAnalysis into classroom activities and homework assignments, and the best strategies to promote active learning strategies using our Great Ideas in Health and Wellness newsletters.

- **Instructor's Resource Manual with Media Guide.** This teaching tool provides student and classroom activities, chapter objectives, lecture outlines, and Companion Website resources to reinforce chapter concepts and develop effective student learning. It also includes ideas for incorporating the *ABC News* video clips into the course and discussion questions for the e-themes articles.

- **Printed Test Bank and Computerized Test Bank.** The questions in the comprehensively revised test bank were reviewed by a panel of instructors for relevance and accuracy. This new test bank incorporates a Bloom's Taxonomy question categorization to indicate the type of learning each question is testing. A Remembering question, for example, tests students' recall of terms. The Understanding, Applying, Analyzing, and Evaluating categories encourage students to think progressively more analytically and critically. The Test Bank includes approximately 2,500 multiple-choice, short-answer, true/false, matching, and essay questions, all with answers and page references. The cross-platform TestGen CD-ROM enables instructors to create tests, edit questions, and add their own material to existing exams.

- **Media Manager.** This cross-platform set of CD-ROMs includes all figures and tables from the book, along with select photos. Lecture outlines that may be customized for presentation are also included, with embedded links to *ABC News* videos and slides with appropriate discussion questions. Word files of the Test Bank and Instructor Resource Manual are available, as well as Active Lecture Questions for in-class clicker systems, and a quiz show game offered in PowerPoint. Media Manager comes packaged with a two-volume CD-ROM with full-screen *ABC News* video clips and the TestGen CD-ROM.

- **Transparency Acetates.** The figures and tables from the text are available as full-color transparencies.

- *Great Ideas: Active Ways to Teach Health and Wellness.* This newly revised publication provides effective, proactive strategies for teaching health topics in a variety of classroom settings, contributed by health educators from around the country.

- **Clickers in the Classroom.** This handbook provides detailed guidance in enhancing lectures using clicker (Classroom Response Systems) technology.

- **Course Management.** In addition to MyHealthLab, WebCT and Blackboard are also available. Contact your Benjamin Cummings sales representative for details.

ACKNOWLEDGMENTS

After writing eight editions of *Health: The Basics,* I can only marvel at the dedication and professionalism of the many fine publishing experts who have helped make such a text successful. With each subsequent edition, their skills in dealing with the complexities and considerations of the publication process have become more apparent. Although the author provides the information and framework for a text, it is really the dedication and skill of the editorial, production, and sales staff that make a book successful. Over the years, I have been extremely fortunate in having a steady stream of fine publishing teams to help me create a text that was responsive to students, creative in approach, and reflective of the most important health trends of the times. I am extremely grateful for all of the contributions that these individuals have made in making *Health: The Basics* a leading text in the field.

Since the acquisition of *Health: The Basics* and *Access to Health* by Benjamin Cummings, I have been extremely pleased by the professionalism, dedication, and attention to detail that this team has displayed as we've progressed through several editions of the books. They are truly outstanding and a pleasure to work with. From the highly skilled and enthusiastic Acquisitions Editor, Sandra Lindelof, to the rest of the superior editorial staff, I have been uniformly amazed at their consistent efforts to produce a great finished product. Although I wouldn't have thought it possible to beat past publishing efforts, I must honestly say that my experiences with Benjamin Cummings have been the best of my publishing years, and remarkably, it just keeps getting better! The team members personify key aspects of what it takes to be successful in the publishing world, from this author's perspective: drive and motivation for hard work and efficient process; commitment to excellence; a vibrant, youthful, and enthusiastic approach that is in tune with college student needs; and personalities that motivate an author to strive continually to produce market-leading texts.

In previous editions of *Health: The Basics*, I was extremely impressed by the superb effort, expertise, and level-headed perspectives that Project Editor Susan Malloy provided in making early editions of the text come alive. In subsequent editions and in the initiation of this edition, I was fortunate to have worked with Alison Rodal, a bright, highly skilled and creative Project Editor who helped bring *Health: The Basics* to the next level. Although I was sorry to see her leave, I was not surprised when Benjamin Cummings followed their tradition of excellence in securing another top-notch Project Editor, Kari Hopperstead. Kari has provided the insight, attention to detail, and creative touches that made this edition especially "tuned in" to student interests. Without undue pressure on me, she was able to keep the book on schedule while paying attention to the countless details and providing direction in what I believe is the best edition of the text to date.

I feel fortunate that Benjamin Cummings invests in their staff and picks outstanding professionals dedicated to producing high quality texts. Without the efforts of people like Kari and her predecessors, in particular, these texts would not have come to fruition or enjoyed the successes that they have achieved. Thank you, Susan, Alison, and Kari!

In addition, I would like to acknowledge the wonderful editorial assistance provided by Developmental Editor Alice E. Fugate, who has been with this project for the last three editions. Her skill in helping merge text from *Health: The Basics* and *Access to Health* has been invaluable. In addition, she has made terrific suggestions on improving each edition of these texts based on reviewer comments and market demands and has provided great ideas for content areas that were "in the news." This was a huge and complicated task, and as usual, Alice did a remarkable job.

Although these women were key contributors to the finished work, there were many other people who worked on this revision of *Health: The Basics*. In particular, I would like to thank Michele Mangelli and Wendy Earl at Wendy Earl Productions for their invaluable assistance in final book development and refinement and Emily Portwood, Assistant Editor, for overseeing the complete supplements package. I would also like to thank the Benjamin Cummings marketing and sales force, particularly Marketing Manager, Neena Bali, who does a superb job of making sure that *Health: The Basics* gets into instructors' hands and that adopters receive the service they deserve. This is an important, often overlooked part of selling texts, and without Neena's direction and the superb work of a dedicated, professional sales force, *Health: The Basics* would not be as successful as it is. In keeping with my overall experiences with Benjamin Cummings, the marketing and sales staff are among the best of the best. I am very lucky to have them working with me on this project and want to extend a special thanks to all of them!

Contributors to the Eighth Edition

Many colleagues, students, and staff members have provided the feedback, reviews, extra time and assistance, and encouragement that have helped me meet the demands of rigorous publishing deadlines over the years. Whether acting as reviewers, generating new ideas, providing expert commentary, or writing chapters, each of these professionals has added his or her skills to our collective endeavor.

I would like to thank specific contributors to chapters in this edition. Dr. Patricia Ketcham (Oregon State University)—Chapter 6, Birth Control, Pregnancy, and Childbirth; Chapter 7, Addictive Behaviors, Licit and Illicit Drugs; Chapter 8, Alcohol, Tobacco, and Caffeine; and Chapter 16, Consumerism—did a superb job of updating key chapters of concern to today's college students. In her position as Director of Health Promotion at OSU, she is in tune with the unique concerns of students and is constantly developing strategies to help students achieve health and success in their college years and beyond. Dr. Peggy Pederson (Western Oregon State University)—Chapter 3, Managing Stress; Chapter 5, Healthy Relationships and Sexuality; and Chapter 14, Life's Transitions—provided both her expertise in this area and an engaging writing style that greatly enhanced the quality and presentation of updates to these chapters; Dr. Amy Eyler (St. Louis University) provided significant expertise and a wealth of teaching and research knowledge to update and expand Chapter 11, Personal Fitness. Dr. Karen Elliott (Oregon State University)—Chapter 17, Complementary and Alternative Medicine—provided important updates for the ever-changing facts about CAM, CAM research, and CAM use in society. Karen also utilized her expertise in teaching courses in HIV/AIDS and STIs to update these discussions within Chapter 13, Infectious and Noninfectious Conditions. Each of these contributors has worked on various chapters of this text over the years. Their expertise and insights help ensure that the specific content oversight of this text is superb and reflects the interests and needs of students on campuses across the country.

Reviewers for the Eighth Edition

Clearly, *Health: The Basics* continues to be an evolving work in progress. With each new edition, we have built on the combined expertise of many colleagues throughout the country who are dedicated to the education and behavioral changes of students. We thank the many reviewers of the past seven editions of *Health: The Basics* who have made such valuable contributions.

For the eighth edition, reviewers who have helped us continue this tradition of excellence include Rachel Abbott, University of West Georgia; Kim Archer, Stephen F. Austin University; Linda Beatty, McLennan Community College; Evonne Bird, Truman State University; Susan Butler, Emory University; Amanda Collings Vann, University of Massachusetts at Amherst; Debra Guenther, Montgomery College at Rockville; Shelley Hamill, Winthrop University; Jody Hart, John A. Logan College; Jessica Hartos, University of North Carolina at Charlotte; Mary Iten, University of Nebraska at Kearney; Mark Kittleson, Southern Illinois University; Justin Laird, Columbia University; Susan Moore, Western Illinois University; Tanya Morgan, Westchester University; Elisha Nixon-Cobb, Kean University; Ann Sebren, Arizona State University; Holly Turner Moses, University of Florida; and Karen Vail-Smith, East Carolina University; and Carolyn Willingham, Philips Community College. Many thanks to all!

Rebecca J. Donatelle, PhD
Health & Kinesiology
Benjamin Cummings
1301 Sansome Street
San Francisco, California 94111

Promoting Healthy Behavior Change

Do my friends and family **influence** my health choices?

What can I do to **change** an unhealthy habit?

How can I **distinguish** a bogus health claim from a real one?

How can I set a realistic health **goal?**

OBJECTIVES

- Discuss health in terms of its dimensions and historical perspectives.
- Explain the importance of a healthy lifestyle in preventing premature disease and in promoting wellness.
- Discuss the health status of Americans and the significance of *Healthy People 2010* and other national initiatives to promote health.
- Understand the importance of a global perspective on health, and recognize how gender and racial and cultural background influence disparities in health status, research, and risk.
- Focus on your current risk behaviors, and realize how they can impact your current and future health.
- Learn how to apply behavior-change techniques to your own lifestyle.

Interested in improving your health? Concerned about the health of a loved one, a particular population, or the state of our global health and not sure what to do about it? If so, you are not alone. At no time in our history have so many individuals, government agencies, community groups, businesses, policymakers, and health organizations focused so intently on a growing list of national and international health concerns. Epidemic rates of obesity, diabetes, and other chronic diseases, a wide range of environmental threats, and other health problems are highlighted daily in the popular media. Fears of terrorist threats, extreme weather events, and a growing list of infectious diseases add to our worries. This widespread focus on health issues makes even the most healthy among us wonder whether there is anything we can do to protect ourselves, our loved ones, and the very future of our planet.

The good news is that in spite of an ever-growing list of threats, the list of actions that we can take to prevent our own premature disease and disability and to help others reduce their risks also grows daily. We're experiencing an unprecedented "wake-up-call" about how our seemingly insignificant actions can ultimately have an affect on life as we know it. There are numerous examples of this rededication to positive change. Consider this: scientists and politicians alike have reached consensus that global warming is real, and all levels of society are calling for change. The food industry is reducing dietary threats to human health, and policies are mandating increased safety in our food supply. Many of us are working hard to change our lifestyles, protect our environment, and be smarter health consumers. So, why isn't the good news even better?

Let's face it: getting and staying healthy is a challenge for most of us and requires knowledge and willpower. We know that we should eat right, exercise more, recycle, and manage stress—but when a pizza with "the works" is placed in front of us, we can't resist. We are creatures of habit, and comfortable habits are often hard to break.

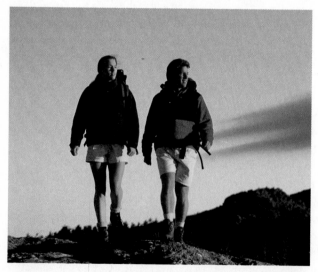

Today, health and wellness mean taking a positive, proactive attitude toward life and living it to the fullest.

Our ability to make wise health choices is complicated by conflicting health claims, faulty research, and scientific reports written in technical language. Even the best scientists struggle to determine which research is valid and which provides only a preliminary indicator of harm or benefit. The average person is left wondering how to wade through the information available on the Internet and in the media and to determine the best course of action.

Not only must we negotiate the variety of information sources available to us, but we also must be aware of how the media often exploits our weaknesses and how businesses profit by catering to our fears and desires through clever ad campaigns. Food advertisements encourage us to consume enormous portions of high-fat foods and to eat when we aren't hungry, are overstressed, or feeling blue.

The struggle to make personal health choices is not just a matter of willpower and knowledge. For some people, making positive lifestyle choices is even more difficult because they lack necessary resources to purchase healthy foods or adequate insurance to have preventive screenings. Social and environmental conditions play an important role in the health choices we make and the options we have. These inequities in health care and information access can make our choices easier or much more difficult.

In spite of the many factors and challenges influencing health, many people have made real strides in reducing personal risks to health. They have become smart and savvy health consumers by successfully negotiating the information available and have taken action to improve their health. Most important, these individuals have found their own unique ways to make small changes to sustain long-term positive behavior change. They have identified unhealthy behavior, planned a course of action, and changed their lifestyle for the better. Have you ever wondered, for example, how one of your friends was able to lose weight and now walks up four flights of stairs to class, while you dash to the nearest elevator? Why do so many good health intentions remain only intentions?

This textbook cannot provide a foolproof recipe for achieving health in all areas. It is designed to provide fundamental knowledge about health topics, to help you use personal and community resources to create your own health profile, and to challenge you to think more carefully before making decisions that affect your health or the health of others at the local, national, and international levels. It shows how policies, programs, media, culture, ethnicity, gender, and socioeconomic status directly and indirectly influence health in the United States and around the world.

It is our hope that you will gain appreciation for the many achievements that have been made in health and the many challenges that lie ahead. Your generation faces an unprecedented number of advances in health, as well as a multitude of challenges. However, you have access to the knowledge, resources, and technology necessary to make positive changes. We hope that you will look at health not in an ethnocentric way, in which you focus only on your own health and that of people who look and talk like you and have habits and customs like yours. Instead, we hope that you consider your actions in the context of your own health, the health of your friends and families, and the health of millions of people in the world who are affected by your decisions.

...r control, ...oday and ...yond your ...opriately, ...ionale for ...ns, you ... life and

Health- is the state of complete physical, mental, & social well-being, not just the absence of disease or infirmity.

...usly, few ... some, ...thers, it ...ist illness. Still others use terms such as **wellness,** or *well-being,* to include a wide array of factors that lead to positive health status. Why all of these variations?

In part, the differences in perception are due to an increasingly enlightened way of viewing health that has taken shape over time. As our understanding of illness has improved, so has our ability to understand what it means to be healthy. Although our current understanding of health has evolved over centuries, we face many challenges in ensuring that everyone has equal opportunities for achieving it.

Health: Yesterday and Today

Prior to the 1800s, if you weren't sick, you were regarded as lucky. When childhood diseases such as diphtheria were virtually unstoppable and deadly epidemics such as bubonic plague, influenza, and cholera killed millions of people, survivors were believed to be of hearty, healthy stock and congratulated themselves on their good fortune. Those in poor health often suffered from the stigma of poor hygiene or being contagious and lived in conditions that harbored illness and spread disease. Not until the late 1800s did researchers recognize that entire populations were victims of environmental factors (such as microorganisms found in contaminated water, air, and human waste) over which they had little control. Public health officials moved swiftly to clean water supplies and enact other policies to help populations at greatest risk. As a result, *health* became synonymous with *good hygiene*. Colleges offered courses in health and hygiene, the predecessors of the course you are taking today.

Investigation into the environment as the primary cause of disease continued into the twentieth century as outbreaks of tuberculosis, pneumonia, and influenza surged in many regions of the world. Continued improvements in sanitation and the development of vaccinations and antibiotics that stopped the spread of infectious diseases brought dramatic changes in life expectancy.

By the 1940s, progressive thinkers began to note that there was more to health than hygiene or disease. At an international conference in 1947, the World Health Organization took the landmark step of clarifying what health truly meant: "Health is the state of complete physical, mental, and social well-being, not just the absence of disease or infirmity."[1]

Today, scientists recognize that health is much more than the absence of disease. It includes the physical, social, and mental elements of life, as well as environmental, spiritual, emotional, and intellectual dimensions. To be truly healthy, a person must be capable of functioning at an optimal level in each of these areas, as well as interacting with others and the greater environment. Rather than simply looking at how long we live, or the number of disease-free years we enjoy, public health researchers know that the quality of those years is also vital. Today, *quality of life* is considered as important as years of life. It's not just how long we live, but also how *well* we live.

Morbidity (illness) rates indicate dramatic decline in common infectious diseases that devastated our ancestors. Today, many childhood diseases, such as measles and pertussis, can be prevented or cured because of improvements in education, socioeconomic conditions, medical technology, vaccinations, and other public health measures. For these reasons, average life expectancy at birth in the United States has risen to 77.85 years. According to **mortality** (death) rate statistics, people are now living longer than at any time in our history.[2]

Will this trend continue? A recent study projects that today's newborns may be the first generation to have a lower life expectancy than that of their parents.[3] Largely attributable to the consequences of obesity, researchers report that life expectancy could decline by as much as 5 years over the course of the next few decades.[4]

The Evolution toward Wellness

René Dubos, biologist and philosopher, aptly summarized the thinking of his contemporaries by defining health as "a quality of life, involving social, emotional, mental, spiritual, and biological fitness on the part of the individual, which results from adaptations to the environment."[5] The concept of adaptability, or the ability to successfully cope with life's ups and downs, became a key element of the overall health definition. Eventually the term *wellness* became popular. It included the previously mentioned elements and also implied that there

health The ever-changing process of achieving individual potential in the physical, social, emotional, mental, spiritual, and environmental dimensions.

wellness The achievement of the highest level of health possible in each of several dimensions.

morbidity The relative incidence of disease.

mortality The proportion of deaths to population.

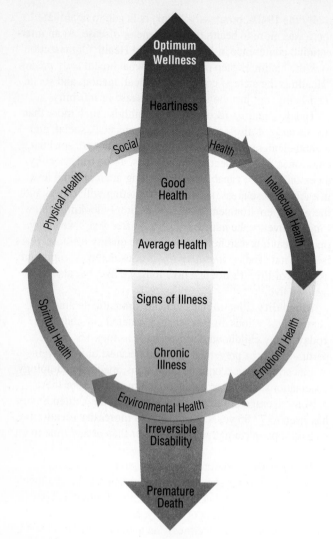

FIGURE 1.1 The Dimensions of Health and the Wellness Continuum

were levels of health within each category. To achieve *high-level wellness,* a person would move progressively higher on a continuum of positive health indicators. People who fail to achieve these levels may move lower on the continuum. Today, the terms *health* and *wellness* are often used interchangeably to mean the dynamic, ever-changing process of achieving one's potential in each of several interrelated dimensions. These dimensions typically include those presented in **Figure 1.1** and described below:

- *Physical health* includes characteristics such as body size and shape, sensory acuity and responsiveness, susceptibility to disease and disorders, body functioning, physical fitness, and recuperative abilities. Newer definitions of

physical health also include our ability to perform normal **activities of daily living (ADLs),** the tasks necessary to normal existence in today's society. Getting out of bed in the morning, bending over to tie your shoes, and other usual daily tasks are examples of ADLs.

- *Social health* refers to the ability to have satisfying interpersonal relationships, including interactions with others, adaptation to social situations, and appropriate daily behaviors in society.
- *Intellectual health* refers to the ability to think clearly, reason objectively, analyze critically, and use brain power effectively to meet life's challenges. It means learning from successes and mistakes and making responsible decisions that take into consideration all aspects of a situation.
- *Emotional health* refers to the ability to express emotions when they are appropriate, controlling them when they are not, and avoiding expressing them inappropriately. Self-esteem, self-confidence, self-efficacy, trust, love, and many other emotional reactions and responses are all part of emotional health.
- *Environmental health* refers to an appreciation of the external environment and the role individuals play to preserve, protect, and improve environmental conditions.
- *Spiritual health* involves subscribing to a way of life or a belief in a supreme being based on a particular religious doctrine or feeling of unity with a greater force and a guiding sense of meaning or value in all life. True spiritual health typically goes well beyond an organized religion and includes many more aspects of living a balanced, introspective and meaningful life.

Although typically not considered a dimension in most wellness continuums, **mental health** is an important concept. Often confused with emotional, social, spiritual, or intellectual

activities of daily living (ADLs) Tasks of everyday living, such as bathing and walking up and down stairs.

mental health The thinking part of psychosocial health; includes your values, attitudes, and beliefs.

TABLE 1.2	What Is *Healthy People 2010?*

Overarching Goals
1. Increase quality and years of healthy life
2. Eliminate health disparities

Focus Areas
1. Access to quality health services
2. Arthritis, osteoporosis, and chronic back conditions
3. Cancer
4. Chronic kidney disease
5. Diabetes
6. Disability and secondary conditions
7. Educational and community-based programs
8. Environmental health
9. Family planning
10. Food safety
11. Health communication
12. Heart disease and stroke
13. Human immunodeficiency virus (HIV)
14. Immunization and infectious diseases
15. Injury and violence prevention
16. Maternal, infant, and child health
17. Medical product safety
18. Mental health and mental disorders

19. Nutrition and overweight
20. Occupational safety and health
21. Oral health
22. Physical activity and fitness
23. Public health infrastructure
24. Respiratory disease
25. Sexually transmitted disease
26. Substance abuse
27. Tobacco use
28. Vision and hearing

Leading Health Indicators
1. Physical activity
2. Overweight and obesity
3. Tobacco use
4. Substance abuse
5. Responsible sexual behavior
6. Mental health
7. Injury and violence
8. Environmental quality
9. Immunization
10. Access to health care

Source: Office of Disease Prevention and Health Promotion, U.S. Department of Health and Human Services, *Healthy People 2010,* 2000, www.health.gov/healthypeople/About/hpfact.htm.

health, it is a broader concept that encompasses all of these dimensions. According to the U.S. surgeon general, this umbrella term refers to the "successful performance of mental function, resulting in productive activities, fulfilling relationships with others, and the ability to adapt to change and cope with adversity. From early childhood until late life, mental health is the springboard of thinking and communication skills, learning, emotional growth, resilience, and self-esteem."[6] What are some behaviors that a healthy individual might practice **(Table 1.1)**?

Many people believe that the best way to achieve wellness is to adopt a *holistic* approach, which emphasizes the integration of and balance among mind, body, and spirit. Achieving wellness means attaining the optimum level of wellness for a person's unique limitations and strengths. A physically disabled person may function at his or her optimum level of performance; enjoy satisfying interpersonal relationships; maintain emotional, spiritual, and intellectual health; and have a strong interest in environmental concerns. In contrast, a person who spends hours lifting weights to perfect the size and shape of each muscle but pays little attention to nutrition may look healthy but not have a good balance in all areas of health. Although we often consider physical attractiveness and other external trappings in measuring overall health, these are only two indicators of wellness and indicate little about the other dimensions.

How healthy are you? Complete the **Assess Yourself** box on page 6 to gain perspective on your own level of wellness in each dimension.

 what do you THINK?

Based on the wellness dimensions discussed, what are your key strengths in each dimension? ▪ What are your key deficiencies? ▪ What one or two things can you do to enhance your strong areas? ▪ To improve your weaknesses?

New Directions for Health

In 1990, the U.S. surgeon general proposed a national plan for promoting health among individuals and groups. Known as *Healthy People 2000,* the plan outlined a series of long-term objectives. Although many communities worked toward achieving these goals, as a nation we still had a long way to go by the new millennium.

Healthy People 2010

The *Healthy People 2010* plan takes the original initiative to the next level. *Healthy People 2010* is a nationwide program with two broad goals: (1) increase life span and quality of life and (2) eliminate health disparities. It includes 28 focus areas and a list of 10 leading health indicators (LHIs) that spell out specific health issues, each representing a public health priority **(Table 1.2).**

(Text continues on page 10.)

ASSESS yourself

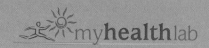

HOW HEALTHY ARE YOU?

Fill out this assessment online at
www.aw-bc.com/MyHealthLab or
www.aw-bc.com/donatelle.

Although we all recognize the importance of being healthy, it can be a challenge to sort out which behaviors are most likely to cause problems or which ones pose the greatest risk. Before you decide where to start, it is important to take a careful look at your health status right now. Think carefully about where you believe that you are today in each of the dimensions of health. Rate your health status in each of the following dimensions by circling the number on the line that comes closest to describing the way you are most of the time.

	Poor Health		Average Health		Excellent Health
Physical health	1	2	3	4	5
Social health	1	2	3	4	5
Emotional health	1	2	3	4	5
Environmental health	1	2	3	4	5
Spiritual health	1	2	3	4	5
Intellectual health	1	2	3	4	5

After completing the above section, how would you rate your *overall* health?

_____

Which area(s), if any, do you think you should work on improving?

_____

If we were to ask your closest friends how healthy they think you are, which area(s) do you think they would say you need to work on and improve?

_____

By completing the following assessment, you will have a clearer picture of health areas in which you excel and those that could use varying degrees of work. Taking this assessment will also help you to reflect on various components of health that you may not have thought about.

Answer each question. Then total your score for each section, and fill it in on the Personal Checklist at the end of the assessment for a general sense of your health profile. Think about the behaviors that influenced your score in each category. Would you like to change any of them? Choose the area that you'd like to improve, and then complete the Behavior Change Contract at the front of your book. Use the contract to think through and implement a behavior change over the course of this class.

Each of the categories in this questionnaire is an important dimension of health, but this is not a substitute for the advice of a qualified health care provider. Consider scheduling a thorough physical examination by a licensed physician or setting up an appointment with a mental health counselor at your school if you think you need help making a behavior change.

For each of the following, indicate how often you think the statements describe you.

	Never	Rarely	Some of the Time	Usually or Always
PHYSICAL HEALTH				
1. I am happy with my body size and weight.	1	2	3	4
2. I engage in vigorous exercises such as brisk walking, jogging, swimming, or running for at least 30 minutes per day, 3–4 times per week.	1	2	3	4
3. I do exercises designed to strengthen my muscles and increase endurance at least 2 times per week.	1	2	3	4
4. I do stretching, limbering up, and balance exercises such as yoga, Pilates, or tai chi to increase my body awareness and to control and increase my overall physical health.	1	2	3	4
5. I feel good about the condition of my body and would be able to respond to most demands placed upon it.	1	2	3	4

	Never	Rarely	Some of the Time	Usually or Always

6. I get at least 7–8 hours of sleep each night.
    1   2   3   4

7. I try to add moderate activity to each day, such as taking the stairs instead of the elevator and walking instead of riding whenever I can.
    1   2   3   4

8. My immune system is strong, and my body heals itself quickly when I get sick or injured.
    1   2   3   4

9. I have lots of energy and can get through the day without being overly tired.
    1   2   3   4

10. I listen to my body; when there is something wrong, I try to make adjustments to heal it or seek professional advice.
    1   2   3   4

Total score for this section: _____

SOCIAL HEALTH

1. When I meet people, I feel good about the impression I make on them.
    1   2   3   4

2. I am open, honest, and get along well with other people.
    1   2   3   4

3. I participate in a wide variety of social activities and enjoy being with people who are different.
    1   2   3   4

4. I try to be a "better person" and work on behaviors that have caused problems in my interactions with others.
    1   2   3   4

5. I get along well with the members of my family.
    1   2   3   4

6. I am a good listener.
    1   2   3   4

7. I am open and accessible to a loving and responsible relationship.
    1   2   3   4

8. I have someone I can talk to about my private feelings.
    1   2   3   4

9. I consider the feelings of others and do not act in hurtful or selfish ways.
    1   2   3   4

10. I try to see the good in my friends and do whatever I can to support them and help them feel good about themselves.
    1   2   3   4

Total score for this section: _____

EMOTIONAL HEALTH

1. I find it easy to laugh, cry, and show emotions such as love, fear, and anger, and I try to express these in positive, constructive ways.
    1   2   3   4

2. I avoid using alcohol or other drugs as a means of helping me forget my problems.
    1   2   3   4

3. When viewing a particularly challenging situation, I tend to view the glass as "half full" rather than "half empty" and perceive problems as opportunities for growth.
    1   2   3   4

4. When I am angry, I try to let others know in nonconfrontational and nonhurtful ways and try to resolve issues rather than stewing about them.
    1   2   3   4

5. I try not to worry unnecessarily and try to talk about my feelings, fears, and concerns rather than letting them become chronic issues.
    1   2   3   4

6. I recognize when I am stressed and take steps to relax through exercise, quiet time, or other calming activities.
    1   2   3   4

7. I feel good about myself and believe others like me for who I am.
    1   2   3   4

8. I try not to be too critical and/or judgmental of others and to understand differences or quirks that I may note in others.
    1   2   3   4

9. I am flexible and adapt or adjust to change in a positive way.
    1   2   3   4

10. My friends regard me as a stable, emotionally well-adjusted person whom they trust and rely on for support.
    1   2   3   4

Total score for this section: _____

(continues)

	Never	Rarely	Some of the Time	Usually or Always
ENVIRONMENTAL HEALTH				
1. I am concerned about environmental pollution and actively try to preserve and protect natural resources.	1	2	3	4
2. I buy recycled paper and purchase biodegradable detergents and cleaning agents whenever possible.	1	2	3	4
3. I recycle my garbage, purchase refillable containers when possible, and try to minimize the amount of paper and plastics that I use.	1	2	3	4
4. I try to wear my clothes for longer periods between washing to reduce water consumption and the amount of detergent in our water sources.	1	2	3	4
5. I vote for pro-environment candidates in elections.	1	2	3	4
6. I write my elected leaders about environmental concerns.	1	2	3	4
7. I turn down the heat and wear warmer clothes at home in winter and use the air conditioner only when necessary or at higher temperatures in summer.	1	2	3	4
8. I am aware of lead pipes in my living area, chemicals in my carpet, and other potential hazards, and I try to reduce my exposure whenever possible.	1	2	3	4
9. I use both sides of the paper when taking class notes or doing assignments.	1	2	3	4
10. I try not to leave the faucet running too long when I brush my teeth, shave, or shower.	1	2	3	4

Total score for this section: _____

	Never	Rarely	Some of the Time	Usually or Always
SPIRITUAL HEALTH				
1. I believe life is a precious gift that should be nurtured.	1	2	3	4
2. I take time to enjoy nature and the beauty around me.	1	2	3	4
3. I take time alone to think about what's important in life—who I am, what I value, where I fit in, and where I'm going.	1	2	3	4
4. I have faith in a greater power, be it a Godlike force, nature, or the connectedness of all living things.	1	2	3	4
5. I engage in acts of caring and goodwill without expecting something in return.	1	2	3	4
6. I feel sorrow for those who are suffering and try to help them through difficult times.	1	2	3	4
7. I look forward to each day as an opportunity for further growth and challenge.	1	2	3	4
8. I work for peace in my interpersonal relationships, in my community, and in the world at large.	1	2	3	4
9. I have a great love and respect for all living things, and regard animals, etc., as important links in a vital living chain.	1	2	3	4
10. I go for the gusto and experience life to the fullest.	1	2	3	4

Total score for this section: _____

	Never	Rarely	Some of the Time	Usually or Always
INTELLECTUAL HEALTH				
1. I carefully consider my options and possible consequences as I make choices in life.	1	2	3	4
2. I learn from my mistakes and try to act differently the next time.	1	2	3	4

	Never	Rarely	Some of the Time	Usually or Always
3. I follow directions or recommended guidelines, avoid risks, and act in ways likely to keep myself and others safe.	1	2	3	4
4. I consider myself to be a wise health consumer and check reliable information sources before making decisions.	1	2	3	4
5. I am alert and ready to respond to life's challenges in ways that reflect thought and sound judgment.	1	2	3	4
6. I have at least one hobby, learning activity, or personal growth activity that I make time for each week: something that improves me as a person.	1	2	3	4
7. I actively learn all I can about products and services before making decisions.	1	2	3	4
8. I manage my time well rather than let time manage me.	1	2	3	4
9. My friends and family trust my judgment.	1	2	3	4
10. I think about my self-talk (the things I tell myself) and then examine the evidence to see whether my perceptions and feelings are sound.	1	2	3	4

Total score for this section: _____

Although each of these six dimensions of health is important, there are some factors that don't readily fit one dimension. As college students, you face some unique risks that others may not. For this reason, we have added an additional section to this self-assessment that focuses on personal health promotion and disease prevention. Answer these questions, and add your results to the Personal Checklist in the following section.

PERSONAL HEALTH PROMOTION/DISEASE PREVENTION

	Never	Rarely	Some of the Time	Usually or Always
1. I know the warning signs of common sexually transmitted infections, such as genital warts (HPV), chlamydia, and herpes, and read new information about these diseases as a way of protecting myself.	1	2	3	4
2. If I were to be sexually active, I would use protection such as latex condoms, dental dams, and other means of reducing my risk of sexually transmitted infections.	1	2	3	4
3. At parties or during happy hours, I find ways other than binge drinking to loosen up and have a good time.	1	2	3	4
4. When I have more than 1 or 2 drinks, I ask someone who is not drinking to drive me and my friends home.	1	2	3	4
5. I have eaten too much in the last month and have forced myself to vomit to avoid gaining weight.	4	3	2	1
6. I have several piercings and have found that I enjoy the rush that comes with each piercing event.	4	3	2	1
7. If I were to have a tattoo or piercing, I would go to a reputable person who follows strict standards of sterilization and precautions against bloodborne disease transmission.	1	2	3	4
8. I engage in extreme sports and find that I enjoy the highs that come with risking bodily harm through physical performance.	4	3	2	1
9. I am careful not to mix alcohol or other drugs with prescription and over-the-counter drugs.	1	2	3	4
10. I practice monthly breast/testicle self-examinations.	1	2	3	4

Total score for this section: _____

(continues)

PERSONAL CHECKLIST

Now, total your scores in each of the health dimensions, and compare them to what would be considered optimal scores. Which areas do you need to work on? How does your score compare with how you rated yourself in the first part of the questionnaire?

	Ideal Score	Your Score
Physical health	40	_____
Social health	40	_____
Emotional health	40	_____
Environmental health	40	_____
Spiritual health	40	_____
Intellectual health	40	_____
Personal health promotion/ disease prevention	40	_____

What Your Scores in Each Category Mean

Scores of 35–40: Outstanding! Your answers show that you are aware of the importance of these behaviors in your overall health. More important, you are putting your knowledge to work for you by practicing good health habits that should reduce your overall risks. Although you received a very high score on this part of the test, you may want to consider areas where your scores could be improved.

Scores of 30–34: Your health practices in these areas are very good, but there is room for improvement. Look again at the items you answered that scored 1 or 2 points. What changes could you make to improve your score? Even a small change in behavior can help you achieve better health.

Scores of 20–29: Your health risks are showing! Find information about the risks you are facing and why it is important to change these behaviors. Perhaps you need help in deciding how to make the changes you desire. Assistance is available from this book, your professor, and student health services at your school.

Scores below 20: You may be taking unnecessary risks with your health. Perhaps you are not aware of the risks and what to do about them. Identify each risk area, and make a mental note as you read the associated chapter in the book. Whenever possible, seek additional resources, either on your campus or through your local community health resources, and make a serious commitment to behavior change. If any area is causing you to be less than functional in your class work or personal life, seek professional help. In this book you will find the information you need to help you improve your scores and your health. Remember that these scores are only indicators, not diagnostic tools.

For each focus area, the plan presents specific objectives for the nation to achieve during the next decade. For instance, nutrition data show that only 42 percent of Americans aged 20 and older are at their healthy weight; the goal is to raise that number to 60 percent. In the focus area of physical activity and fitness, 40 percent of Americans aged 18 and older do not engage in any leisure-time physical activity. The objective is to reduce this number to 20 percent by 2010.[7]

An overarching goal of *Healthy People 2010* is to eliminate **health disparities.** Disparities in health care are often the result of disadvantages faced by minority groups, women, and children, whose health care suffers because of their race,

ethnicity, gender, and/or socioeconomic status. This goal is particularly important as we consider the increasingly diverse population in the United States. According to the 2000 U.S. Census, approximately 30 percent of the population currently belongs to a racial or ethnic minority group. It is projected that by the year 2100, non-Hispanic whites will make up only 40 percent of the U.S. population.[8]

National Changes: Improving Health and Reducing Disparities

Are we making progress? From all indicators, national priorities are shifting, and health professionals and public and private organizations are beginning to work together to help people make better health decisions. For example, cities across the United States are passing legislation that bans

health disparities Differences in the incidence, prevalence, mortality, and burden of diseases and other health conditions among specific population groups.

MAKE it happen!

ASSESSMENT: The Assess Yourself activity gave you the chance to look at the status of your health in several dimensions. Now that you have considered these results, you can begin to take steps toward changing certain behaviors that may be detrimental to your health.

MAKING A CHANGE: To change your behavior, you need to develop a plan. Follow these steps below and complete your Behavior Change Contract to take action.

1. Evaluate your behavior, and identify patterns and specific things you are doing. What can you change now? What can you change in the near future?

2. Select one pattern of behavior that you want to change.

3. Fill out the Behavior Change Contract found at the front of your book. It should include your long-term goals for change, your short-term goals, the rewards you'll give yourself for reaching these goals, potential obstacles along the way, and strategies for overcoming these obstacles. For each goal, list the small steps and specific actions that you will take.

4. Chart your progress in a journal. At the end of a week, consider how successful you were in following your plan. What helped you be successful? What made change more difficult? What will you do differently next week?

5. Revise your plan as needed: Are the short-term goals attainable? Are the rewards satisfying?

EXAMPLE: Felipe assessed his health and discovered that his score in the Personal Health Promotion section was low—25 points—because of some risky behaviors in which he was engaging. In particular, he realized that he had driven several times after drinking and that he was not performing monthly testicle self-examinations. Felipe decided to tackle one of these issues at a time. He completed a Behavior Change Contract to drive only when he had had fewer than 2 drinks. Steps in his contract included finding out about designated driver programs, moderating his drinking so that he was sober and competent to drive at the end of a night out with friends, and finding concerts and other events to attend that did not involve drinking. The rewards he chose for these steps included tickets to a concert and a new computer game. After a few months, Felipe realized that he had been in several situations in which he might previously have driven under the influence. Instead, he had given himself alternatives such as designated drivers, budgeting for a taxi, and moderating his drinking, and thus he had avoided unsafe situations.

Next month, Felipe will get a pamphlet from the health center on testicular self-exams and choose a day of the month to be his self-examination day. Every month that he does the exam, he'll sleep in an extra hour that weekend as a reward.

---

trans fats from restaurant food items. This landmark action and others are designed to improve life span, quality of life, and the state of our environment.

On the flip side, we do still see disparities in health care, such as those evident during the Hurricane Katrina disaster. Some populations are at a distinct disadvantage when it comes to getting healthy and staying healthy. For example, if you are a college student without health insurance and on a limited budget, you may put off a visit to the doctor or not go at all. If you have a serious illness, this delay can lower your chance of successful treatment. Factors such as language barriers can also impact an individual's health negatively. A recent study by the UCLA Center for Health Policy Research reported that people whose primary language is not English or who could not read prescription labels or follow written medical instructions had significant barriers to overall health.[9]

Recognizing the changing demographics of the U.S. population and the vast differences in health status based on racial or ethnic background, *Healthy People 2010* included strong language about the importance of reducing health disparities.[10] Contributors to disparities include the following:

- *Race and ethnicity.* Research indicates dramatic health disparities among people with specific racial and ethnic backgrounds. These differences are believed to be attributed not to race or genetic susceptibility, but rather to socioeconomic differences, poor access to health care, cultural barriers, beliefs, discrimination, and limited education and employment opportunities.

- *Inadequate health insurance.* Large numbers of people are *uninsured* or *underinsured*. Those without adequate insurance coverage may face high co-payments, high deductibles, or limited care in their area (for more on health insurance, see Chapter 16).

- *Lifestyle behaviors.* Persistent poverty may make it difficult to buy healthy food, get enough rest and exercise, cope with stress, and seek preventive medicine. Obesity, smoking, and lack of exercise are examples of health problems related directly to behavioral and cultural patterns we adopt from our families.
- *Transportation.* Whether you live in an urban or rural area and have access to public transportation or your own vehicle can have a huge impact on what you choose to eat and your ability to visit the doctor or dentist. Older people, people with disabilities, and people who lack the financial means to travel for preventive tests such as mammograms are clearly at a health disadvantage.

A New Focus on Health Promotion

The objectives of *Healthy People 2010* have prompted action to promote health and prevent premature disability through social, environmental, policy-related, and community-based programming. There is also a new emphasis on assisting individuals in changing unhealthy behaviors. The term **health promotion** describes the educational, organizational, procedural, environmental, social, and financial supports that help individuals and groups reduce negative health behaviors and promote positive change. Health promotion programs identify healthy people who are engaging in **risk behaviors** (actions that increase susceptibility to negative health outcomes), motivate them to change their actions, and provide support to increase chances of success. Effective stop-smoking programs, for instance, don't simply say, "Just do it." Instead, they provide information about possible consequences to smokers and the people they expose to secondhand smoke (educational support); encourage smokers to participate in smoking cessation classes and allow employees time off to attend or set up buddy systems to help them (organizational support);

establish policies governing smokers' behaviors and supporting their decisions to change, such as banning smoking in the workplace and removing cigarettes from vending machines (environmental support); and provide monetary incentives to motivate people to participate (financial support).

Health promotion programs also encourage people with sound health habits to maintain them. By attempting to modify behaviors, increase skills, change attitudes, increase knowledge, influence values, and improve health decision making, health promotion goes well beyond the simple information campaign. By basing services in communities, organizations, schools, and other places where most people spend their time, health promotion programs increase the likelihood of long-term success on the road to health and wellness.

Whether we use the term *health* or *wellness,* we are talking about a person's overall responses to the challenges of living. Occasional dips into the ice cream bucket and other dietary indulgences, failures to exercise every day, flare-ups of anger, and other deviations from optimal behavior should not be viewed as major failures. Actually, the ability to recognize that each of us is an imperfect being attempting to adapt in an imperfect world signals individual well-being.

We must also remember to be tolerant of others. Rather than be warriors against pleasure in our zeal to change the health behaviors of others, we need to be supportive, nonjudgmental, and helpful to people trying to achieve their own health goals. Ultimately, we all have to find our own best way to make change happen.

Disease Prevention

Most health promotion initiatives include **disease prevention.** Historically, the health literature describes three types of prevention: primary, secondary, and tertiary.

In a general sense, *prevention* means taking positive actions now to avoid becoming sick later. Getting immunized against diseases such as polio, deciding not to smoke cigarettes, and practicing safer sex constitute **primary prevention**—actions designed to reduce risk and avoid health problems before they start. **Secondary prevention** (also referred to as **intervention**) involves recognizing health risks or early problems and taking action (intervening) to stop them before they lead to actual illness. Getting a young smoker to quit is an example of secondary prevention. The third type, **tertiary prevention,** involves treatment and/or rehabilitation after a person is already ill. Typically, health care professionals practice tertiary prevention.

Health Status Report: How Well Are We Doing?

In the United States, chronic diseases account for seven of the ten leading causes of death and are linked to preventable lifestyle behaviors such as tobacco use, poor nutrition and

health promotion   Combined educational, organizational, policy, financial, and environmental supports to help people reduce negative health behaviors and promote positive change.

risk behaviors   Behaviors that increase susceptibility to negative health outcomes.

disease prevention   Actions or behaviors designed to keep people from getting sick.

primary prevention   Actions designed to stop problems before they start.

secondary prevention (intervention)   Intervention early in the development of a health problem.

tertiary prevention   Treatment and/or rehabilitation efforts.

The Centers for Disease Control and Prevention (CDC) has identified six health behaviors that contribute significantly to chronic disease and illness. These habits often begin early in life and are preventable. If you practice any of the behaviors listed below, they may not affect you now, but there is a very high chance they will impact your health down the road. Choosing to make changes now will prevent illness later on.

1. *Tobacco use.* Over 4,000 American youth aged 12–17 start smoking every day. Asthma, respiratory and cardiovascular diseases, gum diseases, cancer, and other chronic health problems increase dramatically in smoking adults.

2. *Unhealthy dietary behavior.* Almost 80% of young adults do not eat the daily recommended serving of fruits and vegetables. Nearly 9 million youth aged 6–19 are overweight.

3. *Inadequate physical activity.* As children age, physical activity declines. Less than one-third of all young adults participate in physical activity on a regular basis.

4. *Unsafe sexual behaviors that lead to HIV, other STIs, and unintended pregnancy.* Nearly 34% of young women become pregnant at least once before they reach the age of 20, and about 19 million become infected with an STI. Almost half of all STIs are in people aged 15–24.

5. *Alcohol and drug use.* Alcohol abuse is the third leading preventable cause of death in the United States and is a factor in approximately 42% of all car crashes.

6. *Injury and violence.* Injury and violence is the leading cause of death among youth aged 10–24.

Source: National Center for Chronic Disease Prevention and Health Promotion, "Healthy Youth! Six Critical Health Behaviors," 2006, www.cdc.gov/HealthyYouth/healthtopics/index.htm.

lack of physical activity leading to obesity, alcohol use, car crashes, risky sexual behavior, and drug use. **Table 1.3** describes the six main preventable risk behaviors identified by the Centers for Disease Control and Prevention (CDC). These preventable risk behaviors not only kill many, but also affect quality of life for nearly 100 million Americans and account for 70 percent of total medical expenditures.[11]

Primary and secondary prevention offers our best hope for reducing the **incidence** (number of new cases), and **prevalence** (number of existing cases) of disease and disability. Model intervention programs for a multitude of health problems have been well tested and have proven effective in the community. If you are interested in learning more about primary prevention programs, check out the CDC website, and search for model prevention programs.

Health educators in our schools and communities offer an effective delivery mechanism for prevention and intervention programs. **Certified Health Education Specialists (CHES)** make up a trained cadre of public health educators with special credentials and competencies in developing prevention programs that offer scientifically and behaviorally sound methods to help individuals and communities increase the likelihood of success in achieving optimal health. These specialists have the skills and experience to greatly enhance the nation's health. A major shift in focus from treatment to prevention is necessary to achieve our national goals.

Improving Quality of Life

In the last decade, the way we look at health has been quietly shifting. This new view will have a profound impact on how we perceive our nation's health status. For decades we have looked at steadily increasing life expectancy rates and proudly proclaimed that the health of Americans has never been better. Recently, however, health organizations and international groups have attempted to quantify the number of years a person lives with a disability or illness compared to the number of healthy years. The World Health Organization summarizes this concept as **healthy life expectancy.** Simply stated, healthy life expectancy refers to the number of years a newborn can expect to live in full health, based on current rates of illness and mortality. For example, if we could delay the onset of diabetes so that a person didn't develop the disease until she was 60 years old, rather than developing it at 30, there would be a dramatic increase in that individual's healthy life expectancy. Several countries are currently working to develop policies to increase healthy life expectancy.[12]

This concept of healthy life expectancy can have tremendous implications for your health and motivation to change behaviors now. Although you know that you should exercise, maintain a healthy weight, and not drink and drive, the threat of heart disease, cancer, or accident-related injuries seems decades away. Recognizing how your present actions will play a role in your future health can motivate you to make behavior changes now to ensure the maximum number of happy, healthy years.

incidence The number of new cases.

prevalence The number of existing cases.

Certified Health Education Specialist (CHES) Academically trained health educator who has passed a national competency examination for prevention and intervention programming.

healthy life expectancy The number of years a newborn can expect to live in full health, based on current rates of illness and mortality.

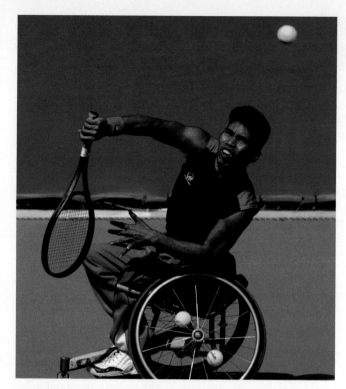

The motivation to improve quality of life within the framework of one's own unique capabilities is crucial to achieving health and wellness.

 what do you THINK?

Think about your own health right now. On a scale from 1 to 10, with 1 being the lowest and 10 the highest, rate your fitness level (going for a run; hiking up a hill), your ability to form and maintain healthy relationships, and your ability to cope with daily stressors.

Achievements in Public Health

Shortcomings aside, for those of us in the field of public health, the saying "We've come a long way, baby" accurately reflects the health achievements of the past 100 years. **Table 1.4** lists the ten greatest public health achievements of the past century according to the CDC.

The more we learn about the remarkable resilience of the human body and spirit, and the more that technology stretches our imagination and enlarges our possibilities, the more likely that the twenty-first century will surpass the twentieth in health-related breakthroughs.

cultural competency A set of congruent attitudes and policies that come together in a system or among individuals and enables effective work in cross-cultural situations.

TABLE 1.4	Ten Greatest Public Health Achievements of the Twentieth Century

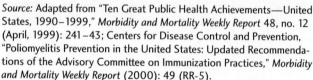
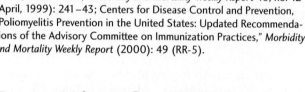

1. Vaccinations
2. Motor vehicle safety
3. Workplace safety
4. Control of infectious diseases
5. Reduction in cardiovascular disease (CVD) and stroke deaths
6. Safe and healthy foods
7. Maternal and infant care
8. Family planning
9. Fluoridated drinking water
10. Recognition of tobacco as a health hazard

Source: Adapted from "Ten Great Public Health Achievements—United States, 1990–1999," *Morbidity and Mortality Weekly Report* 48, no. 12 (April, 1999): 241–43; Centers for Disease Control and Prevention, "Poliomyelitis Prevention in the United States: Updated Recommendations of the Advisory Committee on Immunization Practices," *Morbidity and Mortality Weekly Report* (2000): 49 (RR-5).

Preparing for Better Health in the Twenty-First Century

As the demographics of the U.S. population change, we will need to take action at the federal, state, local, and individual level to reduce health disparities and achieve the goal of health for every person. Although it is important that each of us work to preserve and protect our own health, it is also important to become actively engaged in the health of our communities, our nation, and the global population. Central to this goal is the concept of **cultural competency**, defined as a set of congruent attitudes and policies that come together in a system or among individuals and enables effective work in cross-cultural situations.[13] The mark of a truly healthy person is whether the individual focuses beyond the "me" aspect of human existence and becomes equally concerned with the "we" aspect of health, as well as having a sense of responsibility about the broader environment we live in. As a college student in the twenty-first century, it is important that you understand the cultural differences of America's diverse population, examine your own health-related values and beliefs, and help others navigate the health system and make healthy choices.

A Focus on Global Health Issues

Everyone's health is profoundly affected by economic, social, behavioral, scientific, and technological factors. The world economy has become increasingly interconnected and globalized; every day, millions of people move across national

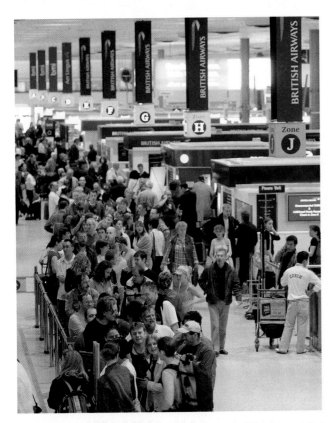

Modern travel has made health and the spread of disease a global issue. The deadly flu pandemic of 1918 took over one year to travel around the globe. Today, modern air travel could spread illness globally in a matter of weeks.

borders, leading to many new challenges for health around the world. Current concern over pandemic flu is a grim reminder of the need for a proactive international response to disease prevention. Health risks are not limited to disease; contaminants to our food, air, and water supplies, global warming, and chemical toxins are modern health threats to the global community.[14]

Likewise, health disparities are not just a national concern. Disparities exist in every nation around the globe, but those that lack adequate resources such as food, water, and shelter, have weak economies, and offer poor access to health care face severe challenges. In developed nations, the leading causes of death are heart disease, stroke, and cancer. In developing nations, people die from infections long eradicated in more prosperous countries.[15]

Attaining global health in the twenty-first century will require each of us to do our part to protect our own health and the health of others, whether at home or abroad. We will need time to understand the vast differences in health status across various social groups and to promote community action that addresses the unique needs of each population.

Gender Differences and Health

When it comes to health-related differences, men and women really do seem to be from Mars and Venus. Though much of the male and female anatomy is identical, researchers are discovering that the same diseases and treatments can affect men and women very differently. Many illnesses—for example, osteoporosis, multiple sclerosis, depression, diabetes, and Alzheimer's disease—are much more common in women, even though rates for these diseases seem to be increasing in men. Why these differences? Is it simply a matter of lifestyle? Clearly, it is much more complicated than that. Consider the following:[16]

- The size, structure, and function of the brain differ in women and men, particularly in areas that affect mood and behavior and in areas used to perform the same tasks. Reaction time is slower in women, but accuracy is higher.
- Bone mass in women peaks in their twenties; in men, it peaks gradually until age 30. At menopause, women lose bone at an accelerated rate, and 80 percent of people with osteoporosis are women.
- Women's cardiovascular systems are different in size, shape, and nervous system impulses, and women have faster heart rates.
- Women's immune systems are stronger than men's, but women are more prone to autoimmune disease (diseases in which the body attacks its own tissues, such as multiple sclerosis, lupus, and rheumatoid arthritis). Women experience pain in ways different from men and may react to pain medications differently.

Differences do not stop there; according to a report by the Society for Women's Health Research:[17]

- Women respond differently to prescription, over-the-counter, and illicit drugs. For example, antidepressants are absorbed, distributed, and eliminated differently in women, and monthly fluctuation in a woman's hormones may also alter drug response. Women are therefore more likely to need dosage adjustments and more follow-up care.
- Women who smoke are at increased risk for elevated LDL (bad) cholesterol and are more likely to die of lung cancer, suffer a stroke, and develop cardiovascular and respiratory disease than men who smoke the same number of cigarettes.
- Women are more likely than men to suffer a second heart attack within one year of their first heart attack.
- Women are two times more likely than men to contract a sexually transmitted infection and ten times more likely to contract HIV (the virus that causes AIDS) when having unprotected intercourse.

Surprisingly, although these and countless other disparities in health have long been recognized, researchers largely ignored the unique aspects of women's health until the 1990s, when the National Institutes of Health (NIH) funded a highly publicized 15-year, $625 million dollar study. Known as the **Women's Health Initiative (WHI),** this study was designed

Women's Health Initiative (WHI) National study of post-menopausal women conducted in conjunction with the NIH mandate for equal research priorities for women's health issues.

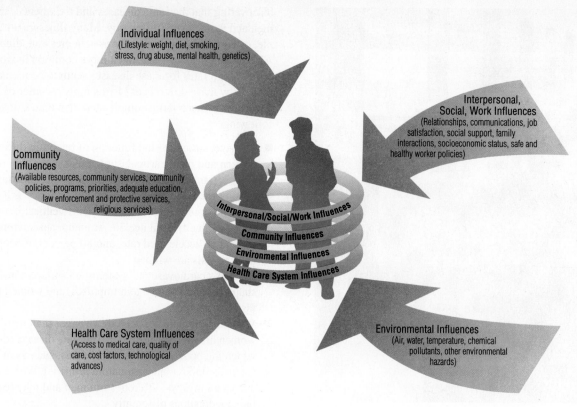

Individual Influences
(Lifestyle: weight, diet, smoking, stress, drug abuse, mental health, genetics)

Interpersonal, Social, Work Influences
(Relationships, communications, job satisfaction, social support, family interactions, socioeconomic status, safe and healthy worker policies)

Community Influences
(Available resources, community services, community policies, programs, priorities, adequate education, law enforcement and protective services, religious services)

Interpersonal/Social/Work Influences
Community Influences
Environmental Influences
Health Care System Influences

Health Care System Influences
(Access to medical care, quality of care, cost factors, technological advances)

Environmental Influences
(Air, water, temperature, chemical pollutants, other environmental hazards)

FIGURE 1.2 Factors That Influence Health Status

to focus research on the uniqueness of women with respect to drug trials, development of surgical instruments, and other health issues rather than assuming that women would respond just like the men previously studied. The WHI and several follow-up studies are providing invaluable information about women's risks and potential strategies for prevention, intervention, and treatment.

 what do you THINK?

Why do you think there are differences between men and women in their risks for certain diseases?
■ Which of the differences highlighted in the previous section could be modified through changes in health behavior?

Improving Your Health

Table 1.5 summarizes the leading causes of death in the United States. Note that Americans aged 15 to 24 are most likely to die from unintentional injuries, followed by homicide and suicide. Alcohol is a leading factor in many of these deaths (see Chapter 8). Unintentional injuries are also the major killer for people aged 25 to 44, followed by malignant neoplasms (cancer) and heart disease.

Individual behavior is a major determinant of good health. Heredity, access to health care, the environment, and many other factors can also influence health status **(Figure 1.2).** When these factors are considered together and form the basis of a person's lifestyle choices, the net effect on health can be great. All of us, no matter where we are on the health and wellness continuum, have to start somewhere.

Changing Your Health Behaviors

As Mark Twain said, "Habit is habit, and not to be flung out the window by anyone, but coaxed downstairs a step at a time." The chances of successfully changing negative habits improve when you identify a key behavior that you want to change and develop a plan for gradual modification that allows you time to unlearn negative patterns and substitute positive ones.

 First, identify what is most important to you or what causes you the greatest immediate and long-term risks. For example, if you are concerned about your weight, assess your eating patterns and decide where you can make changes that you can live with. Too many of us decide on New Year's Day that we are going to lose weight, exercise more, find more friends, and essentially reinvent ourselves overnight! Is it any wonder that we don't keep most of these resolutions?

All Ages

Diseases of the heart	665,089
Malignant neoplasms	556,902
Cerebrovascular diseases	157,689
Chronic lower respiratory diseases	125,382
Unintentional injuries	109,277

Under 1 Year

Congenital anomalies	5,621
Short gestation or low birth weight	4,849
Sudden infant death syndrome	2,162
Maternal complications	1,710
Complications of placenta, cord, membranes	1,099

1–4

Unintentional injuries	1,717
Cogenital anomalies	541
Malignant neoplasms	392
Homicide	376
Diseases of the heart	186

5–14

Unintentional injuries	2,618
Malignant neoplasms	1,076
Congenital anomalies	386
Homicide	324
Suicide	250

15–24

Unintentional injuries	15,272
Homicide	5,368
Suicide	3,988
Malignant neoplasms	1,651
Diseases of the heart	1,133

25–44

Unintentional injuries	29,307
Malignant neoplasms	19,290
Diseases of the heart	16,850
Suicide	11,667
Homicide	7,626

45–64

Malignant neoplasms	145,535
Diseases of the heart	102,792
Unintentional injuries	25,007
Diabetes mellitus	16,389
Cerebrovascular diseases	16,073

65+

Diseases of the heart	563,390
Malignant neoplasms	388,911
Cerebrovascular diseases	138,134
Chronic lower respiratory diseases	109,139
Alzheimer's disease	62,817

Source: D. Hoyert et al., "Deaths: Final Data for 2003," in *National Vital Statistics Reports* 54, no. 13 (Hyattsville, MD: National Center for Health Statistics, 2006).

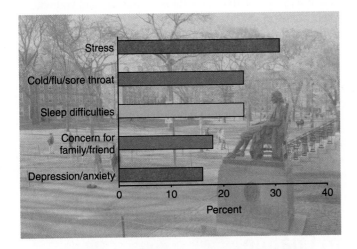

FIGURE 1.3 Effects of Health on Academic Performance
Your personal health and wellness can affect your academic success. In a recent American College Health Association survey, students indicated specific health problems that prevented them from performing at their best.

Source: American College Health Association, "American College Health Association–National College Health Assessment (ACHA–NCHA) Web Summary," 2006, www.acha.org/projects_programs/ncha_sampledata.cfm.

Factors That Influence Behavior Change

Figure 1.4 identifies major factors that influence behavior and behavior-change decisions. They can be divided into three general categories: predisposing, enabling, and reinforcing.

Predisposing Factors Our life experiences, knowledge, cultural and ethnic heritage, and current beliefs and values are all *predisposing factors* that influence behavior. Factors that may predispose us to certain health conditions include age, sex, race, income, family background, educational background, and access to health care. For example, if your parents smoked, you are 90 percent more likely to start smoking than someone whose parents didn't. If your peers smoke, you are 80 percent more likely to smoke than someone whose friends don't.

Enabling Factors Skills and abilities; physical, emotional, and mental capabilities; community and government priorities and commitment to health; and safe and convenient resources and facilities that make health decisions

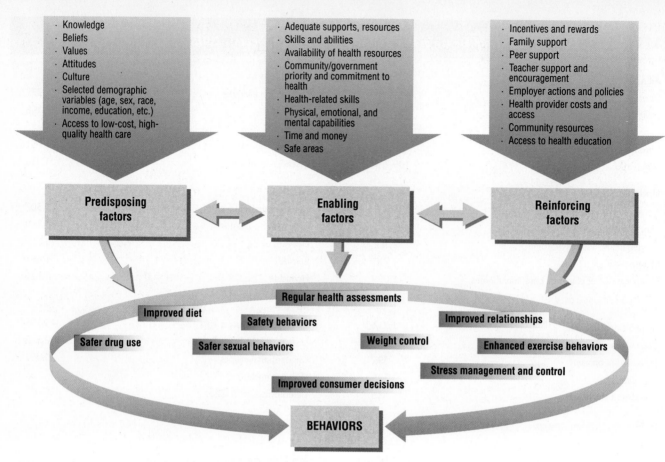

FIGURE 1.4 Factors That Influence Behavior-Change Decisions

easy or difficult are *enabling factors*. Positive enablers encourage you to carry through on your intentions to change. Negative enablers work against your intentions to change. For example, if you would like to join a local fitness center but discover that the closest one is four miles away and the membership fee is $500, those negative enablers may convince you to stay home. By contrast, if your school's fitness center is two blocks away, stays open until midnight, and offers a special student membership, those positive enablers will probably convince you to join. Identifying positive and negative enabling factors and devising alternative plans when the negative factors outweigh the positive are part of planning for behavior change.

Reinforcing Factors *Reinforcing factors* include the presence or absence of support, encouragement, or discouragement that significant people in your life bring to a situation; employer actions and policies; health provider costs and access; community resources; and access to health education. For example, if you decide to stop smoking and your family and friends continue smoking in your presence, you may be tempted to start smoking again. In other words, your smoking behavior is reinforced. If, however, you are overweight, you

lose a few pounds, and all your friends tell you how terrific you look, your positive behavior is reinforced, and you will likely continue your weight-loss plan.

The manner in which you reward or punish yourself in the process of change also plays a role. Accepting small failures and concentrating on your successes can foster further achievements. Berating yourself because you binged on ice cream or argued with a friend may create an internal environment in which failure becomes almost inevitable. Telling yourself that you're worth the extra effort and giving yourself a pat on the back for small accomplishments are often overlooked factors in positive behavior change.

Motivation and Readiness to Change

Wanting to change is a prerequisite of the change process, but there is much more to the process than motivation. *Motivation* must be combined with common sense, commitment, and a realistic understanding of how best to move from point A to point B. *Readiness* is the state of being that precedes behavior change, and people who are ready are likely to make the actual effort.[18] People who are ready to change possess the attitudes, knowledge, skills, and internal and external resources that make change possible.

Some of us need a little boost before we are able to change our behaviors. Rewards, or incentives for successfully reaching goals that we set, are effective ways to keep ourselves on track. For example, you might allow yourself to eat something that you really enjoy after losing 5 pounds, rather than depriving yourself until you lose all 30 of the pounds that you want to lose. The **Skills for Behavior Change** box on page 20 describes the series of stages that a person progresses through in successfully changing a health behavior.

Self-Efficacy

Self-efficacy is one of the most important factors influencing our health status. People who have it are more likely to take action to improve their health, stick to the plan of action, and experiment with other options for making improvements. **Self-efficacy** is defined as an individual's belief that he or she is capable of achieving certain goals or performing at a level that may influence events in life.[19] In general, people who exhibit high self-efficacy are confident they can succeed, and they approach challenges with a positive attitude. Prior success in academics, athletics, or social interactions will lead to expectations of success in the future. Self-efficacious people are more likely to feel a sense of **personal control** over situations. People who approach challenges, such as changing an unhealthy behavior, with confidence may be more motivated to change and achieve a greater level of success. In contrast, someone with low self-efficacy may give up easily or never even try to change a behavior. People with low self-efficacy tend to shy away from difficult challenges. They may have failed before, and when the going gets tough they are more likely to give up or revert to old patterns of behavior. How can one improve self-efficacy? Learning new skills and having successful experiences can help improve confidence and develop a "can-do" attitude.

External versus Internal Locus of Control

 The conviction that you have the ability to change is a powerful motivator. Individuals who feel that they have limited control over their lives often find it more difficult to initiate positive changes.[20] If they believe that someone or something else controls a situation, they may become easily frustrated and give up. People with these characteristics have an *external locus of control,* which can rob them of confidence in their ability to succeed in a particular behavior. Often, they are among the first to follow the crowd and to engage in risky behaviors that they believe will increase their popularity. In contrast, people who are confident that their behavior will influence an outcome in a manner they desire tend to have an *internal locus of control.*

They are more apt to take action because they think it's important, are less motivated by what others think, and feel they are in charge of the situation.

 what do you THINK?

If you were trying to adopt a healthy new behavior—for example, starting to exercise 30 minutes per day—who could you ask to support you?
- What factors could make this change difficult?
- What skills will you need to succeed? ▪ How ready are you?

Beliefs and Attitudes

We often assume that when rational people realize that their actions put them at risk, they will act to reduce that risk—but this is not necessarily true. Consider the number of health professionals who smoke, consume junk food, and act in other unhealthy ways. They surely know better, but their "knowing" is disconnected from their "doing." Why is this so? Two strong influences on behavior are beliefs and attitudes.

A **belief** is an appraisal of the relationship between some object, action, or idea (for example, smoking) and some attribute of that object, action, or idea (for example, smoking is expensive, is dirty, and causes cancer—or, it is relaxing). An **attitude** is a relatively stable set of beliefs, feelings, and behavioral tendencies in relation to something or someone.

Psychologists studying the relationship between beliefs and health habits have determined that although beliefs can subtly influence behavior, they may not actually cause people to behave differently. In 1966, psychologist I. Rosenstock developed a classic theory, the **Health Belief Model (HBM),** to show when beliefs affect behavior change.[21] Although many other models attempt to explain the influence of beliefs on behaviors, the HBM remains one of the most widely accepted. It holds that several factors must support a belief before change is likely:

- *Perceived seriousness of the health problem.* How severe would the medical and social consequences be if the

self-efficacy   Belief in one's ability to perform a task successfully.

personal control   Belief that one's own internal resources allow one to control a situation.

belief   Appraisal of the relationship between some object, action, or idea and some attribute of that object, action, or idea.

attitude   Relatively stable set of beliefs, feelings, and behavioral tendencies in relation to something or someone.

Health Belief Model (HBM)   Model for explaining how beliefs may influence behaviors.

SKILLS FOR *behavior change*

STAGING FOR CHANGE

Many of us resolve to change a given behavior, only to return to the behavior after a short time.

Why do so many good intentions fail? According to Drs. James Prochaska and Carlos DiClemente, we are going about things in the wrong way, and fewer than 20 percent of us are really prepared to take action. Prochaska and DiClemente believe that behavior changes usually fail if they start with the change itself. Instead, we must go through a series of stages to prepare ourselves for that change.

1. *Precontemplation.* People in the precontemplation stage have no current intention of changing. They may have tried to change a behavior before and given up, or they may be in denial and unaware of any problem.
   Strategies for Change: Sometimes a few frank, yet kind, words from friends may be enough to make precontemplators take a closer look at themselves. Recommending readings or making tactful suggestions can help precontemplators consider making a change.
2. *Contemplation.* In this phase, people recognize that they have a problem and begin to contemplate the need to change. People can languish in this stage for years, realizing that they have a problem but lacking the time or energy to address it.
   Strategies for Change: Often, contemplators need a little push to get them started. This may come in the form of helping them set up a change plan (for example, inviting a friend to join you on

your morning walk), buying a helpful gift (such as a low-fat cookbook), sharing articles about a particular problem, or inviting them to go with you to hear a speaker on a related topic.
3. *Preparation.* Most people at this point are close to taking action. They've thought about what they might do and may even have come up with a plan.
   Strategies for Change: People in the preparation stage can benefit from following a few simple guidelines. Set realistic goals (large and small), take small steps toward change, change only a couple of things at once, reward small milestones, and seek support from friends. Fill out the Behavior Change Contract in the front of this book to help you commit to making these changes.
4. *Action.* In this stage, people begin to follow their action plans. Those who have prepared for change, thought about alternatives, engaged social support, and made a realistic plan of action are more ready than those who have given it little thought. Unfortunately, too many people start behavior change here rather than going through the first three stages.
   Strategies for change: Publicly stating the desire to change helps ensure success. Encourage friends who are making a change to share their plans with you. Offer to help, and try to remove potential obstacles from the person's intended action plan.
5. *Maintenance.* Maintenance requires vigilance, attention to detail, and long-term commitment. Many people reach

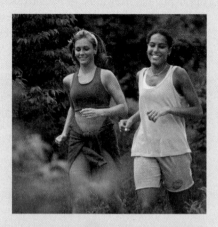

a goal, only to relax and slip back into the undesired behavior. Be aware of the potential for relapses, and develop strategies for dealing with such challenges. Common causes of relapse include overconfidence, daily temptations, stress or emotional distractions, and self-deprecation.
   Strategies for Change: Continue taking the same actions that led to success in the first place. Find fun and creative ways to maintain positive behaviors.
6. *Termination.* By this point, the behavior is so ingrained that the current level of vigilance may be unnecessary. The new behavior has become an essential part of daily living. Can you think of someone you know who has made a major behavior change that has now become an essential part of that person's life?

Source: J. O. Prochaska and C. C. DiClemente, "Stages and Processes of Self-Change of Smoking: Toward an Integrative Model of Change," *Journal of Consulting and Clinical Psychology* 51 (1983): 390–95.

---

health problem were to develop or to be left untreated? The more serious the perceived effects, the more likely that the person will take action.

■ *Perceived susceptibility to the health problem.* What is the likelihood of developing the health problem? People who perceive themselves at high risk are more likely to take preventive action.

■ *Cues to action.* A person who is reminded or alerted about a potential health problem is more likely to take action. For example, having your doctor tell you that your blood sugar levels indicate a prediabetic state may be the cue that pushes you to lose weight and exercise.

Three other factors are linked to perceived risk for health problems: *demographic variables,* including age, gender, race, and ethnic background; *sociopsychological variables,* including personality traits, social class, and social pressure; and *structural variables,* including knowledge about or prior contact with the health problem.

People follow the Health Belief Model many times every day. Take, for example, smokers. Older smokers are likely to know other smokers who have developed serious heart or lung problems. They are thus more likely to perceive tobacco as a threat to their health than is a teenager who has just begun smoking. The greater the perceived threat of health problems caused by smoking, the greater the chance a person will quit.

However, many chronic smokers know the risks yet continue to smoke. Why do they miss these cues to action? According to Rosenstock, some people do not believe that they will be affected by a problem—they act as though they had some kind of immunity to it—and are unlikely to change their behavior. In some cases, they may think that even if they get cancer or have a heart attack, the health care system will cure them. They also may feel that the immediate pleasure outweighs the long-range cost.

Intentions to Change

Our attitudes reflect our emotional responses to situations and follow from our beliefs. The **Theory of Reasoned Action** states that our behaviors result from our intentions to perform actions. An intention is a product of our attitude toward an action and our beliefs about what others may want us to do.[22] A *behavioral intention,* then, is a written or stated commitment to perform an action.

In brief, the more consistent your attitude is towards an action and the more support you receive from others to take that action, the more likely you are to succeed. Verbalizing your intentions is important, but recognize that environmental, physical, and social barriers make even the best laid plans and intentions challenging.

Significant Others as Change Agents

Many of us are highly influenced by the approval or disapproval (real or imagined) of close friends, loved ones, and the social and cultural groups to which they belong. Such influences can support healthy behavior, or they can interfere with even the best intentions.

Your Family From the time of your birth, your parents or other family members have given you strong cues about which actions are and are not socially acceptable. Brushing your teeth, bathing, wearing deodorant, and chewing food with your mouth closed are behaviors that your family probably instilled in you long ago. Your family culture influenced your food choices, religious and political beliefs, and all your other values and actions. If you deviated

Do my friends and family influence my health choices?

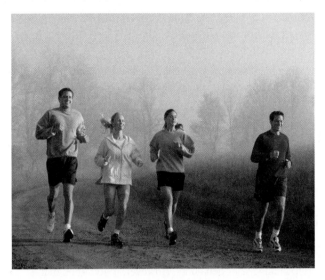

The support and encouragement of friends who have similar goals and interests will strengthen your commitment to develop and maintain positive health behaviors.

from your family's norms, a family member probably let you know fairly quickly. Good family units provide caring, trust, and protection; are dedicated to the healthful development of all family members; and work to reduce problems.

When a loving family unit does not exist, when it does not provide for basic human needs, or when dysfunctional, irresponsible individuals try to build a family under the influence of drugs or alcohol, it becomes difficult for a child to learn positive health behaviors. Often, healthy behaviors get their start in healthy homes; unhealthy homes breed unhealthy habits. Healthy families provide the foundation for a clear and necessary understanding of what is right and wrong, what is positive and negative. Without this fundamental grounding, many young people have great difficulties.

Social Bonds and the Influence of Others

Just as your family influences your actions during your childhood, your friends and significant others influence your behaviors as you grow older. Most of us desire to fit the "norm" and avoid hassles in our daily interactions with others. If you deviate from the actions expected in your hometown, or among your friends, you may suffer ostracism, strange looks, and other negative social consequences. Understanding the subtle and not-so-subtle ways in which other people influence our actions is an important step toward changing our behaviors.

The behavior choices we make can be explained by the *Theory of Planned Behavior.*[23] This theory outlines three reasons for how we choose to behave:

1. *Our attitudes toward the behavior:* what we think about the positive or negative effects of our actions and the importance of each of those

Theory of Reasoned Action Model for explaining the importance of our intentions in determining behaviors.

2. *Our level of perceived behavioral control:* our beliefs about the constraints and/or opportunities we might have concerning the behavior

3. *Our subjective norms:* whether we think our actions will meet the approval or disapproval of people important to us

For example, if you want to lose weight because you believe it will make you more desirable, you'll have strong intentions to begin a weight-loss program (attitudes toward the behavior). Intentions are powerful indicators of successful behavior change. If there is a convenient, affordable fitness center near you, and if the schedule works for you, you'll be even more motivated and believe you can make the change (perceived control). Finally, the influence of others serves as a powerful *social support* for positive change. If friends offer encouragement (subjective norms), you are more likely to remain motivated to change your behaviors. However, if you think that your friends will think you are a "nerd" for going to the gym, or if the gym is inconvenient or expensive, you may quickly lose your motivation. The importance of cultivating and maintaining close *social bonds* with others is an important part of overall health. The key people in our lives play a powerful role in our motivation to change for the better, or for the worse.

 try it NOW!

Stay connected. A broad base of social support is an important part of ensuring overall health. Make an effort to strengthen social bonds. Call a friend right now, and make a date for coffee, lunch, or "fun time" to catch up on each other's lives. Show you care.

Choosing a Behavior-Change Technique

Once you have analyzed all the factors that influence your behaviors, consider what actions you can take to change the negative ones. Behavior-change techniques include shaping, visualization, modeling, controlling the situation, reinforcement, changing self-talk, and problem solving. The options don't stop here, but these are the most common strategies.

> **What can I do to change an unhealthy habit?**

shaping Using a series of small steps to gradually achieve a particular goal.

imagined rehearsal Practicing, through mental imagery, to become better able to perform an event in actuality.

modeling Learning specific behaviors by watching others perform them.

Shaping

Regardless of how motivated you are, some behaviors are almost impossible to change immediately. To reach your goal, you may need to take a number of individual steps, each designed to change one small piece of the larger behavior. This process is known as **shaping.**

For example, suppose that you have not exercised for a while. You decide that you want to get into shape, and your goal is to jog three miles every other day. But you realize that you'd face a near-death experience if you tried to run even a few blocks in your current condition. So you decide to build up to your desired fitness level gradually. During week 1, you will walk for one hour every other day at a slow, relaxed pace. During week 2, you will walk for the same amount of time but speed up your pace and cover slightly more ground. During week 3, you will speed up even more and try to go even farther. You will continue taking such steps until you reach your goal.

Whatever the desired behavior change, all shaping involves the following actions:

- Start slowly, and try not to cause undue stress during the early stages of the program.
- Keep the steps small and achievable.
- Be flexible. If the original plan proves uncomfortable or you deviate from it, don't give up! Start again, and move forward.
- Don't skip steps or move to the next step until you have mastered the previous one.
- Reward yourself for meeting regular, previously-set goals.

Remember, behaviors don't develop overnight, so they won't change overnight.

Visualization

Mental practice can transform unhealthy behaviors into healthy ones. Athletes and others use a technique known as **imagined rehearsal** to reach their goals. By visualizing their planned action ahead of time, they are better prepared when they put themselves to the test.

For example, suppose you want to ask someone out on a date. Imagine the setting (walking together to class). Then practice in your mind and out loud exactly what you want to say. Mentally anticipate different responses ("Oh, I'd love to, but I'm busy that evening. . . .") and what you will say in reaction ("How about if I call you sometime this week?"). Careful mental and verbal rehearsal—you could even try out your scenario on a friend—will greatly improve the likelihood of success.

Modeling

Modeling, or learning behaviors by watching others perform them, is one of the most effective strategies for changing behavior. For example, suppose that you have trouble talking to people you don't know very well. One of the easiest ways to improve your communication skills is to select friends whose social skills you envy. Observe them. Do they talk more or listen more? How do people respond to them? Why are they such good communicators? If you observe behaviors you admire and isolate their components, you can model the steps of your behavior-change technique on a proven success.

Controlling the Situation

Sometimes, the right setting or the right group of people will positively influence your behaviors. Many situations and occasions trigger certain actions. For example, in libraries, houses of worship, and museums, most people talk softly. Few people laugh at funerals. The term **situational inducement** refers to an attempt to influence a behavior by using occasions and social settings to control it.

For example, you may be more apt to stop smoking if you work in a smoke-free office, a positive situational inducement. But working in a smoke-filled bar, a negative situational inducement, may tempt you to resume. By carefully considering which settings will help and which will hurt your effort to change, and by deciding to seek the first and avoid the second, you will improve your chances for change.

Reinforcement

Another way to promote positive behavior change is to reward yourself for it. This is called **positive reinforcement.** Each of us is motivated by different reinforcers.

Most positive reinforcers can be classified into five categories: consumable, activity, manipulative, possessional, and social.

- *Consumable reinforcers* are delicious edibles, such as candy, cookies, or gourmet meals.
- *Activity reinforcers* are opportunities to do something enjoyable, such as watching TV or going on vacation.
- *Manipulative reinforcers* are incentives, such as getting a lower rent in exchange for mowing the lawn or the promise of a better grade for doing an extra-credit project.
- *Possessional reinforcers* are tangible rewards, such as a new TV or a sports car.
- *Social reinforcers* are signs of appreciation, approval, or love, such as loving looks, affectionate hugs, and praise.

When choosing reinforcers, determine what would motivate you to act in a particular way. Research has shown that people can be motivated to change their behaviors, such as not smoking during pregnancy or abstaining from cocaine, if they set up a token economy system whereby they earn tokens or points that can be exchanged for meaningful rewards, such as money.[24] The difficulty often lies in determining which incentive will be most effective. Your reinforcers may initially come from others (extrinsic rewards), but as you see positive changes in yourself, you will begin to reward and reinforce yourself (intrinsic rewards). Although reinforcers should immediately follow a behavior, beware of overkill. If you reward yourself with a movie every time you go jogging, this reinforcer will soon lose its power. It would be better to give yourself this reward after, say, a full week of adhering to your jogging program.

what do you THINK?

What consumable reinforcers would be a healthy reward for your new behavior? ■ If you could choose one activity reinforcer with which to reward yourself after one week of success in your new behavior, what would it be? ■ If you could obtain something (possessional reinforcer) after you reach your goal, what would it be? ■ If you maintain your behavior for one week, what type of social reinforcer would you like to receive from your friends?

Changing Self-Talk

Self-talk, the way you think and talk to yourself, can also play a role in modifying health-related behaviors. Self-talk can reflect your feelings of self-efficacy, discussed earlier in this chapter. When we don't feel self-efficacious, it's tempting to engage in negative self-talk, which can sabotage our best intentions. Here are some strategies for changing self-talk.

Rational-Emotive Therapy Rational-emotive therapy, a form of cognitive therapy or self-directed behavior change, is based on the premise that there is a close connection between what people say to themselves and how they feel. According to psychologist Albert Ellis, most emotional problems and related behaviors stem from irrational statements that people make to themselves when events in their lives are different from what they would like them to be.[25]

For example, suppose that after doing poorly on a test, you say to yourself, "I can't believe I flunked that easy exam. I'm so stupid." By changing this irrational, "catastrophic" self-talk into rational, positive statements about what is really going on, you increase the likelihood that you will make a positive behavior change. Positive self-talk might be phrased as follows: "I really didn't study enough for that exam, and I'm not surprised I didn't do well. I'm certainly not stupid. I just need to prepare better for the next test." Such self-talk will help you to recover quickly and take positive steps to correct the situation.

situational inducement Attempt to influence a behavior through situations and occasions that are structured to exert control over that behavior.

positive reinforcement Presenting something positive following a behavior that is being reinforced.

self-talk The customary manner of thinking and talking to yourself, which can impact your self-image.

CONSUMER health

The Internet can be a wonderful resource for rapid answers. In fact, 72 percent of college students obtain health information from the Web. However, some of the answers are better than others. If you're not careful, you could end up feeling frazzled, confused, and—worst of all—misinformed. How can you maximize your chances of locating high-quality information? Follow these tips:

How can I distinguish a bogus health claim from a real one?

- Look for websites sponsored by an official government agency, a university or college, or a hospital/medical center. These typically offer accurate, up-to-date information about a wide range of health topics. Government sites are easily identified by their .gov extensions (for example, the National Institute of Mental Health is www.nimh.nih.gov); college and university sites typically have .edu extensions (Johns Hopkins University is www.jhu.edu). Hospitals often have a .org extension (Mayo Clinic: www.mayoclinic.org). Major philanthropic foundations, such as the Robert Wood Johnson Foundation, the Legacy Foundation, the Kellogg Foundation, and others, often provide information about selected health topics.

- Search for well-established, professional, peer-reviewed journals such as the *New England Journal of Medicine* (http://content.nejm.org) or the *Journal of the American Medical Association (JAMA)* (http://jama.ama-assn.org). Although some of these sites require a fee for access, often you can locate concise abstracts and information, such as a weekly table of contents, that can help you conduct a search. Other times, you can pay a basic fee for a certain number of hours of unlimited searching. You may also find that your college library subscribes to a number of these online journals.

- Consult the Centers for Disease Control and Prevention (www.cdc.gov) for consumer news, updates, and alerts.

- For a global perspective on health issues, visit the World Health Organization (www.who.int/en/).

- There are many government and education-based sites that are independently sponsored and reliable. The following is just a sample. We'll provide more in each chapter as we cover specific topics.
  - Aetna Intelihealth: www.intelihealth.com
  - Dr. Koop.com: www.drkoop.com
  - Drug Infonet: www.druginfonet.com
  - Health AtoZ.com: www.healthatoz.com

  - WebMD health: http://my.webmd.com

The American Accreditation Healthcare Commission (www.urac.org) has devised over 50 criteria that health sites must satisfy to display its seal. Look for the "URAC Accredited Health Web Site" seal on websites you visit. In addition to policing the accuracy of health claims, URAC evaluates health information and provides a forum for reporting misinformation, privacy violations, and other complaints.

- And finally, don't believe everything you read. Cross-check information against reliable sources to see whether facts and figures are consistent. Be especially wary of websites that try to sell you something. Just because a source claims to be a physician or an expert does not mean that this is true. When in doubt, check with your own health provider, health education professor, or state health division website.

Sources: American College Health Association, "American College Health Association–National College Health Assessment (ACHA–NCHA) Spring 2006 Reference Group Data Report," *Journal of American College Health* 55, no. 4 (2007): 195–206. American Accreditation Healthcare Commission (URAC), "Overview of URAC's Health Web Site Accreditation Review," accessed March 24, 2006, www.urac.org/consumer_review.asp.

Blocking/Thought Stopping By purposefully blocking or stopping negative thoughts, a person can concentrate on taking positive steps toward behavior change. For example, suppose you are preoccupied with your ex-partner, who has recently deserted you for someone else. You consciously stop thinking about the situation and force yourself to think about something more pleasant (perhaps dinner tomorrow with your best friend). By refusing to dwell on negative images and forcing yourself to focus elsewhere, you can avoid wasting energy, time, and emotional resources and move on to positive change.

Problem Solving: The Art of Self-Instruction

Some people seem to naturally take on challenges and deal with stressful life events in positive ways. However, most of us struggle with such challenges. Even so, we can learn to do a better job of tackling and overcoming problems in our lives. According to psychologist Donald Meichenbaum, we can learn to inoculate ourselves against stressful events or control our anger over certain situations. Before a stressful event (for example, going to the doctor for tests for sexually transmitted infection), Meichenbaum encourages his patients to practice coping skills, such as deep breathing or progressive muscle relaxation, or to practice self-instruction ("I'll feel better once I know what is going on here"). He provides a list of strategies that are designed to help each of us cope with stressors and modify anger reactions or other negative behaviors:[26]

- Prepare for the situation by defining your stressor. What is it you have to do? Develop a plan to cope with stress reactions as a problem to be solved.
- Set concrete, realistic goals and specific behaviors you can do to reach goals.
- Try out the most acceptable and practical solution, and generate a wide range of possible alternative courses of action.
- Imagine and consider how others might respond if asked to deal with similar problems.
- Evaluate the pros and cons of each proposed solution, and organize the solutions from least to most practical and desirable.
- Rehearse strategies and behaviors by using imagery or role playing the behavior in advance.
- Confront the situation. Keep the focus on the present. What is it you have to do? Expect fear or anxiety, and use your preparation to cope with it.
- Expect some failures, but reward yourself for having tried.
- Reconsider the original problem in light of your attempt at problem solving.

Changing Your Behavior
Self-Assessment: Antecedents and Consequences

Behaviors, thoughts, and feelings always occur in a context, that is, in a situation. Situations can be divided into two components: the events that come before and those that come after. *Antecedents* are the setting events for a behavior; they stimulate a person to act in certain ways. Antecedents can be physical events, thoughts, emotions, or the actions of other people. *Consequences*—the results of behavior—affect whether a person will repeat that action. Consequences also can consist of physical events, thoughts, emotions, or the actions of other people.

Suppose you are shy and must give a speech in front of a large class. The antecedents include walking into the class, feeling frightened, wondering whether you are capable of doing a good job, and being unable to remember a word of your speech. If the consequences are negative—if your classmates laugh or you get a low grade—your terror about speaking in public will be reinforced, and you will continue to dread this kind of event. In contrast, if you receive positive feedback from the class or instructor, you may actually learn to like speaking in public.

Learning to recognize the antecedents of a behavior and acting to modify them is one method of changing behavior. A diary noting your undesirable behaviors and identifying the settings in which they occur can be a useful tool. **Figure 1.5** identifies factors that can make behavior change more difficult.

If you think... then	try this strategy...
"I don't have enough time"	Chart your hourly activities for one day. What are your highest priorities? What can you eliminate? Plan to make some time for a healthy change next week.
"I'm too stressed"	Assess your major stressors right now. List those you can control and those you can change or avoid. Then identify two things you enjoy that can help you reduce stress now.
"I worry about what others may think"	Ask yourself how much others influence your decisions about drinking, sex, eating habits, etc. What is most important to you? What actions can you take to act in line with these values?
"I don't think I can do it"	Just because you haven't before doesn't mean you can't now. To develop some confidence, take baby steps and break tasks into small pieces.
"It's a habit I can't break"	Habits are difficult to break but not impossible. What triggers your behavior? List ways you can avoid these triggers. Ask for support from friends and family.

FIGURE 1.5 Common Barriers to Behavior Change
What types of things might prevent you from changing a bad habit to a healthy one? If you find that you ask yourself any of these questions, try the suggested strategy to overcome the barrier.

Analyzing Personal Behavior

Successful behavior change requires determining what you want to change. All too often we berate ourselves by using generalities: "I'm lousy to my friends; I need to be a better person." Determining the specific behavior you would like to modify—in contrast to the general problem—will allow you to set clear goals. What are you doing that makes you a lousy friend? Are you gossiping or lying about your friends? Have you been a taker rather than a giver? Or are you really a good friend most of the time?

Let's say the problem is gossiping. You can analyze this behavior by examining the following components.

- *Frequency.* How often do you gossip—all the time or only once in a while?
- *Duration.* How long have you been doing this?
- *Seriousness.* Is your gossiping just idle chatter, or are you really trying to injure other people? What are the consequences for you? For your friends? For your relationships?
- *Basis for problem behavior.* Is your gossip based on facts, perceptions of facts, or deliberate embellishment of the truth?
- *Antecedents.* What kinds of situations trigger your gossiping? Do some settings or people bring it out in you more than others do? What triggers your feelings of dislike or irritation toward your friends? Why are you talking behind their backs?

Once you assess your actions and determine what motivates you, consider what you can do to change your behavior.

Decision Making: Choices for Change

Now it is time to make a decision that will lead to positive health outcomes. Try to anticipate what might occur in a given setting and to think through all possible safe alternatives.

For example, suppose you know that you are likely to be offered a drink when you go to a party. What response could you make that would be okay in your social group? If someone is flirting with you and the conversation takes on a distinct sexual overtone, what might you do to prevent the situation from turning bad? Advance preparation will help you stick to your behavior plan.

Fill out the Behavior Change Contract at the beginning of this book to help you set a goal, anticipate obstacles, and create strategies to overcome those obstacles. Remember that things typically don't "just happen." Making a commitment by completing a contract helps you stay alert to potential problems, be aware of your alternatives, maintain a good sense of your own values, and stick to your beliefs under pressure.

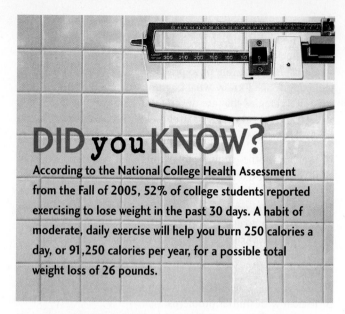

DID you KNOW?

According to the National College Health Assessment from the Fall of 2005, 52% of college students reported exercising to lose weight in the past 30 days. A habit of moderate, daily exercise will help you burn 250 calories a day, or 91,250 calories per year, for a possible total weight loss of 26 pounds.

Source: American College Health Association, "American College Health Association–National College Health Assessment Reference Group Report, Fall 2005," 2006, www.acha.org.

Setting Realistic Goals

How can I set a realistic health goal?

Changing behavior is not easy, but sometimes we make it even harder by setting unrealistic and unattainable goals. To start making positive changes, ask yourself these questions.

1. *What do I want?* What is your ultimate goal—to lose weight? Exercise more? Reduce stress? Have a lasting relationship? Whatever it is, you need a clear picture of the target outcome.

2. *Which change is the greatest priority at this time?* Often people decide to change several things all at once. Suppose that you are gaining unwanted weight. Rather than saying, "I need to eat less, start jogging, and really get in shape," be specific about the current behavior you need to change. Are you eating too many sweets? Too many high-fat foods? Perhaps a realistic goal would be to try to eat less fat during dinner every day. Choose the behavior that constitutes your greatest problem, and tackle that first. You can always work on something else later. Take small steps, experiment with alternatives, and find the best way to meet your goals.

3. *Why is this important to me?* Think through why you want to change. Are you doing it because of your health? To look better? To win someone else's approval? Usually, doing something because it's right for you rather than to win others' approval is a sound strategy. If you are changing for someone else, what happens when that other person isn't around?

4. *What are the potential positive outcomes?* What do you hope to accomplish?

5. *What health-promoting programs and services can help me get started?* Nearly all campuses offer helpful resources. You might buy a self-help book at the campus bookstore, speak to a counselor, or enroll in an aerobics class at the local fitness center.

6. *Are there family or friends whose help I can enlist?* Social support is one of your most powerful allies. Getting a friend to exercise with you, asking your partner to help you stop smoking by quitting at the same time you do, and making a commitment with a friend to never let each other drive if you've been drinking

alcohol—these are all examples of how people can help each other make positive changes.

 what do you THINK?

Why is it sometimes hard to make decisions?
- What factors influence your decision making?
- Select one behavior that you want to change, and refer to the Behavior Change Contract. Using the goal-setting strategies discussed here, outline a plan for change.

TAKING charge

Summary

- Health encompasses the entire dynamic process of fulfilling one's potential in the physical, social, emotional, spiritual, intellectual, and environmental dimensions of life. Wellness means achieving the highest level of health possible in several dimensions.
- Although the average American life span has increased over the past century, we also need to increase the quality of life. Programs such as *Healthy People 2010* have established national objectives for achieving longer life and quality of life for all Americans through health promotion and disease prevention.
- Health disparities have become recognized as contributors to increased disease risks. Factors such as gender, race, and socioeconomic status continue to play a major role in health status and care. Women have longer lives but have more medical problems than do men. To close the gender gap in health care, researchers have begun to include more women in medical research and training.
- For the U.S. population as a whole, the leading causes of death are heart disease, cancer, and stroke. In the 15- to 24-year-old age group, the leading causes are unintentional injuries, homicide, and suicide. Many of the risks associated with cancer, heart disease, and stroke can be reduced

through lifestyle changes. Many of the risks associated with accidents, homicide, and suicide can be reduced through preventive measures, particularly reductions in the use of alcohol and other drugs.
- Several factors contribute to a person's health status, and a number of them are within our control. Beliefs and attitudes, self-efficacy, locus of control, intentions to change, support from significant others, and readiness to change are factors over which individuals have some degree of control. Access to health care, genetic predisposition, health policies that support positive choices, and other factors are all potential reinforcing, predisposing, and enabling factors that may influence health decisions.
- Behavior-change techniques, such as shaping, visualization, modeling, controlling the situation, reinforcement, changing self-talk, and problem solving help people succeed in making behavior changes.
- Decision making has several key components. Each person must explore his or her own problems, the reasons for change, and the expected outcomes. The next step is to plan a course of action best suited to individual needs and fill out a Behavior Change Contract.

Chapter Review

1. Our ability to perform everyday tasks, such as walking up the stairs, is an example of
   a. improved quality of life.
   b. physical health.
   c. health promotion.
   d. activities of daily living.

2. Janice describes herself as confident and trusting, and she displays both high self-esteem and high self-efficacy. The dimension of health this relates to is the
   a. social dimension.
   b. emotional dimension.
   c. spiritual dimension.
   d. intellectual dimension.

3. Which of the following is an example of primary prevention?
   a. attending a smoking cessation program
   b. using a condom during sexual intercourse
   c. receiving radiation therapy for cancer
   d. going to physical therapy for an injury resulting from a skiing accident

4. What statistic is used to describe the number of new cases of AIDS in a given year?
   a. morbidity
   b. mortality
   c. incidence
   d. prevalence

5. Because Craig's parents smoked, he is 90 percent more likely to start smoking than someone whose parents didn't. This is an example of what factor influencing behavior change?
   a. circumstantial factor
   b. enabling factor
   c. reinforcing factor
   d. predisposing factor

6. Suppose you want to lose 20 pounds. To reach your goal, you take small steps to gradually lose weight. You start by joining a support group and counting calories. After 2 weeks, you begin an exercise program and gradually build up to your desired fitness level. What behavior change strategy are you using?
   a. shaping
   b. visualization
   c. modeling
   d. reinforcement

7. After Kirk and Tammy pay their bills, they reward themselves by watching TV together. The type of positive reinforcement that motivates them to pay their bills is
   a. activity reinforcer.
   b. consumable reinforcer.
   c. manipulative reinforcer.
   d. possessional reinforcer.

8. The setting events for a behavior that cue or stimulate a person to act in certain ways are called
   a. antecedents.
   b. frequency of events.
   c. consequences.
   d. cues to action.

9. What strategy for change is advised for an individual in the preparation stage of change?
   a. seeking out recommended readings
   b. finding creative ways to maintain positive behaviors
   c. setting realistic goals
   d. publicly stating the desire for change

10. Spiritual health could best be described as
    a. exclusive to religiosity.
    b. optional for achieving wellness.
    c. related to one's purpose in life.
    d. finding fulfilling relationships.

Answers to these questions can be found on page A-1.

Questions for Discussion and Reflection

1. How are the terms *health* and *wellness* similar? What, if any, are important distinctions between these terms? What is health promotion? Disease prevention?
2. How healthy is the U.S. population today? Are we doing better or worse in terms of health status than we have done previously? What factors influence today's disparities in health?
3. What are some of the major differences in the way men and women are treated in the health care system? Why do you think these differences exist? How do race, sexual orientation, religion, marital status, and age affect how people are treated in the health care system?
4. What is the Health Belief Model? What is the Theory of Reasoned Action? How may each of these models be working when a young woman decides to smoke her first cigarette? Her last cigarette?
5. Explain the predisposing, reinforcing, and enabling factors that might influence a young mother who is dependent on welfare as she decides whether to sell drugs to support her children.
6. Using the stages of change model (described in the Skills for Behavior Change box on page 20), discuss what you might do (in stages) to help a friend stop smoking. Why is it important that a person be ready to change before trying to change?

Accessing Your Health on the Internet

The following websites explore further topics and issues related to personal health. For links to the websites below, visit the Companion Website for *Health: The Basics, Eighth Edition* at www.aw-bc.com/donatelle.

1. *CDC Wonder.* Clearinghouse for comprehensive information from the Centers for Disease Control and Prevention (CDC), including special reports, guidelines, and access to national health data. http://wonder.cdc.gov

2. *Mayo Clinic.* Reputable resource for specific information about health topics, diseases, and treatment options. Easy to navigate and consumer friendly. www.mayo.edu

3. *National Center for Health Statistics.* Outstanding place to start for information about health status in the United States. Links to key documents such as *Health, United States* (published yearly); national survey information; and information on mortality by age, race, gender, geographic location, and other important data. Includes comprehensive information provided by the CDC, as well as easy links to at least ten of the major health resources currently being used for policy and decision making about health in the United States. www.cdc.gov/nchs/default.htm

4. *National Health Information Center.* Excellent resource for consumer information about health. www.health.gov/nhic

5. *World Health Organization.* Excellent resource for global health information. Provides information on the current state of health around the world, such as illness and disease statistics, trends, and illness outbreak alerts. www.who.int/en

Further Reading

Centers for Disease Control and Prevention, *Health, United States: 2005*. Washington, DC: Government Printing Office, 2005.

Provides an up-to-date overview of U.S. health statistics, risk factors, and trends.

Institute of Medicine. *Who Will Keep the Public Healthy? Educating Public Health Professionals for the 21st Century.* Washington, DC: National Academies Press, 2003.

An edited text featuring experts from throughout the country discussing the role that health professionals play in health change. It outlines an ecological approach to improving the nation's health and has served as a catalyst for initiatives focused on current health issues and future plans to improve health and prevent premature death and disability.

Institute of Medicine. *The Future of Public Health in the 21st Century.* Washington, DC: National Academies Press, 2003.

The summary of a national effort to examine the nation's health status and describe how key individuals and organizations can work as a public health system to create conditions in which people can be healthy. In addition, this text recommends the evidence-based actions necessary to make the U.S. health system work effectively.

Lee, P. and C. Estes. *The Nation's Health,* 7th ed. Sudbury, MA: Jones and Bartlett, 2003.

An overview of key writings on public health and issues affecting individuals and populations. Special emphasis on health determinants, emerging threats to health, the health of diverse populations, and issues of health care quality, costs, and access.

U.S. Department of Health and Human Services. *Healthy People 2010: National Health Promotion and Disease Prevention Objectives for the Year 2010.* Washington, DC: Government Printing Office, 1998.

This plan contains the U.S. surgeon general's long-range goals for increasing the life span for all Americans by three years and improving access to health for all Americans, regardless of sex, race, socioeconomic status, and other variables.

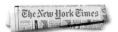

e-themes from *The New York Times*

For up-to-date articles about current health issues, visit www.aw-bc.com/donatelle, select *Health: The Basics,* Eighth Edition, Chapter 1, and click on "e-themes."

References

1. World Health Organization (WHO), "Constitution of the World Health Organization," *Chronicles of the World Health Organization* (Geneva, Switzerland: WHO, 1947).

2. A. M Miniño et al., *Deaths: Preliminary Data for 2004* (Hyattsville, MD: National Center for Health Statistics, 2006), www.cdc.gov/nchs/products/pubs/pubd/hestats/prelimdeaths04/preliminarydeaths04.htm.; Central Intelligence Agency, "The World Factbook: Rank Order—Life Expectancy at Birth," 2007, www.cia.gov/cia/publications/factbook/rankorder/2102rank.html.

3. National Center for Health Statistics, Table 12 from "United States Life Tables, 2002" *National Vital Statistics Reports* 53, no. 6 (November 2005).

4. S. J. Olshansky et al., "A Potential Decline in Life Expectancy in the United States in the 21st Century," *New England Journal of Medicine* 352, no. 11 (2005): 1138–45.

5. R. Dubos, *So Human the Animal* (New York: Scribners, 1968), 15.

6. K. Braithwaite, "Mending our Broken Mental Health Systems," *American Journal of Public Health* 96, no. 10 (2006): 1724.

7. National Center for Health Statistics, "About *Healthy People 2010,*" www.cdc.gov/nchs.

8. Centers for Disease Control and Prevention, Office of Minority Health, Racial and Ethnic Populations, 2007, www.cdc.gov/OMH/Populations/populations.htm.

9. UCLA Center for Health Policy Research, "Language Barrier Puts More than 1 Million Californians in HMOs at Risk for Health Problems," May 10, 2006, www.healthpolicy.ucla.edu/news_05102006.html.

10. National Institutes of Health (NIH), *Strategic Research Plan and Budget to Reduce and Ultimately Eliminate Health Disparities,* vol. 1, *Fiscal Years 2002–2006* (Bethesda, MD: National Institutes of Health, 2006).

11. National Center for Chronic Disease Prevention and Health Promotion, "Healthy Youth! Six Critical Health Behaviors," 2006, www.cdc.gov/HealthyYouth/healthtopics/index.htm.

12. WHO, *The World Health Report 2002: Reducing Risks, Promoting Healthy Life* (Geneva, Switzerland: World Health Organization, 2002), www.who.int/whr/2002/en/; E. Khoman and M. Weale, "Incidence Based Estimates of Healthy Life Expectancy for the United Kingdom: Coherence Between Transition Probabilities and Aggregate Life Tables," *National Institute Discussion Paper* no. 270 (London: National Institute of Economic and Social Research, April 7, 2006).

13. NIH, Office of Minority Health, *What Is Cultural Competency?* (Bethesda, MD: National Institutes of Health, 2006), www.omhrcu.gov/templates/browse.aspx?lv1=1&1v1ID=3%20; A. Kleinman, L. Eisenberg, and B. Good, "Culture, Illness and Care: Clinical Lessons from Anthropologic and Cross-Cultural Research," *Focus: The Journal of Lifelong Learning in Psychiatry* 4, no. 140 (January 2006): 251–58.

14. U.S. Department of Health and Human Services, "The Fifty-Eighth World Health Assembly, Geneva, Switzerland, 2005," www.who.int/mediacentre/events/2005/wha58/en/index.html.

15. A. Lopez et al., "Global and Regional Burden of Disease and Risk Factors: Systematic Analysis of Population Health Data," *The Lancet* 367, no. 9524 (2006): 1747–57.

16. National Heart, Lung and Blood Institute (NHLBI), "News from the Women's Health Initiative" *NIH News,* February 7, 2007, www.nhlbi.nih.gov/new/press/06–02–07.htm; Society for Women's Health Research, "Sex Differences in Cardio- and Cerebrovascular Diseases," 2007, www.womenshealthresearch.org/site?pageServer?pagename=hs_facts_cardio; Society for Women's Health Research, "Top Five Women's Health Stories of 2006," 2006, www.womenshealthresearch.org/site/News2?page=NewsArticle&id=6319.

17. Society for Women's Health Research, "Sex Differences in Response to Pharmaceuticals, Tobacco, Alcohol and Illicit Drugs," 2004, www.womenshealthresearch.org/site/PageServer?pagename=hs-facts-dat.

18. M. Hesse, "The Readiness Ruler as a Measure of Readiness to Change Polydrug Use in Drug Abusers," *Journal of Harm Reduction* 3, no. 3 (2006): 1477–81; M. Cismary, "Using Protection Motivation Theory to Increase the Persuasiveness of Public Service Communications," Saskatchewan Institute of Public Policy, Public Policy Series paper no. 40 (February 2006); A. Fallon et al., "Health Care Provider Advice for African American Adults Not Meeting Health Behavior Recommendations," *Preventing Chronic Disease* 3, no. 2 (2006); M. R. Chacko et al., "New Sexual Partners and Readiness to Seek Screening for Chlamydia and Gonorrhea: Predictors Among Minority Young Women," *Sexually Transmitted Infections* 82 (2006): 75–79.

19. A. Bandura, "Self-Efficacy," in *Encyclopedia of Mental Health,* ed. H. Friedman (San Diego: Academic Press, 1998).

20. J. M. Twenge, et al., "It's Beyond My Control: A Cross-Temporal Meta-Analysis of Increasing Externality in Locus of Control, 1960–2002," *Personality and Social Psychology Review* 8 (2004): 308–20.

21. I. M. Rosenstock, "Historical Origins of the Health Belief Model," *Health Education Monographs* 2 (1974): 328–35.

22. I. Azjen, *Attitudes, Personality and Behavior* (London: Open University Press, 1988); I. Azjen and M. Fishbein, *Understanding Attitudes and Predicting Social Behaviors* (Englewood Cliffs, NJ: Prentice Hall, 1980).

23. I. Ajzen, "The Theory of Planned Behavior," *Organizational Behavior and Human Decision Processes* 50 (1991): 179–211.

24. R. J. Donatelle et al., "Using Incentives and the 5A's in Clinical Practice to Motivate Pregnant Smokers to Quit: The Maternal Intervention to Stop Smoking (MISS) Trial" (forthcoming).

25. A. Ellis, *The Essence of Rational Emotive Behavior Therapy* (New York: The Albert Ellis Institute, 1994).

26. D. Meichenbaum, *Treatment of Patients with Anger Control Problems* (Toronto: Pergamon Press, 2003); D. Meichenbaum, *Stress Inoculation Training* (Toronto: Pergamon Press, 2004).

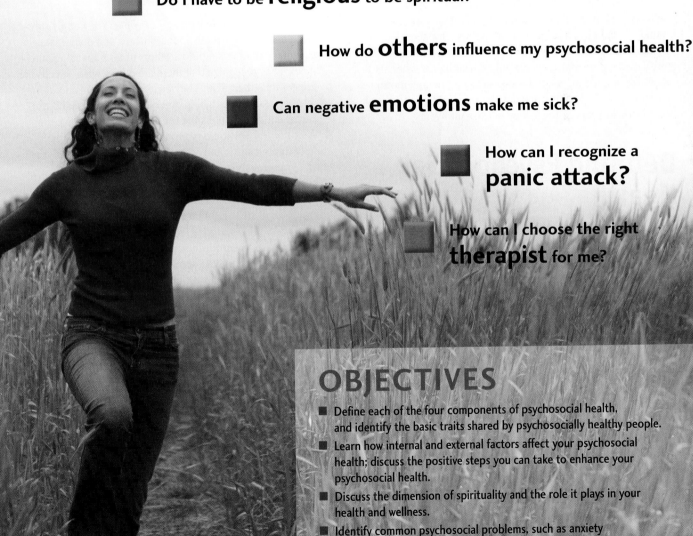

Psychosocial Health

BEING MENTALLY, EMOTIONALLY, SOCIALLY, AND SPIRITUALLY WELL

Do I have to be **religious** to be spiritual?

How do **others** influence my psychosocial health?

Can negative **emotions** make me sick?

How can I recognize a **panic attack?**

How can I choose the right **therapist** for me?

OBJECTIVES

- Define each of the four components of psychosocial health, and identify the basic traits shared by psychosocially healthy people.
- Learn how internal and external factors affect your psychosocial health; discuss the positive steps you can take to enhance your psychosocial health.
- Discuss the dimension of spirituality and the role it plays in your health and wellness.
- Identify common psychosocial problems, such as anxiety disorders and depression, and explain their causes and treatments.
- Explain the methods of different types of health professionals, and examine how they can play a role in preventing specific types of psychosocial health problems.

A lthough the vast majority of college students describe their college years as among the best of their lives, many find the pressure of grades, financial concerns, relationship problems, and the struggle to find themselves to be extraordinarily difficult. Steven Hyman, provost of Harvard University and former director of the National Institutes of Mental Health sounded this alarm about student mental health: "The mental state of many students is so precarious that it is interfering with the core mission of the university."[1] Psychological distress caused by relationship issues, family issues, academic competition, and adjusting to life as a college student is rampant on college campuses today. Experts believe that the anxiety-prone campus environment is a major contributor to poor health decisions such as high alcohol consumption and, in turn, to health problems that ultimately affect academic success and success in life.

Fortunately, even though we often face seemingly insurmountable pressures, human beings possess a resiliency that enables us to cope, adapt, and thrive, regardless of life's challenges. How we feel and think about ourselves, those around us, and our environment can tell us a lot about our psychosocial health and whether we are healthy emotionally, spiritually, and mentally. Increasingly, health professionals recognize that having a solid social network, being emotionally and mentally healthy, and developing spiritual capacity don't just add years to life—they put life into years.

Defining Psychosocial Health

What Is Psychosocial Health?

Psychosocial health encompasses the mental, emotional, social, and spiritual dimensions of what it means to be healthy **(Figure 2.1)**. It is the result of a complex interaction between a person's history and his or her thoughts about and interpretations of the past and what it means to the present. Psychosocially healthy people are emotionally, mentally, socially, intellectually, and spiritually resilient. They respond to challenges and frustrations in appropriate ways most of the time, despite occasional slips **(Figure 2.2)**. When they do slip, they recognize it and take action to rectify the situation. Once they are informed about the resources that are available to help them get through tough situations, they use them. Most authorities identify several basic characteristics shared by psychosocially healthy people.[2]

- *They feel good about themselves.* They typically are not overwhelmed by fear, love, anger, jealousy, guilt, or worry.

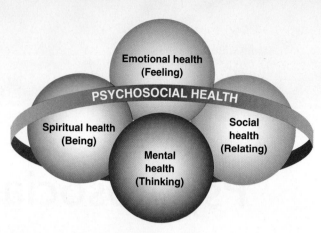

FIGURE 2.1 Psychosocial Health
Psychosocial health is a complex interaction of mental, emotional, social, and spiritual health.

They know who they are, have a realistic sense of their capabilities, and respect themselves even though they realize they aren't perfect.

- *They feel comfortable with other people.* They enjoy satisfying and lasting personal relationships and do not take advantage of others or allow others to take advantage of them. They recognize that there are others whose needs are greater than their own. They can give love, consider others' interests, take time to help others, respect personal differences, and feel responsible for their fellow human beings.

- *They control tension and anxiety.* They recognize the underlying causes and symptoms of stress in their lives and consciously avoid irrational thoughts, hostility, excessive excuse making, and blaming others for their problems. They use resources and learn skills to control reactions to stressful situations.

- *They meet the demands of life.* They try to solve problems as they arise, accept responsibility, and plan ahead. They set realistic goals, think for themselves, and make independent decisions. Acknowledging that change is inevitable, they welcome new experiences.

- *They curb hate and guilt.* They acknowledge and combat tendencies to respond with anger, thoughtlessness, selfishness, vengeful acts, or feelings of inadequacy. They do not try to knock others aside to get ahead but rather reach out to help others—even people they don't particularly like.

- *They maintain a positive outlook.* They approach each day with a presumption that things will go well. They look to the future with enthusiasm rather than dread. Reminders of good experiences brighten their day. Fun and making time for themselves are integral parts of their lives.

- *They value diversity.* They do not feel threatened by people of a different race, gender, religion, sexual orientation, ethnicity, or political party. They are nonjudgmental and do not force their beliefs and values on others.

- *They appreciate and respect nature.* They take the time to enjoy their surroundings, are conscious of their place

psychosocial health The mental, emotional, social, and spiritual dimensions of health.

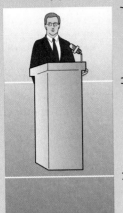

Psychosocially healthy person

— Zest for life, spiritually healthy and intellectually thriving
— High energy, resilient, enjoys challenges, focused
— Realistic sense of self and others, sound coping skills, open-minded
— Adapts to change easily, sensitive to others and environment

— Works to improve in all areas, recognizes strengths and weaknesses
— Healthy relationships with family and friends, capable of giving and receiving love and affection, accepts diversity
— Has strong social support, may need to work on improving social skills/interactions but usually no major problems
— Has occasional emotional "dips" but overall good mental/emotional adaptors

— Shows poorer coping than most, often overwhelmed by circumstances
— Has regular relationship problems, finds that others often disappoint
— Tends to be cynical/critical of others; has friends, but friends tend to be similarly negative/critical
— Lacks focus much of time, hard to keep intellectual acuity sharp
— Quick to anger, a bit volatile in interactions, sense of humor and fun evident less often
— Overly stressed, anxious and pessimistic attitude

— No zest for life; pessimistic/hopeless/cynical most of time; spiritually down
— Laughs, but usually at others, has little fun, no time for self
— Has serious bouts of depression, "down" and "tired" much of time; has suicidal, "life not worth living" thoughts
— A "challenge" to be around, socially isolated
— Developing neurosis/psychosis
— Experiences many illnesses, headaches, aches/pains, gets colds/infections easily

Psychosocially unhealthy person (Illness likely)

FIGURE 2.2 Characteristics of Psychosocially Healthy and Unhealthy People
Where do you fall on this continuum?

in the universe, and act responsibly to preserve their environment.

■ *They enrich the lives of others.* They "tune in," and rather than being narcissistic and self-serving, they often think of others' needs and try to help whenever possible.

Of course, none of us ever achieves perfection in these areas. Attaining psychosocial health and wellness involves many complex processes. This chapter will help you understand not only what it means to be psychosocially well, but also why we may run into problems in our psychosocial health. Learning how to assess your own health and taking action to improve your health are important parts of psychosocial health (see the **Assess Yourself** box).

what do you THINK?

Which psychosocial qualities do you value most in your friends? ■ What area do you think is your greatest psychosocial strength? ■ Your greatest weakness?

Mental Health: The Thinking You

The term **mental health** is often used to describe the "thinking" or "rational" part of psychosocial health. It is defined as the successful performance of mental function and results in productive activities, fulfilling relationships, and the ability to cope with life's challenges. Mental health plays a role in the way we think, communicate, express emotion, and feel about ourselves. A mentally healthy person has the intellectual ability to sort through information, messages, and life events, to attach meaning, and to respond appropriately. This is often referred to as *intellectual health*—a subset of mental health.[3]

(Text continues on page 36.)

mental health   The thinking part of psychosocial health; includes your values, attitudes, and beliefs.

ASSESS yourself

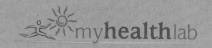

ASSESSING YOUR PSYCHOSOCIAL HEALTH

Fill out this assessment online at www.aw-bc.com/MyHealthLab or www.aw-bc.com/donatelle.

Being psychosocially healthy requires both introspection and the willingness to work on areas that need improvement. Begin by completing the following assessment scale. Use the scale to determine how much each statement describes you. When you've finished, ask someone who is very close to you to take the same test, responding with their perceptions of you. Carefully assess areas where your responses differ from those of your friend or family member. Which areas need some work? Which are in good shape?

	Never	Rarely	Fairly Frequently	Most of the Time	All of the Time
1. My actions and interactions indicate that I am confident in my abilities.	1	2	3	4	5
2. I am quick to blame others for things that go wrong in my life.	1	2	3	4	5
3. I am spontaneous and like to have fun with others.	1	2	3	4	5
4. I am able to give love and affection to others and show my feelings.	1	2	3	4	5
5. I am able to receive love and signs of affection from others without feeling uneasy.	1	2	3	4	5
6. I am generally positive and upbeat about things in my life.	1	2	3	4	5
7. I am cynical and tend to be critical of others.	1	2	3	4	5
8. I have a large group of people whom I consider to be good friends.	1	2	3	4	5
9. I make time for others in my life.	1	2	3	4	5
10. I take time each day for myself for quiet introspection, having fun, or just doing nothing.	1	2	3	4	5
11. I am compulsive and competitive in my actions.	1	2	3	4	5
12. I handle stress well and am seldom upset or stressed out by others.	1	2	3	4	5
13. I try to look for the good in everyone and every situation before finding fault.	1	2	3	4	5
14. I am comfortable meeting new people and interact well in social settings.	1	2	3	4	5
15. I would rather stay in and watch TV or read than go out with friends or interact with others.	1	2	3	4	5
16. I am flexible and can adapt to most situations, even if I don't like them.	1	2	3	4	5
17. Nature, the environment, and other living things are important aspects of my life.	1	2	3	4	5
18. I think before responding to my emotions.	1	2	3	4	5
19. I am selfish and tend to think of my own needs before those of others.	1	2	3	4	5
20. I am consciously trying to be a "better person."	1	2	3	4	5
21. I like to plan ahead and set realistic goals for myself and others.	1	2	3	4	5
22. I accept others for who they are.	1	2	3	4	5
23. I value diversity and respect others' rights, regardless of culture, race, sexual orientation, religion, or other differences.	1	2	3	4	5

	Never	Rarely	Fairly Frequently	Most of the Time	All of the Time
24. I try to live each day as if it might be my last.	1	2	3	4	5
25. I have a great deal of energy and appreciate the little things in life.	1	2	3	4	5
26. I cope with stress in appropriate ways.	1	2	3	4	5
27. I get enough sleep each day and seldom feel tired.	1	2	3	4	5
28. I have healthy relationships with my family.	1	2	3	4	5
29. I am confident that I can do most things if I put my mind to them.	1	2	3	4	5
30. I respect others' opinions and believe that others should be free to express their opinions, even when they differ from my own.	1	2	3	4	5

INTERPRETING YOUR SCORES

Look at items 2, 7, 11, 15, and 19. Add up your score for these five items and divide by 5. Is your average for these items above or below 3? Did you score a 5 on any of these items? Do you need to work on any of these areas? Now look at your scores for the remaining items. (There should be 25 items.) Total these scores and divide by 25. Is your average above or below 3? On which items did you score a 5? Obviously you're doing well in these areas. Now remove these items (scores of 5) from this grouping of 25, and add up your scores for the remaining items. Then divide your total by the number of items included. Now what is your average?

Do the same for the scores completed by your friend or family member. How do your scores compare? Which ones, if any, are different, and how do they differ? Which areas do you need to work on? What actions can you take now to improve your ratings in these areas?

MAKE it happen!

ASSESSMENT: The Assess Yourself activity gave you the chance to look at various aspects of your psychosocial health and compare your self-assessment with a friend's perceptions. Now that you have considered these results, you can change certain behaviors that may be detrimental to your psychosocial health.

MAKING A CHANGE: To change your behavior, you need to develop a plan. Follow these steps below and complete your Behavior Change Contract to take action.

1. Evaluate your behavior, and identify patterns and specific things you are doing. What can you change now? What can you change in the near future?

2. Select one pattern of behavior that you'd like to change.

3. Fill out the Behavior Change Contract found at the front of your book. It should include your long-term goals for change, your short-term goals, the rewards you'll give yourself for reaching these goals, potential obstacles along the way, and strategies for overcoming these obstacles. For each goal, list the small steps and specific actions that you will take.

4. Chart your progress in the journal. At the end of one week, consider how successful you were in following your plan.

5. Revise your plan as needed. Are the short-term goals attainable? Are the rewards satisfying?

EXAMPLE: John assessed himself as a positive and upbeat person, but the assessment his friend gave him rated him as impatient and cynical. John resolved to slow down and become more appreciative of the good things around him. Among his short-term goals: listening to his sister without interrupting her and expressing a sincere compliment to a family member or friend every other day. John found that paying compliments made him stop to think about the qualities he appreciated in friends and family. Although he struggled to listen without interrupting, John found that he was learning a lot about his sister that he had never known before. After several weeks, John's friends commented on his calmer and happier demeanor.

A mentally healthy person is likely to respond to life's challenges constructively. For example, suppose you spend your spring break with friends on the beaches of Mexico, knowing that you have a major term paper due on the first day back from vacation. The night before the paper is due, you quickly throw it together. Rather than falling off the deep end and blaming the instructor if you get a D on the paper, as a mentally healthy student you would accept responsibility for the choices you made, learn from mistakes, and plan differently next time.

When mentally healthy individuals realize that they are getting into trouble with classes, relationships, and life in general, they know when they are still okay and when they are starting to slide. Sadness, unhappiness, fear, and frustration aren't inherently bad and should be acknowledged and dealt with. When the emotions begin to overwhelm you, knowing when to seek help, talk to a trusted friend, or take time out for rest and regrouping are all part of healthy adapting and coping. Unfortunately, far too many of us get caught up in our emotional upheavals and are unable to pull ourselves out of the deep "funks" we can find ourselves in.

Emotional Health: The Feeling You

The term **emotional health** is often used interchangeably with mental health. Although the two are closely intertwined, emotional health more accurately refers to the feeling, or subjective, side of psychosocial health that includes emotional reactions to life. **Emotions** are intensified feelings or complex patterns of feelings that we experience on a regular basis. Love, hate, frustration, anxiety, and joy are only a few of the many emotions we feel. Typically, emotions are described as the interplay of four components: *physiological arousal, feelings, cognitive (thought) processes,* and *behavioral reactions.* Each time you are put in a stressful situation, you react physiologically as you consciously or unconsciously interpret the situation.

Psychologist Richard Lazarus has indicated that there are four basic types of emotions: emotions resulting from harm, loss, or threats; emotions resulting from benefits; borderline emotions, such as hope and compassion; and more complex emotions, such as grief, disappointment, bewilderment, and curiosity.[4] Each of us may experience any of these feelings in any combination at any time. As rational beings, we are responsible for evaluating our individual emotional responses,

emotional health The feeling part of psychosocial health; includes your emotional reactions to life.

emotions Intensified feelings or complex patterns of feelings we constantly experience.

social health Aspect of psychosocial health that includes interactions with others, ability to use social supports, and ability to adapt to various situations.

the environment that is causing them, and the appropriateness of our actions.

Emotionally healthy people usually respond appropriately to upsetting events. Rather than respond in an extreme fashion or behave inconsistently or offensively, they are able to express their feelings, communicate with others, and show emotions in appropriate ways. How many times have you seen someone react with extreme anger by shouting or punching a wall? Ex-lovers who become jealous of new relationships and damage cars or property are classic examples of people exhibiting unhealthy and dangerous emotional reactions. Such violent responses and emotional volatility have become a problem of epidemic proportions in the United States (see Chapter 4).

Emotionally healthy people are usually able to respond in an appropriate manner to upsetting events. Emotionally unhealthy people are much more likely to let their feelings overpower them. They may be highly volatile and prone to unpredictable emotional outbursts and inappropriate, sometimes frightening, responses. An ex-boyfriend who is so jealous of your new relationship that he hits you or tries to manipulate you into spending time only with him is showing an extremely unhealthy and dangerous emotional reaction.

Emotional health also affects *social health.* Someone feeling hostile, withdrawn, or moody may become socially isolated.[5] Because they are not much fun to be around, their friends may avoid them at the very time they are most in need of emotional support. For students, a more immediate concern is the impact of emotional trauma on academic performance. Have you ever tried to study for an exam after a fight with a close friend or family member? Emotional turmoil may seriously affect your ability to think, reason, and act rationally. Many otherwise rational, mentally healthy people do ridiculous things when they are going through a major emotional upset. Mental functioning and emotional responses are intricately connected.

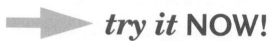

try it NOW!

Seek change! Change is an inevitable part of life, but it can also be a challenge to your psychosocial health. Develop skills to cope with change by making change a regular part of your life. View change as an exciting chance for growth rather than a negative event. Think of the positive things that change will create. Take a different route to class, study at the coffee shop instead of the library, or pick out the people you don't know in class as your project partners. Don't get stuck in a "same old, same old" approach to life.

Social Health: Interactions with Others

Social health, an important part of the broader concept of psychosocial health, includes your interactions with others on an individual and group basis, your ability to use social resources and support in times of need, and your ability to adapt to a variety of social situations. Socially healthy individuals have a wide range of interactions with family, friends, and acquaintances and are able to have a healthy interaction with an intimate partner. Typically, socially healthy individuals are able to listen, express themselves, form healthy attachments, act in socially acceptable and responsible ways, and find the best fit for themselves in society. Numerous studies have documented the importance of positive relationships with family members, friends, and one's significant other in overall well-being and healthy longevity.[6]

As social animals, we grow stronger and learn valuable lessons in groups, whether the interactions are positive or fraught with conflict. From the moment we are born, we rely on families for our care and friends for our sense of "fitting in." We depend on others to learn new skills and develop much of our sense of self-worth as a result of our interactions with others. Our adult lives are spent working with others, developing relationships with family and friends, and participating in our community. In many ways, our value to society is measured by the number of connections we have and even by how many people attend our funerals. Few would disagree that social bonds are the very foundation of human life.

Social bonds reflect the level of closeness and attachment that we develop with individuals. They provide intimacy, feelings of belonging, opportunities for giving and receiving nurturance, reassurance of one's worth, assistance and guidance, and advice. Social bonds take multiple forms, the most common of which are social support and community engagements.

Social support consists of networks of people and services with whom you share ties. These ties can provide tangible support, such as babysitting services or money to help pay the bills, or intangible support, such as encouraging you to share intimate thoughts. Generally, the closer and the higher the quality of the social bond, the more likely a person is to ask for and receive social support. For example, if your car broke down on a dark country road in the middle of a snowy night, who could you call for help and know that they would do everything possible to get there? People who are socially isolated, estranged from their families, and have few social connections will have difficulty thinking of someone to count on when they are in trouble. Often mentally ill and homeless individuals lack the support networks necessary to help them get off the streets and sustain health. Psychosocially healthy people create and maintain a network of friends and family with whom they can give and receive support, and they work hard to maintain those relationships even in difficult times.

Social health also reflects the way we react to others. In its most extreme forms, a lack of social health may be represented by aggressive acts of prejudice toward other individuals or groups. In its most obvious manifestations, **prejudice** is reflected in acts of discrimination, hate, and bias, and in purposeful intent to harm individuals or groups.

Spiritual Health: An Inner Quest for Well-Being

Although mental and emotional health are key factors in overall psychosocial functioning, it is possible to be mentally and emotionally healthy and still not achieve optimal well-being. What is missing? For many people, the difficult-to-describe element that gives zest to life is the spiritual dimension.

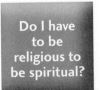

Most experts agree that **spirituality** refers to the personal quest for seeking answers to life's ultimate questions, finding meaning in one's life purpose, and seeking a sense of belonging to something greater than the purely physical or personal dimensions of existence.[7] For some, this unifying force is nature; for others, it is a feeling of connection to other people; for still others, the unifying force is a god or other spiritual symbol.

Dr. N. Lee Smith, internist and associate professor of medicine at the University of Utah, defines spiritual health in the following ways:[8]

- The quality of existence in which one is at peace with oneself and in good standing with the environment

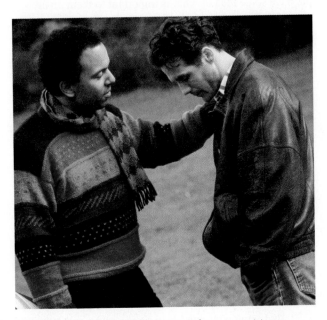

Support from family and friends is a vital component to your social health.

---

social bonds   Degree and nature of interpersonal contacts.

social support   Network of people and services with whom you share ties and get support.

prejudice   A negative evaluation of an entire group of people that is typically based on unfavorable and often wrong ideas about the group.

spirituality   A belief in a unifying force that gives meaning to life and transcends the purely physical or personal dimensions of existence.

- A sense of empowerment and personal control that includes feeling valued and in control of one's responses (but not necessarily in control of one's environment)
- A sense of connectedness to one's deepest self, to other people, and to all that is generally regarded as good
- A sense of meaning and purpose, which provides a sense of mission by finding meaning and wisdom in the here and now

On a day-to-day basis, many of us focus on acquiring material possessions and satisfying basic needs. But there comes a point when we discover that material possessions do not automatically bring happiness or a sense of self-worth. As we develop into spiritually healthy beings, we recognize our identity as unique individuals and gain a better appreciation of our strengths and shortcomings and our place in the universe.

In its purest sense, spirituality addresses four main themes: interconnectedness, the practice of mindfulness, spirituality as a part of everyday life, and living in harmony with the community (**Figure 2.3**).

- *Interconnectedness.* The term **interconnectedness** expresses a sense of harmony with oneself, with others, and with a larger meaning or purpose. Connecting with oneself involves exploring feelings, taking time to consider how you feel in a given situation, assessing your reactions to people and experiences, and taking mental notes when things or people cause you to lose equilibrium. It also involves considering your values and working toward achieving your goals without compromising those values.
- *Practice of mindfulness.* **Mindfulness** is a form of meditation that focuses on one's ability to be fully present in the moment. According to molecular biologist and guru of mindfulness, Jon Kabat-Zinn, PhD, living mindfully means "making more of your ordinary moments notable and noteworthy by taking note of them. . . . When you pay attention to boredom, it gets unbelievably interesting."[9] Mindfulness has been described as a way of nurturing

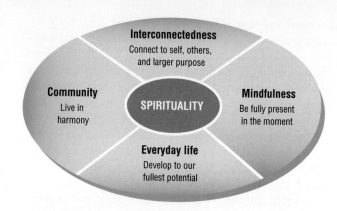

FIGURE 2.3 Four Major Themes of Spirituality

greater awareness, clarity, and acceptance of present-moment reality or a form of inner flow—a holistic sensation you feel when you are totally involved in the moment rather than focused on some distant future event that may or may not happen.[10]

- *Spirituality as a part of daily life.* Spirituality is embodied in the ability to discover and articulate our own basic purpose in life; to learn how to experience love, joy, peace, and fulfillment; and to help ourselves and others achieve our full potential.[11] This ongoing process of growth fosters three convictions: faith, hope, and love. **Faith** is the belief that helps us realize our purpose in life; **hope** is the belief that allows us to look confidently and courageously to the future; and **love** involves accepting, affirming, and respecting self and others, regardless of who they are.[12]
- *Living in harmony with our community.* Our values are an extension of our beliefs about the world and our attitude toward life. They are formed over time through a series of life experiences, and they are reflected in our hopes, dreams, desires, goals, and ambitions.[13] Though most people have some idea of what is important to them, many spend life largely unaware of how their values impact themselves or those around them until a life-altering event shakes up their perspective on life. **Altruism,** the act of giving of oneself out of genuine concern for others, is a key aspect of a spiritually healthy lifestyle.[14] Volunteering to help others, doing charitable work, donating resources to help people in need and other community service venues help you give back to the community and to people who have supported you.

interconnectedness A web of connections, including our relationship to ourselves, to others, and to a larger meaning or purpose in life.

mindfulness Awareness and acceptance of the reality of the present moment.

faith Belief that helps each person realize a unique purpose in life.

hope Belief that allows us to look confidently and courageously to the future.

love Acceptance, affirmation, and respect for the self and others.

altruism The act of giving of oneself out of genuine concern for others.

what do you THINK?

What do social, mental, emotional, and spiritual health mean to you? ■ What are your strengths and weaknesses in each area of psychosocial health? ■ What can you do to enhance your strengths? How can you improve areas that are not strong? ■ Are there community service activities that you could engage in right now to help others?

Spirituality: A Key to Better Health Although the specific impact of spirituality on health remains elusive, many experts affirm the importance of this dimension in achieving health and wellness. Results from studies of spirituality among college students indicate that spirituality may play a role in students' health, their grades, their involvement in student activities, and other aspects of student life.[15] These studies also found a correlation between spirituality and health achievement, with more spiritually oriented students having better health, better grades, more involvement in charitable organizations or volunteerism, and more interest in helping others. Students from different racial and ethnic groups varied in spirituality levels, with African Americans demonstrating more spirituality and being more engaged and benefiting more from spirituality-related behaviors. Other recent studies also indicate a correlation between certain elements of spirituality and positive health outcomes. For example, mindfulness therapies have been used effectively to treat depression, to reduce stress in outpatient therapy and in the nursing profession, to treat anxiety and heart disease, and to address other problems.[16]

A Spiritual Resurgence Over recent decades, studies have shown that most adult Americans, like their student counterparts, believe in God and consider spirituality to be important in their lives, although not necessarily in the form of religion. Many find spiritual fulfillment in music, poetry, literature, art, nature, and intimate relationships.[17] **Table 2.1** details some characteristics that distinguish religion from spirituality. Many religious groups have spawned new philosophies that are more inclusive and often influenced by "New Age" ideas, such as using positive thought to achieve your goals and striving to find your rightful place in the world. A growing body of research focuses on the benefits in quality and quantity of life that optimists—people who maintain a positive and sunny view of the world, even in the face of adversity—experience.[18] Optimists see the good in situations and expect things to go the way they expect them to in life. They always believe the "glass is half full" and focus their energy on the possibilities of life, rather than on their fears.

For some, spirituality means a "quest for self and selflessness"—a form of therapy and respite from a sometimes challenging personal environment. This quest has received much scholarly and popular attention. Self-help books that focus on spirituality consistently top the bestseller lists. Television programs promote the virtues of a spiritual or natural existence. Writers and psychologists such as William James, Carl Jung, Gordon Allport, Erich Fromm, Viktor Frankl, Abraham Maslow, Rollo May, and Jon Kabat-Zinn have made spirituality a major focus of their work.

Spiritual health courses have emerged in public health and medical school training. For example, the Harvard Medical School of Continuing Education offers a course called "Spirituality and Healing in Medicine," which brings together scholars and medical professionals from around the world to

TABLE 2.1	Characteristics Distinguishing Religion and Spirituality

Religion	Spirituality
Community focused	Individualistic
Observable, measurable objective	Less visible and measurable, more subjective
Formal, orthodox, organized	Less formal, less orthodox, less systematic
Behavior oriented, outward practices	Emotionally oriented, inward directed
Authoritarian in terms of behaviors	Not authoritarian, little accountability
Doctrine separating good from evil	Unifying, not doctrine oriented

Source: National Institutes of Health, "Prayer and Spirituality in Health: Ancient Practices, Modern Science," *CAM at the NIH* 12, no. 1 (2005): 1–4.

discuss the role of spirituality in treating illness and chronic pain. Self-help workshops focusing on spiritual elements of health are popular throughout the world.

Putting Spirituality into Practice How can you enhance your spiritual dimension of psychosocial health? Some people seek solace in religion and equate spirituality with religiosity. Although religion and spirituality have some common elements, it is important to note that spirituality and religion are not the same thing. Enhancing your spiritual side takes just as much work as becoming physically fit, improving your diet, or working on your mental health. The **Skills for Behavior Change** box features some strategies you can implement to develop your spiritual side.

Factors Influencing Psychosocial Health

Most of our mental, emotional, and social reactions to life are a direct outcome of our experiences and social and cultural expectations. Our psychosocial health is based, in part, on how we perceive life experiences.

External Factors

Although some life experiences are under our control, others are not. External factors in life are those that we do not control, such as who raised us and where we live.

The Family Families have a significant influence on psychosocial development. Children raised in healthy, nurturing, happy families are more likely to become well-adjusted,

STRATEGIES TO FIND YOUR SPIRITUAL SIDE

Spirituality involves connectedness to others and to the broader community, so it is important that we take time for meaningful interactions with our friends, family, and people within the community with whom we may not interact regularly. What types of actions foster connectedness?

VOLUNTEER

The ability to notice when others are in trouble and reaching out to help them through volunteering is an excellent way to feel connected with others and enhance your own health. In the aftermath of Hurricane Katrina, thousands of people volunteered their time, money, and effort to help an entire population that was suffering. Recognizing that we are all part of the greater system of humanity and that we have roles and responsibilities to help others in times of need is a key part of spirituality. Volunteering by helping your older neighbors clean their home, working at the humane society, or participating in a beach or highway cleanup is all a part of being responsible and finding a place to help in the greater scheme of things. Volunteering can be a huge boost for you when you are feeling down or wondering how you fit in.

TAKE TIME TO REFLECT

Connecting with your self is another method of finding your spiritual side. Make a ritual out of taking a few moments each day to think about who you are, what you value, why you feel good, or what things are troubling you. Setting aside this special time to reflect will become a sacred time meant just for you and can help you relieve tension, seek out answers to problems you are experiencing, or simply empty your mind and enjoy this time to yourself.

GET INVOLVED IN SERVICE LEARNING

Service learning involves making meaningful and productive relationships with the greater community. Students have an opportunity to learn new skills and grow.

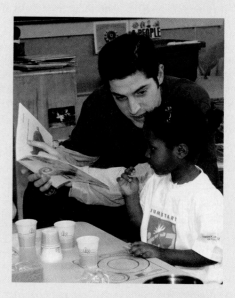

Community agencies and programs benefit from an enthusiastic hardworking group of students. Students will learn to look at the greater community and world around them, rather than remaining absorbed in college life and thoughts of papers due, the party on Friday night, and basketball practice.

How do others influence my psychosocial health?

productive adults. Children raised in **dysfunctional families,** in which there is violence, negative behavior, distrust, anger, dietary deprivation, drug abuse, parental discord, or sexual, physical, or emotional abuse, may have a harder time adapting to life and run an increased risk of psychosocial problems. In dysfunctional families, love, security, and unconditional trust are so lacking that children often become confused and psychologically bruised. Yet, not all people raised in dysfunctional families become psychosocially unhealthy, and not all children from healthy environments become well adjusted. Obviously, more factors are involved in our "process of becoming" than just our family.

The Macro Environment Although isolated negative events may do little damage to psychosocial health, persistent stressors, uncertainties, and threats can cause significant problems. Drugs, neighborhood crime and threats to safety, injury, school failure, unemployment, financial problems, natural disasters and a host of other bad things can happen to good people. But it is believed that certain protective factors, such as having a positive role model in the midst of chaos, or certain positive personality traits can help children from even the worst environments remain healthy and well adjusted (see the next section, Internal Factors). They are often more resilient in the face of adversity and are more likely to have the resources to cope more effectively.

Another important influence is access to health services and programs designed to enhance psychosocial health. Going to a support group or seeing a trained therapist is often a crucial first step in prevention and intervention efforts. Individuals from poor socioeconomic environments who cannot afford such services often find it difficult to secure help in improving their psychosocial health.

dysfunctional families Families in which there is violence; physical, emotional, or sexual abuse; parental discord; or other negative family interactions.

 what do you THINK?

Over which external factors does an individual have the most control? ■ Which factors had the greatest impact on making you who you are today?

Internal Factors

Many internal factors also shape a person's development. These factors include hereditary traits, hormonal function, physical health (including neurological function), physical fitness level, and certain elements of mental and emotional health.

Self-Efficacy and Self-Esteem

During our formative years, successes and failures in school, athletics, friendships, intimate relationships, our jobs, and every other aspect of life subtly shape our beliefs about our own personal worth and abilities. These beliefs in turn become internal influences on our psychosocial health.

Psychologist Albert Bandura used the term **self-efficacy** to describe a person's belief about whether he or she can successfully engage in and execute a specific behavior.

Self-esteem refers to one's sense of self-respect or self-worth. It can be defined as one's evaluation of oneself and one's own personal worth as an individual. People with high self-esteem tend to feel good about themselves and express a positive outlook on life. People with low self-esteem often do not like themselves, constantly demean themselves, and doubt their ability to succeed.

Our self-esteem is a result of the relationships we have with our parents and family during our formative years, with our friends as we grow older, with our significant others as we form intimate relationships, and with our teachers, co-workers, and others throughout our lives. If we felt loved and valued as children, our self-esteem allows us to believe that we are inherently lovable individuals.

How can you build up your self-esteem? **Table 2.2** offers suggestions of small things you can do every day that can have a significant impact on the way you feel about yourself.

Learned Helplessness versus Learned Optimism

Psychologist Martin Seligman has proposed that people who continually experience failure may develop a pattern of responding known as **learned helplessness,** in which they give up and fail to take any action to help themselves. Seligman ascribes this response in part to society's tendency toward victimology, blaming one's problems on other people and circumstances.[19] Although viewing ourselves as victims may make us feel better temporarily, it does not address the underlying causes of a problem. Ultimately, it can erode self-efficacy and foster learned helplessness by making us feel that we cannot do anything to improve the situation.

Today, many people have developed self-help programs that utilize elements of Seligman's principle of **learned optimism.** Foundational to these self-help programs is the thought that just as we learn to be helpless, so can we teach ourselves to be optimistic. By changing our self-talk, examining our reactions and the way we assess what happens to us in life, and blocking negative thoughts, we can "unlearn" negative thought processes that have become habitual. Some programs practice "positive affirmations" with clients, teaching them the sometimes difficult task of learning to write and/or verbalize positive things about themselves.

TABLE 2.2	Tips for Building Self-Esteem

- **Pay attention to your own needs and wants.** Listen to what your body, your mind, and your heart are telling you.
- **Take good care of yourself.** Eat healthy foods, avoid junk foods, exercise, and plan fun activities for yourself.
- **Take time to do things you enjoy.** Make a list of things you enjoy doing. Then do something from that list every day.
- **Do something that you have been putting off.** Cleaning out your closet, going on a diet, or paying a bill that you've been putting off will make you feel like you've accomplished something.
- **Give yourself rewards.** Acknowledge that you are a great person by rewarding yourself occasionally.
- **Wear clothes that make you feel good about yourself.** You don't have to spend a lot to find clothes that make you feel good. Check out local thrift stores and consignment shops for great bargains.
- **Spend time with people.** People who make you feel better about yourself are great self-esteem boosters. Avoid people who treat you badly or make you feel bad about yourself.
- **Display items that you like.** You may have items that remind you of your achievements, your friends, or of special times. Keep those special items close by.
- **Make your meals a special time.** Get rid of distractions such as the television, and really concentrate on enjoying your meal, whether you are by yourself or with others.
- **Learn something new every day.** Take advantage of any opportunity to learn something new every day—you'll feel better about yourself and be more productive.
- **Do something nice for another person.** There is no greater way to feel better about yourself than to help someone in greater need. Check out local volunteer opportunities, or make a special effort to be nice to those around you, such as your parents or siblings.

Sources: A. L. Story, "Self-Esteem and Self-Certainty: A Mediational Analysis," *European Journal of Personality* 18, no. 2 (2004): 115; M. E. Copeland, "Building Self-Esteem: A Self-Help Guide," Center for Mental Health Services [online booklet], accessed March 2007, www.mentalhealth.org/publications/allpubs/SMA-3715/default.asp.

Often we are our own worst critics, and taking praise from others and learning to be kinder to ourselves is difficult.

Personality

Your personality is the unique mix of characteristics that distinguish you from others. Heredity, environment, culture, and experience influence how each person develops. Personality determines how we react to the challenges of life, interpret our feelings, and resolve conflicts.

self-efficacy Belief in one's own ability to perform a task successfully.

self-esteem Sense of self-respect or self-confidence.

learned helplessness Pattern of responding to situations by giving up because of repeated failure in the past.

learned optimism Teaching oneself to think optimistically.

Most of the recent schools of psychosocial theory promote the idea that we have the power not only to understand our behavior, but also to change it and thus mold our own personalities. Although much has been written about the importance of a healthy personality, there is little consensus on what that concept really means. In general, people who possess the following traits often appear to be psychosocially healthy:[20]

- *Extroversion,* the ability to adapt to a social situation and demonstrate assertiveness as well as power or interpersonal involvement
- *Agreeableness,* the ability to conform, be likable, and demonstrate friendly compliance as well as love
- *Openness to experience,* the willingness to demonstrate curiosity and independence (also referred to as inquiring intellect)
- *Emotional stability,* the ability to maintain social control
- *Conscientiousness,* the qualities of being dependable and demonstrating self-control, discipline, and a need to achieve

Life Span and Maturity Our temperaments change as we move through life, as illustrated by the extreme emotions that many young teens experience. Most of us learn to control our emotions as we advance toward adulthood.

The college years mark a critical transition period for young adults as they move away from families and establish themselves as independent adults. The transition to independence will be easier for those who have successfully accomplished earlier developmental tasks, such as learning how to solve problems, make and evaluate decisions, define and adhere to personal values, and establish both casual and intimate relationships. People who have not fulfilled these earlier tasks may find their lives interrupted by recurrent "crises" left over from earlier stages. For example, if they did not learn to trust others in childhood, they may have difficulty establishing intimate relationships as adults.

Resiliency and Developmental Assets

Some people are much better prepared to meet the challenges of life than others. The combination of certain personality traits, coupled with a supportive environment, can equip one to deal effectively with life's many challenges. These

resiliency An individual's capacity for adapting to change and stressful events in healthy and flexible ways.

assets Internal and external resources and community supports that help a person be more resilient in difficult times and more likely to make positive choices and respond in positive, healthful ways.

flourishing Living within an optimal range of human functioning—one that connotes goodness, productivity, growth, and resilience.

individuals are able to cope and even thrive in times of great stress or pressure. **Resiliency,** or *protective factors,* describes those traits or characteristics which protect an individual or community from threat or harm. In a sense, these traits may serve to inoculate one against potential ill health. People with **assets,** whether they be financial, emotional, spiritual, physical, intellectual, or mental, and other positive forces in their lives are more likely to be resilient and bounce back when facing life's challenges.

Flourishing means to live within an optimal range of human functioning—one that connotes goodness, productivity, growth, and resilience. For example, research shows that positive attitudes, such as interest and curiosity, produce more accurate subsequent knowledge than negative attitudes, such as cynicism and boredom. It follows that if you start the first day in a class being "turned off" by the instructor and wondering what you are doing there, it is less likely that you will do well than if you change your attitude and self-talk about the experience.[21]

Strategies to Enhance Psychosocial Health

As we have seen, psychosocial health involves four dimensions. Attaining self-fulfillment is a lifelong, conscious process that involves enhancing each of these components. Strategies include building self-efficacy and self-esteem, understanding and controlling emotions, maintaining support networks, and learning to solve problems and make decisions. In addition to the advice in this chapter, see Chapter 3 for tips on effective stress reduction, relaxation techniques, and other tools for enhancing psychosocial health.

Developing and Maintaining Self-Esteem and Self-Efficacy

There are several ways to build self-esteem and self-efficacy. These include finding a support group, completing required tasks, forming realistic expectations, making time for yourself, maintaining your physical health, and examining your problems and seeking help.

Find a Support Group The best way to promote self-esteem is through a support group—peers who share your values. A support group can make you feel good about yourself and force you to take an honest look at your actions and choices. Although you might seek support in a wholly new group, remember that old ties are often the strongest.

Keeping in contact with old friends and important family members can provide a foundation of unconditional love that will help you through the many life transitions ahead. Try to be a support for others, too. Join a discussion, political action, or recreational group. Write more postcards and "thinking of you" notes to people who matter. This will build your own self-esteem and that of your friends.

Complete Required Tasks A good way to boost your self-efficacy is to learn new skills and develop a history of success. Most college campuses provide study groups and learning centers that can help you manage time, develop study skills, and prepare for tests. Poor grades or grades that do not meet expectations are major contributors to emotional distress among college students.

Form Realistic Expectations Set realistic expectations for yourself. If you expect perfect grades, a steady stream of Saturday-night dates, and the perfect job, you may be setting yourself up for failure. Assess your current resources and the direction in which you are heading. Set small, incremental goals or steps that are possible for you to meet.

Make Time for You Taking time to enjoy yourself is another way to boost your self-esteem and psychosocial health. View a new activity as something to look forward to and an opportunity to have fun. Anticipate and focus on the fun things you have to look forward to each day.

Maintain Physical Health Regular exercise fosters a sense of well-being. Nourishing meals can help you avoid the weight gain that many college students experience. A growing body of research supports the role that exercise plays in improving mental health. (See Chapter 9 for information on nutrition and Chapter 11 for information on the role of exercise on health.)

Examine Problems and Seek Help If Necessary Knowing when to seek help from friends, support groups, family, or professionals is another important factor in boosting self-esteem. Sometimes you can handle life's problems alone; at other times, you need assistance.

Sleep: The Great Restorer

Sleep serves at least two biological purposes: (1) conservation of energy, so that we are rested and ready to perform during high-performance daylight hours; and (2) restoration, so that neurotransmitters that have been depleted during waking hours can be replenished. This process clears the brain of daily minutiae to prepare for a new day. Getting enough sleep to feel ready to meet daily challenges is a key factor in physical and psychosocial health.

All of us can identify with that tired, listless feeling caused by sleep deprivation during periods of high stress. Either we can't find enough hours in the day for sleep, or once we get into bed we can't fall asleep or stay asleep. Sleep, or lack of it, is especially common among college students; in a small survey of students at Notre Dame University, nearly 70 percent of those students surveyed indicated they only receive 5 to 6 hours of sleep each weeknight. College students have a high workload, anxiety, and stress—all factors that may explain the collective lack of sleep among those aged 18 to 24. A recent study of randomly sampled women aged 18 to 65 showed that women in particular suffer from sleep problems:[22]

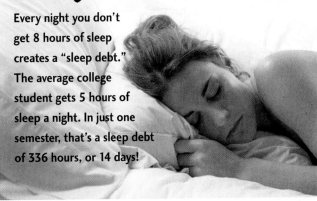

DID you KNOW?

Every night you don't get 8 hours of sleep creates a "sleep debt." The average college student gets 5 hours of sleep a night. In just one semester, that's a sleep debt of 336 hours, or 14 days!

- 67 percent said they frequently experience a sleep problem, and 43 percent said that daytime sleepiness interferes with their daily acivities.
- When pressed for time and tired, 33 percent said they cut back on sex, 39 percent said they cut back on spending time with friends and family, and 37 percent said they stop eating healthy foods.
- 29 percent said they use a sleep aid to help them get to sleep and stay asleep.
- 74 percent of stay-at-home moms reported insomnia, and the numbers were higher among women who work full time and have children at home.
- 31 percent snore, and many have undiagnosed sleep apnea.

How much sleep do we need? This depends on many factors. There is a genetically based need for sleep, and it differs for each species. Sleep duration is also controlled by *circadian rhythms,* which are linked to the hormone *melatonin.* People may also alter sleep patterns by staying up late, drinking coffee, getting lots of physical exercise, eating a heavy meal, or using alarm clocks. In fact, a new syndrome, known as *sleep inertia,* describes the cognitive impairment, disorientation, and grogginess we experience when we first get up in the morning. This sleep inertia may impair our ability to think clearly and function effectively in tasks that occur shortly after we wake up. Coffee in the morning or a quick walk or jog may speed wakefulness, and for people who must wake up fast and be alert—such as physicians, pilots, truck drivers, and students having an 8:00 AM exam—these "jump starts" may be important to performing effectively.[23] Most of us follow characteristic stages of sleep, ranging from *wakefulness* to *drowsiness* to *light sleep,* and then moving to *deeper sleep.* The most important period of sleep, known as the time of *rapid eye movement (REM)* sleep, is essential to feeling rested and refreshed. In REM sleep, heart rate increases, respiration speeds up, and dreaming tends to occur. If we miss REM sleep, we are left feeling groggy and sleep deprived.

Though many people turn to over-the-counter sleeping pills, barbiturates, or tranquilizers, look at **Table 2.3** for more effective and less risky methods for conquering sleeplessness.

- **Establish a consistent sleep schedule.** Go to bed and get up at about the same time every day.
- **Evaluate your sleep environment.** Is there something keeping you awake? If it's noise, wear earplugs or use a white-noise item such as running a fan. If it's light, try room-darkening shades.
- **Exercise regularly.** It's hard to feel drowsy if you have been sedentary all day. Don't exercise right before bedtime, because activity speeds up your metabolism and makes it harder to go to sleep.
- **Limit caffeine and alcohol.** Caffeine can linger in your body for up to 12 hours and cause insomnia. Although alcohol may make you drowsy at first, it interferes with the normal sleep–wake cycle.
- **Avoid eating a heavy meal or drinking large amounts of liquid before bed.**
- **Don't lie in bed tossing and turning.** If you're unable to get to sleep in 30 minutes, get up and do something else. Read, play solitaire, or try other relaxing activities; return to bed when you feel drowsy.
- **Nap only in the afternoon.** This is when our circadian rhythms tend to make us sleepy. Don't let naps interfere with your normal sleep schedule.
- **Establish a relaxing nighttime ritual that puts you in the mood to sleep.** Take a warm shower, relax in a comfortable chair, don your favorite robe. Doing this consistently will cue your mind and body that it's time to wind down.

Insomnia Nearly 70 million Americans suffer from sleep problems and difficulty getting a good night's rest due to a variety of sleep disorders. **Insomnia**—difficulty in falling asleep quickly, frequent arousals during sleep, or early morning awakening—is a common complaint among 20 to 40 percent of Americans. Insomnia is more common among women than men, and its prevalence is correlated with age and low socio-economic status.

Sleep Apnea Some people have difficulty getting a good night's sleep because of *sleep apnea,* an increasingly common and serious disorder. For more on this condition, see Chapter 13.

insomnia Difficulty in falling asleep or staying asleep.

psychoneuroimmunology (PNI) The science that examines the relationship between the brain and behavior and how this affects the body's immune system.

happiness Feeling of contentment created when one's expectations and physical, psychological, and spiritual needs have been met and one enjoys life.

subjective well-being (SWB) That uplifting feeling of inner peace and wonder that we call happiness.

The Mind–Body Connection

Can negative emotions make us physically ill? Can positive emotions and happiness help us stay well? Researchers are exploring the interaction between emotions and health, especially in conditions of uncontrolled, persistent stress. In fact, the National Institutes of Health and other organizations are investing more and more into large research endeavors that will further explore the link between mind and body.

Can negative emotions make me sick?

At the core of the mind–body connection is the study of **psychoneuroimmunology (PNI),** or how the brain and behavior affect the body's immune system. The science of PNI focuses on the relationship between emotions, psychosocial factors, the central nervous system, the immune system, and disease and illness.[24] One emotion that appears to be particularly promising in enhancing physical health is happiness.

Happiness and Physical Health

Happiness is defined as a kind of placeholder for a number of positive states in which individuals actively embrace the world around them.[25] In examining characteristics of happy people, scientists have found that this emotion can have a profound impact on the body. Researchers have found that happiness or related mental states such as hopefulness, optimism, and contentment appear to reduce the risk or limit the severity of cardiovascular disease, pulmonary disease, diabetes, hypertension, colds, and other infections. Laughter can promote increases in heart rate, respiration rate, and reduce levels of stress hormones in much the same way as light exercise. For this reason, it has been promoted as a possible risk reducer for people with hypertension and other forms of cardiovascular disease.[26]

If happiness is good for your health, how do you "get happy"? **Subjective well-being (SWB)** refers to that uplifting feeling of inner peace or overall "feel-good" state, which includes happiness. SWB is defined by three central components:[27]

1. *Satisfaction with present life.* People who are high in SWB tend to like their work and are satisfied with their current personal relationships. They are sociable, outgoing, and willing to open up to others. They also like themselves and enjoy good health and self-esteem.

2. *Relative presence of positive emotions.* People with high SWB more frequently feel pleasant emotions, mainly because they evaluate the world around them in a generally positive way. They have an optimistic outlook, and they expect success in what they undertake.

3. *Relative absence of negative emotions.* Individuals with a strong sense of SWB experience fewer and less severe episodes of negative emotions, such as anxiety, depression, and anger.

How happy are you?

Read the following statements, and then rate your level of agreement with each one using the 1–7 scale.

1	2	3	4	5	6	7
Strongly disagree	Disagree	Slightly disagree	Neither agree nor disagree	Slightly agree	Agree	Strongly agree

1. In most ways, my life is close to my ideal. _____
2. The conditions of my life are excellent. _____
3. I am satisfied with my life. _____
4. So far I have gotten the important things I want in life. _____
5. If I could live my life over, I would change almost nothing. _____

Total score: _____

Scoring:
31–35: You are very satisfied with your life 26–30: Satisfied 21–25: Slightly satisfied
20: You are neither satisfied nor dissatisfied 15–19: Slightly dissatisfied 10–14: Dissatisfied 5–9: Very dissatisfied

FIGURE 2.4 Satisfaction with Life Scale

Source: W. Pavot and E. Diener, "Review of the Satisfaction with Life Scale," *Psychological Assessment* 5 (1993): 164–72.

You do not have to be happy all the time to achieve overall subjective well-being. Everyone experiences disappointments, unhappiness, and times when life seems unfair. But people with SWB are typically resilient, able to look on the positive side, able to get back on track fairly quickly, and less likely to fall into despair over setbacks. Despite what some people may believe, happiness does not depend on age, gender, race, or socioeconomic status.

Scientists suggest that people may be biologically predisposed to happiness. Psychologist Richard Davidson proposes that happiness may, in part, be related to actual differences in brain physiology—that *neurotransmitters,* the chemicals that transfer messages between neurons, may function more efficiently in happy people.[28] Other psychologists suggest that we can develop happiness by practicing positive psychological actions.[29]

How happy are you? Take the quiz in **Figure 2.4** and see how you score.

Using Positive Psychology to Enhance Happiness

The emerging discipline of positive psychology focuses on helping us achieve the happiness we desire, find meaning in life, build our character strengths, and in general, approach life from a more "positivistic" perspective. Currently, researchers are focusing efforts on developing methods that can be used to teach people how to focus on the positive.[30] Though this body of research is still in its early stages, several key aspects have emerged, and you can implement the following strategies to enhance happiness, and employ a more positive outlook on life:[31]

- *Develop gratitude.* **Gratitude** is a sense of thankfulness and appreciation for the good things in your life as well as for life's lessons. In one study, Seligman required individuals to write down three positive occurrences that happened each day for one week, then write an answer to the question, "Why did this good thing happen?" Try this yourself for one week.

- *Use capitalization.* **Capitalization** refers to the process by which we focus on the good things that happen to us and share those things with others. Research in this area says that telling others about a positive experience increases the positive emotion associated with the event and prolongs the good feelings.

- *Know when to say when.* Researchers have found that people who are always trying to do their absolute best and are not meeting their own high expectations may be more prone to depression, frustration, anxiety, and other problems. Researchers have coined the term *satisfice* to describe the ability to know when an outcome is good enough, rather than ideal. We should find a level of achievement that we will be satisfied with, make sure it is realistic, and stick to it.

- *Grow a signature strength.* Traits such as wisdom, courage, humanity, hope, vitality, curiosity, and love are all considered virtues one should work hard to develop. These strengths are believed to be the most important to one's overall health.

gratitude A sense of thankfulness and appreciation for the good things in your life as well as for life's lessons.

capitalization The process by which we focus on the good things that happen to us and share those things with others.

Does Laughter Enhance Health?

Remember the last time you laughed so hard that you cried? Remember how relaxed you felt afterward? Scientists are just beginning to understand the role of humor in our lives and health. For example, laughter has been shown to have the following effects:

- Stressed-out people with a strong sense of humor become less depressed and anxious than those whose sense of humor is less well developed.
- Students who use humor as a coping mechanism report that it predisposes them to a positive mood.
- Telling a joke, particularly one that involves a shared experience, increases our sense of belonging and social cohesion.

Clearly, laughter enhances mental and emotional health. It also promotes social health: people like to be around others who are fun-loving and laugh easily. Learning to laugh puts more joy into everyday experiences and increases the likelihood that fun-loving people will keep company with us.

Psychologist Barbara Fredrickson argued that positive emotions such as joy, interest, and contentment serve valuable life functions. Joy is associated with playfulness and creativity. Interest encourages us to explore our world, which enhances knowledge and cognitive ability. Contentment allows us to savor and integrate experiences, an important step in achieving mindfulness and insight. By building our physical, social, and mental resources, these positive feelings empower us to cope effectively with life's challenges. Subsequent research has demonstrated that although the actual emotions may be transient, their effects can be permanent and provide lifelong enrichment.[32]

Whereas positive emotions appear to benefit physical health, evidence is accumulating that negative emotions can impair it. Studies of widowed and divorced people reveal below-normal immune system functioning and higher rates of illness and death than among married people. Other studies have shown unusually high rates of cancer among depressed people.[33]

Do these studies provide conclusive evidence of a mind–body connection? Not necessarily, because they do not account for other factors known to be relevant to health. For example, some researchers suggest that people who are divorced, widowed, or depressed are more likely to drink and smoke, use drugs, eat and sleep poorly, and be sedentary—all of which may affect the immune system. In fact, the immune system changes measured in studies of the mind–body connection are relatively small. The health consequences of such minute changes are difficult to gauge, and researchers continue to seek the answer to this question.[34]

mental illnesses Disorders that disrupt thinking, feeling, moods, and behaviors and that impair daily functioning.

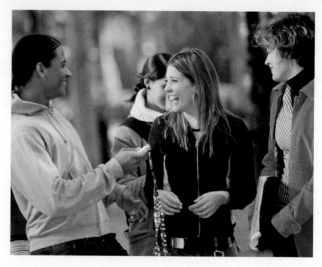

Sharing laughter and having fun with friends improves our social dimension of health and can put more joy into everyday life.

A large body of evidence points to an association between the emotions and physical health, yet we still have much to learn about this relationship. In the meantime, it appears that happiness and an optimistic mind-set don't just feel good—they are also good for you.

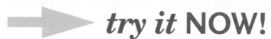 *try it* NOW!

Laugh for health! Laughing not only feels good, but also is good for you. Next time you are in a funk or feeling tired and out of sorts, seek out a laugh or two. Read a funny book, watch a favorite comedy on TV, call a good friend, or play with a pet. You may be surprised how a few chuckles can make you feel better all over!

When Psychosocial Health Deteriorates

Sometimes circumstances overwhelm us to such a degree that we need outside assistance to help us get back on track toward healthful living. Abusive relationships, stress, anxiety, loneliness, financial upheavals, and other traumatic events can sap our spirits, causing us to turn inward or to act in ways that are outside what might be considered normal. Chemical imbalances, drug interactions, trauma, neurological disruptions, and other physical problems also may contribute to these behaviors. **Mental illnesses** are disorders that disrupt thinking, feeling, moods, and behaviors and cause a varying degree of impaired functioning in daily life. They are believed to be caused by life events in some cases and by actual biochemical and/or brain dysfunction in others.[35] As with physical disease, mental illnesses can range from mild to severe and exact a heavy toll on the quality of life, both for people with the illnesses and those who come in contact with them.

Mental illness is universal, affecting all nationalities, ethnicities, and races around the globe. An estimated 26 percent of Americans aged 18 and older suffer from a diagnosed mental disorder in a given year. This is equal to one in every four people. Many individuals suffer from more than one mental disorder at a given time, and there are huge disparities by age, culture, race, ethnicity, and socioeconomic status in the prevalence of mental disorders.[36]

Mental Health Threats to College Students

When it comes to mental health problems, today's students face increasing threats from difficulties in relationships, anxiety, depression, sexual assaults, pressures to take drugs, and a swirling morass of social and environmental problems. The pressures to succeed in an increasingly fast-paced and depersonalized environment often result in significant mental health problems for students. According to a recent American College Health Association Survey of students from across the United States:[37]

- 45.7 percent felt so depressed that they found it difficult to function.
- 93.8 percent had felt overwhelmed.
- 92.2 percent found themselves exhausted (not from physical activity).
- 80.7 percent had felt very sad.
- 63.8 percent had thought things were hopeless.
- 1.2 percent had seriously considered suicide.
- 1.5 percent had attempted suicide.
- 16 percent had been diagnosed with depression, up from 10.3 percent in 2000.

Although there are many types of mental illnesses, we will focus here on those most likely to be experienced by large numbers of college students. For information about other disorders, consult the websites at the end of this chapter, or ask your instructor for local resources.

Mood Disorders

Chronic mood disorders are disorders that affect how you feel, such as persistent sadness or feelings of euphoria. They include depression and bipolar disorder. In any given year, approximately 10 percent of Americans aged 18 or older—about 20.9 million people—suffer from a mood disorder.

Depression: The Full-Scale Tumble

The president of the American Psychological Association once remarked, "Depression has been called the common cold of psychological disturbances, which underscores its prevalence, but trivializes its impact."[38] Depression affects approximately

TABLE 2.4	Are You Depressed?

Sadness and despair are the main symptoms of depression. Other common signs include the following:

- Loss of motivation or interest in pleasurable activities
- Preoccupation with failures and inadequacies; concern over what others are thinking
- Difficulty concentrating; indecisiveness; memory lapses
- Loss of sex drive or interest in close interactions with others
- Fatigue and loss of energy; slow reactions
- Sleeping too much or too little; insomnia
- Feeling agitated, worthless, or hopeless
- Withdrawal from friends and family
- Diminished or increased appetite
- Recurring thoughts that life isn't worth living; thoughts of death or suicide
- Significant weight loss or weight gain

Some depressed people mask their symptoms with a forced, upbeat sense of humor or high energy levels. Communication may cease or seem frantic.

14.8 million American adults, or about 7 percent of the U.S. population each year, and it is the leading cause of disability in the United States for people aged 15 to 44.[39] Although depression can develop at any age, the median age at onset is 32. It is important to recognize that these numbers may reflect just the tip of the iceberg when it comes to determining how many people suffer from depression. Many more are misdiagnosed, underdiagnosed, not receiving treatment, or not treated with the right combinations of therapy.[40]

Some people experience one bout of depression and never have problems again, but others suffer recurrences throughout their lives. (See **Table 2.4**, which lists common symptoms.) Stressful life events are often catalysts for these recurrences.

Types of Depression

Sometimes life throws us down the proverbial stairs. We experience loss, pain, disappointment, and frustration, and we can be left feeling beaten and bruised. How do we know whether those emotions are really signs of a **major depressive disorder**? It's important to note that true depressive disorders are not the same as having a bad day or feeling down after a negative experience. It also isn't something that can be willed or wished away, or just a matter of learning to "grow a thicker

chronic mood disorder Experience of persistent sadness, despair, and hopelessness.

major depressive disorder Severe depression that entails chronic mood disorder, physical effects such as sleep disturbance and exhaustion, and mental effects such as the inability to concentrate.

skin." True depressive disorders are characterized by a combination of symptoms that interfere with work, study, sleep, eating, relationships, and enjoyment of life. Symptoms can last for weeks, months, or years and vary in intensity.[41]

Another type of depression is **bipolar disorder,** also called *manic-depressive illness.* People with bipolar disorder often have severe mood swings, ranging from severe highs (mania) to lows (depression). Sometimes these swings are dramatic and rapid; at other times they are slow and gradual. When in the manic phase, people may be overactive, be talkative, and have tons of energy; in the depressed phase, they may experience some or all of the typical major depressive symptoms.

Although the exact cause of bipolar disorder is unknown, biological, genetic, and environmental factors seem to be involved in causing episodes of the illness. Factors that are believed to trigger episodes include drug abuse and stressful or psychologically traumatic events. Once diagnosed, persons with bipolar disorder have a number of counseling and pharmaceutical options, and most will be able to live a healthy, functional life while being treated.

Causes of Depression

Major depressive disorder is caused by the interaction between biology, learned behavioral responses, cognitive factors, environment, and situational triggers and stressors. Some types of depression, such as bipolar disorder, appear to run in families. People who have low self-esteem, who consistently view themselves and the world with pessimism or who are readily overwhelmed by stress, are also prone to depression. Depression can also be triggered by a serious loss, difficult relationship, financial problems, and pressure to get good grades or succeed in athletics. In recent years, researchers have shown that physical changes in the body can be accompanied by mental changes, particularly depression. Stroke, heart attack, cancer, Parkinson's disease, problems with chronic pain, type 2 diabetes, certain medications, alcohol, hormonal disorders and a wide range of afflictions can cause you to become depressed, frustrated, and angry. When this happens, recovery is often more difficult; adhering to treatment regimens, self-care, and lifestyle behaviors that could help regain strength and vigor tends to slide. A person who feels exhausted and defeated may lack the will to fight the illness and do what needs to be done to optimize recovery.

Depression in Diverse Populations

Depression in College Students
College students—particularly college freshmen, suddenly thrust into a new environment without the support of family,

friends, and their community and confronted with high pressure to succeed—often are at high risk for depressive episodes. The National College Health Assessment revealed that over a 4-year period, from 2000 to 2004, the number of students who reported having been diagnosed with depression increased by nearly 5 percent, from 10.3 percent to 14.9 percent. Updated results from the same National College Health Assessment indicate that 21 percent of students rated depression among their top ten physical and mental problems in the last year. Another 14 percent included anxiety in their top ten problems.[42]

Clearly, the stressors of college life—such as anxiety over relationships, pressure to get good grades and win social acceptance, abuse of alcohol and other drugs, poor diet, and lack of sleep—can create a toxic cocktail that can overwhelm even the most resilient students. Thus, it is no surprise that depression on college campuses is such a huge problem. International students are particularly vulnerable to mental health concerns. Being far from home without the security of family and friends can exacerbate problems and make coping difficult. Those first months of being away from the comfort of home can be devastating to students from all walks of life. Most campuses have counseling centers, cultural centers, and other services available; however, many students do not use them because of persistent stigma about going to a counselor. How serious is the problem?

Overall, nearly 18 percent of college students indicated that they had felt depressed at some time during the last year; moreover, 32.3 percent of men and 39.2 percent of women on U.S. campuses reported that they had felt so depressed that they found it difficult to function one to ten times during the last year. Predictably, students report that stress and depression are among their top five impediments to academic success.[43]

Depression in Women
Women are almost twice as likely as men to experience depression. Hormonal changes related to the menstrual cycle, pregnancy, miscarriage, postpartum period, premenopause, and menopause may be factors in this increased rate.[44] Additionally, women face various stressors in their lives related to multiple responsibilities—work, child-rearing, single parenthood, household work, and caring for older parents—at rates that are higher than those of men. New research indicates that women have more difficulties obtaining restorative sleep, which may contribute to these problems.[45]

Researchers have observed gender differences in coping strategies (responses to certain events or stimuli) and have proposed that some women's strategies make them more vulnerable to depression. Presented with a list of things people do when depressed, college students were asked to indicate how likely they were to engage in each behavior. Men were more likely to assert, "I avoid thinking of reasons why I am depressed," "I do something physical," or "I play sports." Women were more likely to answer, "I try to determine why I am depressed," "I talk to other people about my

bipolar disorder   Form of depression characterized by alternating mania and depression.

MENTAL HEALTH PROBLEMS ON CAMPUS: UNIVERSITIES RESPOND

According to the results of the 2005 National College Health Assessment Survey, 41 percent of the respondents reported they have been diagnosed with depression in the last 12 months, and 9 percent reported they felt too depressed to function nine or more times in the last year.

As students struggle to cope with the escalating pressures of college life, educational administrators are searching for a way to balance their needs with the responsibility of providing a safe learning environment for all. In a recent survey, more than 90 percent of college counseling centers reported seeing an increasing number of students with more serious mental health problems.

Universities are enacting a range of policies to help these students:

- "Student leave" is a growing trend. New York University, Texas A&M, and Cornell University have established various forms of mandatory 6-month or 1-year leave for students who seem to be at highest risk. Because this is a relatively new policy, statistics on the success of student leave are unavailable, and the likelihood that students will return to campus once their problems are

resolved is unknown. Critics argue that such practices are not fair and violate the students' right to an education. For students who do not have health insurance, a 6- to 12-month mandated leave may not be well spent, because access to therapy becomes a serious challenge once they are no longer on campus.

- Some institutions, such as the University of Illinois at Urbana-Champaign, mandate counseling for students who are suicidal, requiring a minimum of four therapy sessions following a suicide attempt.
- Increasing numbers of institutions offer time management workshops, massage and de-stressing sessions during examinations, and workshops on relationships and coping with loss, grief, and other challenges through the academic year.
- Many schools have agreements with off-campus counseling centers, fitness centers, and other community-based resources to provide options for students.
- Most on-campus health services now include counseling centers with easy 24/7 access. Students are encouraged to use them, and increased advertising in new-student orientations let students know what kind of help is available.

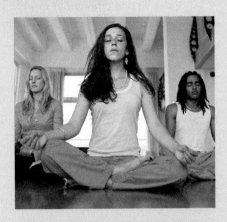

- Many universities, such as Oregon State University, offer extensive orientations at the beginning of each academic year. Students engage in group activities, such as camping trips and movies, to get to know each other in social settings. Professors, upper-class students, and others offer special assistance and lead discussion groups to help students cope with adjusting to life away from home.

Source: Jason Feirman, "New College Drop-Out," *Psychology Today*, May/June 2005. Copyright © 2005 Sussex Publishers, Inc. Reprinted with permission from Psychology Today Magazine; American College Health Association, National College Health Assessment, 2007, www.acha-ncha.org.

---

feelings," and "I cry to relieve the tension." In other words, the men tried to distract themselves from a depressed mood, whereas the women focused on it. If focusing obsessively on negative feelings intensifies these feelings, women who do this may predispose themselves to depression. This hypothesis has not been directly tested recently, but some early supporting evidence suggested its validity.[46]

Depression in Men
Six million men in the United States are currently in treatment for depression, and countless others should be. Depression in men is often masked by alcohol or drug abuse or by the socially acceptable habit of working excessively long hours. Typically, depressed men present not as hopeless and helpless, but as irritable, angry,

and discouraged, often personifying a "tough guy" image. Men are less likely to admit they are depressed, and doctors are less likely to suspect it, based on what men report during doctor's visits.[47]

Depression can also affect men's physical health differently from women's. Although depression is associated with an increased risk of coronary heart disease in both men and women, it is also associated with a higher risk of death by heart disease in men.[48] Men are also more likely to act on suicidal feelings than women, and they are usually more successful at suicide as well; suicide rates among depressed men are four times those of women.[49] Encouragement and support from families and friends may help men recognize symptoms and seek treatment.

what do you THINK?

■ Can you think of reasons why depression rates are so high on college campuses? ■ Why do you think that women experience more depression than men? ■ Do you think men and women cope with depression differently? In what ways? ■ Who is most likely to seek counseling for depression on campus? Why?

Depression in Older Adults Contrary to popular thinking, it is not normal for older people to be depressed; in fact, most older people are satisfied with their lives. However, because they are less likely to discuss feelings of sadness, loss, helplessness or other symptoms, or to attribute their own depression to aging, older people are likely to be undiagnosed or untreated. Additionally, because they often take multiple medications, many of which may result in depression symptoms, they may be at increased risk.

Depression in Children Today, depression in children is an increasingly reported phenomenon, with shocking cases of suicide and other outcomes in children as young as 4 and 5 years old. Depressed children may pretend to be sick, refuse to go to school, sleep incessantly, engage in self-mutilation, get into trouble with drugs or alcohol, feel misunderstood, and attempt suicide. Parents of children who are depressed may find it difficult to find therapists trained in working with kids who are depressed or physicians skilled in determining which adult antidepressants may be best for children.

Treating Depression

The best treatment involves determining the person's type and degree of depression and its possible causes. Both psychotherapeutic and pharmacological modes of treatment are recommended for clinical (severe and prolonged) depression. Drugs often relieve the symptoms of depression, such as loss of sleep or appetite, and psychotherapy can be equally helpful by improving the ability to function. In some cases, psychotherapy alone may be the most successful treatment. The two most common psychotherapeutic treatments for depression are cognitive therapy and interpersonal therapy.

Cognitive Therapy *Cognitive therapy* helps a patient look at life rationally and correct habitually pessimistic thought patterns. It focuses on the here and now rather than analyzing a patient's past. To pull a person out of depression, cognitive therapists usually need 6 to 18 months of weekly sessions consisting of reasoning and behavioral exercises.

Interpersonal Therapy *Interpersonal therapy,* sometimes combined with cognitive therapy, also addresses the present but focuses on correcting chronic relationship problems. Interpersonal therapists focus on patients' relationships with their families and other people.

Pharmacological Treatment Antidepressant drugs offer several options for treating depressive disorders. The most common antidepressants are the selective serotonin reuptake inhibitors (SSRIs), but in the past few years new drugs with different methods of action have also become available. Because any medication can have side effects, it is best to consult with a health care provider experienced in treating depression with medication to determine the right one for you. You may not feel the therapeutic effects of antidepressants for several weeks, so patience is important. Also, you should not stop taking medication all at once, but rather gradually, and always under your doctor's supervision. Countless emergency room visits occur when people misuse antidepressants, try to quit by going "cold turkey," or suffer reactions to the drugs.

The potency and dosage of each drug vary greatly. Antidepressants should be prescribed only after a thorough psychological and physiological examination. It wasn't until 2004 that the U.S. Food and Drug Administration asked the makers of antidepressant drugs to add a warning to the labels advising that patients taking these drugs be monitored for "worsening depression or the emergence of suicidality."[50] Recent reports of suicidal tendencies among some youth taking antidepressants has stirred controversy over the use of these drugs in certain populations.

If your doctor suggests an antidepressant, ask these questions first:

■ What biological indicators are you using to determine whether I really need this drug?
■ What is the action of this drug? When will I start to feel the benefits? What are the side effects of using this drug? What happens if I stop taking it?
■ What is your rationale for selecting this antidepressant over others?

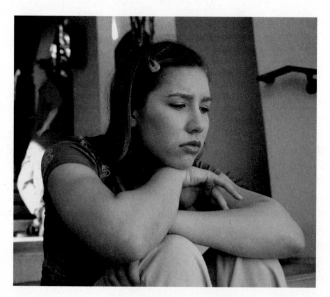

A person experiencing depression should not try to "go it alone." Supportive family and friends and a qualified therapist can help.

- How long can I be on this medication without significant risk to my health?
- How will you follow up or monitor the levels of this drug in my body? How often will I need to be checked?

Beware of the health professional who gives you a 5-minute exam, asks you if you are feeling down or blue, and prescribes an antidepressant to fix your problems.

Anxiety Disorders: Facing Your Fears

Anxiety disorders include generalized anxiety disorder, panic disorders, obsessive-compulsive disorder, and phobic disorders. They are characterized by persistent feelings of threat and worry. Consider John Madden, former head coach of the Oakland Raiders and a true "man's man," who has outfitted his own bus and drives every weekend across the country to serve as commentator on NFL football games. What's the reason behind this exhausting driving schedule? Madden is terrified of getting on a plane.

Anxiety disorders are the number-one mental health problem in the United States, affecting over 40 million people aged 18 to 54 each year, or about 18 percent of all adults.[51] Anxiety is also a leading mental health problem among adolescents, affecting 13 million youngsters aged 9 to 17. Costs associated with an overly anxious populace are growing rapidly; conservative estimates cite nearly $50 billion a year spent in doctors' bills and workplace losses in America. These numbers don't begin to address the human costs incurred when a person is too fearful to leave the house or talk to anyone outside the immediate family.

Generalized Anxiety Disorder

One common form of anxiety disorder, **generalized anxiety disorder (GAD),** is severe enough to significantly interfere with daily life. Generally, the person with GAD is a consummate worrier who develops a debilitating level of anxiety. Often multiple sources of worry exist, and it is hard to pinpoint the root cause of the anxiety. A diagnosis of GAD depends on showing at least three of the following symptoms for more days than not during a period of 6 months.[52]

1. Restlessness or feeling keyed up or on edge
2. Being easily fatigued
3. Difficulty concentrating or mind going blank
4. Irritability
5. Muscle tension
6. Sleep disturbances (difficulty falling or staying asleep or restless sleep)

Often GAD runs in families and is readily treatable with benzodiazepines such as Librium, Valium, and Xanax, which calm the person for short periods. Individual therapy can be a more effective long-term treatment.

Panic Disorders

On a recent trip to a professional conference, Marilyn Erickson (not her real name) boarded a connecting flight at O'Hare International Airport, only to find that her husband John, a professor at a major university, was missing. Marilyn got off the plane and searched frantically throughout the airport for him. Finally, long after the plane had departed, she found John sitting on a bench outside the terminal; he was vomiting, dizzy, and distraught over the mere thought of boarding the plane. When Marilyn suggested catching another flight, he trembled violently and refused to move from the bench. They returned to their home on the West Coast on a bus and missed their scheduled conference appearance.

Professor Erickson suffered a **panic attack,** a form of acute anxiety reaction that brings on an intense physical reaction. This reaction may be so severe that you fear you will have a heart attack and die—or you may dismiss it as the jitters from too much stress. Approximately 6 million Americans aged 18 and older experience panic attacks each year, usually in early adulthood. Although highly treatable, it is also growing in incidence, particularly among young women. Panic attacks may become debilitating and destructive, particularly if they happen often and lead the person to avoid going out in public or interacting with others.

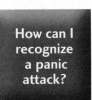

How can I recognize a panic attack?

A panic attack typically starts abruptly, peaks within 10 minutes, lasts about 30 minutes, and leaves the person tired and drained.[53] In addition to those just described, symptoms can include increased respiration rate, chills, hot flashes, shortness of breath, stomach cramps, chest pain, difficulty swallowing, and a sense of doom or impending death.

Although researchers aren't sure what causes panic attacks, heredity, stress, and certain biochemical factors may play a role. Your chances of having a panic attack increase if you have a close family member who has them. Some researchers believe that people who suffer panic attacks are experiencing an overreactive fight-or-flight physical response (see Chapter 3).

anxiety disorders Disorders characterized by persistent feelings of threat and worry in coping with everyday problems.

generalized anxiety disorder (GAD) A constant sense of worry that may cause restlessness, difficulty in concentrating, tension, and other symptoms.

panic attack Severe anxiety reaction in which a particular situation, often for unknown reasons, causes terror.

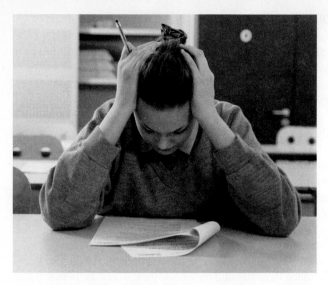

Panic attacks can occur without warning and be precipitated by stressful or uncomfortable situations.

Obsessive-Compulsive Disorder

People who feel compelled to perform rituals over and over again; are fearful of dirt or contamination; have an unnatural concern about order, symmetry, and exactness; or have persistent intrusive thoughts that they can't shake may be suffering from *obsessive-compulsive disorder (OCD)*. Approximately 2 million Americans aged 18 or over have OCD.[54] Not to be confused with being a perfectionist, a person with OCD often knows the behaviors are irrational and senseless yet is powerless to stop them. According to the American Psychiatric Association's *Diagnostic and Statistical Manual of Mental Disorders, DSM-IV-TR,* the obsessions must consume more than 1 hour per day and interfere with normal social and/or life activities. Although the exact cause is unknown, genetics, biological abnormalities, learned behaviors, and environmental factors have all been considered. OCD usually begins in adolescence or early adulthood, and the median age of onset is 19.

As with other anxiety-based disorders, medication and cognitive behavioral therapy are often the keys to treatment. Some individuals are given antidepressants, antianxiety drugs, or other drug combinations, which often prevent future attacks. Cognitive therapy can help sufferers recognize and avoid triggers or deal with triggers through meditation, deep breathing, and other relaxation techniques.

phobia   A deep and persistent fear of a specific object, activity, or situation that results in a compelling desire to avoid the source of the fear.

social phobia   A phobia characterized by fear and avoidance of social situations.

seasonal affective disorder (SAD)   A type of depression that occurs in the winter months, when sunlight levels are low.

Phobic Disorders

In contrast to anxiety disorders, **phobias,** or phobic disorders, involve a persistent and irrational fear of a specific object, activity, or situation, often out of proportion to the circumstances. Phobias result in a compelling desire to avoid the source of the fear. About 13 percent of Americans suffer from phobias, such as fear of spiders, snakes, public speaking, and so on. Social phobias are perhaps the most common phobic response.[55]

Social Phobias   A **social phobia** is an anxiety disorder characterized by the persistent fear and avoidance of social situations. Essentially, the person dreads these situations for fear of being humiliated, embarrassed, or even looked at.[56] These disorders vary in scope. Some cause difficulty only in specific situations, such as speaking in front of a class. In more extreme cases, a person avoids all contact with others.

Sources of Anxiety and Phobic Disorders
Because anxiety disorders vary in complexity and degree, scientists have yet to find clear reasons why one person develops them and another doesn't. The following factors are often cited as possible causes.[57]

- *Biology.* Some scientists trace the origin of anxiety to the brain and brain functioning. Using sophisticated positron emission tomography scans (PET scans), scientists can analyze areas of the brain that react during anxiety-producing events. Families appear to display similar brain and physiological reactivity, so we may inherit our tendencies toward anxiety disorders.
- *Environment.* Anxiety can be a learned response. Although genetic tendencies may exist, experiencing a repeated pattern of reacting to certain situations programs the brain to respond in a certain way. For example, if your mother or father screamed whenever a large spider crept into view or if other anxiety-raising events occurred frequently, you might be predisposed to react with anxiety to similar events later in your life. Interestingly, animals also experience such anxieties—perhaps from being around their edgy owners.
- *Social and cultural roles.* Cultural and social roles also may be a factor in risks for anxiety. Because men and women are taught to assume different roles in society (for example, man as protector, woman as victim), women may find it more acceptable to scream, shake, pass out, and otherwise express extreme anxiety. Men, by contrast, may have learned to hide such anxieties rather than act on them.

Seasonal Affective Disorder

An estimated 6 percent of Americans suffer from **seasonal affective disorder (SAD),** a type of depression, and an additional 14 percent experience a milder form of the disorder known as the *winter blues*. SAD strikes during the winter months and is associated with reduced exposure to sunlight. People with SAD suffer from irritability, apathy, carbohydrate craving and weight gain, increased sleep time, and general sadness. Researchers believe that SAD is caused by a malfunction in the hypothalamus, the gland that regulates responses to external stimuli. Stress also may play a role.

Therapies for SAD are simple but effective. The most beneficial is light therapy, in which patients are exposed to lamps that simulate sunlight. Eighty percent of patients experience relief from their symptoms within 4 days of treatment. Other treatments for SAD include diet change (eating more complex carbohydrates), increased exercise, stress management techniques, sleep restriction (limiting the number of hours slept in a 24-hour period), psychotherapy, and antidepressants.

Schizophrenia

Perhaps the most frightening of all mental disorders is **schizophrenia,** which affects about 1 percent of the U.S. population. Schizophrenia is characterized by alterations of the senses (including auditory and visual hallucinations); the inability to sort out incoming stimuli and make appropriate responses; an altered sense of self; and radical changes in emotions, movements, and behaviors. Victims of this disease often cannot function in society. Contrary to popular belief, schizophrenia is not the same as split personality or multiple personality disorder.

For decades, scientists believed that schizophrenia was an environmentally provoked form of madness. They blamed abnormal family interactions or early childhood traumas. Since the mid-1980s, however, when magnetic resonance imaging (MRI) and positron emission tomography (PET) allowed us to study brain function more closely, scientists have recognized that schizophrenia is a biological disease of the brain. The brain damage occurs early in life, possibly as early as the second trimester of fetal development. However, symptoms most commonly appear in late adolescence.

At present, schizophrenia is treatable but not curable. Treatments usually include some combination of hospitalization, medication, and supportive psychotherapy. Supportive psychotherapy, as opposed to more intensive psychoanalysis, can help the patient acquire skills for living in society.

Even though environmental theories on the causes of schizophrenia have been discarded in favor of biological theories, a stigma remains attached to the disease. Families of people with schizophrenia frequently experience anger and guilt. They often need information, family counseling, and advice on how to meet the schizophrenic person's needs for shelter, medical care, vocational training, and social interaction.

Gender Issues in Psychosocial Health

Unfortunately, gender bias can hinder the correct diagnosis of psychosocial disorders. In one study, 175 mental health professionals of both genders were asked to diagnose a patient based on a summarized case history. Some of the professionals were told that the patient was a man, others that the patient was a woman. The gender of the patient made a substantial difference in the diagnosis (though the gender of the clinician did not). When subjects thought the patient was a woman, they were more likely to diagnose hysterical personality, which is often thought of as a women's disorder. When they believed the patient to be a man, the more likely diagnosis was antisocial personality, often thought of as a men's disorder.

Premenstrual Syndrome: Physical or Mental Disorder?

A major controversy is the inclusion of a provisional diagnosis for premenstrual syndrome (PMS) and premenstrual dysphoric disorder (PMDD) in the *Diagnostic and Statistical Manual of Mental Disorders.* Currently, PMDD, which is considered the more severe form of PMS, is included in the *DSM-IV-TR.* However, the ongoing controversy about its inclusion signals that PMS merits further study.

PMS is characterized by depression, irritability, and other symptoms of increased stress typically occurring just prior to menstruation and lasting for a day or two. Whereas PMS is somewhat disruptive and uncomfortable, it does not interfere with daily function; PMDD does. To be diagnosed with PMDD, a woman must have at least five symptoms of PMS for a week to 10 days, with at least one symptom being serious enough to interfere with her ability to function at work or at home. In these more severe cases, antidepressants may be prescribed.

Suicide: Giving Up on Life

Each year there are over 32,000 reported suicides in the United States.[58] Experts estimate that there may actually be closer to 100,000 cases; the discrepancy is due to the difficulty in determining the causes of many suspicious deaths. More lives are lost to suicide than to any other single cause except cancer and cardiovascular disease. Suicide often results from

schizophrenia A mental illness with biological origins that is characterized by irrational behavior, severe alterations of the senses (hallucinations), and often an inability to function in society.

poor coping skills, lack of social support, lack of self-esteem, and the inability to see one's way out of a bad situation.

College students are more likely than the general population to attempt suicide; suicide is the second leading cause of death on college campuses, and nearly 1.3 percent of students report having attempted suicide at least once during the past year.[59] In fact, this age group now accounts for nearly 20 percent of all suicides.

The pressures, joys, disappointments, challenges, and changes of the college environment are believed to be partially responsible. However, young adults who choose not to go to college but who are searching for direction in careers, relationships, and other life goals are also at risk.

Risk factors for suicide include a family history of suicide, previous suicide attempts, excessive drug and alcohol use, prolonged depression, financial difficulties, serious illness in the suicide contemplator or in his or her loved ones, and loss of a loved one through death or rejection. Societal pressures often serve as a catalyst.

In most cases, suicide does not occur unpredictably. In fact, 75 to 80 percent of people who commit suicide give a warning of their intentions.

Warning Signs of Suicide

Common signs that a person may be contemplating suicide include the following:[60]

- Recent loss and a seeming inability to let go of grief
- Change in personality, such as sadness, withdrawal, irritability, anxiety, tiredness, indecisiveness, apathy
- Change in behavior, such as inability to concentrate, loss of interest in classes or work, unexplained demonstration of happiness following a period of depression
- Diminished sexual interest, such as impotence; menstrual abnormalities
- Expressions of self-hatred, excessive risk taking, or an "I don't care what happens to me" attitude
- Change in sleep patterns and/or eating habits
- A direct statement about committing suicide, such as, "I might as well end it all"
- An indirect statement, such as, "You won't have to worry about me anymore"
- Final preparations, such as writing a will, repairing poor relationships with family or friends, giving away prized possessions, or writing revealing letters
- A preoccupation with themes of death
- Marked changes in personal appearance

? *what do you* THINK?

- If your roommate showed warning signs of suicide, what action would you take? ■ Who would you contact first? ■ Where on campus might your friend get help? ■ What if someone in class whom you hardly know gave warning signs of suicide? What would you do then?

Taking Action to Prevent Suicide

Most people who attempt suicide really want to live but see suicide as the only way out of an intolerable situation. Crisis counselors and suicide hotlines may help temporarily, but the best way to prevent suicide is to get rid of conditions and substances that may precipitate attempts, including alcoholism, drugs, loneliness, isolation, and access to guns.

If someone you know threatens or displays warning signs of suicide, take the following actions.

- *Monitor the warning signals.* Keep an eye on the person, or ensure that there is someone around the person as much as possible.
- *Take threats seriously.* Don't brush them off.
- *Let the person know how much you care about him or her.* State that you are there if he or she needs help.
- *Listen.* Try not to discredit or be shocked by what the person says. Empathize, sympathize, and keep the person talking. Talk about stressors, and listen to the responses.
- *Ask directly.* For example, ask, "Are you thinking of hurting or killing yourself?"
- *Do not belittle the person's feelings.* Don't say that he or she doesn't really mean it or couldn't succeed at suicide. To some people, these comments offer the challenge of proving you wrong.
- *Help the person think about alternatives.* Offer to go for help together. Call your local suicide hotline, and use all available community and campus resources. Recommend a counselor or other person to talk to.
- *Remember that your relationships with others involve responsibilities.* Give of yourself by staying with the person, taking the person to a health care facility, or providing support.
- *Tell your friend's spouse, partner, relatives, or counselor.* Do not keep your suspicions to yourself.

Don't let a suicidal friend talk you into keeping your discussions confidential. If your friend succeeds in a suicide attempt because you kept a promise not to tell others of the danger, you may find that others will question your decision, just as you may blame yourself.

Seeking Professional Help

A physical ailment will readily send most of us to the nearest health professional, but many people view seeking professional help for psychosocial problems as an admission of personal failure. However, increasing numbers of Americans are turning to mental health professionals, and nearly one in five seeks such help. Researchers cite breakdown in support systems, high societal expectations of the individual, and dysfunctional families as three major reasons why more people are asking for assistance than ever before.

Consider seeking help if

- You feel like you need help.
- You experience wild mood swings or inappropriate emotional responses.
- A problem is interfering with your daily life.
- Your fears or feelings of guilt frequently distract your attention.
- You begin to withdraw from others.
- You have hallucinations.
- You feel inadequate or worthless or feel that life is not worth living.
- Your daily life seems to be nothing but repeated crises.
- You feel you can't "get your act together."
- You are considering suicide.
- You turn to drugs or alcohol to escape from your problems.
- You feel out of control.

There are also measures you can take now to feel better and pull yourself out of negative thoughts and feelings **(Table 2.5).**

TABLE 2.5	How to Help Yourself If You Are Depressed

- Set realistic goals in light of the depression, and assume a reasonable amount of responsibility.
- Break large tasks into small ones, set some priorities, and do what you can as you can.
- Try to be with other people and to confide in someone; it is usually better than being alone and secretive.
- Participate in activities that may make you feel better.
- Mild exercise, going to a movie, a ballgame, or participating in religious, social, or other activities may help.
- Expect your mood to improve gradually, not immediately. Feeling better takes time.
- It is advisable to postpone important decisions until the depression has lifted. Before deciding to make a significant transition, change jobs, or get married or divorced, discuss it with others who know you well and have a more objective view of your situation.
- People rarely "snap out of" a depression. But they can feel a little better day by day.
- *Remember*, positive thinking will replace the negative thinking that is part of the depression and will disappear as your depression responds to treatment.
- Let your family and friends help you.

Getting Evaluated for Treatment

If you are considering treatment for a psychosocial problem, schedule a complete evaluation first. Consult a credentialed health professional for a thorough examination, which should include three parts.

1. *A physical checkup,* which will rule out thyroid disorders, viral infections, and anemia—all of which can result in depressive-like symptoms—and a neurological check of coordination, reflexes, and balance to rule out brain disorders
2. *A psychiatric history,* which will attempt to trace the course of the apparent disorder, genetic or family factors, and any past treatments
3. *A mental status examination,* which will assess thoughts, speaking processes, and memory, and will include an in-depth interview with tests for other psychiatric symptoms.[61]

Once physical factors have been ruled out, you may decide to consult a professional who specializes in psychosocial health.

Mental Health Professionals

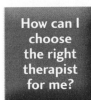

How can I choose the right therapist for me?

Several types of mental health professionals are available to help you; **Table 2.6** compares several of the most common. When choosing a therapist to work with, the most important criterion is not how many degrees this person has, but whether you feel you can work together. A qualified mental health professional should be willing to answer all your questions during an initial consultation. Questions to ask the therapist and yourself include the following:

- *Can you interview the therapist before starting treatment?* An initial meeting will help you determine whether this person will be a good fit for you.
- *Do you like the therapist as a person?* Can you talk to him or her comfortably?
- *Is the therapist watching the clock or easily distracted?* You should be the main focus of the session.
- *Does the therapist demonstrate professionalism?* Be concerned if your therapist is frequently late or breaks appointments, suggests social interactions outside your therapy sessions, talks inappropriately about himself or herself, has questionable billing practices, or resists releasing you from therapy.
- *Will the therapist help you set your own goals?* A good professional should evaluate your general situation and help you set small goals to work on between sessions. The therapist should not tell you how to help yourself, but rather help you discover the steps.

Remember, in most states, the use of the title *therapist* or *counselor* is unregulated. Make your choice carefully.

What to Expect in Therapy

Many different types of counseling exist, ranging from individual therapy, which involves one-on-one work between therapist and client, to group therapy, in which two or more clients meet with a therapist to discuss problems. The first

TABLE 2.6 Mental Health Professionals

What are they called?	What kind of training do they have?	What kind of therapy do they do?	Professional Association
Psychiatrist	Medical doctor degree (MD) followed by 4 years of specialized mental health training	As a licensed MD, a psychiatrist can prescribe medications for various mental or emotional problems and may have admitting privileges at a local hospital. Some psychiatrists are affiliated with hospitals, whereas others are in private practice.	American Psychiatric Association www.psych.org
Psychologist	PhD (doctor of philosophy) or PsyD (doctor of psychology) degree in counseling or clinical psychology followed by several years of supervised practice to earn license	Psychologists are trained in various types of therapy, including behavior and insight therapy. Most can conduct both individual and group counseling sessions. Psychologists may be trained in certain specialties, such as family counseling or sexual counseling.	American Psychological Association www.apa.org
Clinical/psychiatric social worker	Master's degree in social work (MSW) followed by 2 years of experience in a clinical setting to earn license	Social workers may be trained in certain specialties, such as substance abuse counseling or child counseling. Some social workers work in clinical settings, schools, or government agencies, whereas others have private practices.	National Association of Social Workers www.socialworkers.org
Counselor	Master's degree in counseling, psychology, educational psychology, or related human service; generally must complete at least 2 years of supervised practice before obtaining a license	Many counselors are trained to do individual and group therapy. They often specialize in one type of counseling, such as family, marital, relationship, children, drug, divorce, behavioral, or personal counseling.	American Counseling Association www.counseling.org
Psychiatric nurse specialist or psychiatric nurse practitioner	Registered nurse (RN) or licensed nurse practitioner who has gone through additional training and certification to specialize in psychiatric practice	All registered nurses can work in psychiatric settings, but psychiatric nurse specialists and psychiatric nurse practitioners can be certified to specialize in adult, child, or adolescent psychiatric nursing.	American Psychiatric Nurses Association www.apna.org
Psychoanalyst	Postgraduate degree in psychology or psychiatry (PhD or MD), followed by 8 to 10 years of training in psychoanalysis, which includes undergoing analysis themselves	Psychoanalysis is a form of therapy based on the theories of Freud and his successors. It focuses on patterns of thinking and behavior and helps patients remember early traumas that have blocked personal growth. The treatment is intensive—lasting for 5 to 10 years, with 3 or 4 sessions per week.	American Psychoanalytic Association www.apsa.org
Licensed marriage and family therapist (LMFT)	Master's or doctoral degree in psychology, social work, or counseling, specializing in family and interpersonal dynamics; generally must complete at least 2 years of supervised practice before obtaining a license	LMFTs treat individuals or families in the context of family relationships, addressing interpersonal issues. Treatment is typically brief (20 sessions or less) and focused on finding solutions to specific relational problems. Some LMFTs work in clinical settings, schools, or government agencies, whereas others have private practices.	American Association of Marriage and Family Therapists www.aamft.org

trip to a therapist can be difficult. Most of us have misconceptions about what therapy is and what it can do. That first visit is a verbal and mental sizing up between you and the therapist. You may not accomplish much in that first hour. If you decide that this professional is not for you, you will at least have learned how to present your problem and what qualities you need in a therapist.

Before meeting, briefly explain your needs. Ask what the fee is. Arrive on time, wear comfortable clothing, and expect to spend about an hour during your first visit. The therapist will want to take down your history and details about the problems that have brought you to therapy.

Answer as honestly as possible. Many will ask how you feel about aspects of your life. Do not be embarrassed to acknowledge your feelings. It is critical to the success of your treatment that you trust this person enough to be open and honest.

Do not expect the therapist to tell you what to do or how to behave. The responsibility for improved behavior lies with you. Ask if you can set your own therapeutic goals and timetables.

If after your first visit (or even after several visits) you feel you cannot work with this person, say so. You have the right to find a therapist with whom you feel comfortable.

TAKING charge

Summary

- Psychosocial health is a complex phenomenon involving mental, emotional, social, and spiritual health.
- Many factors influence psychosocial health, including life experiences, family, the environment, other people, self-esteem, self-efficacy, and personality. Some of these are modifiable; others are not.
- Developing self-esteem and self-efficacy, making healthy connections, having a positive outlook on life, and getting enough sleep are key to enhancing psychosocial health.
- Many people believe spirituality is important to wellness. Though the exact reasons have not been established, many studies show a connection between the two.
- Happiness is a key factor in determining overall reaction to life's challenges. The mind–body connection is an important link in overall health and well-being.
- Indicators of deteriorating psychosocial health include depression, difficulty sleeping, and emotional volatility.

- College life is a high-risk time for developing depression because of high stress and pressures for grades, financial problems, and other problems. Identifying symptoms of depression is the first step in treating this disorder.
- Other common psychosocial problems include bipolar disorder, anxiety disorders, panic disorders, phobias, seasonal affective disorder, and schizophrenia.
- Suicide is a result of negative psychosocial reactions to life. People intending to commit suicide often give warning signs of their intentions. Such people often can be helped.
- Mental health professionals include psychiatrists, psychoanalysts, psychologists, clinical/psychiatric social workers, counselors, and psychiatric nurse specialists. Many therapy methods exist, including group and individual therapy. It is wise to interview a therapist carefully before beginning treatment.

Chapter Review

1. A person with high self-esteem
   a. possesses feelings of self-respect and self-worth.
   b. believes he or she can successfully engage in a specific behavior.
   c. believes external influences shape one's psychosocial health.
   d. has a high altruistic capacity.

2. Marty flunked a math class twice and does not believe that he is good at math. He has resigned himself to not being able to graduate because he will never pass a required math class. This is known as
   a. external locus of control.
   b. learned helplessness.
   c. post-traumatic stress disorder.
   d. exogenous depression.

3. All of the following traits have been identified as characterizing psychosocially healthy people *except*
   a. conscientiousness.
   b. introversion.
   c. openness to experience.
   d. agreeableness.

4. What hormone is linked to circadian rhythms?
   a. dopamine
   b. serotonin
   c. GABA
   d. melatonin

5. Subjective well-being has all of the following components *except*
   a. psychological hardiness.
   b. satisfaction with present life.
   c. relative presence of positive emotions.
   d. relative absence of negative emotions.

6. The characteristic that describes a person's ability to bounce back in times of difficulty or threats in a healthy way is known as
   a. self-esteem.
   b. self-efficacy.
   c. resiliency.
   d. subjective well-being.

7. What are the two most common psychotherapeutic therapies for depression?
   a. humanistic therapy and gestalt therapy
   b. cognitive therapy and interpersonal therapy
   c. psychodynamic therapy and family therapy
   d. cognitive therapy and psychodynamic therapy

8. What is the number-one mental health problem in the United States?
   a. depression
   b. anxiety disorders
   c. alcohol dependence
   d. schizophrenia

9. Every winter, Stan suffers from irritability, apathy, carbohydrate craving, weight gain, increased sleep time, and sadness. He most likely has
   a. panic disorder.
   b. generalized anxiety disorder.
   c. seasonal affective disorder.
   d. chronic mood disorder.

10. A person with a PhD in counseling psychology and training in various types of therapy is a
    a. psychiatrist.
    b. psychologist.
    c. social worker.
    d. psychoanalyst.

Answers to these questions can be found on page A-1.

Questions for Discussion and Reflection

1. What is psychosocial health? What indicates that you are or aren't psychosocially healthy? Why might the college environment provide a challenge to your psychosocial health?
2. Discuss the factors that influence your overall level of psychosocial health. Which factors can you change? Which ones may be more difficult to change?
3. What steps could you take today to improve your psychosocial health? Which steps require long-term effort?
4. What are four main themes of spirituality, and how are they expressed in daily life?
5. Why is laughter therapeutic? How can humor help you better achieve wellness?
6. What factors appear to contribute to psychosocial difficulties and illnesses? Which of the common psychosocial illnesses is likely to affect people in your age group?
7. What are the warning signs of suicide? Of depression? Why is depression so pervasive among young Americans today? Why are some groups more vulnerable to suicide and depression than are others? What would you do if you heard a friend in the cafeteria say to no one in particular that he was going to "do the world a favor and end it all"?
8. Discuss the different types of health professionals and therapies. If you felt depressed about breaking off a long-term relationship, which professional therapy do you think would be most beneficial? Explain your answer. What services does your student health center provide? What fees are charged to students?
9. What psychosocial areas do you need to work on? Which are most important to you, and why? What actions can you take today?

Accessing Your Health on the Internet

The following websites explore further topics and issues related to personal health. For links to the websites below, visit the Companion Website for *Health: The Basics,* Eighth Edition at www.aw-bc.com/donatelle.

1. *American Foundation for Suicide Prevention.* Resources for suicide prevention and support for family and friends of those who have committed suicide. www.afsp.org
2. *American Psychological Association Help Center.* Includes information on psychology at work, the mind–body connection, psychological responses to war, and other topics. http://apahelpcenter.org/
3. *Anxiety Disorders Association of America.* Offers links to treatment resources, self-help tools, information on clinical trials, and other information. www.adaa.org
4. *National Alliance on Mental Illness.* A support and advocacy organization of families and friends of people with severe mental illnesses. Over 1,200 state and local affiliates; local branches can often help with finding treatment. www.nami.org
5. *National Institute of Mental Health (NIMH).* Overview of mental health information and new research relating to mental health. www.nimh.nih.gov
6. *Mental Health America.* Works to promote mental health through advocacy, education, research, and services. www.nmha.org

Further Reading

Begley, S. *Train Your Mind, Change Your Brain: How a New Science Reveals Our Extraordinary Power to Transform Ourselves.* New York: Ballantine Books, 2007.

> *Reports on how cutting-edge science and the ancient wisdom of Buddhism have come together to show how we all have the power to literally change our brains by changing our minds.*

Dalai Lama and H. C. Cutler. *The Art of Happiness: A Handbook for Living.* New York: Riverhead, 1998.

> *Through a series of interviews, the authors explore questions of meaning, motives, and the interconnectedness of life, including why so many people are unhappy, and offer strategies for becoming happy.*

Karren, K., et al. *Mind/Body Health: The Effects of Attitudes, Emotions, and Relationships,* 3rd ed. San Francisco: Benjamin Cummings, 2006.

> *Details current global findings on the relationships among the mind, body, and health. The authors show that negative emotions such as anger, depression, and anxiety can adversely affect physical health, whereas positive emotions such as humor and optimism can serve to improve health and increase longevity.*

Norem, J. *The Positive Power of Negative Thinking.* New York: Basic Books, 2002.

> *Explores reasons for negative thinking and mechanisms for changing the way you think. Includes self-tests and analysis for helping you retrain your thinking processes.*

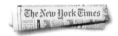

e-themes from *The New York Times*

For up-to-date articles about current health issues, visit www.aw-bc.com/donatelle, select *Health: The Basics,* Eighth Edition, Chapter 2, and click on "e-themes."

References

1. H. Marano, "A Nation of Wimps," *Psychology Today* 37, no. 6 (2004): 58–68.
2. National Institute of Mental Health, 2005, www.nimh.gov.
3. "Executive Summary of the Report of the Surgeon General on Mental Health," June 2006, www.surgeongeneral.gov/library/mentalhealth/summary.html.
4. R. Lazarus, *Stress and Emotion: A New Synthesis* (New York: Springer Publishing Company, 1999).
5. T. M. Chaplin, "Anger, Happiness and Sadness: Associations with Depressive Symptoms in Late Adolescence," *Journal of Youth and Adolescence* 35, no. 6 (2006): 977–86.
6. A. F. Jorm, "Social Networks and Health: It's Time for an Intervention Trial," *Journal of Epidemiology and Community Health* 59 (2005): 537–39; C. Huang, "Elderly Social Support System and Health Status in the Urban and Rural Areas" (Paper presented at the American Public Health Association Annual Meeting, New Orleans, LA, 2005); C. Alarie, *The Impact of Social Support on Women's Health: A Literature Review,* Women's Center of Excellence, www.pwhce.ca/impactDuSupport.htm; A. Sherman, J. Lansford, and B. Volling, "Sibling Relationships and Best Friendships in Young Adulthood: Warmth, Conflict and Well-Being," *Personal Relationships* 13, no. 2 (2006): 151–65; N. Stevens, "Marriage, Social Integration, and Loneliness in the Second Half of Life," *Research on Aging* 28, no. 2 (2006): 713–29.
7. Tufts University Program in Evidence-Based Complementary and Alternative Medicine, "Religion and Spirituality Overview," May 15, 2006, www.tufts.edu/med/ebcam/religion/index.html; H. G. Koenig et al., *Handbook of Religion and Health* (New York: Oxford University Press, 2001), 18.
8. S. R. Hawks et al., "Review of Spiritual Health: Definition, Role, and Intervention Strategies in Health Promotion," *American Journal of Health Promotion* 9, no. 5 (1995): 371–78; K. Karren et al., *Mind/Body Health: The Effects of Attitudes, Emotions, and Relationships,* 3rd ed. (San Francisco: Benjamin Cummings, 2006).
9. J. Kabat-Zinn, *Coming to Our Senses: Healing Ourselves and the World through Mindfulness* (New York: Hyperion, 2005).
10. J. A. Astin et al. "Mind-Body Medicine: State of the Science, Implications for Practice." *Journal of the American Board of Family Practice* 16 (2003): 131–47; J. Bishop et al., "Mindfulness: A Proposed Operational Definition," *Clinical Psychology* 11 (2004): 230–41.
11. National Center for Complementary and Alternative Medicine (NCCAM), *CAM at the NIH: Focus on Complementary and Alternative Medicine,* Winter 2005, http://nccam.nih.gov; K. Karren et al., *Mind/Body Health,* 444–519.
12. Karren et al., *Mind/Body Health.*
13. Ibid.
14. Ibid.
15. A. Astin et al., "Spirituality in Higher Education: A National Study of College Students' Search for Meaning and Purpose," 2004, www.spirituality.ucla.edu; G. D. Kuh and R. M. Gonyea, "Exploring the Relationships between Spirituality, Liberal Learning, and College Student Engagement," *Center for Postsecondary Research—Special Report.* (Bloomington, IN: Indiana University, 2005).
16. C. Shigaki et al., "Mindfulness-Based Stress Reduction in Medical Settings," *Journal of Clinical Psychology in Medical Settings* 13, no. 3 (2006): 209–16; N. Allen et al., "Mindfulness-Based Psychotherapies: A Review of Conceptual Foundations, Empirical Evidence and Practical Considerations," *Australian and New Zealand Journal of Psychiatry* 40, no. 4 (2006): 285–94.
17. Ibid.
18. Karren et al., *Mind/Body Health,* 510–18.

19. M. Seligman and C. Peterson, "Learned Helplessness," in *International Encyclopedia for the Social and Behavioral Sciences,* ed. N. Smelser, vol. 13, 8583–866 (New York: Elsevier, 2002).

20. M. Seligman, *Learned Optimism: How to Change Your Mind and Your Life* (New York: Free Press, 1998); P. Zimbardo, A. Weber, and R. Johnson, *Psychology* (Boston: Allyn & Bacon, 2000), 403; J. H. Martin, "Motivation Processes and Performance: The Role of Global and Facet Personality" (PhD dissertation, University of North Carolina at Chapel Hill, 2002).

21. B. Fredrickson and M. Losada, "Positive Affect and Complex Dynamics of Human Flourishing," *American Psychologist* 60, no. 7 (2005): 678–86.

22. National Sleep Foundation, "NSF's 2007 Sleep in America Poll: Stressed-Out American Women Have No Time for Sleep," March 6, 2007, www.sleepfoundation.org.

23. K. Wright et al, "Effects of Sleep Inertia on Cognition," *Journal of the American Medical Association* 295, no. 2 (2006): 163–65.

24. NCCAM, updated 2007, http://nccam.nih.gov.

25. M. Lemonick, "The Biology of Joy," *Time,* January 17, 2005, A12–A14.

26. J. Kluger, "The Funny Thing about Laughter," *Time,* January 17, 2005, A25–A29.

27. Ibid.

28. R. Davidson et al., "The Privileged Status of Emotion in the Brain," *Proceedings of the National Academy of Sciences of the United States of America* 101, no. 33 (2004).

29. E. Diener and M. E. P. Seligman, "Beyond Money: Toward an Economy of Well-Being," *Psychological Science in the Public Interest* 5 (2004): 1–31; C. Peterson and M. Seligman, *Character Strengths and Virtues* (London: Oxford University Press, 2004).

30. P. Herschberger, "Prescribing Happiness: Positive Psychology and Family Medicine," *Family Medicine* 37, no. 9 (2005): 630–34; M. E. Seligman et al., "Positive Psychology Progress: Empirical Validation of Interventions," *American Psychologist* 60, no. 5 (2005): 410–21.

31. M. Seligman, "Positive Interventions: More Evidence of Effectiveness," *Authentic Happiness Newsletter* (September 2004), www.authentichappiness.org/news/news10.html; S. I. Gable et al., "What Do You Do When Things Go Right? The Intrapersonal and Interpersonal Benefits of Sharing Positive Events," *Journal of Personal and Social Psychology* 87, no. 2 (2004): 228–45; B. Swartz, *The Paradox of Choice: Why More Is Less* (New York: HarperCollins Publishers, 2004); P. C. Seligman, *Character Strengths and Virtues: a Handbook and Classification* (New York: Oxford University Press, 2004).

32. B. Fredrickson, "Cultivating Positive Emotions to Optimize Health and Well-Being," *Prevention and Treatment* 3 (March 7, 2000), Article 0001a; N. Ross, "Health, Happiness, and Higher Levels of Social Organization," *Journal of Epidemiology and Community Health* 59 (2005): 614; A. J. Bishop, P. Martin, and L. Poon, "Happiness and Congruence in Older Adulthood: A Structural Model of Life Satisfaction," *Aging and Mental Health* 10, no. 5 (2006): 445–53.

33. Grady, "Think Right, Stay Well," *American Health* 11 (1992): 50–54.

34. L. Cool, "Is Mental Illness Catching?" *American Health for Women* 16 (1997): 72–75.

35. MayoClinic.com, "Mental Health Definitions," 2006, www.mayoclinic.com.

36. R. C. Kessler et al., "Prevalence, Severity, and Comorbidity of Twelve-Month *DSM-IV* Disorders in the National Comorbidity Survey Replication (NCS-R)," *Archives of General Psychiatry* 62, no. 6 (2005): 617–27; National Institute of Mental Health (NIMH), "The Numbers Count: Mental Disorders in America," updated December 26, 2006, www.nimh.nih.gov/publicat/numbers.cfm; U.S. Office of the Surgeon General, "Executive Summary: Mental Health, Culture, Race and Ethnicity. A Supplement to *Mental Health: A Report of the Surgeon General,*" accessed June 6, 2006, www.surgeongeneral.gov/library/mentalhealth/cre/execsummary-1.html.

37. American College Health Association, *American College Health Association–National College Health Assessment (ACHA–NCHA) Web Summary,* updated April 2006, www.acha.org/projects_programs/ ncha_sampledata.cfm.2006.

38. L. A. Lefton, *Psychology,* 8th ed. (Boston: Allyn & Bacon, 2002), 542.

39. NIMH, "The Numbers Count."

40. Kessler et al, "National Comorbidity Survey Replication," 593–602.

41. NIMH, "Depression," September 13, 2006, www.nimh.nih.gov/publicat/depression.cfm.

42. American College Health Association, *American College Health Association–National College Health Assessment (ACHA–NCHA) Web Summary,* updated April 2006, www.acha-ncha.org/data_highlights.html.2006.

43. American College Health Association, *American College Health Assessment–National College Health Assessment Survey: Reference Group Executive Summary—Spring 2006* (Baltimore: American College Health Association, 2006).

44. NIMH, "Depression"; N. Gavin et al., "Perinatal Depression: A Systematic Review of Prevalence and Incidence," *Obstetrics and Gynecology* 106 (2005): 1071–1083.

45. National Sleep Foundation, "NSF's 2007 Sleep in America Poll."

46. A. K. Ferketick et al., "Depression as an Antecedent to Heart Disease among Women and Men in the NHANES I Study: National Health and Nutrition Examination Survey," *Archives of Internal Medicine* 160, no. 9 (2002): 1261–68.

47. NIMH, "The Numbers Count."

48. Ferketick et al., "NHANES I Study."

49. NIMH, "Depression."

50. U.S. Food and Drug Administration (FDA), "FDA Issues Public Health Advisory on Cautions for Use of Antidepressants in Adults and Children" (FDA Talk Paper, T04–08), March 22, 2004, www.fda.gov/bbs/topics/ANSWERS/2004/ANS01283.html; U.S. FDA, Center for Drug Evaluation and Research, "Antidepressant Use in Children, Adolescents, and Young Adults," March 22, 2004, www.fda.gov/cder/drug/antidepressants/default.htm; NIMH, "The Numbers Count."

51. NIMH, "The Numbers Count."

52. NIMH, "Generalized Anxiety Disorder, GAD." Updated June 28, 2006. www.nimh.nih.gov/healthinformation/gadmenu.cfm.

53. MayoClinic.com, "Panic Attacks," 2006, www.mayoclinic.com

54. NIMH, "The Numbers Count."

55. NIMH, "Generalized Anxiety Disorder, GAD."

56. Ibid.

57. Ibid.

58. NIMH, "Suicide in the U.S.: Statistics and Prevention," April 20, 2007, www.nimh.nih.gov/publicat/harmsway.cfm.

59. American College Health Association, "Campus Violence White Paper," February 5, 2005, www.acha.org/info_resources/campus_violence.pdf.

60. NIMH, "In Harm's Way: Suicide in America," updated December 22, 2006, www.nimh.nih.gov/publicat/harmsway.cfm.

61. L. A. Lefton, *Psychology,* 9th ed., (Boston: Allyn & Bacon, 2005).

3

Managing Stress

COPING WITH LIFE'S CHALLENGES

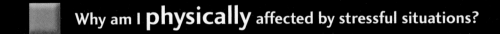 Why am I **physically** affected by stressful situations?

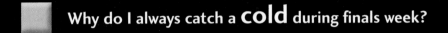 Why do I always catch a **cold** during finals week?

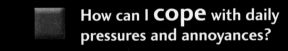 How can I **cope** with daily pressures and annoyances?

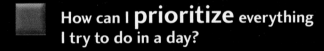 How can I **prioritize** everything I try to do in a day?

OBJECTIVES

- Define *stress*, and examine the potential impact of stress on health, relationships, and success in college.
- Explain the phases of the general adaptation syndrome and the physiological changes that occur.
- Examine the health risks that may occur with chronic stress.
- Discuss sources of stress, and examine the special stressors that affect college students.
- Explore techniques for coping with or reducing exposure to stress and using positive stressors to enrich your life.

It is a common occurrence in today's world to hear people say, "I'm so stressed out," or to describe their job or life as too stressful. Writings and conversations about the impact of stress on our lives are everywhere. You may even have been led to believe that all stress is bad for you. In reality, stress can be our best friend or our worst enemy. Stress can motivate, protect, energize, and excite us. Imagine scoring the winning goal in the championship soccer game, falling in love, meeting a famous person you have always idolized, scoring an A on a tough exam, or reacting quickly to avoid a car accident. Our ability to respond and adapt to these challenges is positive and healthful. Under some conditions, however, stress can overpower us and fatigue our body systems to the point of breakdown and disease.

The negative aspect of stress is a major concern in the United States, and it appears to be getting worse: according to a national survey conducted annually by the Higher Education Research Institute, almost a third of college freshman report feeling "frequently overwhelmed by all they have to do," up from a low of 16 percent when the question was first asked in 1985.[1] If we want stress to be much more a friend than an enemy, there are things we can do. We can begin by learning to anticipate and recognize our personal stressors and to develop skills to reduce or better manage those we cannot avoid or control.

What Is Stress?

Stress may be defined as "the experience of a perceived threat (real or imagined) to one's well-being, resulting from a series of physiological responses and adaptations."[2] This definition has evolved over time as research has advanced our understanding of how the body responds to threats or challenges. A **stressor** is any condition or event that we perceive challenges or threatens us, and a **stress response** is the series of physiological changes and adaptations that result from that stressor. Stressors may be physical, social, emotional, intellectual, economic, or spiritual. They may be tangible or intangible, positive or negative. Key to the whole stress response is our personal perception and interpretation of daily events and situations. These perceptions are filtered by our past experiences, biological factors (e.g., race, age, and gender), characteristics of the event or situation (Can I control it? Is it predictable? Does it occur often?), and by our present set of coping resources. **Coping** is the act of managing events or conditions to lessen the impact of a stressor. Remember that stress is literally in the eyes of the beholder. Each person's unique combination of heredity, life experiences, personality, and ability to cope influences how the person perceives an event and what meaning he or she attaches to it.

Stress can be associated with most daily activities. Generally, positive stress—stress that presents the opportunity for personal growth and satisfaction—is termed **eustress.** Getting married, successfully kayaking Class II rapids, beginning a career, and developing new friends may all give rise to eustress. **Distress,** or negative stress, is caused by events that result in debilitative stress and strain, such as financial problems, the death of a loved one, academic difficulties, and the breakup of a relationship. Prolonged distress can have negative effects on health.

You cannot get rid of distress entirely: like eustress, it is a part of life. However, you can train yourself to recognize the events that cause distress and to anticipate your reactions to them. You can learn coping skills and strategies that will help you manage stress more effectively.

The Body's Response to Stress
The Fight-or-Flight Response

Whenever we're surprised by a sudden stressor, such as someone swerving into our lane of traffic, our emotional reactions trigger the adrenal glands (two almond-sized glands sitting atop the kidneys) to secrete adrenaline and other hormones into the bloodstream. As a result, the heart speeds up, breathing rate increases, blood pressure elevates, and blood flow to the muscles increases with a rapid release of blood sugars into the bloodstream. This sudden burst of energy and strength is believed to provide the extra edge that has helped generations of humans survive during adversity. Known as the **fight-or-flight response,** this physiological reaction is one of our most basic, innate survival instincts.[3] When activated, our bodies go on the alert either to fight danger or to escape from it. The series of behavioral, neurological, and immunological changes are designed to help us; however, if overtaxed, the response can be damaging to our bodies.

WORKSHEET

stress The experience of a perceived threat (real or imagined) to one's well-being, resulting from a series of physiological responses and adaptations.

stressor A physical, social, or psychological event or condition that we perceive challenges or threatens us and that produces a stress response.

stress response The series of physiological changes and adaptations that result from a stressor.

coping The act of managing events or conditions to lessen the physical or psychological effects of excess stress.

eustress Stress that presents opportunities for personal growth; positive stress.

distress Stress that can have a detrimental effect on health; negative stress.

fight-or-flight response Physiological arousal response in which the body prepares to combat or escape a real or perceived threat.

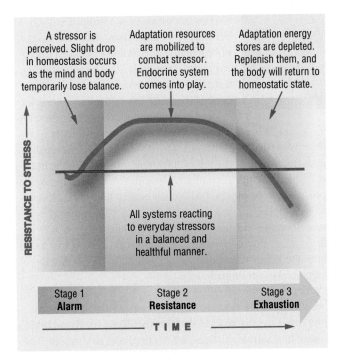

A stressor is perceived. Slight drop in homeostasis occurs as the mind and body temporarily lose balance.

Adaptation resources are mobilized to combat stressor. Endocrine system comes into play.

Adaptation energy stores are depleted. Replenish them, and the body will return to homeostatic state.

RESISTANCE TO STRESS

All systems reacting to everyday stressors in a balanced and healthful manner.

Stage 1 **Alarm** Stage 2 **Resistance** Stage 3 **Exhaustion**

TIME

FIGURE 3.1 **The General Adaptation Syndrome**

The General Adaptation Syndrome

What has just been described in very general terms is a complex physiological response to stress in which our bodies move from **homeostasis,** a level of functioning in which the body's systems operate smoothly and maintain equilibrium, to one of crisis as the body attempts to return to homeostasis after responding to a stressor. This adjustment is referred to as an **adaptive response.** First characterized by Hans Selye in 1936, this internal fight to restore homeostasis is known as the **general adaptation syndrome (GAS) (Figure 3.1).** The GAS has three distinct phases: alarm, resistance, and exhaustion.[4]

Alarm Phase When the body is exposed to a real or perceived stressor, the fight-or-flight response kicks into gear. Stress hormones flow, and the body prepares to do battle. The subconscious perceptions and appraisal of the stressor stimulate the areas in the brain responsible for emotions. This emotional stimulation triggers the physical reactions we associate with stress **(Figure 3.2).** The entire process takes only a few seconds.

Suppose that you are walking to your residence hall after a night class on a dimly lit campus. As you pass a particularly dark area, you hear someone cough behind you, and you sense that this person is fairly close. You walk faster, only to hear the quickened footsteps of the other person. Your senses become increasingly alert, your breathing quickens, your heart races, and you begin to perspire. The stranger is getting closer and closer. In desperation you stop, clutching your

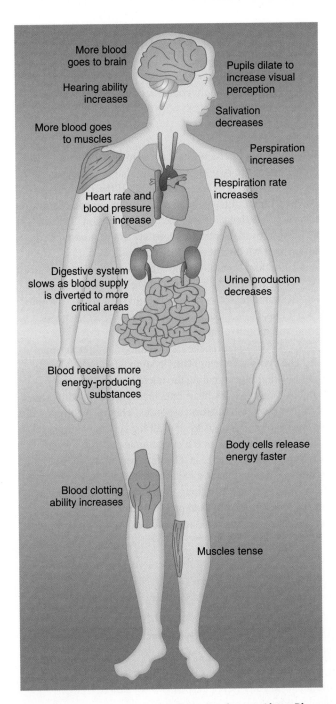

More blood goes to brain

Hearing ability increases

More blood goes to muscles

Heart rate and blood pressure increase

Digestive system slows as blood supply is diverted to more critical areas

Blood receives more energy-producing substances

Blood clotting ability increases

Pupils dilate to increase visual perception

Salivation decreases

Perspiration increases

Respiration rate increases

Urine production decreases

Body cells release energy faster

Muscles tense

FIGURE 3.2 **The General Adaptation Syndrome: Alarm Phase**

homeostasis   A balanced physical state in which all the body's systems function smoothly.

adaptive response   Form of adjustment in which the body attempts to restore homeostasis.

general adaptation syndrome (GAS)   The pattern followed in the physiological response to stress, consisting of the alarm, resistance, and exhaustion phases.

book bag in your hands, determined to use force if necessary to protect yourself. You turn around quickly and let out a blood-curdling yell. To your surprise, the only person you see is your classmate Cindy, who has been trying to stay close to you out of her own anxiety about walking alone in the dark. She screams and jumps back, only to trip and fall. You look at her in startled embarrassment. You have just experienced the alarm phase of GAS.

When the mind perceives a real or imaginary stressor, the cerebral cortex, the region of the brain that interprets the nature of an event, is called to attention. If the cerebral cortex perceives a threat, it triggers an **autonomic nervous system (ANS)** response that prepares the body for action. The ANS is the portion of the central nervous system regulating body functions that we do not normally consciously control, such as heart function, breathing, and glandular function. When we are stressed, the activity rate of all these bodily functions increases dramatically to give us the physical strength to protect ourselves or to make the physiological changes needed to respond and mobilize internal forces.

The ANS has two branches: sympathetic and parasympathetic. The **sympathetic nervous system** energizes the body for fight or flight by signaling the release of several stress hormones that speed the heart rate, increase the breathing rate, and trigger many other stress responses. The **parasympathetic nervous system** functions to slow all the systems stimulated by the stress response—in effect, it counteracts the actions of the sympathetic branch. In a healthy person, these two branches work together in a balance that controls the negative effects of stress. However, long-term stress can strain this balance, and chronic physical problems can occur as stress reactions become the dominant forces in a person's body.

Why am I physically affected by stressful situations?

The responses of the sympathetic nervous system to stress involve a series of biochemical exchanges between different parts of the body. The **hypothalamus,** a structure in the brain, functions as the control center of the sympathetic nervous system and determines the overall reaction to stressors. When the hypothalamus perceives that extra energy is needed to fight a stressor, it stimulates the adrenal glands, located near the top of the kidneys, to release the hormone **epinephrine,** also called *adrenaline*. Epinephrine causes more blood to be pumped with each beat of the heart, dilates the bronchioles (air sacs in the lungs) to increase oxygen intake, increases the breathing rate, stimulates the liver to release more glucose (which fuels muscular exertion), and dilates the pupils to improve visual sensitivity. The body is then poised to act immediately.

As epinephrine secretion increases, blood is diverted away from the digestive system, possibly causing nausea and cramping if the distress occurs shortly after a meal and drying of nasal and salivary tissues, which produces dry mouth. The alarm phase also provides for longer-term reaction to stress. At the same time, the hypothalamus uses chemical messages to trigger the pituitary gland within the brain to release a powerful hormone, *adrenocorticotropic hormone (ACTH)*. ACTH signals the adrenal glands to release **cortisol,** a hormone that makes stored nutrients more readily available to meet energy demands. Finally, other parts of the brain and body release endorphins, the body's naturally occurring opiates, which relieve pain that a stressor may cause.

Resistance Phase The resistance phase of the GAS is similar to the alarm phase in that the same organs and systems are mobilized, but at a less intense level. The body tries to return to homeostasis, but because some perceived stressor still exists, the body does not achieve complete rest. Instead, the body stays activated or aroused at a level that causes a higher metabolic rate in some organ tissues. These organs and systems of resistance are working "overtime" and after prolonged stress will become depleted to the point where they cannot function effectively.

Exhaustion Phase Stress promotes adaptation, but a prolonged response leads to **allostatic load,** or exhaustive wear and tear on the body.[5] In the exhaustion phase of the GAS, the physical and emotional energy used to fight a stressor has been depleted. The toll the stress takes on the body depends on the type of stress or how long it lasts. Short-term stress probably would not deplete all energy reserves in an otherwise healthy person, but chronic stress can create continuous states of alarm and resistance, resulting in total depletion of energy and susceptibility to illness.

As the body adjusts to chronic unresolved stress, the adrenal glands continue to release cortisol, which remains in the bloodstream for longer periods of time due to slower metabolic responsiveness. Over time, without relief, cortisol can reduce **immunocompetence,** or the ability of the

autonomic nervous system (ANS) The portion of the central nervous system regulating body functions that a person does not normally consciously control.

sympathetic nervous system Branch of the autonomic nervous system responsible for stress arousal.

parasympathetic nervous system Branch of the autonomic nervous system responsible for slowing systems stimulated by the stress response.

hypothalamus A structure in the brain that controls the sympathetic nervous system and directs the stress response.

epinephrine Also called *adrenaline,* a hormone that stimulates body systems in response to stress.

cortisol Hormone released by the adrenal glands that makes stored nutrients more readily available to meet energy demands.

allostatic load Wear and tear on the body caused by prolonged or excessive stress responses.

immunocompetence The ability of the immune system to respond to assaults.

immune system to respond to various assaults. Blood pressure can remain dangerously elevated, you may catch colds more easily, or your body's ability to control blood glucose levels can be affected.

Stress and Your Health

Although much has been written about the negative effects of stress, researchers have only recently begun to untangle the complex web of physical and emotional interactions that can break down the body over time. Stress is often described as a "disease of prolonged arousal" that leads to other negative health effects. Nearly all body systems become potential targets, and the long-term effects may be devastating. Look at the stress symptom checklist in **Table 3.1.** Do you have any of these physical symptoms of stress?

Studies indicate that 40 percent of deaths and 70 percent of disease in the United States are related, in whole or in part, to stress.[6] The list of ailments related to chronic stress includes heart disease, diabetes, cancer, headaches, ulcers, low back pain, depression, and the common cold. Chronic stress has also been linked to abdominal fat (see the **Health Headlines** box on page 67). Alarming increases in rates of suicide, homicide, and domestic violence across the United States are additional symptoms of a nation under stress.

Stress and Cardiovascular Disease Risks

Perhaps the most studied and documented health consequence of unresolved stress is cardiovascular disease (CVD). Research on this topic has demonstrated the impact of chronic stress on heart rate, blood pressure, heart attack, and stroke.[7] The largest epidemiological study to date, the INTERHEART Study with almost 30,000 participants in 52 countries, identified stress as one of the key modifiable risk factors for heart attack.[8] Similarly, the National Health Interview Study, conducted annually by the Centers for Disease Control and Prevention (CDC) National Center for Health Statistics, has reported that stress accounts for approximately 30 percent of the attributable risk of myocardial infarction (heart attack).[9]

Historically, the increased risk of CVD from chronic stress has been linked to increased plaque buildup due to elevated cholesterol, hardening of the arteries, alterations in heart rhythm, increased and fluctuating blood pressure, and difficulties in cardiovascular responsiveness due to all of the above. Although these continue to be considered major risks, recent research also points to metabolic abnormalities, insulin resistance, and inflammation in blood vessels (perhaps due to lingering viral effects) as major contributors to heart disease.[10] In the past 15 to 20 years, research has grown exponentially, and direct links have been identified between the incidence and progression of CVD and stressors such as job strain,

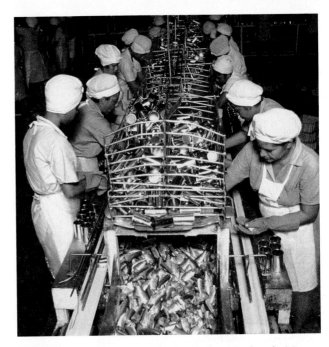

Studies indicate that people who have little control or decision-making powers in their employment are at an increased risk for stress-related cardiovascular disease.

caregiving, bereavement, and natural disasters.[11] Whatever the mechanism, the evidence is clear that stress is a significant contributor to CVD morbidity and mortality. (For more information about CVD, see Chapter 12.)

Stress and Impaired Immunity

As discussed in Chapter 2, a growing area of scientific investigation known as **psychoneuroimmunology (PNI)** analyzes the intricate relationship between the mind's response to stress and the immune system's ability to function effectively. A review of research linking stress to adverse health consequences suggests that too much stress over a long period can negatively regulate various aspects of the cellular immune response.[12] In particular, stress disrupts bidirectional communication networks between the nervous, endocrine, and immune systems. When these networks fail, messenger systems that regulate hormones, blood cell formation, and a host of other health-regulating systems begin to falter or send faulty information. Whereas the acute stress response is essentially protective, prolonged fight-or-flight depresses the immune system, particularly through the actions of cortisol. During prolonged stress, elevated levels of adrenal hormones

> Why do I always catch a cold during finals week?

psychoneuroimmunology (PNI) Science of the interaction between the mind and the immune system.

TABLE 3.1　What Stress Symptoms Do You Have?

Circle the number that indicates the frequency of occurrence of each symptom.

	Never	At least once in the last 6 months	At least once in the last month	At least once in the last week
1. Tension headache	1	2	3	4
2. Migraine (vascular) headache	1	2	3	4
3. Stomachache	1	2	3	4
4. Cold hands	1	2	3	4
5. Acid stomach	1	2	3	4
6. Shallow, rapid breathing	1	2	3	4
7. Diarrhea	1	2	3	4
8. Muscle cramps	1	2	3	4
9. Burping	1	2	3	4
10. Gassiness	1	2	3	4
11. Increased urge to urinate	1	2	3	4
12. Sweaty hands/feet	1	2	3	4
13. Fatigue/exhausted feelings	1	2	3	4
14. Oily skin	1	2	3	4
15. Dry mouth	1	2	3	4
16. Hand tremor	1	2	3	4
17. Backache	1	2	3	4
18. Neck stiffness	1	2	3	4
19. Gum chewing	1	2	3	4
20. Constipation	1	2	3	4
21. Tightness in chest or heart	1	2	3	4
22. Dizziness	1	2	3	4
23. Nausea/vomiting	1	2	3	4
24. Butterflies in stomach	1	2	3	4
25. Skin blemishes	1	2	3	4
26. Heart pounding	1	2	3	4
27. Blushing	1	2	3	4
28. Palpitations	1	2	3	4
29. Indigestion	1	2	3	4
30. Hyperventilation	1	2	3	4
31. Skin rashes	1	2	3	4
32. Jaw pain	1	2	3	4
33. Grinding teeth	1	2	3	4

Evaluating Your Score

<38 = low physiological symptoms
38–50 = moderate physiological symptoms
51–75 = high physiological symptoms
76–99 = excessive physiological symptoms

Source: R. Blonna, Coping with Stress in a Changing World, 4th ed. (New York: McGraw-Hill, 2007), 145.

destroy or reduce the ability of certain white blood cells, known as killer T cells, to aid the immune response. When killer T cells are suppressed and other regulating systems aren't working correctly, illness may occur.

Loss of immune regulation can result in various disease states. The links between stress and physiological features of cancer, arthritis, HIV/AIDS, asthma, and many other ailments have been studied through PNI.[13] Although each of these diseases has distinct clinical consequences, the change in the immune system from balanced and flexible to unbalanced and inflexible suggests increased vulnerability to stress-related immune impairment.

HEALTH headlines

Can chronic stress reshape your body? Research suggests that stress is linked to belly fat and, possibly, that you can keep the inches off your midsection by learning to manage stress.

The exact mechanisms still need clarification, but the hypothesis is that greater vulnerability to stress increases exposure to stress-induced cortisol, a powerful hormone that contributes to increased hunger (which acts as a stimulus to replace fuel used during the fight-or-flight response) and to the deposit of fat in a particularly annoying spot—the waist. When cortisol hits any cell, it activates fat-storing enzymes that cause the cell to enlarge. Fat cells in the belly have the largest number of receptors for cortisol, so the hormone is particularly attracted to this area. The extra calories and the added abdominal fat are both unsightly and dangerous. Experts have identified excess weight around the middle (central fat) as a risk factor for several diseases, including hypertension, coronary heart disease, stroke, and diabetes.

Accumulating evidence from clinical to cellular to molecular studies tend to support the aforementioned hypothesis. For example, in animal studies, stress-induced cortisol secretion has been shown to increase central (abdominal) fat. In human studies, women with central fat distribution have displayed heightened cortisol secretion in response to an acute laboratory stressor and an increase in food consumption following the stressful event. Only longitudinal and genetic studies will determine conclusively whether stress and central fat are causally related, but correlational data suggest that greater life stress and stress reactivity are linked to central fat.

If we want to win the battle of the bulge, we must focus on both stress management and weight-loss strategies. By learning to relax, we can de-stress and prevent excess cortisol secretion. A simple stay-slim solution: engage in regular physical activity. Physical activity will reduce your stress hormones and minimize some of the appetite-triggering and fat-storage effects of cortisol.

Sources: T. Parker-Pope, "Belly Fat May Be the Body's Way of Coping with Stress," *Wall Street Journal,* July 19, 2005; M. F. Dallman et al., "Minireview: Glucocorticoids—Food Intake, Abdominal Obesity, and Wealthy Nations in 2004," *Endocrinology,* 145, no. 6 (2004): 2633–38; E. S. Epel et al., "Stress and Body Shape: Stress-Induced Cortisol Secretion Is Consistently Greater among Women with Central Fat," *Psychosomatic Medicine* 62 (2000): 623–32; E. Epel et al., "Stress May Add Bite to Appetite in Women: A Laboratory Study of Stress-Induced Cortisol and Eating Behavior," *Psychoneuroendocrinology* 26 (2001): 37–49; J. Marniemi et al., "Visceral Fat and Psychosocial Stress in Identical Twins Discordant for Obesity," *Journal of Internal Medicine* 251 (2002): 35–43; M. Duclos et al., "Fat Distribution in Obese Women is Associated with Subtle Alteration of the Hypothalamic-Pituitary-Adrenal Axis Activity and Sensitivity to Glucocorticoids," *Clinical Endocrinology* 55 (2001), 447–54.

How long do you have to be stressed to suffer from impaired immunity? A look at the research yields evidence of impaired immunity following acute stressors, such as arguments, public speaking, and academic examinations. More prolonged stressors, such as the loss of a spouse, exposure to natural disaster, caregiving, living with a handicap, and unemployment, also have been shown to impair the natural immune response among various populations.[14]

Other studies have linked stress with infectious diseases:

- More than 20 years of research examining psychosocial factors in susceptibility to upper-respiratory-tract infections have revealed that higher stress levels are associated with higher rates of viral infection and clinical cold symptoms.[15]
- Psychological stress and loneliness correlate to poorer immune responses following influenza vaccinations in college students.[16]
- Exposure to academic stressors and self-reported stress are associated with increased upper-respiratory-tract infection among students.[17]

Although strong indicators support the hypothesis of a relationship between high stress and increased risk for disease, we are only beginning to understand this link. Some research indicates that other factors, such as genetics and environmental stimuli, may be involved. Even so, studies supporting this relationship outnumber those that don't, and there is convincing evidence that susceptibility to disease is influenced by stress-induced alterations in immune functioning.[18]

Stress and Diabetes

Recent data from large epidemiological studies have provided strong evidence of a link between psychological or physical stress and **diabetes,** a disease in which the pancreas fails to produce enough insulin or to use insulin effectively.[19] The activation of the sympathetic nervous system by the stress response can result in a combination of increased glucose (blood sugars) and inadequate production and release of *insulin,* a hormone that controls blood sugar levels.[20] An occasional stress reaction might not harm you, but high stress in your job; unresolved problems with family, school, or finances; and other sources of chronic stress can contribute

diabetes   Disease in which the pancreas fails to produce enough insulin or to use insulin effectively.

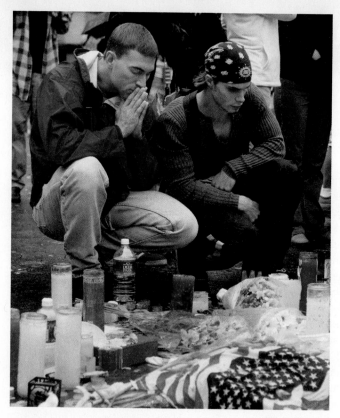

War veterans and other survivors of traumatic events, such as rape, car crashes, and natural disasters, may experience symptoms of post-traumatic stress disorder for months or even years thereafter.

to the onset or progression of diabetes. Over time, high blood sugar levels may begin to damage body organs such as the kidneys and blood vessels in the extremities and eyes.

Controlling stress levels is critical for successful short- and long-term diabetes management.[21] People under lots of stress often don't get enough sleep, don't eat well, and may drink or take other drugs to help them get through a stressful time. All of these behaviors can alter blood sugar levels further, on top of the increased blood sugars the body creates to fuel the fight-or-flight response. Exercise and relaxation techniques are particularly important. Even a short 15-minute walk can cause glucose levels to drop dramatically, as well as yielding other stress-reducing effects. Losing weight is also important. Being at a healthy weight contributes to overall glucose control and prevents the stress that people feel when they are overweight. For more information on diabetes, see Chapter 12.

Stress and the Mind

Stress may be one of the single greatest contributors to mental disability and emotional dysfunction in industrialized

post-traumatic stress disorder (PTSD)   An acute stress disorder caused by experiencing an extremely traumatic event, such as rape or combat.

nations. Studies have shown that the rates of mental disorders, particularly depression and anxiety, are associated with various environmental stressors, including divorce, marital conflict, economic hardship, and stressful life events.[22] In particular, mental disorders are more prevalent among young people aged 15 to 24 than among other age groups. Based on this finding, researchers suggest that as individuals move from adolescence to adulthood, they face stressors of all kinds, from school to employment to relationships, that may challenge their mental health.[23]

Evidence suggests a strong relationship between stress and the potential for negative mental health reactions. Consider the following:[24]

■ Stressful life events and inadequate sources of social support have been identified as predictors of psychiatric morbidity, including anxiety, insomnia, and depression.
■ The high incidence of suicide among college students is assumed to indicate high personal and societal stress in the lives of young people.
■ 85 percent of college counseling centers report an increase in the number of students they see with severe psychological problems—problems largely related to stress and adjustment difficulties.

Post-Traumatic Stress Disorder In severe cases, an individual's response to stress may develop into **post-traumatic stress disorder (PTSD)**. PTSD generally develops within the first hours or days after a traumatic event, but in some cases symptoms do not begin until months or years later. Typically, persons suffering from PTSD have been soldiers returning from war, particularly those who saw friends killed or wounded or who experienced terrible pain themselves. Many of these soldiers continued to suffer from these experiences for decades afterward. Other traumatic events that can cause PTSD include rape or other severe physical attacks, near-death experiences in accidents, witnessing a murder or death, being caught in a natural disaster, or terrorist attacks.

The development of PTSD is based on the hyperresponsive action of the fight-or-flight response. Symptoms include the following:

■ *Dissociation,* or perceived detachment of the mind from the emotional state or even the body. The person may have a sense of the world as a dreamlike or unreal place and have little memory of the events—a form of dissociative amnesia.
■ *Acute anxiety or nervousness,* in which the person is hyper-aroused, may cry easily or experience mood swings, and experience flashbacks, nightmares, and recurrent thoughts or visual images. Some people may sense vague uneasiness or feel as though the event were happening again and again. Others may experience intense physiological reactions, such as shaking or nausea, when something reminds them of the event. In some cases, they may have difficulty returning to areas that remind them of the trauma.

TABLE 3.2   The Student Stress Scale

The Student Stress Scale represents an adaptation of Holmes and Rahe's Social Readjustment Rating Scale (SRRS). The SRRS has been modified for college-aged adults and provides a rough indication of stress levels and health consequences for instructional purposes.

In the Student Stress Scale, each event is given a score that represents the amount of readjustment a person has to make as a result of the life change. To determine your stress score, check each event that you have experienced in the last 12 months, and then add up the number of points corresponding to each event.

1. Death of a close family member	_____	100
2. Death of a close friend	_____	73
3. Divorce between parents	_____	65
4. Jail term	_____	63
5. Major personal injury or illness	_____	63
6. Marriage	_____	58
7. Firing from a job	_____	50
8. Failure of an important course	_____	47
9. Change in health of a family member	_____	45
10. Pregnancy	_____	45
11. Sex problems	_____	44
12. Serious argument with close friend	_____	40
13. Change in financial status	_____	39
14. Change of major	_____	39
15. Trouble with parents	_____	39
16. New girlfriend or boyfriend	_____	37
17. Increase in workload at school	_____	37
18. Outstanding personal achievement	_____	36

19. First quarter/semester in school	_____	36
20. Change in living conditions	_____	31
21. Serious argument with an instructor	_____	30
22. Lower grades than expected	_____	29
23. Change in sleeping habits	_____	29
24. Change in social activities	_____	29
25. Change in eating habits	_____	28
26. Chronic car trouble	_____	26
27. Change in number of family gatherings	_____	26
28. Too many missed classes	_____	25
29. Change of college	_____	24
30. Dropping of more than one class	_____	23
31. Minor traffic violations	_____	20
	Total: _____	

Scoring

If your score is 300 or higher, you may be at high risk for developing a stress-related illness. If your score is between 150 and 300, you have approximately a 50:50 chance of experiencing a serious health problem within the next 2 years. If your score is below 150, you have a 1 in 3 chance of experiencing a serious health change in the next few years.

The following can help you to reduce your risk:
- Watch for early warning signs, such as irritable bowels.
- Avoid negative thinking.
- Exercise regularly and eat nutritiously.
- Practice some form of relaxation regularly.
- Ask for help when necessary.

Source: Reproduced from R. Blonna, "The Social and Spiritual Basis of Stress," in *Coping with Stress in a Changing World,* 4th ed. (New York: McGraw-Hill, 2007), 116. *Original source:* T. Holmes and R. H. Rahe, "The Social Readjustment Rating Scale," *Journal of Psychosomatic Research* 11 (1967): 213. Copyright © 1967 Elsevier, Inc. Used with permission.

 try it NOW!

Write it down! Journal writing is a great method to cleanse the mind, release emotions, and draft strategies for resolution. The next time an event or situation activates your stress response, identify the emotions that accompany it, and then list several options to bring closure to the event.

Sources of Stress

Both eustress and distress have many sources. They include psychosocial factors, environmental stressors, and self-imposed stress.

Psychosocial Sources of Stress

Psychosocial stress refers to the factors in our daily lives that cause stress (see the **Assess Yourself** box on page 70). Interactions with others, the subtle and unsubtle expectations we and others have of ourselves, and the social conditions we live in force us to readjust constantly. Key psychosocial stressors include change, hassles, pressure, inconsistent goals and behaviors, conflict, overload, and other factors.

Change Any time change occurs in your normal routine, whether good or bad, you will experience stress. The more changes you experience and the more adjustments you must make, the greater the stress effects may be. Four decades ago, Drs. Thomas Holmes and Richard Rahe developed the Social Readjustment Rating Scale (SRRS) to identify whether major life events preceded illness onset.[25] They determined that certain events (both positive and negative) were predictive of increased risk for illness. Since this time, the SRRS has served as the model for scales that measure stress levels of certain groups, including students, and research has documented that life events are related to a wide variety of physical and psychological problems. **Table 3.2** shows the Student Stress Scale, one example of a scale based on the SRRS.

(Text continues on page 72.)

ASSESS *yourself*

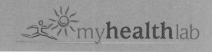

HOW DO YOU RESPOND TO STRESS?

Fill out this assessment online at www.aw-bc.com/myhealthlab or www.aw-bc.com/donatelle.

Each of us reacts differently to life's little challenges. Faced with a long line at the bookstore, most of us will get anxious for a few seconds before we start grumbling or shrug and move on. For others—the one in five of us whom researchers call hot reactors—such incidents are part of a daily health assault. These individuals may get outwardly angry or appear calm and collected. It is what is going on under the surface that affects health. Surges in blood pressure, increases in heart rate, nausea, sweating, and other hot-reactor indicators may occur. Completing the following assessment will help you think about how you respond to daily stressors. Although this survey is just an indicator of what your stress levels might be, it will help you focus on areas that you may need to work on.

Respond to each of the following statements with a rating of how likely you are to react to a given stressful event.

	Never	Rarely	Some of the Time	Usually or Always
SCENARIO 1				
You've been waiting 20 minutes for a table in a crowded restaurant, and the hostess seats a group that arrived after you.				
1. You feel your anger rise as your face gets hot and your heart beats faster.	1	2	3	4
2. You yell, "Hey! I was here first," in an irritated voice to the hostess.	1	2	3	4
3. You angrily confront the people who are being seated in front of you and tell them you were there first.	1	2	3	4
4. You say, "Excuse me," in a polite voice and inform the other group and/or the hostess that you were there first.	1	2	3	4
5. You note it, but don't react. It's no big deal, and the hostess obviously didn't notice the order of arrival.	1	2	3	4
SCENARIO 2				
You get to a movie theater early so that you and a friend can get great seats. You strategically pick a seat that will give you a good view. Although the theater is nearly empty, a large, tall man plops himself in the seat directly in front of you. Try as you might, you cannot see the screen.				
1. You say in a very loud voice, "There's a whole theater, and he has to sit right in front of us!"	1	2	3	4
2. You yell directly at the man, saying, "Can't you sit somewhere else? I can't see!"	1	2	3	4
3. You tap the man on the shoulder and say, "Excuse me, I wonder if you could slide down a seat. I can't see."	1	2	3	4
4. You calmly nudge your friend and decide to move.	1	2	3	4
5. You aren't bothered by the person in front of you. This is just part of going to the movies, and it is no big deal.	1	2	3	4
OTHER SCENARIOS				
How would you respond to the following?				
1. Your sister calls out of the blue and starts to tell you how much you mean to her. Uncomfortable, you change the subject without expressing what you feel.	1	2	3	4
2. You come home to find the kitchen looking like a disaster area and your spouse/roommate lounging in front of the TV. You tense up and can't seem to shake your anger, but you decide not to bring it up.	1	2	3	4
3. Faced with a public speaking event, you get keyed up and lose sleep for a day or more, worrying about how you'll do.	1	2	3	4

4. Your boyfriend/girlfriend/partner is seen out with another person and appears to be acting quite close to the person. You are a trusting person and decide not to worry about it. If your significant other has anything to tell you, you know he/she will talk to you.

    1   2   3   4

5. You aren't able to study as much as you'd like for an exam, yet you think that you really "nailed" the exam once you take it. When you get it back, you find that you did horribly. You make an appointment to talk with the professor and determine what you can do to improve on the next exam. You acknowledge that you are responsible for the low grade this time but vow to do better next time. You are disappointed, but you don't let it bother you.

    1   2   3   4

ANALYZING THIS SECTION

Look carefully at each of these scenarios. Obviously, none of us is perfect, and we sometimes react in ways that we later regret. The key here is to assess how you react the majority of the time.

If stressful events occur and you remain calm, do not experience increases in heart rate or blood pressure, or avoid excess anxiety, anger, or frustration, you are probably a cool reactor who tends to roll with the punches when a situation is out of your control. This usually indicates a good level of coping; overall, you will suffer fewer health consequences when stressed. The key here is that you really are not stressed, and you really are calm and unworried about the situation.

If you fret and stew about a stressor, can't sleep, or tend to react with hostility, anger, or other negative physiological over-reactions, you probably are a hot reactor who responds to mildly stressful situations with a fight-or-flight adrenaline rush that drives up blood pressure and can lead to heart rhythm disturbances, accelerated clotting, and damaged blood vessel linings. Some hot reactors can seem cool on the outside, but inside their bodies are silently killing them. They may be on edge, jumpy, or unable to sleep, even though most people would never suspect that they are in trouble. Before you honk or make obscene gestures at the guy who cuts you off in rush hour traffic, remember that getting angry can destroy thousands of heart muscle cells within minutes. Robert S. Eliot, author of *From Stress to Strength*, says hot reactors have no choice but to calm themselves down with rational thought. Look at ways to change your perceptions and cope more effectively. Ponder the fact that the only thing you'll hasten by reacting is a decline in health.

MAKE it happen!

ASSESSMENT: The Assess Yourself activity gave you the chance to look at your stress levels and identify situations in your life that particularly cause stress. Now that you are aware of these patterns, you can change a behavior that leads to increased stress.

MAKING A CHANGE: To change your behavior, you need to develop a plan. Follow these steps below, and complete your Behavior Change Contract to take action.

1. Evaluate your behavior, and identify patterns.

2. Select one pattern of behavior that you want to change.

3. Fill out the Behavior Change Contract found at the front of your book. It should include your long-term goals for change, your short-term goals, the rewards you'll give yourself for reaching these goals, potential obstacles along the way, and strategies for overcoming these obstacles. For each goal, list the small steps and specific actions that you will take.

4. Chart your progress in a journal.

5. Revise your plan as needed: Are the short-term goals attainable? Are the rewards satisfying?

EXAMPLE: Kim discovered that much of her stress was caused by school deadlines. She wanted to learn how to manage her time more efficiently. Kim filled out a Behavior Change Contract, with a goal of finishing her history term paper 5 days before its due date to give herself enough time to study for her biology final. She broke the paperwriting process into manageable steps of research, writing, revising, and proofreading. Each time she finished a stage, she rewarded herself with a movie or a trip to the local coffeehouse. She fell behind when her sister unexpectedly visited her for 2 days, but she got back on schedule when she worked on her paper instead of watching her afternoon soap opera. Kim completed her paper in plenty of time, was able to study efficiently for her biology exam, and didn't come down with her usual finals-period cold.

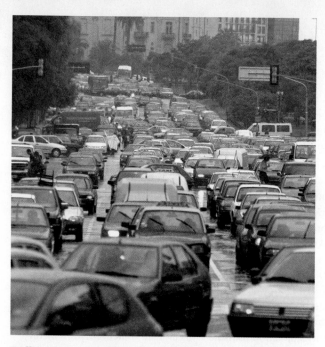
Traffic jams are a modern stressor and an example of the daily strains that can add up and jeopardize our health.

Hassles While Holmes and Rahe focused on major stressors, psychologists such as Richard Lazarus and Susan Folkman pioneered research in the 1980s that focused on petty annoyances and frustrations, collectively referred to as *hassles*.[26] Minor hassles—losing your keys, slipping and falling in front of everyone as you walk to your seat in a new class, finding that you went through a whole afternoon with spinach stuck in your front teeth—seem unimportant. However, their cumulative effects have been shown to be harmful in the long run. In fact, hassles are related to subsequent illness and disease to a greater degree than are major life events.[27]

Pressure Pressure occurs when we feel forced to speed up, intensify, or shift the direction of our behavior to meet a higher standard of performance.[28] Pressures can be based on our personal goals and expectations, concern about what others think, or outside influences. Among the most significant outside influences are society's demands that we compete and be all that we can be. The forces that push us to compete for the best grades, nicest cars, most attractive significant others, and highest-paying jobs create significant pressure to be the personification of success.

Inconsistent Goals and Behaviors For many of us, negative stress effects are magnified when there is a disparity between our goals (what we value or hope to obtain in life) and our behaviors (actions that may or may not lead to these goals). For instance, you may want good grades, and your family may expect them. But if you party and procrastinate throughout the term, your behaviors are inconsistent with your goals, and significant stress in the form of guilt, last-minute frenzy before exams, and disappointing grades may result. By contrast, if you dig in, work, and remain committed to getting good grades, your behaviors will be consistent with your goals and may eliminate much of your negative stress. Thwarted goals can lead to frustration, and frustration has been shown to be a significant disrupter of homeostasis.

Determining whether behaviors are consistent with goals is an essential component of maintaining balance in life. If we consciously strive to attain our goals in a direct manner, we greatly improve our chances of success.

Conflict Conflict occurs when we are forced to make difficult decisions between competing motives, behaviors, or impulses, or when we are forced to face incompatible demands, opportunities, needs, or goals. What if your best friends all choose to smoke marijuana and you don't want to smoke but fear rejection? Conflict often occurs as our values are tested. College students who are away from home for the first time often face conflict between parental values and their own set of developing beliefs.

Overload Excessive time pressure, too much responsibility, high expectations of yourself and those around you, and lack of support can lead to **overload,** a state of being overburdened. Have you ever felt you had so many responsibilities that you couldn't possibly begin to fulfill them all? Have you longed for a weekend when you could just take time out with friends and not feel guilty? These feelings are symptoms of overload. Students suffering from overload may experience anxiety about tests, poor self-esteem, a desire to drop classes or drop out of school, and other problems. In severe cases, in which they are unable to see any solutions to their problems, students may suffer from depression or turn to substance abuse. Binge drinking (see Chapter 8) is one of the leading problems on college campuses today, and numerous studies have linked periods of academic overload with increased consumption of alcohol among college students.[29]

Burnout People who regularly suffer from overload, frustration, and disappointment may eventually experience **burnout,** a state of physical and mental exhaustion caused by excessive stress. People involved in the "helping professions," such as teaching, social work, drug counseling, nursing, and psychology, experience high levels of burnout, as do police officers, air-traffic controllers, and other people who work in high-pressure, dangerous jobs. Accumulated evidence suggests that burnout resulting from prolonged exposure to stress is associated with increased risk of cardiovascular disease.[30]

overload   A condition in which a person feels overly pressured by demands.

burnout   A state of physical and mental exhaustion caused by excessive stress.

Other Forms of Psychosocial Stress Other forms of psychosocial stress include problems with overcrowding, discrimination, and socioeconomic difficulties such as unemployment and poverty. People of different ages or ethnic backgrounds may face a disproportionately heavy impact from these sources of stress. In addition to all of these we face increasing threats from technological stressors. For more information, see the **Spotlight on Your Health** box on page 74.

Stress and "-isms"

Today's racial and ethnic diversity of students, faculty members, and staff enriches everyone's educational experience yet also challenges everyone to deal with differences. Students come from vastly different contexts and life experiences. Imagine what it would be like to come to campus and find yourself isolated, lacking friends, and ridiculed on the basis of who you are or how you look. Often, those who act, speak, or dress differently face additional pressures that do not affect students considered more typical. Students perceived as different may become victims of subtle and not-so-subtle forms of bigotry, insensitivity, harassment, or hostility. Race, ethnicity, religious affiliation, age, sexual orientation, or other "-isms"—different viewpoints and backgrounds—may hang like a dark cloud over these students.

Evidence of the health effects of excessive stress in minority groups abounds. For example, African Americans suffer higher rates of hypertension, CVD, and most cancers than do white people. Although poverty and socioeconomic status have been blamed for much of the spike in hypertension rates for African Americans and other marginalized groups, chronic, physically debilitating stress may reflect real and perceived status in society more than it reflects actual poverty. Feeling that you occupy a position of low status because of your living conditions, financial security, or job status can be a source of stress. The problem is exacerbated for people who are socially disadvantaged early in life and grow up without a nurturing environment.[31]

Environmental Stress

Environmental stress results from events occurring in the physical environment. Environmental stressors include natural disasters, such as floods and hurricanes, and human-made disasters, such as chemical spills and explosions. Often as damaging as one-time disasters are **background distressors,** such as noise, air, and water pollution, although we may be unaware of them and their effects may not become apparent for decades. As with other challenges, our bodies respond to environmental stressors with the GAS. People who cannot escape background distressors may exist in a constant resistance phase, which can contribute to stress-related disorders.

Internal Sources of Stress

Appraisal and Stress We encounter many different types of life demands and potential stressors—some biological, some psychological, and others sociological. In any case, it is our appraisal of these demands, not the demands themselves, that results in the experience of stress. **Appraisal** is defined as the interpretation and evaluation of information provided to the brain by the senses. Appraisal is not a conscious activity, but rather a natural process that the brain constantly performs. As new information becomes available, appraisal helps us recognize stressors, evaluate them on the basis of past experiences and emotions, and decide how to cope with them. When you perceive that your coping resources are sufficient to meet life's demands, you experience little or no stress. By contrast, when you perceive that life's demands exceed your coping resources, you are likely to feel strain and distress. Several coping resources influence how you appraise stress. Two of the most important ones, self-esteem and self-efficacy, are discussed below.

Self-Esteem As we learned in Chapter 2, self-esteem refers to a sense of positive self-regard, or how you feel about yourself. Self-esteem varies; it can and does continually change.[32] When you feel good about yourself, you are less likely to respond to or interpret an event as stressful. Conversely, if you place little or no value on yourself and believe you have inadequate coping skills, you become susceptible to stress and strain.[33]

Self-esteem is closely related to the emotions engendered by past experiences. Low self-esteem can lead to helpless anger. People suffering helpless anger usually have learned that they are wrong to feel anger, so instead of expressing it in healthy ways they turn it inward. They may swallow their rage in food, alcohol, or other drugs, or they may act in other self-destructive ways. Of particular concern, research with high school and college students has found that low self-esteem and stressful life events significantly predict **suicidal ideation,** a desire to die and thoughts about suicide. On a more positive note, research has also indicated that it is possible to increase an individual's ability to cope with stress by increasing self-esteem.[34] Chapter 2 discussed several ways to develop and maintain self-esteem.

Self-Efficacy Self-efficacy, also introduced in Chapter 2, is another important factor in the ability to cope with life's

---

background distressors Environmental stressors of which people are often unaware.

appraisal The interpretation and evaluation of information provided to the brain by the senses.

suicidal ideation A desire to die and thoughts about suicide.

SPOTLIGHT on your health

TAMING TECHNOSTRESS

If you are like millions of people today, you find that technology is often a daily terrorizer that raises your blood pressure, frustrates you, and prevents you from ever really getting away from it all. In short, you may be a victim of stressors that previous generations only dreamed (or had nightmares) about. Known as *technostress,* this problem is defined as stress created by a dependence on technology, the constant state of being "plugged in," and the fear of technology failure. When technostress grabs you, it may interact with other forms of stress to create a never-ending form of stimulation that keeps your stress response reverberating all day.

Part of the problem, ironically, is that technology enables us to be so productive. Because it encourages polyphasic activity, or "multitasking," people are forced to juggle multiple thoughts and actions at the same time, such as driving and talking on cell phones or checking handheld devices for appointments. People who multitask, however, are actually less efficient than

those who focus on one project at a time. Moreover, there is clear evidence that multitasking contributes to auto accidents and other harmful consequences, including short-term memory loss. What is less clear is what happens to someone who is always plugged in.

What are the symptoms of technology overload? It evokes typical stress responses by increasing heart rate and blood pressure and causing irritability and memory disturbances. Over time, many stressed-out people lose the ability to relax and find that they feel nervous and anxious when they are supposed to be having fun. Headaches, stomach and digestive problems, skin irritations, frequent colds, difficulty in wound healing, lack of sleep, ulcers, and other problems may result. Other red flags include gaps in your attentiveness and changes in your ability to concentrate. A study conducted by Yale University indicates that chronic stress may even thicken the waistline; increased secretions of cortisol caused even slender women to store added fat in the abdomen.

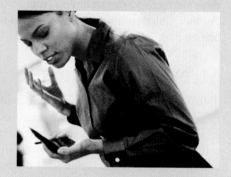

Authors Michelle Weil and Larry Rosen describe *technosis,* a syndrome in which people get so immersed in technology that they risk losing their own identity. If you answer yes to questions such as, "Do you rely on preprogrammed systems to contact others?" and "Do you feel stressed if you haven't checked your e-mail within the last 12 hours?" you may be too dependent on technology. A small, but growing, number of people are choosing to reduce or eliminate their reliance on technology. Termed "tech-no's," these individuals limit their connectivity (e.g., no sending or checking e-mail more than once a week; no

---

challenges. Self-efficacy refers to belief or confidence in personal skills and performance abilities.[35] Self-efficacy is considered one of the most important personality traits that influence psychological and physiological stress responses, and it has been found to predict a number of health behaviors in college students.[36]

Type A Personality and Hostility Personality may contribute to the kind and degree of self-imposed stress we experience. In 1974, physicians Meyer Friedman and Ray Rosenman identified two stress-related personality types: Type A and Type B.[37] Type A personalities are hard-driving, competitive, time-driven perfectionists. Type B personalities are relaxed, noncompetitive, and more tolerant

hostility The cognitive, affective, and behavioral tendencies toward anger and cynicism.

of others. According to Rosenman and Friedman, people with Type A characteristics are more prone to heart attacks than are their Type B counterparts. Because some Type A behavior is learned, it can be modified. Some Type A individuals are able to slow down and become more tolerant and patient. Unfortunately, many people do not decide to modify their Type A habits until after they become ill or suffer a heart attack. Preventing stress-related health problems requires recognizing and changing dangerous behaviors before damage is done.

Researchers today believe that more needs to be discovered about personality types. Most people are not one personality type all the time, and other unexplained variables must also be explored. For example, researchers at Duke University contend that the Type A personality may be more complex than previously described. They have identified a "toxic core" in some Type A personalities, which makes them angry, distrustful of others, and cynical—a collection of characteristics commonly referred to as **hostility**.[38] It may

YouTube, Facebook, or MySpace; no cell phone; no Blackberry). Tech-no's don't view limiting their connectivity as missing out, but rather as regaining sanity in tech-crazed world.

TIPS FOR FIGHTING TECHNOSTRESS

- *Become aware of what you are doing.* Log the time you spend on e-mail, voicemail, and so on. Set up a schedule to limit your use of technology. For example, spend no more than a half-hour per day answering e-mails.
- *Give yourself more time.* If you are surfing the Web for resources for a term paper, start early rather than the night before the paper is due.
- *Manage the telephone—don't let it manage you.* Rather than interrupting what you're doing to answer, screen calls with an answering machine or caller ID. Get rid of call waiting, which forces you to juggle multiple calls, and subscribe to a voicemail service that takes messages when you're on the phone.

- *Take regular breaks.* Even when you're working, every hour get up, walk around, stretch, do deep breathing, or get a glass of water.
- *If you are working on the computer, look away from the screen and focus on something far away every 30 minutes.* Stretch your shoulders and neck periodically as you work. Playing soft background music can help you relax.
- *Resist the urge to buy the newest and fastest technology.* Such purchases not only cause financial stress, but also add to stress levels with the typical glitches that occur when you are installing and adjusting to new technology.
- *Do not take laptops, PDAs, or other technological gadgets on vacation.* If you must take a cell phone for emergencies, turn it and your voice messaging system off, and use the phone only in true emergencies.
- *Back up materials on your computer at regular intervals.* Writing a term paper

only to lose it during a power outage will send you into hyperstress very quickly.
- *Expect technological change.* The only constant with technology is improvement and change. No matter how at ease you are with your current computer, cell phone, PDA, and so on, at some point you will need to move on to a new one.

Sources: D. Zielinski, "Techno-stressed?" *Presentations* 18, no. 2 (2004): 28–34; Dr. Larry D. Rosen and Dr. Michelle M. Weil, *TechnoStress: Coping with Technology @Work@Home@Play* (New York): John Wiley & Sons, 1997). Copyright © 1997. Material used by permission of John Wiley & Sons; J. Kornblum, "No Cellphone? No Blackberry? No Email? No Way? (It's true.)," *USA Today,* January 11, 2007, M. Weil and L. Rosen, "Technostress: Are You a Victim of Technosis?" 2004, www.technostress.com/tstechnosis.htm; Yale University, "Stress May Cause Excess Abdominal Fat in Otherwise Slender Women, Study Conducted at Yale Shows," *ScienceDaily,* November 23, 2000; MayoClinic.com, "Are You a Slave to the Telephone?" November 1, 2000, www.mayoclinic.com.

be this toxic core rather than their hard-driving nature that makes Type A individuals more vulnerable to self-imposed stress. People who are hostile often have below-average levels of self-esteem and social support and other increased risks for ill health.

Hostility: The Lethal Reaction The tendency toward hostility can have severe effects on cardiovascular health. Hostility has three components: (1) *cognitive*—negative beliefs about and attitudes toward others, including cynicism and mistrust; (2) *affective*—anger, which can range from irritation to rage and be assessed with regard to frequency, intensity, and target; and (3) *behavioral*—actions intended to harm others, either verbally or physically, usually in an aggressive way. A wide range of studies has identified hostility as an independent risk factor for coronary heart disease (CHD), hypertension, and premature mortality. Hostility is thought to harm individuals by influencing health behaviors that themselves confer risk, such as smoking or fast driving, or by being associated

with sociodemographic characteristics and physiological states that in turn increase the risk of heart disease.[39] White men and people with low socioeconomic status appear to be at highest risk for hostility, along with people who are overweight or obese, who smoke, who consume excessive amounts of alcohol, or who have a sedentary lifestyle, hypertension, or high total cholesterol levels.

Psychological Hardiness According to psychologist Susanne Kobasa, **psychological hardiness** may negate self-imposed stress associated with Type A behavior. Psychologically hardy people are characterized by control, commitment, and an embrace of challenge.[40] People with a sense of control are able to accept responsibility for their

psychological hardiness A personality trait characterized by control, commitment, and the embrace of challenge.

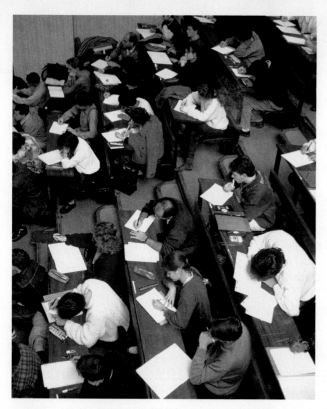

College can be a stressful time for students, whether they are young people choosing a career path or older adults returning to school to change directions later in life.

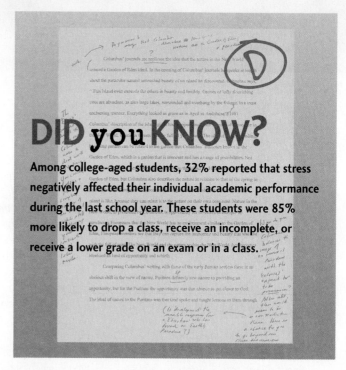

DID you KNOW?

Among college-aged students, 32% reported that stress negatively affected their individual academic performance during the last school year. These students were 85% more likely to drop a class, receive an incomplete, or receive a lower grade on an exam or in a class.

Source: American College Health Association, *National College Health Assessment,* 2005, www.acha.org.

behaviors and change those that they discover to be debilitating. People with a sense of commitment have good self-esteem and understand their purpose in life. People who embrace challenge see change as a stimulating opportunity for personal growth. The concept of hardiness has been studied extensively, and many researchers believe it is the foundation of an individual's ability to cope with stress and remain healthy.[41]

Stress and the College Student

College students thrive under a certain amount of stress, but excessive stress can leave them overwhelmed and less than enthusiastic about their classes and social interactions. Students can experience numerous distressors, including changes related to being away from home, pressure to make friends, the feeling of anonymity imposed by large classes, and academic pressures and test-taking anxiety. (For tips on how to overcome test-taking anxiety, see **Table 3.3.**) Some

psychological stress Stress caused by being in an environment perceived to be beyond one's control and endangering one's well-being.

32 percent of students surveyed for the National College Health Assessment reported that stress was the number-one factor affecting their individual academic performance, followed closely by stress-related problems such as cold/flu/sore throats (26 percent) and sleep difficulties (23.9 percent; see Did You Know?).[42]

A 2005 study by UCLA's (University of California–Los Angeles) Higher Education Research Institute reported that the year's current college freshmen were more stressed than any class of freshmen before them. These researchers define **psychological stress** as a relationship between a person and the environment that the person judges to be beyond his or her resources and jeopardizes his or her well-being.[43] Freshmen seem to be the most vulnerable to the negative effects of psychological stress; relationships, school events, safety, and feelings that they fail to meet school norms have been noted as particularly distressful. Freshmen have reported not only more problems with these issues, but also more emotional reactivity in the form of anger, hostility, frustration, and a greater sense of being out of control. Sophomores and juniors reported fewer problems with these issues, and seniors reported the fewest problems. These results may indicate students' progressive emotional growth through experience, maturity, increased awareness of support services, and more social connections.

Male and female students also report different stressors. Women indicate that among their most frequent stressors are being overweight, trying to diet, and managing an overload of schoolwork. Men, in contrast, tend to identify the following items as major stressors: being underweight, not having

TABLE 3.3   Overcoming Test-Taking Anxiety

Doing well on a test is an ability needed far beyond college. Here are some helpful hints to try on your next exam.

Before the Exam

1. **Manage your time.** Plan to start studying a week before your test (longer if it's a professional exam required for your career). Being prepared will reduce anxiety. Do a limited review the night before, get a good night's sleep, and arrive for the exam early. This will ease your anxiety and increase your confidence.

2. **Build your test-taking self-esteem.** On a 3 × 5 inch card write down three reasons why you will pass the exam. Carry the card with you, and look at it whenever you study. When you get the test, write your three reasons on the test or on a piece of scrap paper. Positive affirmations such as this will help you succeed.

3. **Eat a balanced meal before the exam.** Avoid sugar and rich or heavy foods, as well as foods that might upset your stomach. You want to feel your best.

During the Test

1. **Manage your time during the test.** Decide how much time you need to take the test, review your answers, and go back over questions you might be stuck on. Hold to this schedule. If you feel that you are a slow reader and need more time, talk to your teacher or test administrator before the exam.

2. **Slow down.** When you open your test book, always write RTFQ (Read the Full Question) at the top. Make sure you understand the question before answering.

3. **Stay on track.** If you begin to get anxious, reread your three reasons for success.

someone to date, not having enough sex, being behind in schoolwork, not having enough friends, and concerns about drug or alcohol use.

Differences in coping behaviors also have been identified. Women report greater use of time management techniques to deal with stress, whereas men tend to engage in more leisure activities to lessen academic stress. Students generally report using health-enhancing methods to combat stress, but research has found that students sometimes resort to health-compromising activities, such as procrastination, avoidance, and substance use to escape the stress and anxiety of college.[44]

If you experience any of the stressors listed in the Student Stress Scale in Table 3.2, explore constructive ways to reduce their impact. Most colleges offer stress management workshops through health centers or student counseling departments. Do not ignore the symptoms of stress overload, such as those listed in Table 3.1. If stress is not dealt with, it can lead to long-lasting problems. Numerous researchers have identified stress among college students to be correlated to unhealthy behaviors such as substance abuse, lack of physical activity, poor psychological and physical health, lack of social problem solving, and low utilization of social support

networks.[45] Many mental health problems may be traced to stress-related trauma that occurs at key periods of life, particularly the college years.

Managing Your Stress

Recognizing your personal stressors is the first step toward making positive changes. Being on your own in college poses many challenges; however, it also lets you evaluate your unique situation and take steps that fit your own schedule and lifestyle to reduce negative stressors in your life.

One of the most effective ways to combat stressors is to build skills and coping strategies that will help inoculate you against them. Such efforts are known collectively as stress management techniques. They range from doing something as simple as taking 20 minutes each day to be alone, to developing an elaborate time management plan for eating, socializing, and exercising.

Recall the process of shaping described in Chapter 1, which involves taking a number of smaller steps to achieve a larger behavior change. Be careful not to change too many things at once, or your new stress management program could stress you out!

Building Skills to Reduce Stress

Dealing with stress involves assessing all aspects of a stressor, examining your response and how you can change it,

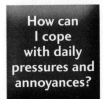

and learning to cope. Often we cannot change the requirements at our college, assignments in class, or unexpected stressors. Inevitably, we will be stuck in classes that bore us and for which we find no application in real life. We feel powerless when a loved one dies. Although we cannot alter the facts, we can change our reactions to them.

Assess Your Stressors After recognizing a stressor, evaluate it. Can you alter the circumstances to reduce the amount of distress you are experiencing, or must you change your behavior and reactions to reduce stress levels? For example, you may have five term papers due for five different courses during the semester, but your professors are unlikely to drop such requirements. However, you can change your behavior by beginning the papers early and spacing them over time to avoid last-minute panic.

Change Your Responses Changing your responses requires practice and emotional control. For example, suppose your roommate is habitually messy, and this causes you stress. You can choose from among several responses: you can express your anger by yelling; you can pick up the mess and leave a nasty note; or you can defuse the situation with humor. The first reaction that comes to mind is not always the best. Stop before reacting, so that you gain the time you need to find an appropriate response. Ask yourself, "What is to be gained from my response?"

Many people change their responses to potentially stressful events through cognitive coping strategies. These strategies help them prepare through gradual exposure to increasingly higher stress levels.

Learn to Cope

Everyone copes with stress in different ways. Some people drink or take drugs; others seek help from counselors; and still others try to forget about it or engage in positive activities, such as exercise. **Stress inoculation** helps people prepare for stressful events ahead of time. For example, suppose speaking in front of a class petrifies you. Practicing in front of friends or in front of a video camera may inoculate you and prevent your freezing up on the day of the presentation. The assumption is that by dealing with smaller fears, a person develops resistance, so that larger fears do not seem so overwhelming. Some health experts compare stress inoculation to a vaccine given to protect against a disease. Regardless of how you cope with a situation, your conscious effort to deal with it is an important step in stress management.

Consider Downshifting

Today's lifestyles are hectic and pressure-packed, and stress often comes from trying to keep up. Many people are questioning whether "having it all" is worth it, and they are taking a step back and simplifying their lives. This trend has been labeled *downshifting* or *voluntary simplicity*. Moving from a large urban area to a smaller town, leaving a high-paying, high-stress job for one that makes you happy, and a host of other changes in lifestyle typify downshifting.

Downshifting involves a fundamental alteration in values and honest introspection about what is important in life. When you consider any form of downshift or perhaps even start your career this way, it's important to move slowly and consider the following.

- *Determine your ultimate goal.* What is most important to you, and what will you need to reach that goal? What can you do without?
- *Make both short-term and long-term plans for simplifying your life.* Set up your plan in doable steps, and work slowly toward each step. Begin saying no to requests for your time, and identify which people it is important for you to spend time with. Clear out clutter or material items you don't need or use.

- *Complete a financial inventory.* How much money will you need to do the things you want to do? Will you live alone or share costs with roommates? Do you need a car, or can you rely on public transportation? Pay off your debt, and get used to paying with cash. If you don't have the cash, don't buy. Remember, your lifestyle as a student will be different from living at home.
- *Plan for health care costs.* Make sure that you budget for health insurance and basic preventive health services if you're not covered under your parents' plan. Understand your coverage. This should be a top priority.
- *Select the right career.* Look for work that you enjoy. Can you be happy taking a lower-paying job that is less stressful and allows you the opportunity to have a life?
- *Consider options for saving money.* Downshifting doesn't mean you renounce money; it means you choose not to let money dictate your life. It's still important to save. If you're just getting started, you need to prepare for emergencies and for future plans.

Managing Social Interactions

As you plan a stress management program, don't underestimate the importance of social networks and social bonds. Consider the nature and extent of your friendships. Do you have someone with whom you can share intimate thoughts and feelings? Do you trust your friends to be supportive? Will your friends be honest with you if you are doing something risky or inappropriate? Friendships are an important aspect of inoculating yourself against harmful stressors. Studies have demonstrated the importance of social support in buffering individuals from the effects of stress.[46] It isn't necessary to have a large number of friends. However, different friends often serve different needs, so having more than one is usually beneficial. As you work to develop and cultivate friendships, look for individuals who

- Have values and interests that are similar to your own (as well as those with different interests that force you to grow and explore new ideas).
- Are good listeners, give and share freely, are tolerant, and do not rush to judgment.
- Are trustworthy and have your best interests at heart.
- Are not unusually critical, negative, or selfish and don't bring you down. Avoid people who enjoy "stirring things up" and always seem to be in some crisis themselves; they often precipitate rather than reduce stress responses.
- Are responsible and value doing well in school, but also know when and how to have fun.
- Are willing to be exercise and diet buddies or study partners with a mutual interest in a healthy lifestyle.
- Know how to laugh, cry, engage in meaningful conversation, and feel comfortable with silence.

Just as it is important to find these characteristics in your friends, it is also important for you to bring these qualities to

---

stress inoculation Stress management technique in which a person consciously tries to prepare ahead of time for potential stressors.

HEALTH IN A *diverse world*

STRESS AMONG INTERNATIONAL STUDENTS

Academic stress may pose a particular problem for the more than 400,000 international students who have left support networks of family and friends in their native countries to study in the United States. Accumulating evidence suggests that seeking emotional support from others is among the most effective ways to cope with stressful and upsetting situations. Unfortunately, many international students refrain from seeking emotional support because of cultural norms, feelings of shame, and the belief that seeking support is a sign of weakness that calls inappropriate attention to both the individual and the respective ethnic or cultural group. This reluctance to seek support, coupled with language barriers, cultural conflicts, racial prejudices, and other stressors, is the reason why international students suffer significantly more stress-related illnesses than their American counterparts, researchers theorize. There are no easy solutions to the numerous stressors that international students encounter, yet there are things we can do to make one person's life (or maybe two or three persons' lives) a little less stressful: share companionship and communication, and lend a hand to help others. To paraphrase a popular Hindu proverb: "Help thy neighbor's boat across, and thine own boat will also reach the shore."

Sources: Institute of International Education, "Open Doors on the Web," 2005, http://opendoors.iienetwork.org; M. R. Cunningham and A. P. Barbee, "Social Support," in *Close Relationships: A sourcebook,* ed. C. Hendrick and S. S. Hendrick (Thousand Oaks, CA: Sage, 2000), 272–85; K. J. Edwards, P. J. Herschberger, R. K. Russell, and R. J. Market, "Stress, Negative Social Exchange, and Health Symptoms in University Students," *Journal of American College Health* 50 (2001): 75–79; S. T. Mortenson, "Cultural Differences and Similarities in Seeking Social Support as a Response to Academic Failure: A Comparison of American and Chinese College Students," *Communication Education* 55, no. 2 (2006): 127–46.

your friendships. Sometimes, focusing on others can help you get your own problems into better focus and control.

If you do not have a close friend or support group, find out where to turn when the pressures of life seem overwhelming. Family members are often a steady base of support on which you can rely. But if friends or family are unavailable, most colleges and universities offer counseling services at no cost for short-term crises. Clergy, instructors, and residence hall supervisors also may be excellent resources. If university services are unavailable, or if you are concerned about confidentiality, most communities offer low-cost counseling through mental health clinics.

Taking Mental Action

Stress management calls for mental action in two areas. First, positive self-esteem, which can help you cope with stressful situations, comes from learned habits and responses to people and events. Successful stress management involves mentally developing and practicing self-esteem skills, focusing on positive thinking about yourself, and examining self-talk to reduce irrational responses. Focus on the here and now rather than on past problems.

Second, because you can't always anticipate what the next stressor will be, you need to develop the mental skills necessary to manage your reactions after it has occurred. The ability to react productively and appropriately comes with time, practice, patience, and experience with a variety of stressful situations.

Change the Way You Think As noted earlier, our appraisals, thoughts, and ideas of people and situations are what make these things stressful, not the people or situations themselves. To combat negative self-talk, we must first become aware of it, then stop it, and finally replace the negative thoughts with positive ones—a process referred to as **cognitive restructuring.** Several types of negative self-talk exist, but among the most common are pessimism, or focusing on the negative; perfectionism, or expecting superhuman standards; "should-ing," or reprimanding yourself for items that you should have done; blaming yourself or others for circumstances and events; and dichotomous thinking, in which everything is either black or white (good or bad) instead of gradations.[47] Once you realize that some of your thoughts may be irrational or overreactive, interrupt this self-talk by saying, "Stop" (under your breath or out loud), and make a conscious effort to adjust your thinking. Focus on more positive patterns. If you can learn to view potential stressors more positively, you can reduce your stress levels without having to remove the potential stressors. Here are other actions you can take to develop these mental skills:

■ *Reframe a distressing event from a positive perspective.* Reframing is a stress management technique that assists

---

cognitive restructuring The modification of thoughts, ideas, and beliefs that contribute to stress.

you to reconstruct or draft a "reframed" perspective to a situation from a positive vantage point.

- *Worry constructively.* Don't waste time and energy worrying about things you can't change or events that may never happen.
- *Look at life as being fluid.* If you accept that change is a natural part of living and growing, the jolt of changes will become less stressful.
- *Consider alternatives.* Remember, there is seldom only one appropriate action. Anticipating options will help you plan for change and adjust more rapidly.
- *Moderate your expectations.* Aim high, but be realistic about your circumstances and motivation.
- *Weed out trivia.* Cardiologist Robert Eliot offers two rules for coping with life's challenges: "Don't sweat the small stuff," and remember, "It's all small stuff."
- *Don't rush into action.* Think before you act.
- *Tolerate mistakes by yourself and others.* Rather than getting angry or frustrated by mishaps, evaluate what happened and learn from them.
- *Live simply.* Eliminate unnecessary things and obligations. Learn to say no. Prioritize. Make commitments only to things you have to or want to do.

Once you have improved your mental outlook and gained a more positive perspective on life, you will find it easier to cope with stressors.

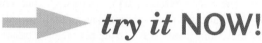 *try it* NOW!

A penny for your thoughts! Negative self-talk can contribute to feelings of stress. Try this exercise now to see how often you have negative emotional responses. Place a handful of pennies in your right-hand pocket, and each time you catch yourself having a negative thought, remove a penny from your right pocket and place it in your left pocket. After this exercise, resolve to replace negative thoughts with a positive or optimistic statement that boosts your self-esteem.

Managing Emotional Responses

Have you ever gotten all worked up about something only to find that your perceptions were totally wrong? We often get upset not by realities, but by our faulty perceptions. For example, suppose you found out that everyone except you is invited to a party. You might easily begin to wonder why you were excluded. Does someone dislike you? Have you offended someone? Such thoughts are typical. However, the reality of the situation may have absolutely nothing to do with your being liked or disliked. Perhaps, for example, you were sent an invitation and it didn't reach you.

In Chapter 1 we introduced the concept of self-talk. Stress management requires that you examine your self-talk and your emotional responses to interactions with others. With

any emotional response to a stressor, you are responsible for the emotion and the resultant behaviors. Learning to tell the difference between normal emotions and those based on irrational beliefs can help you stop the emotion or express it in a healthy and appropriate way.

Learn to Laugh and Cry Have you noticed that you feel better after a good laugh or cry? It isn't your imagination. Laughter and crying stimulate the heart and temporarily rev up many body systems. Heart rate and blood pressure then decrease significantly, allowing the body to relax. The positive psychological and physiological responses of laughter and crying have been demonstrated in a variety of settings. Laughing and crying have been shown to reduce stress hormone levels, improve mood, enhance creativity, reduce pain, and improve immunity.[48]

Fight the Anger Urge Anger usually results when we feel we have lost control of a situation and/or are frustrated by a situation that we can do little about. The five main sources of anger are related to threats to (1) safety and well-being, (2) power, (3) perfectionism and pride, (4) self-sufficiency and autonomy, and (5) self-esteem and status.[49]

Anger may vary in intensity from mild irritation to rage and may be acted out as cynicism, sarcasm, intimidation, frustration, impatience, quick flaring of temper, distrust, or anxiety. Not all anger is inherently bad. Sometimes, it can give us the energy we need to fight back if attacked or the resolve to work even harder to accomplish a goal. It is unresolved anger, the kind that festers and clouds our reasoning and our reactions, that we need to control.

Each of us has learned by this point in our lives that we have three main approaches to dealing with anger: expressing it, suppressing it, or calming it. You may be surprised to find out that *expressing* your anger is probably the healthiest thing to do in the long run, particularly if you express anger in an assertive rather than aggressive way. However, it's a natural reaction to want to respond aggressively, and that is what we must learn to keep at bay. See **Table 3.4** to review strategies for managing anger in your life.[50]

Taking Physical Action

Physical activities can complement the emotional and mental strategies of stress management.

Exercise It is important to remember that the human stress response is intended to end in physical activity (fight or flight). The outpouring of sugar and fats into the blood is meant to nourish the muscles and brain. The heart and respiration rates speed up to meet the impending physical demands of the threat. If the threat persists, hormones are released into the bloodstream to maintain the response. Historically, most threats required physical responses. Today that is not true, yet our stress response has not changed to fit with the times. When we are stressed, this is not the time to sit and feel all those fight-or-flight sensations tearing away at our body's

TABLE 3.4 | Strategies for Anger Management

1. **Identify your anger style.** Do you express anger passively or in an active style? Are you the type of person who holds anger in, or are you the kind of person who explodes? Take mental notes of what ticks you off and how you typically react.

2. **Learn to recognize patterns in your anger responses and how to de-escalate your anger.** Keep track of everything that angers you for a week's time. What patterns do you see? What thoughts or feelings lead up to your "boiling point"? Explore how you can interrupt patterns of anger, such as walking around the block, counting to 10, getting a drink of water, taking some deep breaths, or taking a short time-out.

3. **Plan ahead.** Some situations can be foreseen as potentially provoking anger. Identify these situations (family get-togethers, long lines at the post office, traffic backups at 5:00 PM, finding a parking spot on campus) and identify options to minimize your exposure to them.

4. **Develop a support system.** Find a few close friends you can confide in or vent your frustrations to. Don't force a person to agree with you, but allow him or her to listen and perhaps provide insight or another perspective that your anger has blinded you to.

5. **Develop realistic expectations of yourself and others.** Anger is often the result of unmet expectations. Are the expectations you have of yourself and others realistic? If you have expectations of others, have you verbally shared those expectations with them?

6. **Turn complaints into requests.** Anyone can complain, whine, or moan. When frustrated or angry with someone, try reworking the problem into a request. Instead of screaming and pounding on the floor because your neighbor's music is blaring and woke you up at 2:00 AM, have a conversation with your neighbors. Try to reach an agreement that everyone will keep music turned down after 11:00 PM.

7. **Make past anger past.** Learn to resolve issues that have caused pain, frustration, or stress. If you need to seek the counsel of a professional to make that happen, do so. Set a "statute of limitations" on your anger, and move on.

Source: Adapted from B. L. Seaward, "The Stress Emotions: Anger and Fear," from *Managing Stress: Principles and Strategies for Health and Well-Being,* 4th ed. Copyright © 2006 Jones & Bartlett Publishers, Sudbury, MA. Reprinted with permission.

systems. This is the time to move and use up those products of the stress response. Exercise "burns off" existing stress hormones by directing them toward their intended metabolic function.[51] In addition, exercise can help combat stress by raising levels of endorphins—mood-elevating, pain-killing hormones—in the bloodstream, increasing energy, reducing hostility, and improving mental alertness.

Most of us have relieved stress by engaging in vigorous physical activity: joining a kickboxing class is one example. Exercise performed as an immediate response can help alleviate stress symptoms. However, a regular exercise program yields even more substantial benefits. Try to engage in at least 25 minutes of aerobic exercise three or four times a week. Although it may not improve your aerobic capacity, a quiet walk can refresh your mind, calm your stress response, and replenish your adaptation energy stores. Plan walking breaks alone or with friends, or stretch after prolonged periods of study at your desk. A short period of physical exercise may provide the break you really need. For more information on the beneficial effects of exercise, see Chapter 11.

Relax Like exercise, relaxation can help you cope with stress- ful feelings, preserve adaptation energy stores, and refocus your energies. Relaxation techniques that involve both the mind and body are great stress reducers for college students. Yoga and other exercises that increase flexibility also aid in relaxation (see Chapter 11). Practice relaxation daily until it becomes a habit. You will probably find that you enjoy it.

Once you have learned simple relaxation techniques, you can use them at any time—before or during a tough exam or when faced with a stressful confrontation or assignment, for example. As your body relaxes, your heart rate slows, your blood pressure and metabolic rate decrease, and many other body-calming effects occur, all of which allow you to channel energy appropriately. (See the **Skills for Behavior Change** box on page 82 for more on relaxation techniques.)

Eat Right Is food really a de-stressor? Whether foods can calm us and nourish our psyches is a controversial question. High-potency supplements that are supposed to boost resistance against stress-related ailments are nothing more than gimmicks. However, it is clear that eating a balanced, healthful diet will help provide the stamina you need to get through problems and will stress-proof you in ways that are not fully understood. It also is known that undereating, overeating, and eating the wrong kinds of foods can create distress in the body. In particular, avoid **sympathomimetics,** food substances that produce (or mimic) stress-like responses. The most common sympathomimetic is caffeine, commonly found in sodas, coffee, tea, and chocolate. Sugar is often considered a sympathomimetic, but much of what has been published about hyperactivity and its relation to the consumption of sweets has been shown to be scientifically invalid. For more information about the benefits of sound nutrition, see Chapter 9.

Managing Your Time

Time. Everybody needs more of it, especially students trying to balance the demands of classes, social life, earning money for school, and family obligations. Keep a journal for one week to become aware of your time patterns, and use the following time management tips in your stress management program.

How can I prioritize everything I try to do in a day?

sympathomimetics Food substances that can produce stress-like responses.

SKILLS FOR *behavior change*

RELAXATION TECHNIQUES FOR STRESS MANAGEMENT

Relaxation techniques to reduce stress have been practiced for centuries, and there is a wide selection from which to choose. In addition to those discussed in the chapter, five to consider are yoga, qigong, tai chi, deep breathing, and progressive muscle relaxation.

YOGA

An estimated 20 million adults in America actively engage in yoga, an ancient tradition that combines meditation, stretching, and breathing exercises designed to relax, refresh, and rejuvenate. There are several popular versions.

Classical yoga is the ancestor of nearly all forms of yoga practiced today. Breathing, poses, and verbal mantras are often part of classical yoga.

Kripalu is a gentle, introspective practice in which much emphasis is placed on breathing techniques and releasing emotional blockages. Initially practitioners concentrate mainly on poses and deep breathing, followed by emotional exercises. In later stages, practitioners focus primarily on poses. Kripalu is particularly suited for people who want to go slowly and gently or who have underlying injuries or problems.

Popularized by Madonna, *Ashtanga yoga* is designed to improve sport performance with deep breathing and a progressive series of postures. Less familiar than other forms, this type of yoga is growing in popularity.

Hot yoga, also known as *Bikram yoga,* differs from traditional yoga in that classes are held in rooms where the temperatures reach up to 105 degrees Fahrenheit. After going through up to 26 poses, students emerge from these classes drained of energy, drenched in sweat, and feeling cleansed. Although bikram centers have sprung up across the country, there have been reports of heat exhaustion, dehydration, and other problems. This style of yoga is risky for people with hypertension, certain respiratory conditions, and other cardio-vascular risks. If you feel weak, dizzy, nauseated, or have other ill effects, use caution. Before attending a class, speak with your doctor if you have questions or concerns, and make sure you go to a reputable facility with qualified staff.

QIGONG

Qigong (pronounced "chee-kong") is one of the fastest-growing and most widely accepted forms of mind–body health exercises. Even some of the country's largest health care organizations, such as Kaiser

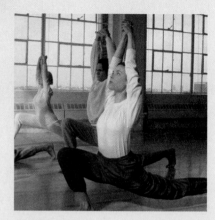

Permanente, have incorporated this relaxation technique into their system, particularly for people suffering from chronic pain or stress. Like acupuncture, qigong taps into a complex system of internal pathways called meridians, which are thought to run along the length of the body. According to Chinese medicine, meridians carry qi (pronounced "chee"), or vital energy, throughout your body. If your qi becomes stagnant or blocked, you'll feel sluggish or power-less. Thus, a series of flowing movements, mental visualization exercises, and vocalizations of healing sounds such as "shhhuuu" are designed to integrate and refresh the mind and body through easy-to-perform techniques.

- *Take on only one thing at a time.* Don't try to pay bills, wash clothes, and write your term paper all at once. Stay focused.
- *Clean off your desk.* Go through the things on your desk, toss the unnecessary papers, and put into folders the papers for tasks that you must do. When bills come in, take care of them immediately. Write a check and hold it for mailing. Read your mail, and file it or toss it.
- *Find a clean, comfortable place to work.* Go someplace where you won't be distracted.
- *Prioritize your tasks.* Make a daily "to do" list, and try to stick to it. Categorize the things you must do today, the things that you have to do but not immediately, and the things that it would be nice to do. Consider the "nice to do" items only if you finish the others or if they include something fun. Give yourself a reward as you finish each task.

- *Don't be afraid to say no.* All too often, we do things out of fear of what someone may think. Set your school and personal priorities, and live according to your own agenda, values, and goals.
- *Avoid interruptions.* When you have a project that requires total concentration, schedule uninterrupted time. Don't answer the phone; close your door, and post a "Do Not Disturb" sign; go to a quiet room in the library or student union where no one will find you.
- *Reward yourself for work completed.* Did you finish a task on your list? See a movie or go for a walk. Differentiate between rest breaks and work breaks. Work breaks simply mean switching tasks for awhile. Rest breaks give you time to yourself to help you recharge and refresh your energy levels.

TAI CHI

Tai chi (pronounced "ty-chee") is sometimes described as "meditation in motion." Originally developed in China as a form of self-defense, this graceful form of exercise has existed for about 2,000 years. Tai chi is noncompetitive and self-paced. To do tai chi, you perform a defined series of postures or movements in a slow, graceful manner. Each movement or posture flows into the next without pause. Tai chi is becoming increasingly popular around the world, both as a basic exercise program and as a complement to other health care methods. Health benefits include stress reduction, greater balance, and increased flexibility.

DIAPHRAGMATIC OR DEEP BREATHING

Typically, we breathe only using the upper chest and thoracic region rather than involving the abdominal region. Simply stated, diaphragmatic breathing is deep breathing that maximally expands the chest by involving the movement of the lower abdomen. This technique is commonly used in yoga exercises. The diaphragmatic breathing process occurs in three stages.

Stage 1: Assume a comfortable position. Whether sitting or lying down on your back, find the most natural position to be in. Close your eyes, unbutton your shirt or binding clothes, remove your belt, and unbutton your pants. Often it works best to fold your hands over your abdomen and get used to feeling the rise and fall of your stomach.

Stage 2: Concentrate on the act of breathing. Shut out external noise. Focus on inhaling, exhaling, and the route the air is following. Try saying to yourself, "Feel the warm air coming into my nose, warming my windpipe, and flowing into my lungs. Feel my stomach rise and fall as I inhale slowly and exhale slowly, and feel the air flow out of my nose." Repeat this action several times.

Stage 3: Visualize. The above stages seem to work best when combined with visualization. A common example is to visualize clean, fresh, invigorating air slowly entering the nose and being exhaled as gray, stale air that has accumulated in the body. Such processes, particularly when they involve the whole body, seem to help deep breathers become more refreshed from their experience.

PROGRESSIVE MUSCLE RELAXATION

Progressive muscle relaxation involves systematically contracting and relaxing each of several muscle groups; proper breathing and concentration are part of this process. Again, find a comfortable position, and begin a deep-breathing cycle. The difference from diaphragmatic breathing is that as you concentrate on inhaling, you also contract a particular muscle group (for example, the hand and fingers). Hold that position for a short period. Then, as you exhale, slowly release the muscles that you have been contracting. Repeat and add more muscle groups. You might start with a hand, then move to the forearm, the entire arm, the neck, to the shoulders, back, buttocks, foot, and thigh. You can add components of other relaxation techniques to this experience by saying, "My hands are getting warmer, my arm is getting warmer," and so on as you work to gain maximum control of blood flow and muscle tension in a region.

Sources: Mayo Clinic Staff, "Tai Chi: Stress Reduction, Balance, Agility and More," December 7, 2005, www.mayoclinic.com/health/tai-chi/SA00087; paragraph on qigong from C. Dold, "The New Yoga," *Health* (May 2004): 73–77.

- *Use time to your advantage.* If you're a morning person, schedule activities to coincide with the time when you're at your best. Take a short nap or break when you need it.
- *Break overwhelming tasks into small pieces, and allocate a certain amount of time to each.* If you are floundering in a task, move on and come back to it when you're refreshed.
- *Remember that time is precious.* Many people learn to value their time only when they face a terminal illness. Try to value each day. Time spent not enjoying life is a tremendous waste of potential.

Managing Your Finances

Higher education can involve a considerable financial burden. A recent study conducted by the Higher Education Research Institute (HERI) reported that 64.1% of students indicated that they have "some" or "major" concerns regarding their ability to finance the costs of their college education.[52] Many students work increasingly long hours to pay their way through school, and others incur large consumer debt—both of which are related to decreased academic performance and psychological well-being.[53] The pressure to succeed in college needs to be understood in the context of students' financial circumstances and the related implications for their health. Follow these tips to manage your money and reduce finance related stress:

- *Develop a realistic budget.* What are your monthly expenses? What types of "luxuries" do you regularly splurge on?
- *When bills come in, take care of them immediately.* Write a check and hold it for mailing, or send it right away so you don't forget and pay late fees.

- *Consider electronic banking.* This can make the process of paying bills faster and easier.
- *Become knowledgeable about how to manage your money.* Take advantage of campus workshops on financial aid, money management, and part-time jobs.
- *Avoid those tempting credit cards.* If you get offers in the mail, toss them. You only need one or two credit cards.
- *Don't get into debt.* If you don't have the money for an item now, don't buy it on credit and expect to pay for it later. If you want to buy a pricey item or take a trip, create a savings plan.

Alternative Stress Management Techniques

Popular stress fighters include visualization, hypnosis, massage therapy, meditation, and biofeedback.

Visualization Often it is our own thoughts and imagination that provoke distress by conjuring up worst-case scenarios and exaggerating the significance of situations. Our imagination, however, can be an asset as well as a liability. **Visualization,** or the creation of mental scenes, works by engaging one's imagination of the physical senses of sight, sound, smell, taste, and feel to replace stressful stimuli with peaceful or pleasurable thoughts. The choice of mental images is unlimited, but natural settings such as ocean beaches and mountain lakes are often used because they simulate vacation locations where people typically go to escape the stress of home, school, or work environments. So the next time you are feeling stressed, close your eyes, imagine yourself at some tranquil location full of color, fresh air, soothing sounds, and other elements of nature, and take a mini mental vacation to allow your mind and body a chance to unwind.

Massage Therapy If you have ever had someone massage your stiff neck or aching feet, you know that massage is an excellent way to relax. Massage techniques vary from vigorous Swedish massage to the gentler acupressure and Esalen massage.

Before selecting a massage therapist, check his or her credentials carefully. The therapist should have training from a reputable program that teaches scientific principles for anatomic manipulation and should be certified through the American Massage Therapy Association. Chapter 17 provides more information about the benefits of massage as well as other body-based methods, such as acupressure and shiatsu.

Meditation There are many different forms of **meditation.** Most involve sitting quietly for 15 to 20 minutes, focusing on a particular word or symbol, controlling breathing, and getting in touch with the inner self. Practiced by Eastern religions for centuries, meditation is believed to be an important form of introspection and personal renewal. As a stress management tool, it can calm the body and quiet the mind, creating a sense of peace.

Biofeedback **Biofeedback** involves self-monitoring, by machine, of physical responses to stress and attempts to control these responses. The machine may record perspiration, heart rate, respiration rate, blood pressure, surface body temperature, muscle tension, or other stress responses. Various relaxation techniques are employed while the person is hooked up to a biofeedback machine and, through trial and error and signals from the machine, the person learns to lower the stress response. Eventually, the person develops the ability to recognize and lower stress responses without using the machine.

Developing Your Spiritual Side: Mindfulness

In discussions of spirituality, the concept of mindfulness often emerges. As a meditative technique, **mindfulness**—the ability to be fully present in the moment—can aid relaxation; reduce emotional and physical pain; and help us connect more effectively with ourselves, with others, and with nature.[54] The practice of mindfulness includes strategies and activities that contribute to overall health and wellness. In fact, mindfulness and wellness are interconnected and can be developed concurrently, each reinforcing the other. In addition to the themes of spirituality discussed in Chapter 2, we can think of spirituality as encompassing four dimensions: physical, emotional, social, and intellectual.

The Physical Dimension: Moving in Nature

Want an enjoyable way to strengthen your body, build endurance, and bring peace of mind? Interact with the natural environment. Activities such as walking, jogging,

visualization   The creation of mental images to promote relaxation.

meditation   A relaxation technique that involves deep breathing and concentration.

biofeedback   A technique that involves using a machine to self-monitor physical responses to stress.

mindfulness   The ability to be fully present in the moment.

biking, and swimming foster this interaction, providing sensory experience (feeling, smelling, touching, listening, and hearing) while strengthening muscles and the cardiovascular system. Appreciating and absorbing the beauty of nature allow us to unwind emotionally even as our bodies are at work. Our relationship with the earth and our natural environment is as important as our relationship to the people in our lives.

The Emotional Dimension: Dealing with Negative Feelings

Each of us has positive and negative emotions that govern moods and behaviors throughout the day. We often take joy, happiness, and contentment for granted, because we tend not to notice the *absence* of stress and distress. However, we typically are aware of negative emotions, such as jealousy, hatred, and anger, because they deplete our energy reserves and cause us problems in interacting with others.

To improve our emotional health and access our spiritual side, we must take notice of the situations that trigger negative emotions. By stopping in the midst of anger and concentrating on physical reactions, we realize the full extent of the damage we inflict on ourselves when we allow negativity to get the best of us. We might ask ourselves, "Is it worth it?" And probably we will conclude: "I don't like allowing this kind of hit on my body. I've got to get a handle on this before I hurt myself or someone else." By practicing thought-stopping, blocking negative thoughts, and focusing on positive emotions via self-talk and other methods of diversion, we can help ourselves through a negative experience.

Just as important as controlling negative emotions is developing spiritual wholeness characterized by faith, hope, and love, the beliefs mentioned in Chapter 2. These beliefs contribute to spiritual growth and also lessen the negative effects of stress.

The Social Dimension: Interacting, Listening, and Communicating

Developing the spiritual side is not just an internal process. It is also a social process that enhances relationships with others. The ability to give and take, speak and listen, forgive and move on are all integral to spiritual development.

Today, life is busier than ever. While we are constantly juggling responsibilities, it is easy to get so caught up in the stresses of our own lives that we find it difficult to give to others. Being too self-enmeshed can affect relationships and the ability to communicate with others. Communication is a two-way process in which listening is every bit as important as speaking. The ability to *listen actively* is a potent asset. Active listeners take note of content, intent, and feelings being expressed. They listen to all levels of the communication. Sensitivity and honesty are also essential to the give-and-take of communication. Ask questions, rephrase the speaker's ideas, and focus genuine attention on the speaker. Through such active participation, you gain a greater insight into the other person, who in turn will be encouraged to share more. Sharing becomes more intimate and relationships more connected when people feel that others care and are genuinely interested in their well-being. Both parties benefit from such an interchange. For more on communication, see Chapter 5.

The Intellectual Dimension: Sharpening Intuition

Take the time to assess events in life, their causes, and your own involvement in them. This often involves putting aside the emotional dimension for a moment to reflect, read, and ponder. Sometimes this process leads to startling new insights. Such moments mean so much, but few people include this mental activity in daily rituals. Examining the past, how we've gotten to where we are in the present, and what actions might have changed the course of events is a critical element of spiritual growth. By using our minds for objective reasoning, we develop the intellectual dimension of spiritual health.

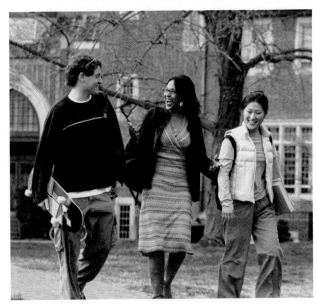

Spending time with friends is an important part of stress reduction.

TAKING charge

Summary

- Stress is an inevitable part of our lives. *Eustress* refers to stress associated with positive events, *distress* to negative events.
- The alarm, resistance, and exhaustion phases of the general adaptation syndrome involve physiological responses to both real and imagined stressors and cause a complex cascade of hormones to rush through the body. Prolonged arousal due to stress may be detrimental to health.
- Undue stress for extended periods of time can compromise the immune system and result in serious health consequences. Psychoneuroimmunology is the science that analyzes the relationship between the mind's reaction to stress and the function of the immune system. Although increasing evidence links disease susceptibility to stress, much of this research remains controversial. However, stress has been linked to numerous health problems, including CVD, diabetes, cancer, and increased susceptibility to infectious diseases.
- Multiple factors contribute to stress and the stress response. Psychosocial factors include change, hassles, pressure, inconsistent goals and behaviors, conflict, overload, and burnout. Other factors are environmental stressors and self-imposed stress. Persons subjected to discrimination or bias due to "-isms" may face unusually high levels of stress.
- College can be especially stressful. Recognizing the signs of stress is the first step toward better health. Learning to reduce test anxiety and cope with multiple stressors is also important.
- Managing stress begins with learning simple coping mechanisms: assessing stressors, changing responses, and learning to cope. Finding out what works best for you—probably some combination of managing emotional responses, taking mental or physical action, downshifting, learning time management, or using alternative stress management techniques—will help you better cope with stress in the long run.
- Developing the spiritual side involves practicing mindfulness and its many dimensions. These include the physical dimension (moving in nature); the emotional dimension (identifying and controlling negative feelings); the social dimension (interacting, listening, and communicating); and the intellectual dimension (sharpening intuition).

Chapter Review

1. Even though André experienced stress when he graduated from college and moved to a new city, he viewed these changes as an opportunity for growth. What is André's stress called?
   a. strain
   b. distress
   c. eustress
   d. adaptive response

2. The branch of the autonomic nervous system that is responsible for energizing the body for either fight or flight and for triggering many other stress responses is the
   a. central nervous system.
   b. parasympathetic nervous system.
   c. sympathetic nervous system.
   d. endocrine system.

3. During what phase of the general adaptation syndrome has the physical and psychological energy used to fight the stressors been depleted?
   a. alarm phase
   b. resistance phase
   c. endurance phase
   d. exhaustion phase

4. A state of physical and mental exhaustion caused by excessive stress is called
   a. conflict.
   b. overload.
   c. hassles.
   d. burnout.

5. Losing your keys is an example of what psychosocial source of stress?
   a. pressure
   b. inconsistent behaviors
   c. hassles
   d. conflict

6. After 5 years of 70-hour work weeks, Tom decided to leave his high-paying, high-stress law firm and lead a simpler lifestyle. What is this trend called?
   a. adaptation
   b. conflict resolution
   c. burnout reduction
   d. downshifting

7. Which of the following test-taking techniques is *not* recommended to reduce test-taking stress?
   a. Plan ahead and study over a period of time for the test.
   b. Take regular breaks to refresh the over stimulated brain.
   c. Do all of the studying the night before the exam so it is fresh in your mind.
   d. Practice by testing yourself with other classmates' sample test questions.

8. Which of the following is *not* an example of a time management technique?
   a. scheduling one's time with a calendar or day planner
   b. identifying time robbers
   c. practicing procrastination in completing homework assignments
   d. developing a game plan

9. Which of the following is an example of a chronic stressor?
   a. giving a talk in public
   b. meeting a deadline for a big project
   c. dealing with a permanent disability
   d. death of a family member or close friend

10. In which stage in the general adaptation syndrome does the fight-or-flight response occur?
    a. the exhaustion stage
    b. the alarm stage
    c. the resistance stage
    d. the response stage

Answers to these questions can be found on page A-1.

Questions for Discussion and Reflection

1. Describe the alarm, resistance, and exhaustion phases of the general adaptation syndrome and the body's physiological response to stress. Does stress lead to more irritability or emotionality, or does emotionality lead to stress? Provide examples.
2. What are some of the health risks that result from chronic stress? How does the study of psychoneuroimmunology link stress and illness?
3. Why are some students more vulnerable to stress than others? What services are available on your campus to help you deal with excessive stress?
4. What can college students do to inoculate themselves against negative stress effects? What actions can you take to manage your stressors? How can you help others manage their stressors more effectively?
5. How does anger affect the body? Discuss the steps you can take to manage your own anger and help your friends control theirs.
6. What can you do to develop the dimensions of spirituality in your life? How can you apply the social dimension of spirituality to your current relationships?

Accessing Your Health on the Internet

The following websites explore further topics and issues related to personal health. For links to the websites below, visit the Companion Website for *Health: The Basics,* Eighth Edition at www.aw-bc.com/donatelle.

1. *American College Counseling Association.* The website of the professional organization for college counselors; offers useful links and articles. www.collegecounseling.org
2. *American College Health Association.* Provides information and data from the National College Health Assessment survey. www.acha.org
3. *American Psychological Association.* Current information and research on stress and stress-related conditions. www.apa.org/topics/topicstress.html
4. *National Institute of Occupational Safety and Health.* Excellent source for information and resources on workplace stress. www.cdc.gov/niosh/topics/stress
5. *National Institute of Mental Health.* A resource for information on all aspects of mental health, including the effects of stress. www.nimh.nih.gov

Further Reading

Blonna, R. *Coping with Stress in a Changing World*, 4th ed. New York: McGraw-Hill, 2007.

A comprehensive overview of current perspectives on stress and stress management across the life span.

Romas, J. A., and M. Sharma. *Practical Stress Management,* 4th ed. San Francisco: Benjamin Cummings, 2007.

An accessible text that combines theory and principles with hands-on exercises to manage stress. Includes an audio CD with guided relaxation techniques, such as progressive muscle relaxation, deep breathing, and visual imaging.

Seaward, B. *Managing Stress: Principles and Strategies for Health and Well-Being,* 5th ed. Sudbury, MA: Jones and Bartlett, 2006.

Spirituality and stress expert provides complete overview of stress and health effects, as well as strategies for reducing risk.

The New York Times

e-themes from *The New York Times*

For up-to-date articles about current health issues, visit www.aw-bc.com/donatelle, select *Health: The Basics,* Eighth Edition, Chapter 3, and click on "e-themes."

References

1. L. J. Sax et al., *The American Freshman: National Norms for Fall 2004* (Los Angeles: Higher Education Research Institute, 2005).
2. B. Seaward, *Managing Stress: Principles and Strategies for Health and Well-Being,* 5th ed. (Sudbury, MA: Jones and Bartlett, 2006), 3.
3. W. B. Cannon, *The Wisdom of the Body* (New York: W. W. Norton, 1932).
4. H. Selye, *Stress without Distress* (New York: Lippincott, 1974), 28–29.
5. B. S. McEwen, "Mood Disorders and Allostatic Load," *Biological Psychiatry* 54 (2003): 200–207.
6. A. Mokdad et al., "Actual Causes of Death in the United States 2000," *Journal of the American Medical Association* 291 (2004): 1238–45.
7. S. Das and J. H. O'Keffe, "Behavioral Cardiology: Recognizing and Addressing the Profound Impact of Psychosocial Stress on Cardio-vascular Health," *Current Atherosclerosis Reports* 8, no. 2 (2006): 111–18; A. K. Ferketich and P. F. Binkley, "Psychological Distress and Cardiovascular Disease: Results from the 2002 National Health Interview Study," *European Heart Journal* 26, no. 18 (2005): 1923–29.
8. S. Yusef et al., "Effect of Potentially Modifiable Risk Factors Associated with Myocardial Infarction in 52 Countries (The INTERHEART Study): Case-Control Study," *The Lancet* 364, no. 9438 (2004): 937–52.
9. Ferketich and Binkley, "Psychological Distress and Cardiovascular Disease," 1923–29.
10. J. R. Hapuarachchi et al., "Changes in Clinically Relevant Metabolites with Psychological Stress Parameters," *Behavioral Medicine* 29 (2003): 52–60; C. N. Merz et al., "Psychosocial Stress and Cardiovascular Disease: Pathophysiological Links," *Behavioral Medicine* 27 (2002): 141–48; S. Das and J. H. O'Keffe, "Behavioral Cardiology," 111–18.
11. S. A. Everson-Rose and T. T. Lewis, "Psychosocial Risk Factors and Cardiovascular Disease," *Annual Review of Public Health* 26 (2005): 469–500.
12. S. C. Segerstrom and G. E. Miller, "Psychological Stress and the Human Immune System," *Psychological Bulletin* 130, no. 4 (2004): 601–30.
13. E. M. Reiche et al., "Stress, Depression, the Immune System, and Cancer," *The Lancet Oncology* 5, no. 10 (2004): 617–25; Segerstrom and Miller, "Psychological Stress and the Human Immune System," 601–30.
14. Segerstrom and Miller, "Psychological Stress and the Human Immune System," 601–30.
15. S. Cohen, keynote presentation at the Eighth International Congress of Behavioral Medicine: "The Pittsburgh Common Cold Studies: Psychosocial Predictors of Susceptibility to Respiratory Illness," *International Journal of Behavioral Medicine* 12, no. 3 (2005): 123–31; S. Cohen et al., "Reactivity and Vulnerability to Stress-Associated Risk for Upper Respiratory Illness," *Psychosomatic Medicine* 64 (2002): 302–10; B. Takkouche et al., "A Cohort Study of Stress and the Common Cold," *Epidemiology* 12, no. 3 (2001): 345–49.
16. S. D. Pressman et al., "Loneliness, Social Network Size, and Immune Responses to Influenza Vaccinations in College Freshman," *Health Psychology* 24, no. 3 (2005): 297–306.
17. E. R. Volkman and N. Y. Weekes, "Basal SigA and Cortisol Levels Predict Stress-Related Health Outcomes," *Stress and Health* 22 (2006): 11–23.
18. E. V. Yang and R. Glaser, "Stress-Induced Immunomodulation and the Implications for Health," *International Immunopharmacology* 2 (2002): 315–24; R. Glaser, "Stress-Associated Immune Dysregulation and Its Importance for Human Health: A Personal History of Psychoneuroimmunology," *Brain, Behavior, and Immunity* 19 (2005): 3–11.
19. E. Shiloah and M. J. Rapoport, "Psychological Stress and New Onset Diabetes," *Pediatric Endocrinology Reviews* 3, no. 3 (2006): 272–75; American Diabetes Association, "Stress," 2004, www.diabetes.org/type-1-diabetes/stress.jsp.
20. R. Rosmond, "Role of Stress in the Pathogenesis of the Metabolic Syndrome," *Psychoneuroendocrinology* 30 (2005): 1–10.
21. M. Scollan-Koliopoulos, "Managing Stress Response to Control Hypertension in Type 2 Diabetes," *The Nurse Practitioner* 30, no. 2 (2005): 46–49.
22. D. A. Katerndahl and M. Parchman, "The Ability of the Stress Process Model to Explain Mental Health Outcomes," *Comprehensive Psychiatry* 43 (2002): 351–60; R. C. Kessler et al., "The Epidemiology of Major Depressive Disorder," *Journal of the American Medical Association* 289 (2003): 3095–3105.
23. R. L. Turner and D. A. Lloyd, "Stress Burden and the Lifetime Incidence of Psychiatric Disorder in Young Adults: Racial and Ethnic Contrasts," *Archives of General Psychiatry* 61 (2004): 481–488.
24. V. R. Wilburn and D. E. Smith, "Stress, Self-Esteem, and Suicidal Ideation in Late Adolescents," *Adolescence* 40 (2005): 33–46; A. Väänänen et al., "Sources of Social Support as Determinants of Psychiatric Morbidity After Severe Life Events: Prospective Cohort Study of Female Employees," *Journal of Psychosomatic Research* 58 (2005); 459–67.
25. T. Holmes and R. Rahe, "The Social Readjustment Rating Scale," *Journal of Psychosocial Research* (1967): 213–17; B. P. Dohrenwend, "Inventorying Stressful Life Events as Risk Factors for Psychopathology: Toward Resolution of the Problem of Intracategory Variability," *Psychological Bulletin* 132, no. 3 (2006): 477–95.

26. R. Lazarus, "The Trivialization of Distress," in *Preventing Health Risk Behaviors and Promoting Coping with Illness,* ed. J. Rosen and L. Solomon (Hanover, NH: University Press of New England, 1985), 279–98.

27. D. J. Maybery and D. Graham, "Hassles and Uplifts: Including Interpersonal Events," *Stress and Health* 17 (2001): 91–104; R. Blonna, *Coping with Stress in a Changing World,* 4th ed. (New York: McGraw-Hill, 2007).

28. L. Lefton, *Psychology,* 9th ed. (Boston: Allyn & Bacon, 2005).

29. C. L. Park, S. Armeli, and H. Tennen, "The Daily Stress and Coping Process and Alcohol Use Among College Students," *Journal of Studies on Alcohol* 65, no. 1 (2004): 126–30; B. E Miller et al., "Alcohol Misuse among College Athletes: Self-Medication for Psychiatric Symptoms?" *Journal of Drug Education* 32 (2002): 41–52.

30. J. M Peiró et al., "Does Role Stress Predict Burnout Over Time Among Health Care Professionals?" *Psychology and Health* 16 (2001): 511–25; S. Melamed et al., "Burnout and Risk of Cardiovascular Disease: Evidence, Possible Causal Paths, and Promising Research Directions," *Psychological Bulletin* 132, no. 3 (2006): 327–53.

31. T. LaVeist, *Minority Populations and Health: An Introduction to Health Disparities* (San Francisco: Jossey-Bass, 2006); T. Lewis, "Discrimination, Black Americans, and Health: Results of the SWAN Study," paper presented at the annual meeting of the American Heart Association, Washington, D.C., 2005.

32. K. J. Karren et al., *Mind/Body Health: The Effects of Attitudes, Emotions, and Relationships,* 3rd ed. (San Francisco: Benjamin Cummings, 2006).

33. Seaward, *Managing Stress;* Wilburn and Smith, "Stress, Self-Esteem, and Suicidal Ideation," 33–46.

34. Wilburn and Smith, "Stress, Self-Esteem, and Suicidal Ideation," 33–46; D. Robotham and C. Julian, "Stress and the Higher Education Student: A Critical Review of the Literature," *Journal of Further and Higher Education* 30, no. 2 (2006): 107–17.

35. K. Glanz, B. Rimer, and F. Levis, eds., *Health Behavior and Health Education: Theory, Research, and Practice,* 3rd ed. (San Francisco: Jossey-Bass, 2002).

36. A. D. Von et al., "Predictors of Health Behaviors in College Students," *Journal of Advanced Nursing* 48, no. 5 (2004): 463–74.

37. M. Friedman and R. H. Rosenman, *Type A Behavior and Your Heart* (New York: Knopf, 1974).

38. Karren et al., *Mind/Body Health.*

39. R. Niaura et al., "Hostility, Metabolic Syndrome, and Incident Coronary Heart Disease," *Health Psychology* 21, no. 6 (2002): 588–93.

40. S. Kobasa, "Stressful Life Events, Personality, and Health: An Inquiry into Hardiness," *Journal of Personality and Social Psychology* 37 (1979): 1–11.

41. B. J. Crowley, B. Hayslip, and J. Hobdy, "Psychological Hardiness and Adjustment to Life Events in Adulthood," *Journal of Adult Development* 10 (2003): 237–48; S. R. Maddi, "The Story of Hardiness: Twenty Years of Theorizing, Research, and Practice," *Consulting Psychology Journal: Practice and Research* 54 (2002): 173–86.

42. American College Health Association, *American College Health Association–National College Health Assessment: Reference Group Executive Summary—Spring 2005. Part C, Academic Impacts* (Baltimore: American College Health Association, 2005), www.acha.org/projects_programs/NCHA_docs/ACHANCHA _Reference_Group_ExecutiveSummary_Spring2005.pdf

43. J. H Pryor et al., *The American Freshman: National Norms for Fall 2005* (Los Angeles: Higher Education Research Institute, 2006).

44. M. E. Pritchard and G. S. Wilson, "Do Coping Styles Change During the First Semester of College?" *Journal of Social Psychology* 146, no. 1 (2006): 125–27; C. L. Broman, "Stress, Race, and Substance Use in College," *College Student Journal* 39, no. 2 (2005), 340–52; D. Kariv, D. Heilman, and T. Heilman, "Task-Oriented versus Emotion-Oriented Coping Strategies: The Case of College Students," *College Student Journal* 39, no. 1 (2005): 72–84; K. M. Kieffer et al., "Test and Study Worry and Emotionality in the Prediction of College Students' Reasons for Drinking: An Exploratory Investigation," *Journal of Alcohol and Drug Education* 50, no. 1 (2006): 57–81.

45. P. A. Bovier, E. Chamot, and T. V. Perneger, "Perceived Stress, Internal Resources, and Social Support as Determinants of Mental Health Among Young Adults," *Quality of Life Research* 13, no. 1 (2004): 161–70; E. Largo-Wright, P. M. Peterson, and W. W. Chen, "Perceived Problem Solving, Stress, and Health Among College Students," *American Journal of Health Behavior* 29, no. 4 (2005): 360–70; C. L. Park et al., "The Daily Stress and Coping Process and Alcohol Use Among College Students," *Journal of Studies on Alcohol* 65, no. 1 (2004): 126–35.

46. Bovier, Chamot, and Perneger, "Perceived Stress, Internal Resources, and Social Support," 161–70; A. DeLongis and S. Holtzman, "Coping in Context: The Role of Stress, Social Support, and Personality in Coping," *Journal of Personality* 73, no. 6 (2005): 1633–56.

47. Seaward, *Managing Stress.*

48. C. Hassed, "How Humor Keeps You Well," *Australian Family Physician* 30, no. 1 (2001): 25–28.

49. P. Holmes, "Managing Anger: Understanding the Dynamics of Violence, Abuse and Control," SIUC Mental Health Web Site, 2004, siu.edu/offices/counsel/anger.htm.

50. Ibid.

51. D. A. Girdano, D. E. Dusek, and G. S. Everly, *Controlling Stress and Tension,* 7th ed. (San Francisco: Benjamin Cummings, 2005), 371.

52. Higher Education Research Institute (HERI), *The American Freshman, National Norms for 2006,* www.gseis.ucla.edu/heri/ norms06.php.

53. B. Andrews and J. M. Wilding, "The Relations of Depression and Anxiety to Life-Stress and Achievement in Students," *British Journal of Psychology* 95 (2004): 509–21; J. M. Norvilitis et al., "Personality Factors, Money Attitudes, Financial Knowledge, and Credit-Card Debt in College Students," *Journal of Applied Social Psychology* 36, no. 6 (2006): 1395–1413.

54. N. B. Allen, R. Chambers, and W. Knight, "Mindfulness-Based Psychotherapies: A Review of Conceptual Foundations, Empirical Evidence, and Practical Considerations," *Australian and New Zealand Journal of Psychiatry* 40 (2006): 285–94.

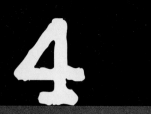

Preventing Violence and Abuse

CREATING HEALTHY ENVIRONMENTS

Is **America** really more violent than other countries?

Is there anything I can do to **protect** myself from terrorism?

Are men ever **victims** of domestic violence?

What can I do if I think I am being **stalked?**

OBJECTIVES

- Dicuss factors that contribute to homicide, domestic violence, sexual victimization, and other intentional acts of violence.
- Explain how terrorism can affect individuals and populations, and summarize practical steps to lower your risk from terrorist attacks.
- Discuss strategies to prevent intentional injuries and reduce their risk of occurrence.
- Explain potential risks to students on campus and potential strategies that campus leaders, law enforcement officials, and individuals can develop to prevent students from becoming victims.

Across the land, waves of violence seem to crest and break, terrorizing Americans in cities and suburbs, in prairie towns, and mountain hollows.

To millions of Americans few things are more pervasive, more frightening, more real today than violent crime. . . . The fear of being victimized by criminal attack has touched us all in some way.

Among urban children ages 10–14, homicides are up 150 percent, robberies are up 192 percent, assaults are up 290 percent.

You might think these are statements from today's newspapers or television news. They're not. The first quotation comes from President Herbert Hoover's 1929 inauguration speech, the second from the 1860 Senate report on crime, and the third from a 1967 report on children's violence.[1] Clearly, violence has been a part of U.S. history since our country's early days.

The term **violence** indicates a set of behaviors that produce injuries, either **intentional injuries** (committed with intent to harm) or **unintentional injuries** (committed without intent to harm, often accidentally), as well as the outcome of these behaviors. In this chapter, we focus on the various types of violence, the underlying causes of or contributors to these problems, strategies to reduce risk of encountering violence, and possible methods to prevent violence. Although certain indicators of violence, such as murders and deadly assaults, seem to be on the decline, other forms of violence, such as rape, suicide, and hate crimes, are on the increase. Even more important is that, despite all we know about the incidence and prevalence of violence, a great deal remains unknown. Just how many people suffer in silence, failing to report violent acts because of fear of repercussions or because they accept violence as part of life, remains unknown.

Violence in the United States

Although violence has long been a concern in American society, not until 1985 did the U.S. Public Health Service formally identify violence as a leading public health problem that contributes significantly to death and disability rates. The Centers for Disease Control and Prevention (CDC) created the Division of Violence Prevention and considers violence a *chronic disease that is pervasive at all levels of American society.* Vulnerable populations, such as children, women, African American men, and older adults, are identified as being at high risk for certain types of crime. Older teens and young adults have the highest rates of violent crime, both as victims and as offenders.[2]

Since 1973, statistics from the Federal Bureau of Investigation (FBI) had shown that, overall, crime and certain types of violent crime have decreased each year. However, between

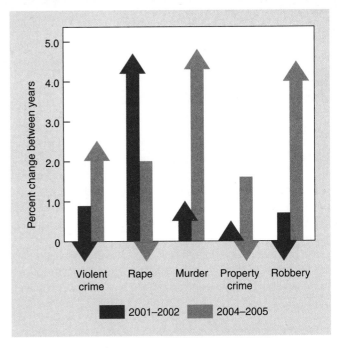

FIGURE 4.1 Changes in Violent Crime Rates, 2001–2002 and 2004–2005

Source: Federal Bureau of Investigation, "Preliminary Uniform Crime Report," 2005, Table 3: Percent Change for Consecutive Years, June 12, 2006, www.fbi.gov.ucr/2005preliminary.

January and June 2006, violent crime was up by 3.7 percent when compared to the same period in 2005 in all major regions of the country. Robbery increased dramatically; up by almost 13 percent in cities with populations of 10,000 to 25,000. Murders were up nationally, particularly in larger cities of 500,000 to 1 million residents, where rates soared by over 8 percent. Aggravated assaults were also up in 2005; overall rates of violent crime actually increased by 2.5 percent overall, and murder specifically increased by nearly 5 percent in 2005 over the previous year **(Figure 4.1).**[3]

Is crime an issue on college campuses? Specific crime rates vary tremendously from region to region across the United States, and over the years data have indicated that college campuses are not immune. However, many people question the accuracy of such campus crime reports because petty theft, date rape, fighting, and other common campus incidents are not always reported to police. Some people also criticize campus administrators' reluctance to report incidents

violence A set of behaviors that produce injuries, as well as the outcomes of these behaviors (the injuries themselves).

intentional injuries Injuries committed on purpose with intent to harm.

unintentional injuries Injuries committed without intent to harm.

Any definition of violence implicitly includes the use of force, regardless of the intent; however, it is important to realize that some forms of violence are unintentional. Unintentional injuries, injuries that occur without planning or intending to harm, are the fifth leading cause of death in America today. They include a variety of accidental deaths from automobile crashes and sporting events, accidental shootings, drownings, and so on—often situations where drinking and risk taking are involved. Accidents are the leading cause of death in the United States for young adults aged 15 to 24. Most efforts to prevent unintentional injuries and accidental deaths focus on changing something about the person, the environment, or the circumstances (policies, procedures) that put people in harm's way. You can learn how to avoid these types of injuries in Chapter 8, which addresses the prevention of alcohol abuse and subsequent injuries, and in the Injury Prevention and Emergency Care section within the Health Resources section at the back of this text.

Source: Centers for Disease Control and Prevention, "Leading Causes of Death by Age, Sex and Race," *Health—United States, 2006,* www.cdc.gov/nchs/hus.htm.

---

due to concerns over reputation and other difficulties that could affect overall enrollment. Most schools are intensely aware, though, of the potential for violent crime on campus, especially given the high stress prevalent in this environment, where alcohol often plays a role. For this reason, schools do take steps to protect students. It is important to note that 70.8 percent of all deaths among persons aged 10 to 24 have violent elements and stem from just four causes: motor vehicle crashes (particularly where alcohol is involved), other unintentional injuries, homicide, and suicide.[4]

Why should we be concerned about a violence-prone society? Violence affects everyone, directly or indirectly. Although the direct victims of violence and those close to them obviously suffer the most, others suffer in various ways because of the climate of fear that violence generates.

> **Is America really more violent than other countries?**

Women are afraid to walk alone at night. Older people are often afraid to go out even in the daytime. After terrorist episodes such as the 2001 World Trade Center attack and the Madrid and London subway attacks, some people are afraid to fly, use mass transit, work in tall buildings, or travel to popular international destinations. The cost of homeland security is staggering.

You might be surprised to learn that international travelers often fear coming to the United States in much the same way that some Americans fear traveling to other regions of the world where attacks on U.S. citizens have taken place. Tourists from foreign countries are afraid of being brutalized in many of our nation's cities, and they worry about being caught in the crosshairs of gang violence or other forms of violent assault or robbery. Many of these reports are carried in the international news media, depicting the United States as a violent nation. Even people who live in supposedly safe areas can become victims of violence within their own homes or at the hands of family members. Statistics on total crime and homicides in different nations of the world can be found at www.nationmaster.com/cat/cri-crime.

Societal Causes of Violence

Several social, cultural, and individual factors increase the likelihood of violent acts:[5]

- *Poverty.* Low socioeconomic status and poor living conditions can create an environment of hopelessness; people view violence as the only way to obtain what they want.
- *Unemployment.* It is a well-documented fact that when the economy goes sour, violent and nonviolent crimes increase.
- *Parental influence.* Children raised in environments in which shouting, hitting, and other forms of violence are commonplace are more apt to act out these behaviors as adults. Recent research has substantiated this cycle of violence.
- *Cultural beliefs.* Cultures that objectify women and empower men to be tough and aggressive show higher rates of violence in the home.
- *The media.* A daily dose of murder and mayhem can take a toll on even resistant minds.
- *Discrimination or oppression.* Whenever one group is oppressed or perceives that its members are oppressed by those of another group, seeds of discontent are sown, and violence against others is more likely.
- *Religious beliefs and differences.* Religious persecution has been a part of the human experience since earliest times. Strong beliefs can lead people to think violence against others is justified by religious doctrine. Such beliefs also foster martyrdom, often expressed in such actions as suicide bombings.

- *Political differences.* Civil unrest and differences in political party affiliations and beliefs have historically been triggers for violent acts.
- *Breakdowns in the criminal justice system.* Overcrowded prisons, lenient sentences, early releases from prison, and trial errors subtly encourage violence in a number of ways.
- *Stress.* People who are in crisis or under stress are more apt to be highly reactive, striking out at others or acting irrationally.
- *Heavy use of alcohol and other substances.* Alcohol and drug abuse are often catalysts for violence and other crimes.[6]

In addition to these broad, societally based factors, many personal factors also can lead to violence.[7]

what do you THINK?

Why do you think rates of violence in the United States are so much higher than that of other nations, such as Great Britain and Japan? ■ How do you react when you note that a country has particularly high or low rates of various types of crime? ■ What actions can each of the following do to lower risks from crime: National governments? Communities? Campus administrators? Individuals?

Personal Precipitators of Violence

We as a nation are often shocked by the unanticipated violence of incidents such as the April 2007 massacre at Virginia Tech. Even so, we must realize that individuals do not suddenly become violent without any cause or precursors. Many factors contribute to the eventual violent acts. How they learn to respond to frustration, how others around them cope, how they learn to perceive the events around them, their self-esteem, and a host of other life experiences lead people to act in the ways that they do. Also, societal rules and cultural background influences certain behaviors. Usually, you learn behavior that is appropriate and inappropriate from a very young age. If you are like most people, you probably acted out your anger more readily as a child than you do today. With increasing maturity, most people learn to control outbursts of anger in a socially acceptable and rational manner. However, some people go through life acting out their aggressive tendencies in much the same ways they did as children or as their families did. Why do two children from the same neighborhood, or even from the same family, go in different directions when it comes to violence? There are several predictors of future aggressive behavior.[8]

Anger

Anger is a spontaneous, usually temporary, biological feeling or emotional state of displeasure that occurs most frequently during times of personal frustration. Because life is stressful, anger becomes a part of daily experience. Anger can range from slight irritation to *rage,* a violent and extreme form of anger. When a person acts out on his or her rage at home or on the road, the consequences can be deadly.

What makes some people flare up at the slightest provocation? Often, people who are quick to anger have a low tolerance for frustration, believing that they should not have to put up with inconvenience or petty annoyances. They feel entitled and seek instant gratification. The cause may be genetic or physiological; there is evidence that some people are born unstable, touchy, or easily angered. Another cause of anger is sociocultural. People who are taught not to express anger in public do not know how to handle it when it reaches a level where they can no longer hide it. Family background may be the most important factor. Typically, anger-prone people come from families that are disruptive, chaotic, and unskilled in emotional expression.[9]

Aggressive behavior is often a key aspect of violent interactions. **Primary aggression** is goal-directed, hostile self-assertion that is destructive in nature. **Reactive aggression** is more often part of an emotional reaction brought about by frustrating life experiences. Whether aggression is reactive or primary, it is most likely to flare up in times of acute stress, during relationship difficulties or loss, or when a person is so frustrated that he or she feels the only recourse is to strike out at others.

what do you THINK?

Think of two examples where you or a loved one became very angry over some life event. If the setting for the anger had been different, do you think the anger event would have been different? Why? ■ What factors make people more likely to "act out" their anger? ■ What is an example of an appropriate way to deal with frustration or anger? ■ Is anger ever justified?

Substance Abuse

Much has been written about a link between substance abuse and violence. In fact, drinking is a major contributor to the fifth leading cause of death in America today: accidents—particularly auto accidents. Substance abuse is

---

primary aggression Goal-directed, hostile self-assertion that is destructive in character.

reactive aggression Emotional reaction brought about by frustrating life experiences.

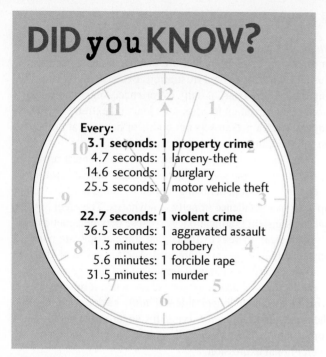

DID you KNOW?

Every:
3.1 seconds: 1 property crime
4.7 seconds: 1 larceny-theft
14.6 seconds: 1 burglary
25.5 seconds: 1 motor vehicle theft

22.7 seconds: 1 violent crime
36.5 seconds: 1 aggravated assault
1.3 minutes: 1 robbery
5.6 minutes: 1 forcible rape
31.5 minutes: 1 murder

Source: Federal Bureau of Investigation, "Crime in the United States," 2005, www.fbi.gov/ucr/05cius/about/crime_clock.html.

also linked to many other forms of violence, even though we have yet to show that substance abuse actually causes violence. In fact, many violent episodes are carefully planned actions that involve no alcohol or drug abuse. In some situations, however, psychoactive substances appear to be a form of ignition for violence:[10]

■ Consumption of alcohol—by perpetrators of the crime, the victim, or both—immediately preceded over half of all violent crimes, including murder.
■ Chronic drinkers are more likely than others to have histories of violent behavior.
■ Criminals using illegal drugs commit robberies and assaults more frequently than nonusing criminals and do so especially during periods of heavy drug use.
■ In domestic assault cases, more than 86 percent of the assailants and 42 percent of victims reported using alcohol at the time of the attack. Nearly 15 percent of victims and assailants reported using cocaine at the time of the attack.
■ 92 percent of assailants and 42 percent of victims reported using alcohol or other drugs on the day of the assault.
■ Mentally ill patients who fail to adhere to prescription drug regimens and abuse alcohol and/or other drugs are significantly more likely to be involved in a serious violent act.
■ Substance abuse markedly increases the risk of both homicide and suicide. Problems at work due to drinking, hospitalization for a drinking problem, use of illicit drugs, and

homicide Death that results from intent to injure or kill.

arrest for use of illicit drugs all place subjects at risk for violent death by homicide. The combination of depression and alcohol or other drugs increases homicide and suicide rates threefold.

Intentional Injuries

Any time someone sets out to harm other people or their property, the incident may be referred to as *intentional* violence. Though nonviolent crime is more common, violent crime occurs all too often. The resulting intentional injuries cause pain and suffering at the very least, and death and disability at the worst.

Gratuitous Violence

Violence can manifest itself in many ways. Often the most gratuitous and shocking crimes gain the greatest attention, such as stories of innocent victims of drive-by shootings or situations like the Columbine and Virginia Tech shootings, where young students turn their rage on family, classmates, and teachers. Many people question whether the major network coverage of these events actually makes would-be assailants more likely to act in ways that may give them a moment of fame. Mass shootings capture our national attention, even though every day in the United States and throughout other regions of the world, people die in large numbers at the hands of others.

Homicide **Homicide,** defined as murder or non-negligent manslaughter, is the 15th leading cause of death in the United States, but the second leading cause of death for persons aged 15 to 24.[11] It accounts for nearly 18,000 premature deaths in the United States annually.[12] Homicide rates reveal particularly clear disparities among races. For an American, the average lifetime probability of being murdered is 1 in 153—but this average masks large differences for specific segments of the population. Asian/Pacific Islanders, Hispanic or Latino, and African American groups all list homicide among the top ten causes of death, but homicide is not among the top ten killers of white Americans. Homicide rates for African American men are higher than those for any other group.[13] For African American men of any age, the risk of murder is 1 in 28; for a black man aged 20 to 22 years the risk is 1 in 3.

Most homicides are not random acts of violence. Over half of all homicides occur among people who know one another. In two-thirds of these cases, the perpetrator and the victim are friends or acquaintances; in one-third, they belong to the same family.[14]

Bias and Hate Crimes A hate or bias crime is a crime committed against a person, property, or a group of people that is motivated by the offender's bias against a race, religion, disability, sexual orientation, or ethnicity.[15] In spite of national efforts in workplaces, schools, and communities to promote understanding and diversity-related appreciation, intolerance of differences continues to smolder in many parts of U.S. society. The 2002 murder of Gwen Araujo, a transgendered teen in California, and arson attacks on Alabama churches in 2006 remind Americans that violence based on sexuality, race, and other "-isms" still occurs. International terrorist acts often reflect the hatred of one religious or political group toward another. Recent acts of violence by police against different racial groups, racially motivated gang beatings in public schools and on the streets, and other hate crimes are common events on the nightly news. According to the Federal Bureau of Investigation's most recent Hate Crime Statistics Report, 7,163 bias-motivated crimes were reported in 2005 (**Figure 4.2**).[16]

Since the 2001 terrorist attacks in the United States and the conflicts in Iraq and Afghanistan, reports of hate-related incidents, beatings, and other physical and verbal assaults have escalated. In particular, persons of Muslim or Middle-Eastern descent reported civil rights violations at work, in mass transit, and in communities throughout the United States. Many believe that the reported incidents are only the tip of the iceberg and that actual numbers of bias- or hate-related crimes are much higher because people do not report them out of fear of possible retaliation.

Hate crimes vary along two dimensions: (1) the way they are carried out and (2) their effects on victims. Vicious gossip, nasty comments, and devilish pranks may not make headlines, but they can hurt nonetheless. Generally, about 30 percent of all hate crimes are against property, and the other 70 percent are against the person. Recent studies have identified three additional characteristics of hate crimes:[17]

- Excessively brutal
- Perpetrated at random on total strangers
- Perpetrated by multiple offenders

In addition, the perpetrators tend to be motivated by thrill, defensive feelings, or a hate-mongering mission.

Academic settings are not immune to hatred and bias. Campuses have responded to reports of hate crimes by offering courses that emphasize diversity, training faculty appropriately, and developing policies that strictly enforce punishment for hate crimes.[18] Sadly, many minor assaults do go unreported because the victims fear retaliation or continued stigmatization for being different; underreporting is a major impediment to reducing the rate of hate crimes on campus.

The tendency toward violent acts on campus might best be defined as campus **ethnoviolence,** a term that describes violence among groups in the larger society that is based on prejudice and discrimination. Although ethnoviolence often is directed randomly at persons affiliated with a particular group, the group itself is specifically targeted apart from other people, and that differentiation is usually ethnic in nature. Typically, the perpetrators agree that the group is an acceptable target, and amid fears of terrorism and war, this type of violence may increase.

Prejudice and discrimination are always at the base of ethnoviolence. **Prejudice** is a set of negative attitudes toward a group of people. To say that a person is prejudiced against some group is to say that the person holds a set of beliefs about the group, has an emotional reaction to the

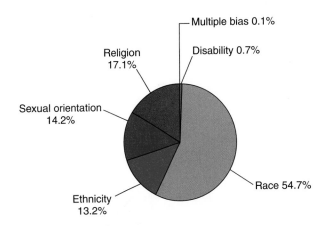

FIGURE 4.2 Bias-Motivated Crimes, 2005

Source: Federal Bureau of Investigation, "Hate Crime Statistics," 2005, www.fbi.gov/ucr/hc2005.

group, and is motivated to behave in a certain way toward the group. **Discrimination** constitutes actions that deny equal treatment or opportunities to a group of people, often based on prejudice.

Often intolerance stems from a fear of change and a desire to blame others when forces such as the economy and crime seem to be out of control. What can you do to be part of the solution rather than the problem?

- Support educational programs and campus groups that foster understanding and appreciation for differences in people. Many colleges now require diversity classes as part of their academic curriculum.
- Examine your own values, attitudes, and behaviors. Are you intolerant of others? Do you engage in racist, sexist, or similar behaviors meant to demean a group of individuals? Do you judge people on appearances? If you have problems with a particular group, why?
- Do you discourage hurtful jokes and other forms of social or ethnic bigotry? Do not participate in such behaviors, and express your dissatisfaction with those who do.
- Educate yourself. Read, interact with, and attempt to understand people who appear to be different from you. Remember that you do not have to like everything about them, but respecting people's right to be different is a part of being a healthy, integrated individual.
- Encourage your legislators to support legislation against hate and bias. Vote for those who support antidiscrimination policies and programs.

ethnoviolence Violence directed randomly at persons affiliated with a particular, usually ethnic, group.

prejudice A negative evaluation of an entire group of people that is typically based on unfavorable and often wrong ideas about the group.

discrimination Actions that deny equal treatment or opportunities to a group, often based on prejudice.

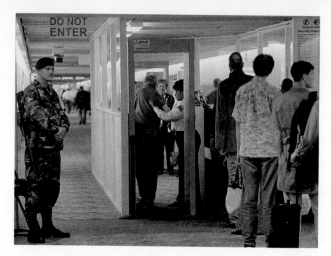

The threat of terrorism has affected many aspects of our daily lives.

? *what do you* THINK?

Think about the bias and hate crimes that you have heard about. Who were the victims? ▪ Did you know any of them? ▪ Why do you think people are motivated to initiate such crimes against strangers? ▪ What can you do to reduce the risk of such crimes in your area? ▪ What should be done nationally?

Gang Violence The growing influence of street gangs has had a harmful impact on our country, even though gang violence has not been highlighted in the popular media as often recently as it was some years ago. Drug abuse, gang shootings, beatings, thefts, carjackings, and the possibility of being caught in the crossfire have caused entire neighborhoods to be held hostage by gang members. Once thought to occur only in urban areas, gang violence now also appears in rural and suburban communities, particularly in southeastern, southwestern, and western states.

Why do young people join gangs? Although the reasons are complex, gangs seem to meet many of their needs. Gangs provide a sense of belonging to a family that gives them self-worth, companionship, security, and excitement. In other cases, gangs provide economic security through criminal activity, drug sales, or prostitution. Once young people become involved in the gang subculture, it is difficult for them to leave. Threats of violence or fear of not making it on their own dissuade even those who are most seriously trying to get out.

Who is at risk for gang membership? The age range of gang members is typically 12 to 22 years. Risk factors include low self-esteem, academic problems, low socioeconomic status, alienation from family and society, a history of family violence, and living in gang-controlled neighborhoods.[19]

Terrorism: Increased Risks from Multiple Sources

Not so long ago, Americans thought terrorism occurred only in distant cities, seldom amounting to more than a blip on the evening news. Since September 11, 2001, times have changed dramatically. Terrorist attacks on the World Trade Center and Pentagon revealed our nation's vulnerability to domestic and international threats. Today, the specter of a terrorist attack looms ever present. On national holidays or any other occasion where many Americans gather, we worry about a terrorist event.

According to the Code of Federal Regulations, **terrorism** is "the unlawful use of force or violence against persons or property to intimidate or coerce a government, the civilian population, or any segment thereof, in furtherance of political or social objectives."[20] Typically, terrorism is of two major types:

1. *Domestic terrorism,* which involves groups or individuals whose terrorist activities are directed at elements of our government or population without foreign direction
2. *International terrorism,* which involves groups or individuals whose terrorist activities are foreign-based, transcend national boundaries, and are directed by countries or groups outside the United States

Clearly, terrorist activities may have immediate impact in loss of lives and resources. However, the 2001 attacks also had far-reaching effects on the U.S. economy, airlines, and transportation systems. Perhaps most damaging in the aftermath of the attacks was the fear, anxiety, and altered behavior of countless Americans. How many people will fear working in skyscrapers for years to come? How many will fear climbing on a plane, crossing a bridge, or getting on the subway? Will worry about biological weapons and future terrorist attacks disrupt our lives and our interactions with others?

The CDC has a wide range of ongoing programs and services to help Americans respond to terrorist threats and prepare for possible attacks. Information is available on the CDC website and is updated regularly. A newer government entity, the Department of Homeland Security, has been established to prevent future attacks, and the FBI and other government agencies have also prepared a sweeping set of procedures and guidelines for ensuring citizen safety. Here are some things you can do to help reduce anxiety and harm related to terrorist attacks.

> Is there anything I can do to protect myself from terrorism?

▪ *Be aware of your own reactions to stress, anxiety, and fear.* Try to assess how much of your fear is justifiable in a given

---

terrorism The unlawful use of force or violence against persons or property to intimidate or coerce a government, the civilian population, or any segment thereof, in furtherance of political or social objectives.

situation and how much is a product of media sensationalism. Practice stress reduction techniques, determine the source of your stressors, and react as prudently as possible.

- *Be conscious of your surroundings.* If you notice suspicious activities or irregularities, report them to a person in authority. Being a passive observer and not speaking up when warranted may put you and others at risk.
- *Stay informed.* Try to stay on top of the news and understand the underlying roots of violent activity. Persistent poverty, pervasive religious or political fanaticism, and political situations that involve an imbalance of power can provide fodder for violent acts. Consider when self-righteous contempt for others may lead to persecution and violation of human rights. Be skeptical of acts perpetrated in the name of some cause, and intervene if possible to defuse violence.
- *Seek understanding.* Whenever two opposing groups stop engaging with each other mentally or communication breaks down, hatred, bigotry, and anger may result. Knowing about each other's customs, cultures, and beliefs and keeping the lines of communication open are good steps to avoid separation.
- *Seek information.* When political parties fight for power in election years, know your candidates. What are their underlying beliefs regarding national defense, spending for consumer protection, immigration policies, human rights violations, diversity issues, hate crimes, gun control, and so forth? Are they more aligned with one ideology than another? What is their stance on government interference and control, punishment of offenders, and other key issues?
- *Know what to do in an emergency.* Who would you call? How would you access local and regional assistance? Do you have the necessary provisions for basic survival—food, water, prescription medications, first aid? What happens when your electricity is off, your phone and communication systems are down, and your access to health care is limited?

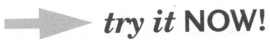 *try it* NOW!

Create an emergency plan. An emergency plan can make you feel more at ease and eliminate anxiety. Get together with your family, friends, or roommates and make a plan for emergencies such as natural disasters or terrorist attacks. Keep an emergency kit on hand containing several days' worth of food and water, flashlights, batteries, and even a small radio. Determine a meeting spot in case there are no phones or other ways to get in touch with each other.

Domestic Violence

In the 1970s a popular country-western song crooned, "No one knows what goes on behind closed doors." Domestic violence shows us just how true that refrain can be. **Domestic violence** refers to the use of force to control and maintain power over

another person in the home environment. It can occur between parent and child, between spouses, or between siblings and may involve emotional abuse, verbal abuse, threats of physical harm, and actual physical violence ranging from slapping and shoving to beatings, rape, and homicide. Today, domestic violence is at epidemic levels in America. It is the number-one cause of injury to women aged 15 to 44, and annually 2 to 4 million women are battered, 2,000 of whom are beaten to death.[21]

Women as Victims Although young men are more apt to become victims of violence from strangers, women are much more likely to become victims of violent acts perpetrated by spouses, lovers, ex-spouses, and ex-lovers. This aggression often includes pushing, slapping, and shoving, but it can take more severe forms. In reported assaults, only 31 percent of the men who attack women are "strangers." In fact, six of every ten women in the United States will be assaulted at some time in their lives by someone they know.[22] Every year, according to a national survey, approximately 12 percent of married women are the victims of physical aggression perpetrated by their husbands.[23]

On college campuses, relationship violence is a serious problem and includes emotional, physical, and sexual abuse. In the most recent American College Health Survey, 16 percent of women and 10 percent of men reported being emotionally abused in the last 12 months by a significant other. Nearly 5 percent of survey respondents reported physical abuse during this time period.[24] The following U.S. statistics indicate the seriousness of this long-hidden problem.[25]

- African American women aged 25 to 29 have 11 times the risk for being murdered while pregnant than white women of the same age.
- Homicide is the second leading cause of injury-related death among pregnant women and new mothers.
- Every 15 seconds, someone batters a woman; only 1 in every 250 such assaults is reported to the police.
- More than one-third of female victims of domestic violence are severely abused on a regular basis.
- About five women are killed every day in domestic violence incidents.

Although the ultimate result of these assaults can be murder, there are other devastating effects as well. Depression, panic attacks, disordered eating, chronic neck or back pain, migraine and other headaches, sexually transmitted infections, ulcers, and social isolation can all result from domestic violence.

How many times have you heard of a woman who is repeatedly beaten by her partner and wondered, "Why

domestic violence The use of force to control and maintain power over another person in the home environment, including both actual harm and the threat of harm.

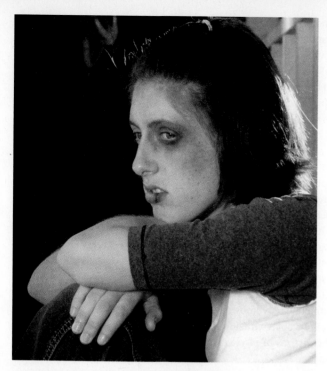

Despite obvious physical and psychological injury, it can be difficult for a person to leave an abusive partner.

doesn't she just leave him?" There are many reasons why some women find it difficult to break their ties with their abusers. Many women, particularly those with small children, are financially dependent on their partners. Others fear retaliation against themselves or their children. Some hope the situation will change with time (it rarely does), and others stay because cultural or religious beliefs forbid divorce. Finally, some women still love the abusive partner and are concerned about what will happen to him if they leave.

Psychologist Lenore Walker developed a theory known as the *cycle of violence* to explain how women can get caught in a downward spiral without realizing it.[26] The cycle has three phases:

1. *Tension building.* In this phase, minor battering occurs. To forestall further violence, the woman may become more nurturing, more pleasing, and more intent on anticipating the abuser's needs. She assumes guilt for doing something to provoke him and tries hard to avoid doing it again.

2. *Acute battering.* At this stage, pleasing her man doesn't help, and she can no longer control or predict the abuse. Usually, the spouse is trying to "teach her a lesson," and when he feels he has inflicted enough pain, he'll stop. When the acute attack is over, he may respond with shock and denial about his own behavior. Both batterer and victim may soft-pedal the seriousness of the attacks.

3. *Remorse/reconciliation.* During this "honeymoon" period, the batterer may be kind, loving, and apologetic, swearing he will never act violently again. He may

"behave" for several weeks or months, and the woman may come to question whether she overreacted. However, when the tension that precipitated past abuse resurfaces, the man beats her again. Unless some form of intervention breaks this downward cycle of abuse, contrition, further abuse, denial, and contrition, it will repeat itself again and again—perhaps ending only in the woman's (or, rarely, the man's) death.

Most women who get caught in this cycle (which may include forced sexual relations and psychological and economic abuse as well as beatings) find it very hard to summon the resolution to extricate themselves. Most need effective outside intervention.

Men as Victims Are men also victims of domestic violence? Some women do abuse and even kill their partners. The difference between male and female batterers is twofold. First, although the frequency of physical aggression may be similar, the impact is drastically different: women are injured in domestic incidents two to three times more often than men.[27] These injuries tend to be more severe and have resulted in significantly more deaths. Second, a woman who is physically abused by a man is generally intimidated by him: she fears that he will use his power and control over her in some fashion. Men, however, generally report that they do not live in fear of their wives.

> Are men ever victims of domestic violence?

Causes of Domestic Violence There is no single explanation for why people tend to be abusive in relationships. Although alcohol abuse is often associated with such violence, marital dissatisfaction is also a predictor.[28] Numerous studies also point to differences in the communication patterns between abusive and nonabusive relationships.[29] Although some researchers argue that the hormone testosterone causes male aggression, studies have failed to show a strong association between physical abuse in relationships and this hormone.[30] Many experts believe that men who engage in severe violence are more likely than other men to suffer from personality disorders.[31] Clearly, more research is needed to understand abusive relationships.

Regardless of the cause, it is the dynamics that both people bring to a relationship that result in violence and allow it to continue. Community support and counseling services can help determine underlying problems and allow the victim and batterer to break the cycle. The **Assess Yourself** box on page 100 may help you determine whether you are involved in an abusive relationship.

Child Abuse and Neglect Children raised in families in which domestic violence and/or sexual abuse occur are at great risk for damage to personal health and well-being. The effects of such violent acts are powerful and long-lasting.

Child abuse refers to the systematic harm of a child by a caregiver, generally a parent.[32] The abuse may be sexual, psychological, physical, or any combination of these. Although exact figures are lacking, many experts believe that nearly 1 million cases of child abuse and neglect occur every year in the United States, involving severe injury, permanent disability, or death.[33]

Neglect includes failure to provide for a child's basic needs for food, shelter, clothing, medical care, education, or proper supervision. How serious is the problem (see **Figure 4.3**)? In 2004, 2.6 million reports concerning the welfare of approximately 4.5 million children were made to child protective services agencies in the United States.[34] In about two-thirds of these cases, sufficient abuse was detected to prompt investigation—resulting in over 896,000 cases, or 2,450 cases per day![35] Of these cases, 60 percent of victims experienced neglect.

There is no single profile of a perpetrator of fatal child abuse. Frequently, the perpetrator is a young adult in his or her mid twenties without a high school diploma, living at or below the poverty level, depressed, socially isolated, with a poor self-image, and with difficulty coping with stressful situations. In many instances, the perpetrator has experienced violence and is frustrated by life. Most fatalities from *physical abuse* are caused by fathers and other male caretakers. Mothers are most often held responsible for deaths resulting from *neglect*. However, in some cases the reason may be that it is women who spend the most time with the children and whom society deems responsible for their care. Although it is difficult to measure long-term consequences of abuse, an average of nearly four children die every day as a result of abuse or neglect.[36]

Not all violence against children is physical. Health can be severely affected by psychological violence—assaults on personality, character, competence, independence, or general dignity as a human being. The negative consequences of this kind of victimization can be harder to discern and therefore harder to combat. They include depression, low self-esteem, and a pervasive fear of offending the abuser.

 what do you THINK?

■ What factors in society lead to child abuse and neglect? ■ What actions can be taken to prevent such behaviors?

Sexual Victimization

As with all forms of violence, men and women alike are susceptible to sexual victimization. However, sexual violence against women is of epidemic proportions, so we will focus on women. Physical battering and emotional abuse often leave psychological as well as physical scars. One-quarter to one-third of high school and college stu-

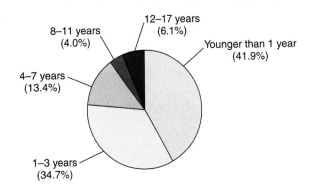

FIGURE 4.3 Child Abuse and Neglect Fatalities, by Age, 2005
Source: U.S. Department of Health and Human Services, Administration on Children, Youth and Families, *Child Maltreatment 2005* (Washington, DC: U.S. Government Printing Office, 2007), www.acf.hhs.gov/programs/cb/pubs/cm05/index.htm.

dents report involvement in dating violence, as perpetrators, victims, or both.[37]

Sexual Assault and Rape

Sexual assault is any act in which one person is sexually intimate with another person without that person's consent. This act may range from simple touching to forceful penetration and may include, for example, ignoring indications that intimacy is not wanted, threatening force or other negative consequences, and actually using force. According to victims' reports, nearly six out of ten rapes and sexual assaults occur in their own or a friend's home.[38]

Rape The most extreme form of sexual assault, **rape** is defined as "penetration without the victim's consent."[39] Whether committed by an acquaintance, a date, or a stranger, rape is a criminal activity that usually has serious emotional, psychological, social, and physical consequences for the victim. Typically, victims are young females; 29 percent are under 11 years of age, 32 percent are between the ages of 11 and 17; and 22 percent are between ages of 18 and 24.[40] Women aged 16 to 19 are four times as likely as the general population to be rape victims.[41]

One of the most startling aspects of sex crimes is how many go unreported, usually out of a belief that this is a private matter, fear of reprisal by the assailant, or unwar-

child abuse The systematic harming of a child by a caregiver, typically a parent.

neglect Failure to provide for a child's basic needs such as food, shelter, medical care, and clothing.

sexual assault Any act in which one person is sexually intimate with another person without that person's consent.

rape Sexual penetration without the victim's consent.

ASSESS yourself

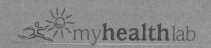

RELATIONSHIP VIOLENCE: ARE YOU AT RISK?

Fill out this assessment online at www.aw-bc.com/myhealthlab or www.aw-bc.com/donatelle.

Although we all want healthy relationships, many of us get caught in patterns of behavior that are a direct result of things we've learned or haven't learned in our past. Sometimes we don't even recognize that we are acting inappropriately; other times we know we should act in a particular way but get caught up in our own emotions and act out in ways that are physically or emotionally abusive. To prevent violence, we have to be able to recognize it, deal with it in appropriate ways, and/or take action to avoid it. Answer the following questions about your current or past relationships.

How often does your partner:

	Never	Sometimes	Often
1. Criticize you for your appearance (weight, dress, hair, and so on)?	☐	☐	☐
2. Embarrass you in front of others by putting you down?	☐	☐	☐
3. Blame you or others for his or her mistakes?	☐	☐	☐
4. Curse at you, say mean things, or mock you?	☐	☐	☐
5. Demonstrate uncontrollable anger?	☐	☐	☐
6. Criticize your friends, family, or others who are close to you?	☐	☐	☐
7. Threaten to leave you if you don't behave in a certain way?	☐	☐	☐
8. Manipulate you to prevent you from spending time with friends or family?	☐	☐	☐
9. Express jealousy, distrust, and anger when you spend time with other people?	☐	☐	☐
10. Tell you that you are crazy, irrational, or paranoid?	☐	☐	☐
11. Call you names to make you lose confidence in yourself?	☐	☐	☐
12. Make all the significant decisions in your relationship?	☐	☐	☐
13. Intimidate or threaten you, making you fearful or anxious?	☐	☐	☐
14. Make threats to harm others you care about?	☐	☐	☐
15. Prevent you from going out by taking your car keys?	☐	☐	☐
16 Control your telephone calls, listen in on your messages, or read your e-mail?	☐	☐	☐
17. Punch, hit, slap, or kick you?	☐	☐	☐
18. Gossip about you to turn others against you or make them think bad things about you?	☐	☐	☐
19. Make you feel guilty about something?	☐	☐	☐
20. Use money or possessions to control you?	☐	☐	☐
21. Force you to have sex or perform sexual acts that make you uncomfortable?	☐	☐	☐
22. Threaten to kill himself or herself if you leave?	☐	☐	☐
23. Control your money and make you ask for what you need?	☐	☐	☐
24. Set many rules that you must abide by?	☐	☐	☐
25. Follow you, call to check on you, or demonstrate a constant obsession with what you are doing?	☐	☐	☐

ranted feelings of guilt and responsibility. It is thought that one out of every three women is the victim of an attempted or completed rape in her lifetime. Although as many as

aggravated rape   Rape that involves one or multiple attackers, strangers, weapons, or physical beating.

two-thirds of all rapes are never reported, there were over 683,000 reported cases of rape, attempted rape, or sexual assault in 2003.[42]

Incidents of rape generally fall into one of two types—aggravated or simple. An **aggravated rape** involves one or multiple attackers, strangers, weapons, or physical beatings.

ANALYZING YOUR RESPONSES

Now look at your responses to the list of questions. If you answered "sometimes" to one or more of these questions, you may be at risk for emotional or physical abuse. If you answered "often" to any question, you may need to talk with someone about immediate threats to your emotional or physical health. Typically, such potentially abusive patterns only get worse over time as a person gains control and power in a relationship. If you are anxious about talking to your partner, seek counseling through your campus counseling center, student health center, or community services. If you don't know where to go, ask your professor for possible options.

After you have completed the test about your partner's behavior, you should ask the same questions about your own behavior. If any of the questions describe your actions in a relationship, you should seek help to change these behavioral patterns. These actions are not conducive to healthy relationships and may result in harm to you or your loved ones. Seek help now to insure healthier relationships in the future.

MAKE it happen!

ASSESSMENT: The Assess Yourself activity gave you a chance to consider symptoms of abuse. If any of the symptoms describe a relationship you or someone you know is involved in, you should consider taking action.

MAKING A CHANGE: To change your behavior, you need to develop a plan. Follow these steps below and complete your Behavior Change Contract to take action.

1. Evaluate your behavior, and identify patterns and specific things you are doing. What can you change now? What can you change in the near future?

2. Select one pattern of behavior that you want to change.

3. Fill out the Behavior Change Contract found at the front of your book. It should include your long-term goals for change, your short-term goals, the rewards you'll give yourself for reaching these goals, potential obstacles along the way, and strategies for overcoming these obstacles. For each goal, list the small steps and specific actions that you will take.

4. Chart your progress in a journal. At the end of a week, consider how successful you were in following your plan. What helped you be successful? What made change more difficult? What will you do differently next week?

5. Revise your plan as needed. Are the short-term goals attainable? Are the rewards satisfying?

EXAMPLE: Sondra thought that her roommate, Jessie, was experiencing several symptoms of abuse. Jessie's boyfriend, Carl, sometimes belittled her in front of her friends. He once broke her cell phone by throwing it against a wall toward Jessie and seemed resentful when she spent time with anyone but him. When Sondra talked to Jessie about her perceptions, Jessie was surprised and very defensive at first. The more she thought about it, though, she realized that sometimes she was afraid of Carl's actions. She started to consider what she could do about the situation. As a first step, Sondra helped Jessie make immediate appointments at the school counseling center, one for herself and one for her and Carl together.

A **simple rape** is perpetrated by one person, whom the victim knows, and does not involve a physical beating or use of a weapon. Most incidents are classified as simple rapes. One report suggests that 82 percent of female rape victims have been victimized by acquaintances (53 percent), current or former boyfriends (16 percent), current or former spouses (10 percent), or other relatives (3 percent). With almost half of all rape charges dismissed before the cases reach trial, and with a perceived lack of men's understanding of how rape affects women, it's easy to understand why experts feel that so-called simple rape is seriously underreported and ignored.

simple rape Rape by one person, usually known to the victim, that does not involve a physical beating or use of a weapon.

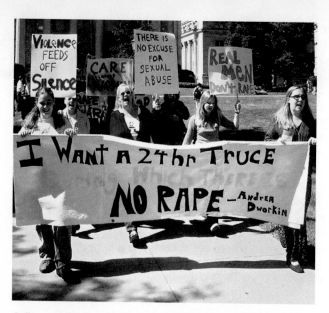

College students can organize vigils, marches, and educational programs to raise awareness about violence against women.

Acquaintance or Date Rape

Although the terms *date rape, friendship rape,* and *acquaintance rape* have become standard terminology, they are typically misused. Not all rapes occur on dates, not all the relationships are friendships, and sometimes the term *acquaintance* is used all too loosely. Many acquaintance rapes occur as the result of incidental contact at a party or when groups of people congregate at one person's house. These are crimes of opportunity, not necessarily a prearranged date. This is an important distinction because the term *date* suggests some type of reciprocal interaction arranged in advance. Although most date or acquaintance rapes happen to women aged 15 to 24 years, the 18-year-old new college student is the most likely victim.[43]

Consider the following:[44]

- 84 percent of rape on college campuses is acquaintance rape. Fifty-seven percent of these assaults occurred while the victim and offender were on a date.
- Sexual coercion and aggression may occur at any stage of a relationship.
- Acquaintance rape tends to occur on weekends, on the rapist's "turf," and it may include verbal and physical force.
- Alcohol and drugs are often involved.

Date rape is not simply miscommunication; it is an act of violence. Well-known expert on interpersonal relationships Susan Jacoby puts it this way:

> Some women (especially the young) initially resist sex not out of real conviction, but as part of the elaborate persuasion and seduction rituals accompanying what was once called courtship. And it is true that many men (again, especially the young) take pride in their ability to coax a woman further than she intended to go. But these mating rituals do not justify or even explain date rape. Even the most callow youth is

capable of understanding the difference between resistance and genuine fear; between a halfhearted "no, we shouldn't" and tears or screams.[45]

Marital Rape

Although the legal definition varies within the United States, *marital rape* can be defined as any unwanted intercourse or penetration (vaginal, anal, or oral) obtained by force, by threat of force, or when the wife is unable to consent.[46] Some researchers estimate that marital rape may account for 25 percent of all rapes; rape in marriage may be an extremely prevalent form of sexual violence.

Although this problem has undoubtedly existed since the origin of marriage as a social institution, it is noteworthy that marital rape did not become a crime in all 50 states until 1993. Even more noteworthy is the fact that 30 states still allow exemptions from rape prosecution, meaning that the judicial system may treat it as a lesser crime.

Who is most vulnerable to marital rape? In general, women under the age of 25 and those from lower socioeconomic groups are at highest risk. Women from homes where other forms of domestic violence are common and where alcoholism and/or substance abuse are prevalent also tend to be victimized at greater rates. Women who are subjected to marital rape often report multiple offenses over a period of time; these events are likely to be forced anal and oral experiences.[47]

Again, abuse of power and a need to control and dominate seem to be key factors in the husband-rapist profile. Marital rape can have devastating short- and long-term consequences for women, including injuries to the vaginal and anal areas, lacerations, soreness, bruising, torn muscles, fatigue, panic attacks, sexually transmitted infections, broken bones, wounds, and other emotional and physical scars.

Social Contributors to Sexual Assault

According to many experts, certain common assumptions in our society prevent both the perpetrator and the wider public from recognizing the true nature of sexual assault.[48] These assumptions include the following:

- *Minimization.* It is often assumed that sexual assault of women is rare because official crime statistics, including the Uniform Crime Reports of the FBI, show very few rapes per thousand population. However, rape is the most underreported of all serious crimes. Researchers have found that one out of every six women in the United States has been a victim of sexual assault.[49]
- *Trivialization.* Incredibly, sexual assault of women is still often viewed as a jocular matter. During a gubernatorial election in Texas a few years back, one of the candidates reportedly compared a bad patch of weather to rape: If there's nothing you can do about it, just lie back and enjoy it. (He lost the election—to a woman.)
- *Blaming the victim.* Many discussions of sexual violence against women display a sometimes unconscious assumption

that the woman did something to provoke the attack—that she flirted or dressed revealingly, for example.

- *"Boys will be boys."* According to this assumption, men just can't control themselves once they become aroused.

Over the years, psychologists and others have proposed several theories to explain why many men sexually victimize women. In one of the first major studies to explore this issue, almost two-thirds of the male respondents had engaged in intercourse unwanted by the woman, primarily because of male peer pressure.[50] By all indicators, these trends continue today. Peer pressure is certainly a strong factor, but a growing body of research suggests that sexual assault is encouraged by the socialization processes that men experience daily, including the belief that rape is something women secretly desire, and by norms that often portray women as the targets of male aggression.[51]

Child Sexual Abuse

Sexual abuse of children by adults or older children includes sexually suggestive conversations; inappropriate kissing; touching; petting; oral, anal, or vaginal intercourse; and other kinds of sexual interaction. The most frequent abusers are a child's parents or the parents' companions or spouses. The next most frequent abusers are grandfathers and siblings. Girls are more commonly abused than boys, although young boys are also frequent victims, usually of male family members. Between 20 and 30 percent of all adult women report having had an unwanted childhood sexual encounter with an adult male, usually a father, uncle, brother, or grandfather.[52] Perpetrators appear to be normal people and are impossible to pick out by sight or behavior alone. There is much controversy surrounding sex offender databases, which make the offender's identity known to neighbors, prospective employers, and other individuals.

Most sexual abuse occurs in the child's home. The following situations raise the risk:[53]

1. The child lives without one of his or her biological parents.

2. The mother is unavailable because she is disabled, ill, or working outside the home.

3. The parents' marriage is unhappy.

4. The child has a poor relationship with his or her parents or is subjected to extremely punitive discipline.

5. The child lives with a stepfather.

People who were abused as children bear spiritual, psychological, and/or physical scars. To appreciate the impact of child abuse on later life, studies have shown that children who experience maltreatment and abuse are at increased risk later in life for smoking, alcoholism, drug abuse, eating disorders, mental health problems, and suicide.[54]

Parents and caretakers of children should be aware of behavioral changes that may signal sexual abuse:[55]

- Noticeable fear of a certain person or place
- Unusual or unexpected response when the child is asked whether he or she has been touched by someone
- Unreasonable fear of a physical exam
- Drawings that show sexual acts
- Abrupt changes in behavior, such as bed-wetting
- Sudden or unusual awareness of genitals or sexual acts
- Attempts to get other children to perform sexual acts

what do you THINK?

What factors make a person likely to commit sexual assault? ■ Why are family members often the perpetrators of child sexual abuse? ■ What measures might be effective in preventing sexual assault and abuse?

Crime on Campus: Victims and Perpetrators

On April 16, 2007, Americans were horrified by news of the most deadly mass shooting in U.S. history at Virginia Tech (VT) University. Later, when the full number of fatalities and injuries and the emotional toll were assessed, many would comment on the seemingly obvious shooter profile: a loner student who had had enough trouble in classes that he was sent to counseling, who had interactions with law enforcement for his behavior, and who displayed an abnormal amount of anger in his written work and interactions with others, so that his instructors and classmates feared him. Why didn't someone do something to help this student earlier? Why did faculty and student concerns about this student go largely unnoticed? Why didn't administrators and members of the law enforcement community act more quickly in a case like this to prevent large numbers of fatalities? The tragedy shocked the nation and will leave an indelible mark on our collective thoughts, but it also sparked dialogue and action on campuses across the nation and throughout the world. How safe are our campuses? What policies and procedures must be in place to control such emergencies more effectively and to minimize risks to students, faculty, and staff? What can each of us do to help ensure our own safety and the safety of others?

In truth, college has long been regarded as a safe haven for parents to send their sons and daughters. Parents may

sexual abuse of children Sexual interaction between a child and an adult or older child. Includes, but is not limited to, sexually suggestive conversations; inappropriate kissing; touching; petting; and oral, anal, or vaginal intercourse.

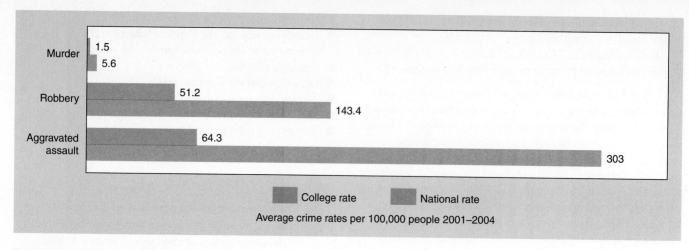

FIGURE 4.4 Crime in the Quad

Despite some high-profile tragedies, data reported by U.S. colleges suggest campuses are among the safest places in America. But though murder is rare, alcohol and sexual assault pose big risks.

Source: A. Kingsbury, "Toward a Safer Campus," *U.S. News and World Report*, April 16, 2007, 49. Copyright © 2007 U.S. News and World Report. Used with permission.

worry that their children will have trouble adjusting to college life, drink too much and party too hard, connect with bad influences, and not eat right or sleep enough. However, few realize that the 16 million students enrolled in some 4,200 colleges and universities in the United States face risks of violence from a variety of threats, both on campus and in the outlying community. Campuses may be relatively safe, but they are by no means immune from acts of violence **(Figure 4.4)**. In the wake of the VT shootings, university officials compared the campus community to a small city, with all of the typical problems that one might see in a city and similar issues in trying to respond to major emergencies. Just like other communities, campuses have their share of violent acts that can cause significant physical and mental problems. The term *campus violence* typically includes acts of physical violence such as homicide, suicide, rape, assault, dating violence, harassment and stalking, hazing, and hate crimes.[56] Consider the following facts on campus violence:[57]

- Simple assault (that is, attack without a weapon resulting either in no injury or in minor injuries) accounted for about two-thirds of college student violent crimes (63 percent). Rape or sexual assault accounted for 6 percent.
- Only about 5 percent of completed and attempted rapes committed against students are ever reported to the police.
- Nearly 80 percent of all rapes on campus are committed by persons the victim knows.
- Alcohol and other drugs are implicated in 55 to 74 percent of sexual assaults on campus.

sexual harassment Any form of unwanted sexual attention.

- Approximately 93 percent of crimes against students occurred at off-campus locations.
- More than 36 percent of lesbian, gay, bisexual, and transgender (LGBT) students have experienced harassment within the last year.
- White college students experience higher rates of violent victimization than students of other races.

However, these statistics represent only a glimpse of the big picture. The sad fact is that fewer than 25 percent of campus crimes are reported to *any* authority.[58] Why would students fail to report such crimes? Typical reasons include concerns over privacy, embarrassment or shame, lack of support, perception that the crime was too minor, or uncertainty that it was a crime.

In 1992, Congress passed the Campus Sexual Assault Victim's Bill of Rights, known as the Ramstad Act. The act gives victims the right to call in off-campus authorities to investigate serious campus crimes. In addition, it requires universities to set up educational programs and notify students of available counseling. More recent provisions of the act specify received notification procedures and options for victims, rights of victims and the accused perpetrators, and consequences if schools do not comply. It also requires the Department of Education to publish campus crime statistics annually.

Sexual Violence on Campus

Sexual Harassment **Sexual harassment** is defined as unwelcome sexual conduct that is related to any condition of employment or evaluation of student performance. It includes unwarranted sex-related comments, sexually explicit comments or graphics, or unwelcome touching.[59] Harassment can take other forms that some people may not have considered: making derogatory jokes based on sex or appearance, speaking in crude or offensive language, spreading rumors about a person's sexuality, placing compromising photos on the Web, or ogling are common forms of sexual harassment. Commonly, people think of harassment as involving only faculty members or persons in power, where sex is used to exhibit control of a situation. However, peers can harass one another too. Harassment can occur at many levels and can be extremely detrimental. Although exact numbers of cases of sexual harassment are difficult to determine, it is widely perceived to be a major problem on college campuses, forcing administrators to enact strict guidelines about interpersonal relationships between students and instructors or co-workers.

It's always important to watch what you say and how you say it. Learning now what constitutes sexual harassment may save you embarrassment or worse in the future. A simple compliment on someone's appearance can be offensive if stated without sensitivity, regardless of the intent. "You look very nice today" can become offensive if stated as, "That dress looks great on your body." Also, the context in which such comments are made can make a huge difference in interpretation. Even inadvertant mannerisms, such as gazing at a woman's chest while speaking with her, can make others feel sexually harrassed.

Most schools and companies have sexual harassment policies in place, as well as procedures for dealing with harrassment problems. If you feel you are being harassed, the most important thing you can do is be assertive. Immediately after the incident occurs, follow the guidelines in **Table 4.1.**

? *what do you* THINK?

What policies does your school have regarding consensual relationships between faculty members and students? ■ Should consenting adults have the right to become intimate or interact socially, regardless of their positions within a system or workplace? ■ What are the potential dangers of such interactions? ■ Are there ever situations when such interactions are okay?

Sexual Assault on Campus

Earlier in this chapter, you learned about rape and sexual assault. Rape, acquaintance rape, sodomy, unwanted touching, and other forms of sexual assault occur daily on campuses throughout the United States, and, like other forms of violence, these crimes have particularly high rates of going unreported. In fact, it is believed that as few as 8 percent of college women who have been date raped reported the crime to the police.[60] According to the U.S. Department of Justice, rape is the most underreported violent crime in the United States.[61]

Sexual assault often involves force sufficient to cause serious injury, and psychological trauma may be substantial.

TABLE 4.1	Strategies for Preventing or Stopping Harassment
Tell the harasser to stop.	Be clear and direct about what is bothering you and why you are upset.
Document the harassment.	Make a record of the incident. If the harassment becomes intolerable, a record of exactly what occurred (and when and where) will help make your case.
Complain to a higher authority.	Talk to your instructor, adviser, or counseling center about what happened. If they don't take you seriously, investigate your school's internal grievance procedures.
Remember that you have not done anything wrong.	You will likely feel awful after being harassed (especially if you have to complain to superiors). However, feel proud that you are not keeping silent. The person who is harassing you is wrong, not you.

Results of sexual assaults studies vary considerably; however, over the years, consistently 5 to 15 percent of college men have acknowledged that they have forced intercourse, and 5 to 25 percent have acknowledged that they have been sexually aggressive.[62] A recent survey of college women found that the incidence of unwanted sexual contact ranging from kissing and petting to oral, anal, or vaginal intercourse was as high as 27 percent. Participants reported that most often, a boyfriend was the sexual aggressor (41 percent); a friend was the sexual aggressor in 30 percent of cases, and an acquaintance was the aggressor in about 21 percent of cases. Strangers, husbands, and others (such as professors and supervisors) made up the remaining numbers of assailants. Usually the first 2 years on campus were the riskiest for students.[63] Reports show little consistency in the profile of the victims; some studies have shown that white women experience higher numbers of sexual assaults on campus, whereas other studies have shown that African American women are more likely to be victimized.[64] Regardless of the study, alcohol use by either the victim or the perpetrator is typically an issue.

? *what do you* THINK?

Why do you think so few college women ever report date rape or other forms of sexual assault to the police? ■ What actions might be taken to encourage women who are sexually assaulted to step forward and file complaints against their assailants?

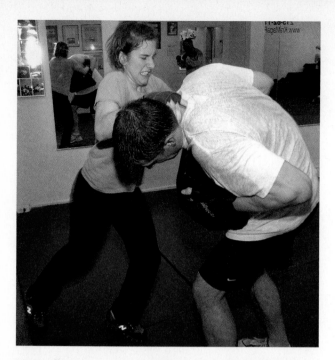

More college campuses are offering safety workshops to equip students with skills to protect themselves from violent acts.

Stalking Conduct directed at a specific person that involves repeated visual or physical proximity, features non-consensual written or verbal communication, and may imply threats is known as **stalking.**[65] The typical victim of stalking tends to be the same age as the stalker, knows the stalker, lives alone, and is an undergraduate student. The most common form of stalking—and that which poses the greatest risk of violence—occurs following the termination of a romantic relationship.[66] However, stalking may be more subtle, particularly with the use of modern technology. For example, cell phone–stalkers can keep track of a victim's actions by calling repeatedly, asking questions about what the person is doing, who the person is with, and other seemingly harmless checks on activity. If this happens to you, let the person know it's not appropriate behavior, and tell him or her to stop calling. Although stalking occurs in virtually all populations, research suggests that stalking rates may be higher among college students than in the general population.[67]

Researchers suggest several reasons for stalking: (1) Stalkers may have deficits in social skills; (2) they are young and have not yet learned how to deal with complex social relationships and situations; (3) they may not realize

> **What can I do if I think I am being stalked?**

stalking   The willful, repeated, and malicious following, harassing, or threatening of another person.

their behavior is stalking; (4) they have a flexible schedule and free time; and (5) they are not accountable to authority figures for their daily activities.[68] How prevalent is stalking on campus? As with other violent acts, stalking behaviors are believed to be widely underreported; however, it is estimated that between 25 and 30 percent of college women and between 11 and 17 percent of college men have been stalked.[69]

Campus Dating Violence Actual or threatened physical or sexual violence or psychological and emotional abuse directed toward a current or former dating partner is known as campus *dating violence.* **Table 4.2** offers tips for safe dating. Intimate partners may be heterosexual, bisexual, or homosexual.[70] Often, violence involving an intimate partner is repetitive, and victims do not readily seek help. Studies of campus dating violence indicate that 15 percent of women and 9.2 percent of men reported being in emotionally abusive relationships during the previous year, and 2.4 percent of women and 1.3 percent of men reported physically abusive relationships. Sexually abusive relationships were reported by 1.7 percent of women and 1 percent of men.[71] As with many forms of campus violence, alcohol use is frequently involved. See the **Spotlight on Your Health** box for more on drug use and rape.

Reducing Your Risk

After a violent act is committed against someone we know, we acknowledge the horror of the event, express sympathy, and go on with our lives—but the person who has been brutalized may take months or years to recover. It is far better to prevent a violent act than to recover from it.

DRUG-FACILITATED CRIMES: ALCOHOL, ROHYPNOL, AND OTHER DANGERS

The biggest risk of crime on campus results from abuse of alcohol. Alcohol-related injuries led to more than 1,700 deaths on campus in 2001. Although deaths capture media attention, sexual assault is one of the most underreported and potentially damaging crimes on campus. In the same year, 97,000 students were victims of alcohol-related rape or sexual assaults, and 696,000 were assaulted by a student who had been binge drinking, according to the National Center on Addiction and Substance Abuse's most recent statistics.

Usually, alcohol serves as a catalyst for aggressive behavior in perpetrators and lowers normal resistance behaviors in victims. Sometimes specific drugs are used to immobilize victims and make them unable to defend themselves. These drugs are typically slipped into the drinks of unsuspecting people, who wake up later and can remember few details of the assault. Three of the most common drugs used are Rohypnol, GHB, and Burundanga. Although these drugs are often called "date rape" drugs, their use typically has nothing to do with a date and may serve to downplay what really happened. As such, the term *drug-facilitated rape or crime* is a much more accurate way to discuss these crimes. Many times, these drugs are slipped into the drinks of women whose only meeting with the male perpetrator is to be bought a drink at a bar or handed a drink at a party.

Although not approved for sale in the United States, Rohypnol (flunitrazepam) is widely available in other countries as a sleep aid. Street names for it include Roaches, LaRocha, rope, Rib Roche, Roches, roofies, Ruffies, Mexican Valium, and roach-2. When dissolved in a drink, Rohypnol produces a sedative-hypnotic effect that includes muscle relaxation and amnesia. Generally, sedative effects occur within 20 to 30 minutes and incapacitation within 1 to 2 hours, often lasting for hours. People who take it may appear drunk or sleepy, dizzy, or confused. Tablets are white and contain the name "Roche" and an encircled "1" or "2" on one side indicating dosage. The manufacturer has now released a new, lower-dose blue tablet designed to be impossible to slip into a drink without detection. Tests are available at rape crisis centers and emergency rooms and through law enforcement agencies to determine whether Rohypnol has been administered.

GHB (gamma-hydroxybutyrate) is known as Liquid E, Liquid Ecstasy, Liquid X, Grievous Bodily Harm, and Easy First. Illicitly used for its euphoric, sedative, and anabolic (body-building) effects, today GHB is more commonly used than Rohypnol in sexual assaults. GHB is usually a colorless, odorless liquid that may taste salty. Used as a surgical anesthetic in Europe, it is not legal in the United States and can induce short-term coma, slowed heart rate, decreased breathing, seizures, and death.

A drug that has recently appeared and that causes similar reactions is Burundanga, a tasteless yellow powder that has an immediate effect. Burundanga affects the central nervous system and can be highly dangerous.

Each year, several deaths result from these crime-facilitating drugs. Survivors must cope with the fact that they have been violated without a chance to defend themselves. To reduce your risk, follow these guidelines:

- Do not accept drinks from strangers. In fact, do not take any beverages or open-container drinks from anyone you do not know well and trust. At a bar or club, accept drinks only from the bartender or wait staff.
- Never leave a drink or food unattended. If you get up, have someone watch your drink or food, or take it with you.
- Go with friends and leave with friends. Never leave a bar or party with someone you don't know well.
- If you think you may have been slipped something in a drink, tell a friend, and have him or her get you to an emergency room. If friends seem disproportionately "out of it" in relation to what they've had to drink, stay with them and watch them carefully. Call 911 if anyone experiences seizures, vomits, passes out, has difficulty breathing, or experiences other complications.

Sources: A. Kingsbury, "Toward a Safer Campus," *U.S. News and World Report,* April 16, 2007, 48–51. National Institute of Drug Abuse, "NIDA Info Facts: Rohypnol and GHB," May 5, 2006, www.nida.nih.gov/infofax/RohypnolGHB.html.

Self-Defense against Personal Assault and Rape

Assault can occur no matter what preventive actions you take, but commonsense self-defense tactics can lower the risk. Self-defense is a process that includes increasing your awareness, developing self-defense skills, taking reasonable precautions, and having the judgment necessary to respond to different situations. The **Skills for Behavior Change** box on page 108 identifies practical tips for preventing personal assaults.

Most attacks by unknown assailants are planned in advance. Sexual assault frequently begins with a casual, friendly conversation. Although many women have said that they started to feel uneasy during such a conversation, they denied the possibility of an assault until it was too late.

SKILLS FOR behavior change

TIPS FOR PROTECTING YOURSELF

There are many steps you can take to protect yourself from personal assault. Follow these tips to increase your awareness and reduce your risk of a violent attack.

WHEN DATING

- Set limits. If the situation feels like it is getting out of control, stop and talk, say "no" directly, and don't be coy or worry about hurting feelings. Be firm, and avoid drinking too much.
- Most rapes are committed by someone you know. If you feel uncomfortable, protect yourself or get away.
- Date in couples or groups when dating someone new.
- Pay attention to your date's actions. If there is too much teasing and all of the decisions are made for you, it may mean trouble.
- Trust your intuitions. Talk to the person, and try to get a sense of the person's history with others, what issues with past relationships the person mentions, and so on.
- Stick with your friends. Agree to keep an eye out for one another at parties, and have a plan for leaving together and checking in with each other. Never leave a bar or party alone with a stranger.

WHEN YOU'RE OUTSIDE ALONE

- Carry a cell phone, but stay off it. Many people are attacked when they are talking on their phones and not paying attention.

- Be aware of what is happening around you. Look, listen, and notice what is happening and how close people are to you.
- If you are being followed, don't go home. Head for a location where there are other people. If you decide to run, run fast and scream loudly to alert attention.
- Vary your routes; walk or jog with others at a steady pace. Stay close to others.
- Park near lights; avoid dark areas where people could hide.
- Carry pepper spray or other deterrents. Consider using your campus escort service.
- Tell others where you are going and when you expect to be back.

WHILE IN YOUR CAR

- Lock your doors.
- Purchase cars with alarm systems and remote entry with a light that goes on. Have your keys ready as you approach your car.
- If someone hits you while you are driving, drive to the nearest gas station or other public place. Call the police or road service for help, and stay in your car until help comes. Do not open your doors or windows to strangers.
- Be alert to cars that appear to be following you. Do not drive home. Drive to the nearest police station.

WHILE AT HOME

- Install dead-bolt locks on all doors, including screen doors, and locks on all windows. Make sure locks work, and

don't leave a spare key outside. Consider installing a home alarm system.
- Lock doors when at home, even during the day. Close blinds and drapes whenever you are away and in the evening when you are home.
- Rent apartments that require a security code or clearance to gain entry, and avoid easily accessible apartments, such as first-floor units. When you move into a new residence, pay a locksmith to change the keys and locks.
- Don't let repair people in without asking for their identification, and have someone else with you when repairs are being made in your home or apartment.
- Avoid dark parking structures, laundry rooms, and so on. Try to use these areas only when others are around.
- Use initials for first names on mailboxes and in phone listings. Keep your address out of phone books.
- Keep a cell phone near your bed, and program it to dial 911. Intruders commonly pick up the receiver in another room, thereby disabling a bedroom phone.
- Get to know your neighbors. Organize a neighborhood watch.
- If your residence is broken into, don't enter—and call the police. If you encounter an intruder, it is far better to give up your money than to fight.

Listen to your feelings, and trust your intuition. Be assertive and direct to someone who is getting out of line or threatening—this may convince the would-be rapist or attacker to back off. Stifle your tendency to be nice, and don't fear making a scene. Let him know that you mean what you say and are prepared to defend yourself. Consider the following.

- *Speak in a strong voice.* Use statements such as, "Leave me alone" rather than questions such as, "Will you please

leave me alone?" Avoid apologies and excuses. Sound like you mean it.
- *Maintain eye contact with the would-be attacker.* This keeps you aware of the person's movements and conveys an aura of strength and confidence.
- *Stand up straight, act confident, and remain alert.* Walk as though you owned the sidewalk.

Many rapists use certain ploys to initiate their attacks. Examples include asking for help; offering help; staging a deliberate "accident," such as bumping into you; or posing as a police officer or other authority figure.

If you are attacked, act immediately. Draw attention to yourself and your assailant. Scream, "Fire!" loudly. Research has shown that passersby are much more likely to help if they hear the word *fire* rather than just a scream. Your attacker also may be caught off-balance by the action.

What to Do If Rape Occurs

If you are a rape victim, report the attack. This gives you a sense of control. Follow these steps.

- Call 911 (if a phone is available).
- Do not bathe, shower, douche, clean up, or touch anything the attacker may have touched.
- Save the clothes you were wearing, and do not launder them. They will be needed as evidence. Bring a clean change of clothes to the clinic or hospital.
- Contact the rape assistance hotline in your area, and ask for advice on therapists or counseling if you need additional help.

If a friend is raped, here's how you can help.

- Believe her, and don't ask questions that may appear to implicate her in the assault.
- Recognize that rape is a violent act and that the victim was not looking for this to happen.
- Encourage your friend to see a doctor immediately because she may have medical needs but feel too embarrassed to seek help on her own. Offer to go with her.
- Encourage her to report the crime.
- Be understanding, and let her know you will be there for her.
- Recognize that this is an emotional recovery, and it may take 6 months to a year for her to bounce back.
- Encourage your friend to seek counseling.

A Campus-Wide Response to Violence

Increasingly, campuses have become microcosms of the greater society, complete with the risks, hazards, and dangers people face in the world. Many college administrators have been proactive in establishing violence prevention policies, programs, and services. They have also begun to examine the culture that promotes violent acts and tolerance for them.[72]

Changing Roles of Campus Law Enforcement
To increase student protection, campus law enforcement has changed over the years in both numbers and authority to prosecute student offenders. Campus police are responsible for emergency responses to situations that threaten safety, human resources, the general campus environment, traffic and bicycle safety, and other dangers. They have the power to enforce laws with students in the same

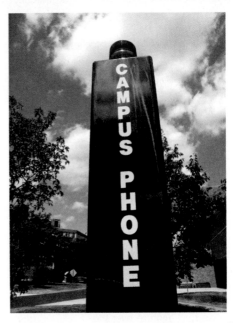

Emergency call boxes are becoming a common sight on college campuses as school administrators beef up their safety and emergency alert systems.

way they are handled in the general community. In fact, many campuses now hire state troopers or local law enforcement officers to deal with campus issues rather than maintain a separate police staff.

Many of these law enforcement groups follow a community policing model in which officers have specific responsibilities for certain areas of campus, departments, or events. By narrowing the scope of each officer's territory, officers get to know people in the area and are better able to anticipate and prevent risks. This differs from earlier safety policies, in which campus security typically swooped down only in times of trouble.

Prevention Efforts
Many universities now hire crime prevention and safety specialists. In light of the Virginia Tech incident, vast restructuring of existing policies, methods of notifying students of risk, and strategies for prevention have been enacted (see the **Health Headlines** box on page 110). Historically, prevention efforts have focused on rape awareness programs, safety workshops, anti-theft programs, and grounds safety measures such as good lighting, escort services, and emergency call boxes. Future programs will undoubtedly use mass communication strategies, cell phone and e-mail response systems, and a host of early alert and behavioral response strategies. What types of resources are available to you on your campus? Does your school now have a system for sending campus alerts to all students? Does it have an emergency plan in the event of a biological or physical threat to students?

The Role of Student Affairs
Although there may be some overlap with law enforcement activities, student affairs offices need to play a vital role in all on-campus programs, both to prevent trouble and to resolve problems

POST VIRGINIA TECH: AN EPILOGUE OF ACTION

In the wake of tragedy, it is always easy to look back and say, "If only we'd done things differently." Why didn't the campus administrators at Virginia Tech close the campus after the first shootings? Why did it take over 2 hours to let students know that a shooting had occurred on campus? Why didn't someone report the strange actions of this student and stop him beforehand? Did law enforcement respond appropriately?

Although we may agonize over the needless deaths of young adults in the prime of life, we should also be aware that the Virginia Tech tragedy was the latest in history of publicized gun violence on U.S. college campuses (see the figure). If there is a bright spot in all of the horror, it is that administrators at educational institutions throughout the United States and internationally have been forced to ask themselves, "Are we prepared in the event this happens at our school?"

Since the VT shootings, campuses are reexamining their policies, programs, and emergency response networks. Examples of "change in action" are everywhere:

- On the Oregon State campus, campus police, members of the community law enforcement, and emergency medical teams staged their "first ever" emergency response drill, essentially practicing how they would respond in the event of a shooter on campus.
- Campuses throughout the country report special training for officers and issuing stun guns and other equipment meant to disable potential offenders.
- Campuses are reviewing the effectiveness of campus e-mail for emergency messaging. Although these e-mail warnings are great in theory, they do little to protect those who aren't at their computers.
- Cell phone alerts are likely to become even more common, with REVERSE 911 systems in place to notify campus police in the event of problems. Companies such as RAVE wireless are working to develop a system for students to receive official university text alerts. Some campuses are giving all incoming freshmen phones with numbers programmed into the university system. In the event of a threat, students need only hit a button on their phones, whereupon tracking devices will pinpoint their location.
- Gun-toting students? A tremendous amount of controversy exists about whether lives might have been saved if students had carried guns with them to class. Most authorities question this practice and indicate that gun-toting students, particularly on campuses where binge drinking is prevalent, could spell disaster. Nevertheless, as of this date, Utah has voted to allow concealed weapons on campus—an act that may signal more change in the days ahead.

For an up-to-date listing of how campuses throughout the country are responding to the threat of violence, particularly violence caused by alcohol abuse, see the following website: www.higheredcenter.org/ideasamplers. In the days ahead, you can become part of the solution by becoming involved in the discussion on your campus and helping to insure that violent events of all kinds are prevented.

Sources: N. Shute, "What Went Wrong," *U.S. News and World Report,* April 16, 2007, 43–46; A. Kingsbury, "Toward a Safer Campus," *U.S. News and World Report,* April 16, 2007, 48–52; B. Shute, "Dialing 911 . . . in Reverse," *U.S. News and World Report,* April 16, 2007, 52.

that do occur. Student groups should monitor progress, identify potential threats, and advocate for improvements in any areas found to be deficient. A student affairs office can play a key role in making sure that mental health services, student assistance programs, and other services are high in quality, are easily accessible, and meet student needs. A human services or student affairs office should seek to involve the entire student body and ensure that all are aware of its services. Any programs that are not visible or proactive in ensuring campus safety should be evaluated carefully. Student leaders can play a major role in shaping such services and advocating for the campus population.

Community Strategies for Preventing Violence

Because the causes of homicide and assaultive violence are complex, community strategies for prevention must be multidimensional. Successful strategies include the following:

- Developing and implementing educational programs to teach communication, conflict resolution, and coping skills.
- Working with individuals to help them develop self-esteem and respect for others.

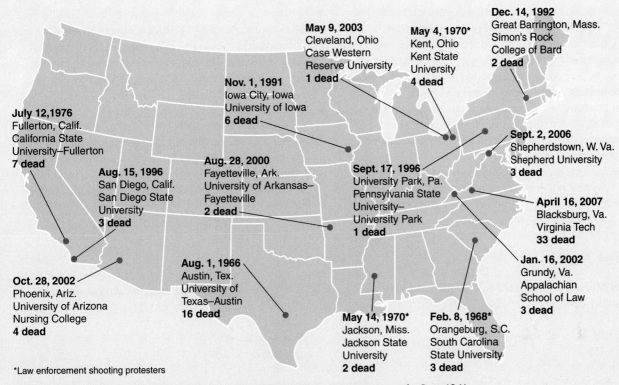

July 12,1976
Fullerton, Calif.
California State
University–Fullerton
7 dead

Aug. 15, 1996
San Diego, Calif.
San Diego State
University
3 dead

Oct. 28, 2002
Phoenix, Ariz.
University of Arizona
Nursing College
4 dead

Aug. 28, 2000
Fayetteville, Ark.
University of Arkansas–
Fayetteville
2 dead

Aug. 1, 1966
Austin, Tex.
University of
Texas–Austin
16 dead

Nov. 1, 1991
Iowa City, Iowa
University of Iowa
6 dead

May 9, 2003
Cleveland, Ohio
Case Western
Reserve University
1 dead

Sept. 17, 1996
University Park, Pa.
Pennsylvania State
University–
University Park
1 dead

May 14, 1970*
Jackson, Miss.
Jackson State
University
2 dead

Feb. 8, 1968*
Orangeburg, S.C.
South Carolina
State University
3 dead

May 4, 1970*
Kent, Ohio
Kent State
University
4 dead

Dec. 14, 1992
Great Barrington, Mass.
Simon's Rock
College of Bard
2 dead

Sept. 2, 2006
Shepherdstown, W. Va.
Shepherd University
3 dead

April 16, 2007
Blacksburg, Va.
Virginia Tech
33 dead

Jan. 16, 2002
Grundy, Va.
Appalachian
School of Law
3 dead

*Law enforcement shooting protesters

Campus Violence Across the United States: Gun Deaths on College Campuses over the Past 40 Years

Source: A. Kingsbury, "Toward a Safer Campus," *U.S. News and World Report,* April 16, 2007, 52.
Copyright © 2007 *U.S. News and World Report.* Used with permission.

- Rewarding youngsters for good behavior and never spanking a child when angry. Children need to know that anger is sometimes acceptable, but violence never is. Use family meetings to resolve conflicts.
- Establishing and enforcing policies that forbid discrimination on the basis of gender, religious affiliation, race, sexual orientation, marital status, or age.
- Increasing and enriching educational programs for family planning.
- Increasing efforts by health care and social service programs to identify victims of violence.
- Improving treatment and support for victims.
- Treating the psychological as well as the physical consequences of violence.

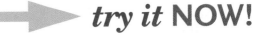 *try it* NOW!

Make a safety plan. Take safety precautions in your home or dorm to prevent intruders. Check your living space to identify places where an intruder could enter your dorm or apartment. Be more attentive to unusual behaviors, and find out whom to call if you see someone behaving suspiciously. Keep a list of emergency phone numbers by the phone. Get your roommates in on the plan, and spend a day "safety proofing."

TAKING charge

Summary

- Intentional injuries result from actions committed with intent to harm. Many factors lead people to be violent. Among them are anger, substance abuse, discrimination, mental health problems, and economic difficulties. To prevent violence, these underlying causes often must be dealt with before they ignite into a major event.

- Acts of terrorism are becoming more common in the United States. In addition to their immediate impact, terrorist activities can exert damaging long-term effects by fostering an atmosphere of fear and anxiety.

- Violence affects everyone in society—from the direct victims to those who live in fear of it. Over half of all homicides are committed by people who know their victims.

- Bias and hate crimes divide people, but teaching tolerance can reduce risks. Gang violence continues to grow but can be combated by programs that reduce the problems that lead to gang membership. Violence on campus may be increasing, but victims' rights also have increased as a result of major legislation.

- Preventing violent acts begins with avoiding potentially dangerous situations. There are several avenues available for reducing risks, including community, school, workplace, and individual strategies. Many crimes committed in general society are now commonplace at colleges, including personal assaults, sexual assaults, harassment, hate crimes, and even murder.

Chapter Review

1. For an African American man aged 20 to 22 years, the probability of being murdered is
   a. 1 in 3.
   b. 1 in 28.
   c. 1 in 153.
   d. 1 in 450.

2. Emotional reaction brought about by frustrating life experiences is called
   a. reactive aggression.
   b. primary aggression.
   c. secondary aggression.
   d. tertiary aggression.

3. When Jane began her new job with all male co-workers, her supervisor told her that he enjoyed having an attractive woman in the workplace, and he winked at her. His comment constitutes
   a. acquaintance rape.
   b. sexual assault.
   c. sexual harassment.
   d. sexual battering.

4. Psychologist Lenore Walker developed a theory known as the
   a. aggression cycle.
   b. sexual harassment cycle.
   c. cycle of child abuse.
   d. cycle of violence.

5. What is the single greatest cause of injury to women?
   a. rape
   b. mugging
   c. auto accidents
   d. domestic violence

6. In a sociology class, a group of students was discussing sexual assault. One student commented that some women dress too provocatively. The social assumption this student made is
   a. minimization.
   b. trivialization.
   c. blaming the victim.
   d. "boys will be boys."

7. Rape by a person known to the victim and that does not involve a physical beating or use of a weapon is called
   a. simple rape.
   b. sexual assault.
   c. simple assault.
   d. aggravated rape.

8. Which of the following is not a cause of violence?
   a. cultural beliefs
   b. poverty
   c. lack of education
   d. unemployment

9. Which of the following is an example of stalking?
   a. making intimate and personal sexually charged comments to another person
   b. repeated visual or physical seeking out of another person
   c. an unwelcome sexual conduct by the perpetrator
   d. sexual abuse upon a child

10. Jack beats his wife Melissa "to teach her a lesson." Afterward, he denies attacking her. The phase of the cycle of violence that this illustrates is
    a. acute battering.
    b. chronic battering.
    c. remorse/reconciliation.
    d. tension building.

Answers to these questions can be found on page A-1.

Questions for Discussion and Reflection

1. What major types of crimes are committed in the United States? What is the difference between primary and reactive aggression?
2. What is terrorism, and why does it occur? What can you do to protect yourself against terrorist attacks?
3. Compare domestic violence against men and against women. What are the differences? What are the similarities? What causes domestic violence?
4. What conditions put a child at risk for abuse? What can be done to prevent or decrease child abuse?
5. What is sexual harassment, and what factors contribute to it in the workplace?
6. What are the most effective violence prevention strategies on your campus?

Accessing Your Health on the Internet

The following websites explore further topics and issues related to personal health. For links to the websites below, visit the Companion Website for *Health: The Basics,* Eighth Edition at www.aw-bc.com/donatelle.

1. *Communities against Violence Network.* An extensive, searchable database for information about violence against women, with articles, legal information, and statistics. www.cavnet2.org
2. *Higher Education Center for Alcohol and Other Drug Abuse and Violence Prevention.* This division of the U.S. Department of Education helps college and community leaders create and implement programs and policies to address problems of violence and substance abuse on campuses. www.higheredcenter.org
3. *Men Can Stop Rape.* Practical suggestions for men interested in helping to protect women from sexual predators and assault. www.mencanstoprape.org
4. *National Center for Injury Prevention and Control.* The WISQARS database of this Centers for Disease Control and Prevention (CDC) section provides statistics and information on fatal and nonfatal injuries, both intentional and unintentional. www.cdc.gov/ncipc
5. *National Center for Victims of Crime.* Provides information and resources for victims of crimes ranging from hate crimes to sexual assault. www.ncvc.org
6. *National Sexual Violence Resources Center.* An excellent resource for victims of sexual violence. www.nsvrc.org

Further Reading

Hines, D., and K. Malley-Morrison. *Family Violence in the United States: Defining, Understanding, and Combating Abuse.* Thousand Oaks, CA: Sage Publications, 2005.

> *Overview of violence statistics, risk factors for various types of violence, and strategies for control and prevention.*

Karjane, H., B. Fisher, and F. Cullen. *Sexual Assault on Campus: What Colleges and Universities Are Doing about It.* NCJ Publication no. 205521. Washington, DC: National Institute of Justice, 2005.

> *Overview of trends, causes, and contributors to violence on campus, as well as policies and programs designed to prevent violence.*

Kruttschnitt, C., B. McLauglin, and C. Petrie. *Advancing the Federal Research Agenda on Violence Against Women.* Washington, DC: National Research Council, 2004.

> *Provides key statistics on the epidemic of violence against women, suspected contributors, and areas where more research is needed.*

Wellford, C., J. Pepper, and C. Petrie. *Firearms and Violence: A Critical Review.* Washington, DC: National Academies Press, 2004.

> *Overview of firearm violence and exploration of key issues to violence.*

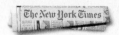

e-themes from *The New York Times*

For up-to-date articles about current health issues, visit www.aw-bc.com/donatelle, select *Health: The Basics.* Eighth Edition, Chapter 4, and click on "e-themes."

References

1. D. Zucchio, "Today's Violent Crime Is an Old Story with a New Twist," *San Jose Mercury News,* November 21, 1994.
2. Bureau of Justice Statistics, "Homicide Trends in the U.S.," September 2004, www.ojp.usdoj.gov/bjs/homicide/teens.htm.
3. Federal Bureau of Investigation, "Preliminary Crime Statistics for January–June, 2006," www.fbi.gov/ucr/ucr.htm.
4. Centers for Disease Control and Prevention, "Youth Risk Behavioral Surveillance U.S.," vol. 53/SS-2: 3, 2003, www.cdc.gov/mmwr.
5. D. P. Barash, *Understanding Violence* (Boston: Allyn & Bacon, 2001), 118–22.
6. K. Maguire and A. L. Pastore, eds. *Sourcebook of Criminal Justice Statistics,* 2002, www.albany.edu/sourcebook.
7. Federal Bureau of Investigation, "National and Regional Crime Statistics from 1970–2003: Summary Findings," 2005, www.fbi.gov.
8. M. Teicher, et al., "Sticks, Stones and Hurtful Words: Relative Effects of Various Forms of Childhood Maltreatment," *American Journal of Psychiatry,* 163 (2006): 993–1000.
9. Ibid.
10. National Center for Health Statistics, "Deaths, Final Data," *National Vital Statistics Report* 54, no. 13 (2006), www.cdc.gov/nchs/data/nvsr/nvsr54/nvsr54_13.pdf.
11. Centers for Disease Control and Prevention, "Leading Causes of Death by Age, Sex and Race," *Health–United States, 2006,* www.cdc.gov/nchs/hus.htm.
12. National Center for Health Statistics, "Deaths, Final Data."
13. Ibid.
14. Federal Bureau of Investigation, "Preliminary Uniform Crime Report," 2005, Geographic Trends in Crime, June 12, 2006, www.fbi.gove.ucr/2005preliminary.
15. Federal Bureau of Investigation, "Hate Crime Statistics—2005, Report Summary," 2006, www.fbi.gov/ucr/hc2005/index.html.
16. Ibid.
17. C. Berlet, "Hate, Repression and the Apocalyptic Style: Facing Complex Questions and Challenges," *Journal of Hate Studies* 3 (2004): 145–58.
18. J. Carr, *American College Health Association Campus Violence White Paper* (Baltimore, MD: American College Health Association, 2005), 11.
19. National Youth Violence Prevention Resource Center, "Youth Gangs and Violence," 2006, www.safeyouth.org/scripts/faq/youthgang.asp.
20. U.S. Code of Federal Regulations, Title 28CFRO. 85.
21. American College of Emergency Physicians, "Fact Sheet on Domestic Violence," 2006, www.acep.org/Webportal/PatientsConsumers/HealthSubjectsByTopic/Violence/domviolence.htm.
22. L. Rosen and J. Fontaine, *Compendium of Research on Violence Against Women, 1993–2005* (Washington, DC: National Institute of Justice, 2006).
23. National Coalition Against Domestic Violence, "Domestic Violence Facts 2006," www.ncadv.org.
24. American College Health Association, "Abusive Relationships—Last 12 Months," in *National College Health Assessment,* Fall 2005, www.acha-ncha.org.
25. National Center for Injury Prevention and Control, "Domestic Violence Fact Sheet," 2005, www.cdc.gov/ncdv/factsheets.htm; J. Chang et al., "Homicide: A Leading Cause of Injury Deaths Among Pregnant and Postpartum Women in the United States, 1991–1999," *American Journal of Public Health* 95, no. 3 (2005): 471–77.
26. N. West, "Crimes Against Women," *Community Safety Quarterly* 5 (1992): 3.
27. National Coalition Against Domestic Violence, "2005 Domestic Violence Statistics," 2006, www.ncadv.org/files/DV_Facts.pdf.
28. Rosen and Fontaine, *Compendium of Research on Violence Against Women.*
29. Ibid.
30. Ibid.
31. Ibid.
32. National Center for Injury Prevention and Control, "Child Maltreatment: Fact Sheet," 2006, www.cdc.gov/ncipc/factsheets/cmfacts.htm.
33. Ibid.
34. Administration for Children and Families, "An Issue Facing All Communities: The National Scope of the Problem," 2005, nccanch.acf.hhs.gov/topics/prevention/childabuse_neglect/scope.cfm.
35. Ibid.
36. Ibid.
37. American College of Emergency Physicians, 2006.
38. National Women's Health Information Center, "Sexual Assault," 2005, www.4woman.gov/faq/sexualassault.htm.
39. National Center for Injury Prevention and Control, "Sexual Violence Fact Sheet," 2007, www.cdc.gov/ncipc/factsheets/svfacts.htm.
40. D. Elliot et al., "Adult Sexual Assault: Prevalence, Symptomology, and Sex Differences in the General Population," *Journal of Traumatic Stress* 17, no. 3 (2004): 203–11.
41. National Women's Health Information Center, "Sexual Assault."
42. Ibid.
43. J. Carr, *Campus Violence White Paper,* 12.
44. University of Chicago, "Sexual Violence," 2006, sexualviolence.uchicago.edu/resources.shtml.
45. J. Butcher, S. Mineka, and J. Hooley, *Abnormal Psychology,* 13th ed. (Boston: Allyn & Bacon, 2007).
46. R. K. Bergen, "Violence Against Women Online Resources," University of Minnesota, 2005, www.vaw.umn.edu.
47. Ibid.
48. P. Benson et al., "Acquaintance Rape on Campus," *Journal of American College Health* 40 (1992): 157–65.
49. Rape, Abuse, and Incest National Network, "The Victims of Sexual Assault," 2006, www.rainn.org/statistics/victims-of-sexual-assault.html.
50. A. Berkowitz, "College Men as Perpetrators of Acquaintance Rape and Sexual Assault," *Journal of American College Health* 40 (1992): 175–81.
51. Bergen, "Violence Against Women Online Resources."
52. World Health Organization, "Injuries and Violence Prevention: Child Abuse and Neglect," 2006, www.who.int/violence_injury_prevention/violence/neglect/en.

53. National Center for Injury Prevention and Control, "Sexual Violence: Fact Sheet," 2006, www.cdc.gov/ncipc/factsheets/cmfacts.htm.

54. National Center for Injury Prevention and Control, "Sexual Violence Fact Sheet"; D. Rungan et al., "Child Abuse and Neglect by Parents and Caregivers," in *World Health Report on Violence and Health*, ed. E. Krug et al., 59–86 (Geneva, Switzerland: World Health Organization, 2002).

55. American Academy of Pediatrics, "Children's Health Topics: Child Abuse and Neglect," 2007, www.aap.org/healthtopics/childabuse.cfm.

56. A. Hoffman et al., eds., *Violence on Campus: Defining the Problems, Strategies for Action* (Gaithersburg, MD: Aspen Publishers, 1998), 1–40.

57. J. Carr, *Campus Violence White Paper*, 4.

58. Hoffman et al., *Violence on Campus*, 1–40.

59. Ibid.

60. A. Gross et al., "An Examination of Sexual Violence Against College Women," *Violence Against Women* 12, no. 3 (2006): 240–50.

61. S. Catalano, *National Crime Victimization Survey: Criminal Victimization 2005*, NCJ Publication no. 214644 (Washington, DC: U.S. Department of Justice, 2006).

62. American College Health Association, "Sexual Abuse and Assault," in *National College Health Assessment*, Fall 2005, www.acha-ncha.org.

63. A. Gross, et al., "An Examination of Sexual Violence," 240–50.

64. Ibid.

65. National Center for Victims of Crime, Stalking Resource Center, 2007, www.ncvc.org/src/Main.aspx.

66. J. Carr and K. Van Deusen, "Risk Factors for Male Sexual Aggression on College Campuses," *Journal of Family Violence* 19, no. 5 (2004): 279–89.

67. Ibid.

68. Ibid.

69. Ibid.

70. Ibid.

71. K. Baum and P. Klaus, *Violent Victimization of College Students, 1995–2002*, NCJ Publication no. 206836 (Washington, DC: U.S. Department of Justice, 2005).

72. J. Carr, *Campus Violence White Paper*, 10. (Baltimore. MD: American College Health Association, 2005).

5

Healthy Relationships and Sexuality

MAKING COMMITMENTS

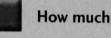 Does an **intimate** relationship have to be sexual?

How can I communicate **better?**

Is it good to **live** together before getting married?

What is "**normal**" sexual behavior?

How much **sex** do my peers have?

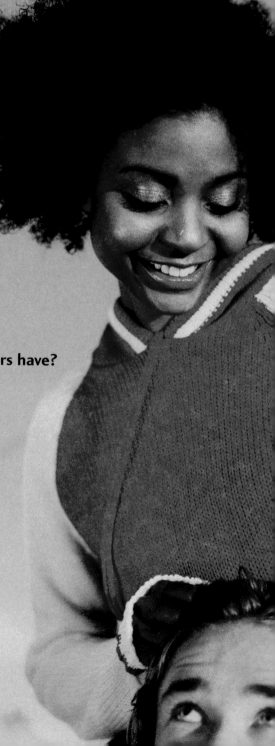

OBJECTIVES

- Discuss ways to improve communication skills and interpersonal interactions.
- Identify the characteristics of successful relationships, including how to maintain them and overcome common barriers.
- Examine factors that affect life decisions, such as whether to have children.
- Define *sexual identity,* and discuss its major components, including biology, gender identity, gender roles, and sexual orientation.
- Identify major features and functions of sexual anatomy and physiology.
- Classify sexual dysfunctions, and describe major disorders.

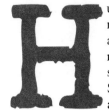umans are social beings—we have a basic need to belong and to feel loved, appreciated, and wanted. We can't live without relating to others in some way. In fact, a study done by researchers at the Harvard School of Public Health shows that the ability to relate well with people, as well as give and receive love and support throughout your life, can have almost as much impact on your health as exercise and good nutrition.[1]

All relationships involve a degree of risk. However, only by taking these risks can we grow and truly experience all that life has to offer. By looking at our intimate and non-intimate relationships, components of sexual identity, gender roles, and sexual orientation, we will come to better understand who we are.

Characterizing and Forming Intimate Relationships

We can define **intimate relationships** in terms of four characteristics: behavioral interdependence, need fulfillment, emotional attachment, and emotional availability. Each of these characteristics may be related to interactions with family, close friends, and romantic partners.

Behavioral interdependence refers to the mutual impact that people have on each other as their lives and daily activities intertwine. What one person does influences what the other person wants to do and can do. Behavioral interdependence may become stronger over time to the point that each person would feel a great void if the other were gone.

Intimate relationships also fulfill psychological needs and so are a means of *need fulfillment*. Through relationships with others, we fulfill our needs for

- *Intimacy*—someone with whom we can share our feelings freely
- *Social integration*—someone with whom we can share worries and concerns
- *Nurturance*—someone whom we can take care of and who will take care of us
- *Assistance*—someone to help us in times of need
- *Affirmation*—someone who will reassure us of our own worth and tell us that we matter

In intimate relationships that are mutually rewarding, partners and friends meet each other's needs. They disclose feelings, share confidences, and provide support and reassurance. Each person comes away from interactions feeling better for the experience and validated by the other person.

Does an intimate relationship have to be sexual?

In addition to behavioral interdependence and need fulfillment, intimate relationships involve strong bonds of *emotional attachment,* or feelings of love. When we hear the word *intimacy,* we often think of a sexual relationship. Although sex can play an important role in emotional attachment, a relationship can be very intimate and yet not sexual. Two people can be emotionally intimate (share feelings) or spiritually intimate (share spiritual beliefs and meanings), or they can be intimate friends. With such a range of possibilities, the intimacy level two people experience cannot be judged easily by those outside the relationship (**Figure 5.1**).

Emotional availability, the ability to give to and receive from others emotionally without fear of being hurt or rejected, is the fourth characteristic of intimate relationships. At times, all of us may limit our emotional availability. For example, after a painful breakup we may decide not to jump into another relationship immediately, or we may decide not to talk about it with every friend. Holding back can offer time

> **intimate relationships** Relationships with family members, friends, and romantic partners, characterized by behavioral interdependence, need fulfillment, emotional attachment, and emotional availability.

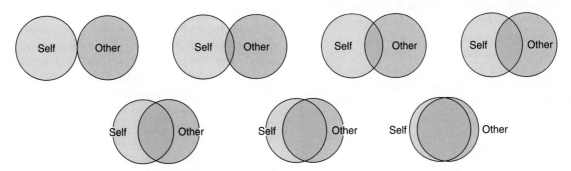

FIGURE 5.1 How Intimate Is a Relationship?
Relationships can exist on a continuum of closeness and inclusion. Asking people to choose the diagram that best portrays a particular relationship of theirs does a remarkably good job of assessing the closeness they feel.

Source: A. Aron, D. J. Mashek, and E. N. Aron, "Closeness as Including the Other in the Self," in *Handbook of Closeness and Intimacy,* ed. D. J. Mashek and A. Aron (Mahwah, N. J.: Erlbaum, 2004), 27–41.

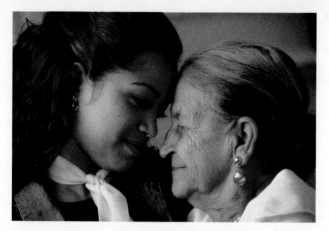

The emotional bonds that characterize intimate relationships often span the generations and help individuals gain insight and understanding into each other's worlds.

for introspection and healing, as well as for considering the lessons learned. However, some people who have experienced intense trauma find it difficult ever to be fully available emotionally. This limits their ability to experience intimate relationships.

In the early years of life, families provide the most significant relationships. Gradually, the circle widens to include friends, co-workers, and acquaintances. Ultimately, most of us develop romantic or sexual relationships with significant others. Each of these relationships plays a significant role in psychological, social, spiritual, and physical health.

Families: The Ties That Bind

A family is a recognizable group of people with roles, tasks, boundaries, and personalities whose central focus is to protect, care for, love, and socialize one another. Because the family is a dynamic institution that changes as society changes, the definition of *family,* and those individuals believed to constitute family membership, changes over time as well. Who are members of today's families? Historically, most families have been made up of people related by blood, marriage or long-term committed relationships, or adoption.[2] Yet today, many other groups of people are being recognized and are functioning as family units (**Table 5.1**). Although there is no "best" family type, we do know that a healthy family's key roles and tasks are to nurture and support. Healthy families foster a sense of security and feelings of belonging that are central to growth and development. It is from our **family of origin,** the people present in our household during our first years of life, that we initially learn about feelings, problem solving, love, intimacy, and gender roles. We learn to negotiate relationships and have opportunities to communicate effectively; develop attitudes, beliefs, and

family of origin   People present in the household during a child's first years of life—usually parents and siblings.

TABLE 5.1   Today's Changing Families

The United States is a melting pot of family types. The estimated percentages of school-aged children living in various family structures is listed below.

Family structure	School-aged children living in identified family structure (%)
Nuclear family: husband and wife plus biological offspring	58
Stepparent family: one biological parent plus one stepparent	10
Blended family: parents plus children born to several families	5
Adoptive family: two parents	2
Single mother, never married	10
Single mother, divorced	10
Single father, divorced and never remarried	5

Source: Based on data from the U.S. Census Bureau, 2000.

values; and explore spiritual belief systems. It is not uncommon when we establish relationships outside the family to rely on these initial experiences and on skills modeled by our family of origin.

Establishing Friendships

Good friends—they can make a boring day fun, a cold day warm, or a gut-wrenching worry disappear. They can make us feel that we matter and that we have the strength to get through just about anything. They can also make us angry, disappoint us, or seriously jolt our comfortable ideas about right and wrong.

Friendships are relationships between two or more people that involve mutual respect, trust, support, and intimacy that may or may not include sexual intimacy. Like our family relationships, our friendships should have identified roles and boundaries. Persons in friendships should communicate their understandings, needs, expectations, limitations, and affections.[3]

Psychologists believe that people are attracted to and form relationships with people who give them positive reinforcement and that they dislike those who punish or overcriticize them. The basic idea is simple: you like people who like you. Another factor that affects the development of a friendship is a real or perceived similarity in attitudes, opinions, and background.[4] In addition, true friends have a sense of equity in which they share confidences, contribute fairly and equally to maintaining the friendship, and consistently try to give as much as they get back from the interactions.[5]

Take a few minutes to examine one of your current friendships. What characteristics can you identify in that relationship that keep your friendship intact?

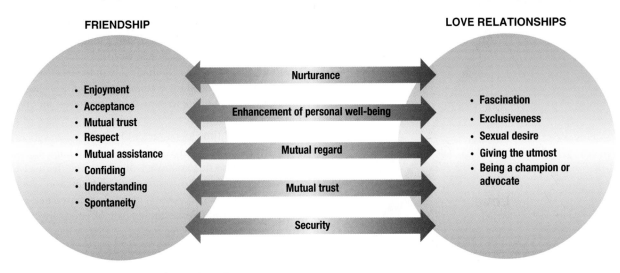

FIGURE 5.2 **Common Bonds of Friends and Lovers**

Significant Others, Partners, and Couples

Most people choose at some point to enter into an intimate sexual relationship with another person. Most committed partners fit into one of four categories: married heterosexual couples, cohabitating heterosexual couples, lesbian couples, and gay male couples. These groups are discussed in greater detail later in this chapter.

Love relationships in each of these four groups typically include all the characteristics of friendship as well as the following characteristics related to passion and caring **(Figure 5.2)**.[6]

- *Fascination.* Lovers tend to pay attention to the other person even when they should be involved in other activities. They are preoccupied with the other and want to think about, talk to, or be with the other.
- *Exclusiveness.* Lovers have a special relationship that usually precludes having the same relationship with a third party. The love relationship often takes priority over all others.
- *Sexual desire.* Lovers desire physical intimacy and want to touch, hold, and engage in sexual activities with the other.
- *Giving the utmost.* Lovers care enough to give the utmost when the other is in need, sometimes to the point of extreme sacrifice.
- *Being a champion or advocate.* Lovers actively champion each other's interests and attempt to ensure that the other succeeds.

This Thing Called Love

What is love? This four-letter word has been written about and engraved on walls; it has been the theme of countless novels, movies, and plays. There is no single definition of *love,* and the word may mean different things to people,

depending on cultural values, age, gender, and situation. Yet, we all know what it is when it strikes.

Many social scientists maintain that love may be of two kinds: companionate and passionate. Companionate love is a secure, trusting attachment, similar to what we may feel for family members or close friends. In companionate love, two people are attracted, have much in common, care about each other's well-being, and express reciprocal liking and respect. Passionate love, in contrast, is a state of high arousal filled with the ecstasy of being loved and the agony of being rejected.[7] In this next section, we will explore what passionate love is.

Theories of Love

How and why love develops are not easy questions to answer. Several theories have been proposed to help provide insight into the process. Sternberg's classic Triangular Theory of Love **(Figure 5.3)** suggests that there are three key components to loving relationships.[8]

1. *Intimacy*—the emotional component, which involves closeness, sharing, and mutual support

2. *Passion*—the motivational component, which includes lust, attraction, sexual arousal, and sharing

3. *Commitment*—the cognitive component, which includes the decision to be open to love in the short term and the commitment to the relationship in the long term

The quality of love relationships is reflected by the level of intimacy, passion, and commitment each person brings to the relationship over time.

A second theory of love and attraction, based on brain circuitry and chemistry, is quite different from that of Sternberg. Anthropologist Helen Fisher, among others, hypothesizes that attraction and falling in love follow a fairly predictable pattern based on (1) *imprinting,* in which our evolutionary patterns, genetic predispositions, and past experiences trigger

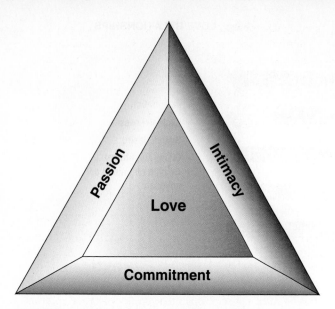

FIGURE 5.3 Sternberg's Triangular Theory of Love

Source: R. Sternberg, "Construct Validation of a Triangular Love Scale," *European Journal of Social Psychology* 27 (1997): 313–35. Copyright © Robert Sternberg.

a romantic reaction; (2) *attraction,* in which neurochemicals produce feelings of euphoria and elation; (3) *attachment,* in which endorphins—natural opiates—cause lovers to feel peaceful, secure, and calm; and (4) *production of a cuddle chemical,* in which the brain secretes the chemical *oxytocin,* thereby stimulating sensations during lovemaking and eliciting feelings of satisfaction and attachment.[9]

Lovers who claim that they are swept away by passion may not be far from the truth. Why? Because the love-smitten person's endocrine system secretes chemical substances such as dopamine, norepinephrine, and phenylethylamine (PEA), which are chemical cousins to amphetamines.[10] Although attraction may in fact be a "natural high," this hit of passion loses effectiveness over time as the body builds up tolerance. Many people may become attraction junkies, seeking the intoxication of love much as the drug user seeks a chemical high.[11] Fisher speculates that PEA levels drop significantly over a 3- to 4-year period, leading to the "4-year itch" that shows up in the peaking fourth-year divorce rates present in over 60 cultures. Romances that last beyond the 4-year mark are influenced by another set of chemicals, known as endorphins, soothing substances that give lovers a sense of security, peace, and calm.[12]

Communicating: A Key to Good Relationships

From the moment of birth, we struggle to be understood. We flail our arms, cry, scream, smile, frown, and make sounds and gestures to attract attention, get a reaction from someone we care about, or have someone understand what we want or need from him or her. By the time we enter adulthood, each of us has developed a unique way of communicating to others with gestures, words, expressions, and body positions. No two of us communicate in the exact same way or have the same need for connecting with others. Some of us are outgoing and quick to express our emotions and thoughts. Others are quiet, are reluctant to talk about feelings, and may prefer to spend time alone rather than with others.

Different cultures have not only different languages and dialects, but also different ways of expressing themselves and using body language to communicate information. Some cultures gesture wildly; others maintain a closed and rigid means of speaking. Some cultures are offended by apparent "fixed and dilated" staring, whereas others welcome a steady look in the eyes.

Although people differ in the way they communicate, this doesn't mean that one sex, culture, or group is better or should be a model for the others. We have to be willing to accept differences and work to keep communication lines open and fluid. Appearing interested, actively engaged in the interaction, and open and willing to exchange ideas and thoughts is something that we typically learn with practice and hard work.

Communicating How You Feel

Do you find it easy to convey how much you care about friends and family members with hugs and verbal expressions of appreciation and love? If you are comfortable telling them you love them and that they mean a lot to you, chances are that you also will be able to tell them when you are feeling bad, disappointed, angry, or frustrated. However, it's important to realize that some people were not raised in openly affectionate families, do not readily discuss feelings or emotions, and sometimes may struggle to find the right words for expressing what they feel.

When two people begin a relationship, they bring their past communication styles with them. How often have you heard someone say, "We just can't communicate," or "You're sending mixed messages"? These exchanges occur regularly as people start relationships or work through ongoing communication problems in an existing relationship. Because communication is a process, our every action, word, facial expression, gesture, or body posture becomes part of our shared history and part of the evolving impression we make on others. If we are angry in our responses, others will be reluctant to interact with us. If we bring "baggage" from past bad interactions to new relationships, we may be cynical, distrustful, and guarded in our exchanges with others. If we are positive, happy, and share openly with others, they will be more likely to communicate openly with us. This ability to communicate assertively is an important skill in relationships (see the **Assess Yourself** box on page 122). Assertive communicators are in touch with their feelings and values and are able to communicate their needs directly and honestly and to defend choices in a positive manner.

Improving Your Communication Skills

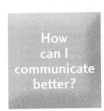

How can I communicate better?

Because people have such different ways of communicating, there is no recipe for how to communicate best in a given situation. At times, silence may be the best approach. However, there are things that each of us can do to become a better communicator and to encourage and assist others in their attempts to interact with us.

Learning Appropriate Self-Disclosure Sharing personal information with others is called **self-disclosure.** If you are willing to share personal information with others, they will likely share personal information with you. In other words, if you want to learn more about someone, you have to be willing to share parts of your personal self with that person. Self-disclosure is not storytelling or sharing secrets; rather, it is revealing how you are reacting to the present situation and giving any information about the past that is relevant to the other person's understanding of your current reactions.

Self-disclosure can be a double-edged sword, for there is risk in divulging personal insights and feelings. If you sense that sharing feelings and personal thoughts will result in a closer relationship, you will likely take such a risk. But if you believe that the disclosure may result in rejection or alienation, you may not open up so easily. If the confidentiality of previously shared information has been violated, you may hesitate to disclose yourself in the future.

However, the risk in not disclosing yourself to others is that you will lack intimacy in relationships. Psychologist Carl Rogers stressed the importance of understanding yourself and others through self-disclosure. Rogers believed that weak relationships were characterized by inhibited self-disclosure.[13]

If self-disclosure is a key element in creating healthy communication, but fear is a barrier to that process, what can we do? The following suggestions can help:

- *Get to know yourself.* Remember that your self includes your feelings, beliefs, thoughts, and concerns. The more you know about yourself, the more likely you will be able to communicate with others about yourself. Think about who you are, what you are passionate about, and what your strengths and limitations are. Which of these do you feel good about? Which cause you concern?
- *Become more accepting of yourself.* No one is perfect or has to be. Even the people you look up to have their flaws. Only by accepting your imperfections can you expect others to accept them, too.
- *Be willing to discuss your sexual history.* In a culture that puts many taboos on discussions of sex in everyday conversation, it's no wonder we find it hard to disclose our sexual feelings to those with whom we are intimate. However, with the soaring rate of sexually transmitted infections and the ever-looming threat of AIDS, there has never been a more important time to disclose sexual feelings and history. The life-altering effects of an unwanted pregnancy or contracting HIV underscore the need to communicate about sex before you become intimate.
- *Choose a safe context for self-disclosure.* Context refers to the setting in which the self-disclosure occurs. When and where you make such disclosures and to whom may greatly influence the response. Choose a setting in which you feel safe to let yourself be known.

Becoming a Better Listener

Listening is a vital part of interpersonal communication; it allows us to share feelings, express concerns, communicate wants and needs, and let our thoughts and opinions be known. We must do the necessary work to improve both our speaking and listening skills, which will enhance our relationships, improve our grasp of information, and allow us to interpret more effectively what others say. We listen best when (1) we believe that the message is somehow important and relevant to us; (2) the speaker holds our attention through humor, dramatic effect, use of media, or other techniques; and (3) we are in the mood to listen (free of distractions and worries). When we really listen effectively, we try to understand what people are thinking and feeling from their perspective. We not only hear the words, but also try to understand what is really being said. How many times have you been caught pretending to listen when you were not? After several moments of nodding and saying, "Uh-huh," your friend finally asks you a question, and you haven't a clue what she has been saying. Sometimes this tuned-out behavior is due to lack of sleep, stress overload, being preoccupied, having had too much to drink, or being under the influence of drugs. Other times the reason is that the speaker is a motormouth who talks for the sake of talking, or that you find the speaker or topic of conversation boring. Some of the most common listening difficulties are things that we can work to improve. See the **Skills for Behavior Change** box on page 124 for suggestions to improve your listening.

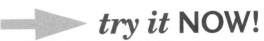

try it NOW!

Change the "you" to "I." Think about the last time you had an argument with a friend, sibling, or roommate. On a piece of paper, rewrite your stance in this disagreement using an "I" message (such as "I feel . . .") instead of a "you" message implying blame or criticizing the other person. The next time you have a similar disagreement with the same person, use the "I" message. Notice how the other person's response changes and how the conversation becomes less hostile and more solution oriented.

self-disclosure Sharing personal feelings or information with others.

ASSESS *yourself*

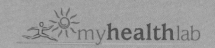

STANDING UP FOR YOURSELF

You know that sinking feeling. Someone asks you to do something, and your stomach lurches. You don't want to go along, but you can't come up with a good excuse not to do so.

It's hard to say no. How often are you caught in the "I can't say no" trap? Read the following situations, and assess your response according to the following 5-point scale.

	Never	Seldom	Sometimes	Frequently	Always
1. Friends ask you to ride home with them after they've all been drinking. You know you shouldn't go, but you don't want to seem like a prude. You take the ride.	1	2	3	4	5
2. Your decisions can be easily swayed by a strong argument from someone else pushing you in the opposite direction.	1	2	3	4	5
3. You feel strongly about a political issue, but it is the opposite of the opinion your parents hold. You remain silent rather than getting into an argument.	1	2	3	4	5
4. You start out by saying no to something but get talked into doing it after a short time.	1	2	3	4	5
5. You're stressed out with too much to do and too little time, but you can't seem to say no when someone asks for a favor.	1	2	3	4	5
6. Someone says something really nasty about a person you like. You jump to the defense of the person being criticized, even though you are in the minority opinion.	1	2	3	4	5
7. You would describe yourself as assertive and tend to quickly let others know your thoughts about certain issues.	1	2	3	4	5
8. Someone is critical of something you do. You quickly defend your actions by explaining why you did what you did.	1	2	3	4	5

INTERPRETING YOUR SCORE

Think about your responses to each statement. Do your responses indicate an assertive communication style in which you stand up for your feelings or beliefs? What factors cause you to hold back when you should probably speak up? How can you work to improve your communication behaviors in this area? For statements 1 through 5, do you have several "5" responses? If yes, you should consider what skills you could develop to help you communicate more assertively.

Gender Issues in Relationships

When it comes to relationships, are men really from Mars and women from Venus? If they are not planets apart, how far apart are they, and what are the implications of the disparities? In her landmark book *You Just Don't Understand: Women and Men in Conversation,* psychologist Deborah Tannen coined the term **genderlect** to characterize differences in word choices, interruption patterns, questioning patterns, language interpretations and misinterpretations, and vocal influences based on gender.[14] Tannen is not alone in her research; communication patterns between women and men have been studied for generations with similar results. Recent research validates much of this work and indicates that women tend to be more expressive, relationship oriented, and concerned with creating and maintaining intimacy; men tend to be more instrumental, task oriented, and concerned with gathering information or establishing and maintaining social status or power.[15] Unlike women, men tend to believe that they are not supposed to show emotions and are brought up to believe that "being strong" is often more important than having close friendships. As a result, men are generally less likely to share their innermost thoughts.

genderlect The "dialect," or individual speech pattern and communication style, of each gender.

MAKE it happen!

ASSESSMENT: The Assess Yourself activity gave you the chance to look at how you communicate in certain situations. It is important to be able to communicate assertively and to feel that you can stand up for yourself. Now that you have considered your responses to the statements, you may want to take steps toward becoming a more assertive communicator. **MAKING A CHANGE:** To change your behavior, you need to develop a plan. Follow these steps below and complete your Behavior Change Contract to take action.

1. Evaluate your behavior, and identify patterns. What can you change now? What can you change in the near future?

2. Select one pattern of behavior that you want to change.

3. Fill out the Behavior Change Contract found at the front of your book. It should include your long-term goal for change, your short-term goals, the rewards you'll give yourself for reaching these goals, potential obstacles along the way, and strategies for overcoming these obstacles. For each goal, list the small steps and specific actions that you will take.

4. Chart your progress in a journal. At the end of a week, consider how successful you were in following your plan.

What helped you be successful? What made change more difficult? What will you do differently next week?

5. Revise your plan as needed: Are the short-term goals attainable? Are the rewards satisfying?

EXAMPLE: When Stacey assessed her responses to the statements about assertiveness, she realized that she tended to say yes when someone asked her for a favor, no matter how busy or stressed out she was. Stacey decided she wanted to learn to say no when necessary. She set a goal of imagining certain situations that she had faced recently and how she would handle them more assertively. The first week, she imagined her older sister asking her to babysit her son at the last minute and her roommates asking her for car rides while she was in the middle of studying. She planned what she would say and how she would explain her reasons for saying no. The second week, when her roommates asked for a ride to the movies, Stacey calmly stated that she was busy and needed 2 hours more for studying before she could take a break. Her roommates decided to walk to the video store instead and rented a movie they could all watch together when Stacey was ready for a break.

what do you THINK?

Who are the people with whom you feel most comfortable talking about personal issues? ■ Do you talk with both men and women about these issues, or do you tend to gravitate toward just one sex? ■ Why do you think you do this?

Picking Partners

For both men and women, the choice of relationship partners is influenced by more than just chemical and psychological processes. One important factor is *proximity,* or being in the same place at the same time. The more you see a person in your hometown, at social gatherings, or at work, the more

likely that you will interact with him or her. Thus, if you live in New York, you'll probably end up with another New Yorker. With the advent of the Internet, however, geographic proximity has become less important.

You also pick a partner based on *similarities* (attitudes, values, intellect, interests); the old adage that "opposites attract" usually isn't true. If your potential partner expresses interest or liking, you may react with mutual regard known as *reciprocity.* The more you express interest, the safer it is for someone else to return the regard, and the cycle spirals onward.

A final factor that plays a significant role in selecting a partner is *attraction.* Whether such attraction is caused by a chemical reaction or a socially learned behavior, men and women appear to have different attraction criteria. When selecting mates, men tend to be attracted primarily to youth and beauty. Although physical attractiveness is an important

SKILLS FOR behavior change

LEARNING TO REALLY LISTEN

Most of us have lamented the fact that someone "never listens" and seems to monopolize the entire conversation. Although we are quick to recognize such flaws in others, we are often less likely to spot listening problems of our own. If the truth be told, most of us are only mediocre listeners. What does it take to be an excellent listener? Try practicing the following skills and consciously using them on a daily basis.

- *Be present in the moment.* Good listeners don't just sit back with their mouths shut. They participate and acknowledge what the other person is saying. Nodding, smiling, saying "yes" or "uh-huh," and asking questions at appropriate times are all part of this. Take care, however, not to numbly reply, "uh-huh" to every word, which is distracting and conveys insincerity.
- *Use positive body language and voice tone.* Voice tone, posture, and an attitude that conveys interest are all key. Avoid barrier gestures such as shaking your head no, making negative faces, or folding your arms. Smile at appropriate times, and maintain appropriate eye contact (deadpan stares can also be distracting).
- *Show empathy and sympathy.* Watch for verbal and nonverbal clues to the other person's feelings and try to relate. For example, saying, "That must have been really hard for you," can encourage the speaker to talk and feel more comfortable with you.
- *Ask for clarification.* If you aren't sure what the speaker means, indicate that you're not sure you understand, or paraphrase what you think you heard.
- *Control that deadly desire to interrupt.* Some people start nodding and gesturing before you ever get a word out of your mouth. If you are like that, squelch it, even if you have to put an inconspicuous hand over your mouth. Try taking a deep breath for two seconds, then hold your breath for another second and really listen to what is being said as you slowly exhale. Don't be so enthusiastically empathetic that you finish speakers' sentences or put words in their mouths.
- *Avoid snap judgments based on what other people look like or are saying.* If you notice some strange mannerism, try to focus on what is being said, not how it is being said.
- *Resist the temptation to "set the other person straight".* Control your urge to correct errors or react defensively.
- *Try to focus on the speaker.* Sometimes it is very tough to listen to someone who is trying to talk about a painful situation, especially if we have experienced the same thing. Hold back the temptation to fly off into your own rendition of a similar situation. Give the speaker the moment, and later, after he or she is done talking, you may want to discuss your own experience as a way of validating the feelings expressed. Don't tell him how he is feeling or how he should feel.
- *Be tenacious.* Stick with the speaker, and try to stay on the topic. If the speaker seems to wander, gently nudge the person back by saying, "You were just saying . . ." Offer your thoughts and suggestions, but remember that you should advise only up to a certain point. Clarify statements by saying, "This is my opinion," as a reminder that it is only opinion, rather than fact.

---

criterion for women in mate selection, they tend to find older mates more attractive and to place higher emphasis on partners who have good financial prospects and who appear to be dependable and industrious.[16]

Sharing Feelings

Although men tend to talk about intimate issues with women more frequently than with other men, many women still complain that men do not communicate enough about what is really on their minds. This may reflect the different socialization processes experienced by women and men, which influence their communication styles. Throughout their lives, women are offered opportunities to practice sharing their thoughts and feelings with others. In contrast, men often receive strong societal messages to withhold their feelings. The classic example of this training in very young boys is the familiar saying, "Big boys don't cry." Men learn early that certain emotions are not to be shared, with the result that they are more information-focused and businesslike in their conversations. Understandably, such differences in communication styles contribute to misunderstandings and conflict.

Although men are sometimes perceived as being less emotional than women, do they really feel less, or do they just have more difficulty expressing their emotions? In one study in which men and women were shown scenes of people in distress, the men exhibited little outward emotion, whereas the women communicated feelings of concern and distress. However, physiological measures of emotional arousal (such as heart rate and blood pressure) indicated that the male subjects were as affected emotionally as the female subjects but inhibited the expression of their emotions; the women openly expressed them. In other studies, men and women responded very differently to the same test.[17]

When men are angered, they tend to interpret the cause of their anger as something or someone in their environment and are likely to turn their anger outward in an aggressive manner.

Women, by contrast, tend to see themselves as the source of the problem and turn their anger inward, suppressing direct expression of it.[18]

what do you THINK?

Do you believe that men and women really communicate in different styles? ■ What can you do to improve your communication with members of the other sex?

Overcoming Barriers to Intimacy

Obstacles to intimacy include lack of personal identity, emotional immaturity, and a poorly developed sense of responsibility. The fear of being hurt, low self-esteem, mishandled hostility, chronic "busyness" (and its attendant lack of emotional presence), a tendency to "parentify" loved ones, and a conflict of role expectations may be equally detrimental. Individual insecurities and difficulties in recognizing and expressing emotional needs also can create obstacles. These barriers to intimacy may have many causes, including miscommunication, a dysfunctional family background, and jealousy.

Barriers to Communication

In today's world of instant messages, cell phones, pagers, and technologically advanced information systems, communication problems have grown exponentially. Our current means of communication differ greatly from those of our ancestors. In addition, people around the world must increasingly interact with others of vastly different backgrounds and values. Finding a means of communicating that accommodates everyone can be difficult. Barriers to communication take many forms.

Differences in Background
Age, education, social status, gender, culture, political beliefs, and many other variables can lead to differences between communicators. Your closest friends from high school, with whom you grew up, shared many similar experiences with you. Shared experiences contribute to shared meaning and understanding. At college, however, you may suddenly find yourself among people having few shared experiences. Remember that the goal of good communication is not necessarily to have everyone agree with you; rather, it is to have others understand you.

Alcohol and Drugs
Perhaps nothing stands in the way of effective communication more than alcohol and drugs. With an inhibited ability to express yourself clearly, you may not be understood correctly. With an inhibited

ability to comprehend another's communication, you may misinterpret someone else's message. Is it any wonder that 90 percent of campus rapes take place under the influence of alcohol? Avoiding date rape depends on a woman's ability to be clear in her own mind about what she wants and then to make herself clearly understood, as well as on a man's ability to listen and hear what the woman is saying rather than what he thinks she is saying. In most college campus sexual encounters that lead to date rape complaints, alcohol and drugs have played a role.

Dysfunctional Families

As noted earlier, the ability to sustain genuine intimacy is largely developed in the family of origin. If you were to examine even the most pristine family under a microscope, you would likely find some problems. No group of people can interact perfectly all the time, but this does not necessarily make them dysfunctional. In a truly **dysfunctional family,** interaction between family members inhibits psychological growth, self-love, emotional expression, and individual development. Negative interactions are the norm rather than the exception. It is important to note that dysfunctional families are found in every social, ethnic, religious, economic, and racial group.

Learning new and healthful communication and relationship skills takes time. However, with support from loved ones, and counseling when needed, children from even the most dysfunctional homes have proven to be remarkably resilient. Many are able to move beyond the past, focus on the future, and develop into healthy, well-adjusted adults.

Jealousy in Relationships

"Jealousy is like a San Andreas fault running beneath the smooth surface of an intimate relationship. Most of the time, its eruptive potential lies hidden. But when it begins to rumble, the destruction can be enormous."[19] **Jealousy** has been described as an aversive reaction evoked by a real or imagined relationship involving one's partner and a third person.

Contrary to what many of us may believe, jealousy is not a sign of intense devotion. Instead, jealousy often indicates underlying problems that may prove to be a significant barrier to a healthy intimate relationship. Often, jealousy in a relationship is rooted in a past relationship in which an individual experienced deception, or from observing

dysfunctional family   A family in which the interaction between family members inhibits rather than enhances psychological growth.

jealousy   An aversive reaction evoked by a real or imagined relationship involving a person's partner and a third person.

patterns among friends. Causes of jealousy typically include the following.

- *Overdependence on the relationship.* People who have few social ties and rely exclusively on their significant others tend to be fearful of losing them.
- *High value on sexual exclusivity.* People who believe sexual exclusivity is a crucial indicator of love are more likely to become jealous.
- *Severity of the threat.* People may feel uneasy if someone with stunning good looks and a great personality appears interested in their partners.
- *Low self-esteem.* The underlying question that torments people with low self-esteem is "Why would anyone want me?" People who feel good about themselves and believe that they are a good "catch" are less likely to fear that someone else is going to snatch their partners.
- *Fear of losing control.* Some people need to feel in control of the situation. Feeling that they may be losing the attachment of or control over a partner can cause jealousy.

In both sexes, jealousy is related to the expectation that it would be difficult to find another relationship if the current one ends. For men, jealousy is positively correlated with self-evaluative dependence, the degree to which the man's self-esteem is affected by his partner's judgments. Though a certain amount of jealousy can be expected in any loving relationship, it doesn't have to threaten a relationship as long as partners communicate openly about it.[20]

 what do you THINK?

"Jealousy is not a barometer by which the depth of love can be read. It merely records the depth of the lover's insecurity," observed anthropologist Margaret Mead. ■ Do you agree or disagree with this statement? ■ What other factors may play a role in jealousy?

Committed Relationships

Commitment in a relationship means that one intends to act over time in a way that perpetuates the well-being of the other person, oneself, and the relationship. Polls show that the majority of Americans—as many as 96 percent—strive

monogamy Exclusive sexual involvement with one partner.

serial monogamy A series of monogamous sexual relationships.

open relationship A relationship in which partners agree that sexual involvement can occur outside the relationship.

to develop a committed relationship, even though many have difficulty maintaining them. These relationships can take several forms, including marriage, cohabitation, and gay and lesbian partnerships.

Marriage

In many societies around the world, traditional committed relationships take the form of marriage. In the United States, marriage means entering into a legal agreement that includes shared financial plans, property, and responsibility for raising children. Many Americans also view marriage as a religious sacrament that emphasizes certain rights and obligations for each spouse.

Historically, close to 90 percent of Americans marry at least once during their lifetime. In recent years, Americans have become less likely to marry. From 1970 to 2004, annual marriages of adult women declined by 50 percent.[21] This decrease may be due to several factors, including delay of first marriages, increase in cohabitation, and a small decrease in the number of divorced persons who remarry. In 1970, the median age for first marriage was 22.5 years for men and 20.6 years for women; in 2004, the median age of first marriage had risen to 26 for females and 27 for males.[22]

Many Americans believe that marriage involves **monogamy,** or exclusive sexual involvement with one partner. In fact, the lifetime pattern for many Americans appears to be **serial monogamy,** which means that a person has a monogamous sexual relationship with one partner before moving on to another monogamous relationship. However, some people prefer to have an **open relationship,** or open marriage, in which the partners agree that there may be sexual involvement for each person outside their relationship.

Marriage is socially sanctioned and highly celebrated in our culture, so there are numerous incentives for couples to formalize their relationship with a wedding ceremony. A healthy marriage provides emotional support by combining the benefits of friendship and a loving committed relationship. A happy marriage also provides stability for both the couple and for those involved in the couple's life. Considerable research indicates that married people live longer, feel happier, remain mentally alert longer, and suffer fewer physical and mental health problems.[23] Couples in healthy marriages have less stress, which in turn contributes to better overall health. Healthy marriage contributes to lower levels of stress in three important ways: financial stability, expanded support networks, and improved personal behaviors. Married adults are about half as likely to be smokers as are single, divorced, or separated adults. They are also less likely to be heavy drinkers or to engage in risky sexual behavior. The one negative health indicator for married people is body weight. Married adults, particularly men, weigh more than do single adults.[24]

However, traditional marriage does not work for everyone, and it is not the only path to a happy and successful committed relationship.

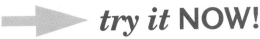

try it NOW!

Create an ideal partner checklist. List the factors you have used or think would be useful in choosing a partner for a committed relationship. Then go to the **Spotlight on Your Health** box on page 128 to review the information on common myths associated with marriage and choosing a partner. Were you surprised when you compared your list with current research findings?

Cohabitation

Cohabitation is defined as a relationship in which two unmarried people with an intimate connection live together in the same household. For a variety of reasons, increasing numbers of Americans are choosing cohabitation. In some states, cohabitation that lasts a designated number of years (usually 7) legally constitutes a **common-law marriage** for purposes of purchasing real estate and sharing other financial obligations.

Between 1960 and 2004, the number of cohabiting adults in America increased by over 1,000 percent. In fact, today over half of all first marriages are preceded by cohabitation.[25] Cohabitation can serve as a prelude to marriage, but for some people it is an alternative to marriage. Cohabitation is more common among people of lower socioeconomic status, who are less religious, who have been divorced, and who have experienced parental divorce or high levels of parental conflict during childhood. Many people believe that living together before marriage is a good way to find out how compatible you are with your partner and possibly avoid a bad marriage; however, current data does not support this belief. The long-term outcomes or implications of living together may be related more to who chooses to cohabit rather than the experience of cohabiting itself.

Although cohabitation has its advantages, it also has some drawbacks. Perhaps the greatest disadvantage is the lack of societal validation for the relationship, especially if the couple then has children. Many cohabitors must deal with pressures from parents and friends, difficulties in obtaining insurance and tax benefits, and legal issues over property. In 1996, the U.S. Congress reaffirmed tax advantages for married couples and effectively blocked cohabiting heterosexual and homosexual couples from these benefits through the Defense of Marriage Act (DOMA). The purpose of DOMA was to normalize heterosexual marriage on a federal level and permit each state to decide for itself whether to recognize same-sex unions or not.

Gay and Lesbian Partnerships

Most adults want intimate, committed relationships, whether they are gay or straight, men or women. Lesbians and gay men seek the same things in primary relationships that heterosexual partners do: friendship, communication, validation, companionship, and a sense of stability.

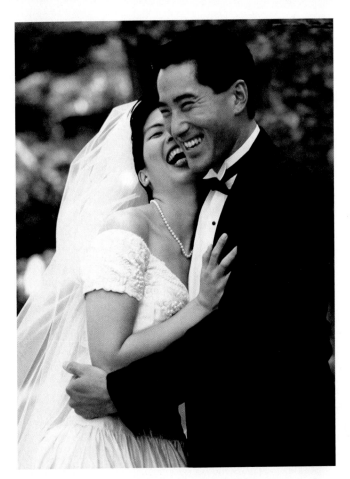

For many people, marriage or commitment ceremonies serve as the ultimate symbol of commitment between two people and validate their love for each other.

The 2000 U.S. Census revealed a significant increase in the number of same-sex partner households across the country—more than three times the total reported in the 1990 Census. The states with the most reported same-sex households are California, New York, Florida, Illinois, and Georgia. According to Lee Badgett, research director of the Institute for Gay and Lesbian Strategic Studies, the actual number of households is probably much higher. Many gay and lesbian partners hesitate to report their relationship because of concerns about discrimination.[26]

Studies of lesbian couples indicate high levels of attachment and satisfaction and a tendency toward monogamous, long-term relationships. Much like their heterosexual counterparts, gay men tend to form committed, long-term relationships, especially as they age.

Challenges to successful lesbian and gay relationships often stem from discrimination and difficulties dealing with

cohabitation   Living together without being married.

common-law marriage   Cohabitation lasting a designated period of time (usually 7 years) that is considered legally binding in some states.

MARRIAGE DEMYSTIFIED: HELPFUL FACTS AND COMMON MYTHS

What does marriage mean to you? Do you wonder when Mr. or Ms. Right will come along, where you'll find your lifetime partner, or whether there is such a thing as the "perfect" marriage?

The National Marriage Project, a research initiative at Rutgers University in New Jersey, is researching the attitudes of young adults toward marriage and working to educate them on how to prepare for marriage in the future. Here is a sampler of the Project's research findings.

Fact—*The most likely way to find a marriage partner is through an introduction by family, friends, or acquaintances.* Despite the romantic notion that people meet and fall in love through chance or fate, the evidence suggests that social networks are important in bringing together individuals of similar interests and backgrounds. According to a large-scale national survey, almost 60 percent of married people were introduced by family, friends, co-workers, or other acquaintances.

Myth—*Marriage benefits men much more than women.* Contrary to earlier and widely publicized reports, recent research finds men and women benefit about equally from marriage, although in different ways. Both men and women

live longer, happier, healthier, and wealthier lives when they are married. Husbands typically gain greater health benefits, whereas wives gain greater financial advantages.

Fact—*The more similar people are in their values, backgrounds, and life goals, the more likely they are to have a successful marriage.* Opposites may attract, but they may not live together harmoniously as married couples.

Myth—*Couples who live together before marriage, and are thus able to test how well suited they are for each other, have more satisfying and longer-lasting marriages than couples who do not.* Many

> **Is it good to live together before getting married?**

studies have found that couples who live together before marriage have less satisfying marriages and a considerably higher chance of eventually breaking up. One reason is that people who cohabit may be more skittish of commitment and more likely to call it quits when problems arise. (An important exception: cohabiting couples who already plan to marry each other in the near future have just as good a chance at staying together as couples who don't live together before marriage.)

Fact—*For large segments of the population, the risk of divorce is far below 50 percent.* Although the overall divorce rate in America remains close to 50 percent of all marriages, it has been dropping gradually over the past 20 years. The risk of divorce is far below 50 percent for educated people going into their first marriage and lower still for people who wait to marry until at least their mid-twenties, haven't lived with many different partners prior to marriage, or are strongly religious and marry someone of the same faith.

Myth—*Married people have less satisfying sex lives and less sex than single people.* According to a large-scale national study, married people have both more and better sex than do their unmarried counterparts. Not only do they have sex more often, but they also enjoy it more, both physically and emotionally.

Source: Popenoe, David, "Top Ten Myths of Marriage," 2002. Copyright © 2002 by the National Marriage Project at Rutgers University and Popenoe, David and Barbara Dafoe Whitehead, "Ten Important Reasearch Findings on Marriage and Choosing a Marriage Partner," 2004. Copyright © 2004 by the National Marriage Project at Rutgers University. Reprinted by permission of the National Marriage Project.

social, legal, and religious doctrines. For lesbian and gay couples, obtaining the same level of "marriage benefits," such as tax deductions, power-of-attorney rights, child custody rights, and other rights, continues to be a challenge. Currently, Massachusetts is the only state to grant same-sex couples marriage equality. Six other states currently have broad family recognition laws that extend to same-sex couples all, or nearly all, the state rights and responsibilities extended to married heterosexual couples. More limited rights and protections for same-sex couples are legislated in three additional states and the District of Columbia.[27] Worldwide, same-sex marriages are legal in the Netherlands, Belgium, Spain, Canada, and South Africa.

Staying Single

Increasing numbers of adults of all ages are electing to marry later or to remain single altogether. Data from 2004 indicate that the percentage of women aged 20 to 24 who have never been married is 75 percent. Likewise, men in this age group postponed marriage in increasing numbers, with over 86 percent of this group remaining unmarried in 2004.[28] According to the most recent figures from the U.S. Census Bureau and National Center for Health Statistics, the number of unmarried women aged 15 and older will soon surpass the number of married women.[29] The number of unmarried men is also increasing.

Today, large numbers of people prefer to remain single or to delay marriage. Singles clubs, social outings arranged by communities and religious groups, extended family environments, and many social services support the single lifestyle. Many singles live rich, rewarding lives and maintain a large network of close friends and families. Although sexual intimacy may or may not be present, the intimacy achieved through other interactions with loved ones is a key aspect of the single lifestyle.

? *what do you* THINK?

What are the advantages to remaining single? ■ What are the potential disadvantages? ■ What societal or organizational supports are available for the single lifestyle?

Success in Relationships

Our definition of success in a relationship tends to be based on whether a couple stays together over the years. Learning to communicate, respecting each other, and sharing a genuine fondness are crucial to relationship success. Many social scientists agree that the happiest committed relationships are flexible enough to allow the partners to grow throughout their lives.

Partnering Scripts

Parents often believe that their children will achieve happiness by living much as they have. Accordingly, most children are reared with a very strong script for what is expected of them as adults. Each group in society has its own partnering script that prescribes standards regarding sex, age, social class, race, religion, physical attributes, and personality types. By adolescence, people generally know exactly what type of person they are expected to befriend or date. By which partnering script were you raised? Just picture whom you could or couldn't bring home to meet your family.

Society provides constant reinforcement for traditional couples, but it may withhold this reinforcement from couples of the same sex, mixed race, mixed religion, or mixed age. People who have not chosen a traditional partner are subject to a great deal of external stress. In addition to denying recognition to such couples, friends and family often blame the nontraditional nature of the couple if the relationship fails.

Nonetheless, many nontraditional relationships survive and flourish. For example, the number of interracial marriages has quadrupled since the late 1960s, and the number of same-sex partner households has grown from 145,130 to almost half a million over the past 10 years.[30]

Being Self-Nurturant

It is often stated that you must love yourself before you can love someone else. What does this mean? Learning how you function emotionally and how to nurture yourself through all

life's situations is a lifelong task. You should certainly not postpone intimate connections with others until you have achieved this state. However, a certain level of individual maturity helps in maintaining a committed relationship. For example, divorce rates are much higher for couples under age 30 than for older couples.

Two concepts that are especially important to a good relationship are accountability and self-nurturance. **Accountability** means that both partners in a relationship see themselves as responsible for their own decisions, choices, and actions. They don't hold the other person responsible for positive or negative experiences.

Self-nurturance, which goes hand in hand with accountability, means developing individual potential through a balanced and realistic appreciation of self-worth and ability. To make good choices in life, a person needs to balance many physical and emotional needs, including sleeping, eating, exercising, working, relaxing, and socializing. When the balance is disrupted, as it will inevitably be, self-nurturing people are patient with themselves and try to put things back on course. It is a lifelong process to learn to live in a balanced and healthy way. Two people who are on a path of accountability and self-nurturance together have a much better chance of maintaining a satisfying relationship.

Confronting Couples Issues

Couples seeking a long-term relationship have to confront a number of issues that can enhance or ruin their chances of success. Some of these issues involve gender roles and power sharing.

Changing Gender Roles Throughout history, women and men have taken on various roles in their relationships. In agricultural America, gender roles were determined by tradition, and each task within a family unit held equal importance. Our modern society has very few gender-specific roles. Women and men alike drive cars, care for children, operate computers, manage finances, and perform equally well in the tasks of daily living. Rather than taking on traditional female and male roles, many couples find it makes more sense to divide tasks on the basis of schedule, convenience, and preference. However, it rarely works out that the division is equal. Today's working woman, living in a dual-career family and coping with the responsibilities of being a partner, a mother, and a professional, is often stressed and frustrated. Men, who may have expected a more traditional role for their partners, may experience difficulties. Even when women work full time, they tend to bear heavy family and household responsibilities. Over time, if couples

accountability Accepting responsibility for personal decisions, choices, and actions.

self-nurturance Developing individual potential through a balanced and realistic appreciation of self-worth and ability.

are unable to communicate how they feel about performing certain tasks, the relationship may suffer.

Sharing Power **Power** can be defined as the ability to make and implement decisions. There are many ways to exercise power, but powerful people are those who know what they want and have the ability to attain it. In traditional relationships, men were the wage earners and consequently had decision-making power. Women exerted much influence, but in the final analysis they needed a man's income for survival. As women became wage earners in increasing numbers and began enjoying their own financial resources, the power dynamics between women and men have shifted considerably. Part of the increase in the divorce rate undoubtedly reflects the recognition by working women that they can leave bad relationships in which they previously felt trapped. In general, successful couples have power relationships that reflect their unique needs rather than popular stereotypes.

Having Children … Or Not?

When a couple decides to raise children, their relationship changes. Resources of time, energy, and money are split many ways, and the partners no longer have each other's undivided attention. Babies and young children do not time their requests for food, sleep, and care to the convenience of adults. Therefore, individuals or couples whose own basic needs for security, love, and purpose are already met make better parents. Any stresses existing in a relationship will be further accentuated when parenting is added to the responsibilities. Having a child does not save a bad relationship— in fact, it seems only to compound the problems that already exist. A child cannot and should not be expected to provide the parents with self-esteem and security.

Changing patterns in family life affect the way children are raised. In modern society, it is not always clear which partner will adjust his or her work schedule to provide the primary care of children. Nearly half a million children each year become part of a blended family when their parents remarry; remarriage creates a new family of stepparents and stepsiblings. In addition, increasing numbers of individuals are choosing to have children in a family structure other than a heterosexual marriage (see Table 5.1 on page 118). Single women or lesbian couples can choose adoption or alternative insemination as a way to create a family. Single men or gay couples can choose to adopt or obtain the services of a surrogate mother. According to the 2000 census, over 25 percent of all school-aged children were living in families headed by a man or woman raising a child alone, reflecting a growing trend in America and in the international community.

power The ability to make and implement decisions.

Regardless of the structure of the family, certain factors remain important to the well-being of the unit: consistency, communication, affection, and mutual respect.

Finally, potential parents must consider the financial implications of deciding to have a child. Today, many families find that they need two incomes just to make ends meet. For more on family planning and financial evaluation, see Chapter 6.

Some people become parents without a lot of forethought. Some children are born into a relationship that was supposed to last and didn't. This does not mean it is too late to do a good job of parenting. Children are amazingly resilient and forgiving if parents show respect and communicate about household activities that affect their lives. Even children who grew up in a household of conflict can feel loved and respected if the parents treat them fairly. This means that parents must take responsibility for their own emotions and make it clear to children that they are not the reason for the conflict.

When Relationships Falter

Breakdowns in relationships usually begin with a change in communication, however subtle. Either partner may stop listening and cease to be emotionally present for the other. In turn, the other feels ignored, unappreciated, or unwanted. Unresolved conflicts increase, and unresolved anger can cause problems in sexual relations.

When a couple who previously enjoyed spending time together find themselves continually in the company of others, spending time apart, or preferring to stay home alone, it may be a sign that the relationship is in trouble. Of course, the need for individual privacy is not a cause for worry—it's essential to health. If, however, a partner decides to change the amount and quality of time spent together without the input or understanding of the other, it may be a sign of hidden problems.

College students, particularly those who are socially isolated and far from family and hometown friends, may be particularly vulnerable to staying in unhealthy relationships. They may become emotionally dependent on a partner for everything from eating meals to spending recreational and study time; mutual obligations, such as shared rental arrangements, transportation, and child care, can make it tough to leave.

It's also easy to mistake sexual advances for physical attraction or love. Without a network of friends and supporters to talk with, to obtain validation for feelings, or to share concerns, a student may feel stuck in a relationship that is headed nowhere.

Honesty and verbal affection are usually positive aspects of a relationship. In a troubled relationship, however, they can be used to cover up irresponsible or hurtful behavior. "At least I was honest" is not an acceptable substitute for acting in a trustworthy way. "But I really do love you" is not a license for acting inconsiderate or rude.

Most communities have trained therapists who specialize in relationship difficulties, and most student health centers offer these services at reduced fees for students. If you are unaware of such services, ask your instructor for suggestions.

When and Why Relationships End

Often we hear in the news that 50 percent of American marriages end in divorce. This number is based on the annual marriage rate compared with the annual divorce rate. This is misleading because in any given year, the people who are divorcing are mostly not the same as those who are marrying. The preferred method to determine the divorce rate is to calculate how many people who have ever married subsequently divorce. Using this calculation, the divorce rate in the U.S. has never exceeded 41 percent.[31] Although this number is still high, the divorce rate in this country has declined slightly from previous decades. This decrease may be related to an increase in the number of cohabiting couples, or to an increase in the age at which persons first marry and to a higher level of education among those who are marrying—both of the latter contribute to marital stability.[32]

The divorce rate represents only a portion of the actual number of failed relationships. Many people never go through a legal divorce process so are not counted in these statistics. Cohabitors and unmarried partners who raise children, own homes together, and exhibit all the outward appearances of marriage without the license are also not included.

Why do relationships end? There are many reasons, including illness, financial concerns, and career problems. Other breakups arise from unmet expectations. Many people enter a relationship with certain expectations about how they and their partner will behave. Failure to communicate these beliefs can lead to resentment and disappointment. Differences in sexual needs may also contribute to the demise of a relationship.

Under stress, communication and cooperation between partners can break down. Conflict, negative interactions, and a general lack of respect between partners can erode even the most loving relationship. One of the greatest predictors of divorce appears to be the husband's dissatisfaction in the first 5 years of marriage.

Coping with Failed Relationships

No relationship comes with a guarantee, no matter how many promises partners make to be together forever. Losing a love is as much a part of life as falling in love. That being said, the uncoupling process can be very painful. Whenever we risk getting close to another, we also risk being hurt if things don't work out. Remember that knowing, understanding, and feeling good about oneself before entering the relationship is

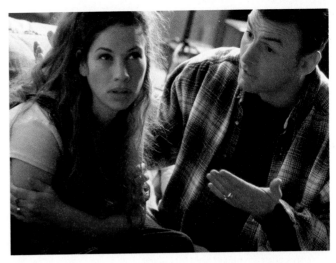

Open communication is key in addressing relationship problems. When one person shuts down, the argument can spin out of control.

very important. Consider these tips for coping with a failed relationship.[33]

- *Recognize and acknowledge your feelings.* These may include grief, loneliness, rejection, anger, guilt, relief, or sadness. Seek professional help and support as needed.
- *Find healthful ways to express your emotions, rather than turning them inward.* Go for a walk, talk to friends, listen to music, work out at the gym, volunteer with a community organization, or write in a journal.
- *Spend time with current friends, or reconnect with old friends.* Get reacquainted with yourself, what you enjoy doing, and the people whose company you enjoy.
- *Don't rush into a "rebound" relationship.* You need time to resolve your past experience rather than escape from it. You can't be trusting and intimate in a new relationship if you are still working on getting over a past relationship.

Building Better Relationships

Most relationships start with great optimism and true love. So why do so many run into trouble? One contributing factor is the message (or myth) that many of us grew up with about relationships. We were often told that if we found the right person, we would "live happily ever after." What was missing in that message is that healthy relationships don't just happen—they require psychosocial skills and continued effort.

Satisfying and stable relationships share certain identifiable traits, such as good communication, intimacy, friendship, and other factors discussed in this chapter **(Table 5.2).** A key ingredient is **trust,** the degree of confidence partners feel in a

trust The degree of confidence partners feel in a relationship.

TABLE 5.2 Healthy versus Unhealthy Relationships

Being in a *healthy relationship* means . . .	If you are in an *unhealthy relationship* . . .
Loving and taking care of yourself before and while in a relationship.	You care for and focus on another person only and neglect yourself or you focus only on yourself and neglect the other person.
Respecting individuality, embracing differences, and allowing each person to "be themselves."	You feel pressure to change to meet the other person's standards, you are afraid to disagree, and your ideas are criticized. Or, you pressure the other person to meet your standards and criticize his or her ideas.
Doing things with friends and family and having activities independent of each other.	One of you has to justify what you do, where you go, and who you see.
Discussing things, allowing for differences of opinion, and compromising equally.	One of you makes all the decisions and controls everything without listening to the other's input.
Expressing and listening to each other's feelings, needs, and desires.	One of you feels unheard and is unable to communicate what you want.
Trusting and being honest with yourself and each other.	You lie to each other and find yourself making excuses for the other person.
Respecting each other's need for privacy.	You don't have any personal space and have to share everything with the other person.
Sharing sexual histories and sexual health status with a partner.	Your partner keeps his or her sexual history a secret or hides a sexually transmitted infection from you, or you do not disclose your history to your partner.
Practicing safer sex methods.	You feel scared of asking your partner to use protection, or he or she has refused your requests for safer sex. Or, you refuse to use safer sex methods after your partner has requested, or you make your partner feel scared to ask.
Respecting sexual boundaries and being able to say no to sex.	Your partner has forced you to have sex or you have had sex when you don't really want to. Or, you have forced or coerced your partner to have sex.
Resolving conflicts in a rational, peaceful, and mutually agreed-upon way.	One of you yells and hits, shoves, or throws things at the other in an argument.
Having room for positive growth and learning more about each other as you develop and mature.	You feel stifled, trapped, and stagnant. You are unable to escape the pressures of the relationship.

Source: Advocates for Youth, "Healthy versus Unhealthy Relationships." Reprinted with permission of Advocates for Youth from www.advocatesforyouth.org. © 2000, Washington D.C. 20036.

relationship. Without trust, intimacy will not develop, and the relationship could fail. Trust includes three fundamental elements:

1. *Predictability* means that you can predict your partner's behavior, based on the knowledge that your partner acts in consistently positive ways.

2. *Dependability* means that you can rely on your partner to give support in all situations, particularly those in which you feel threatened with hurt or rejection.

3. *Faith* means that you feel absolutely certain about your partner's intentions and behavior.

Trust can develop even when it is initially lacking. This requires opening yourself to others, which carries the risk of hurt or rejection.

sexual identity   Recognition of oneself as a sexual being; a composite of biological sex characteristics, gender identity, gender roles, and sexual orientation.

intersexuality   Not exhibiting exclusively male or female primary and secondary sex characteristics.

Your Sexual Identity: More Than Biology

Sexual identity, the recognition and acknowledgment of oneself as a sexual being, is determined by a complex interaction of genetic, physiological, environmental, and social factors. The beginning of sexual identity occurs at conception with the combining of chromosomes that determine sex. The biological father determines whether a baby will be a boy or a girl. All eggs carry an X sex chromosome; sperm may carry either an X or a Y chromosome. If a sperm carrying an X chromosome fertilizes an egg, the resulting combination of sex chromosomes (XX) provides the blueprint to produce a female. If a sperm carrying a Y chromosome fertilizes an egg, the XY combination produces a male.

Not all people, however, have XX or XY chromosomes, nor do they all necessarily exhibit exclusively female or male sexual anatomy. **Intersexuality** may occur as often as 1 in 100 live births. Intersexuality is a biological condition in which a person is born with sex chromosomes, external genitalia, and/or an internal reproductive system that have both male and female components.

The genetic instructions included in the sex chromosomes lead to the differential development of male and female **gonads** (reproductive organs) at about the eighth week of fetal life. Once the male gonads (testes) and the female gonads (ovaries) develop, they play a key role in all future sexual development because the gonads are responsible for the production of sex hormones. The primary female sex hormones are estrogen and progesterone. The primary male sex hormone is testosterone. The release of testosterone in a maturing fetus signals the development of a penis and other male genitals. If no testosterone is produced, female genitals form.

At the time of **puberty,** sex hormones again play major roles in development. Hormones released by the **pituitary gland,** called *gonadotropins,* stimulate the testes and ovaries to make appropriate sex hormones. The increase of estrogen production in females and testosterone production in males leads to the development of **secondary sex characteristics.** Male secondary sex characteristics include deepening of the voice, development of facial and body hair, and growth of the skeleton and musculature. Female secondary sex characteristics include growth of the breasts, widening of the hips, and the development of pubic and underarm hair.

Thus far, we have described sexual identity only in terms of a person's biology. Although biology is an important facet of sexual identity, the relationship between biology and culture is much more complicated than the popular notion that *sex* refers to biology and *gender* to social issues. Biological factors are themselves always understood and interpreted within the cultural framework that gives meaning to those facts.

Gender is the practice of behaving in masculine or feminine ways as defined by the society in which one lives and as a component of one's identity. Sex, in contrast, is more related to physical form and function. In this sense, gender is a performance, something we do rather than something we have, and we learn gender through the process of **socialization.** Through interactions with family, peers, teachers, media, and other social organizations, we learn to act in ways that society deems appropriate. Think about the television shows you watch. Do the characters play out traditional gender roles?

Each of us expresses our maleness or femaleness to others on a daily basis by the **gender roles** we play. **Gender identity** refers to the personal sense or awareness of being masculine or feminine, a male or a female. A person's gender identity does not always match his or her biological sex—this is called being **transgendered.** There is a broad spectrum of expression among transgendered persons that reflects the degree of dissatisfaction they have with their sexual anatomy. Some trangendered persons are very comfortable with their bodies and are content simply to dress and live as the other gender. At the other end of the spectrum are **transsexuals,** who feel extremely trapped in their bodies and may opt for therapeutic interventions, such as sex reassignment surgery. Being

transgendered or transsexual is not related to sexual orientation, nor should it be confused with transvestism, or cross-dressing.

It may sometimes be difficult to express one's true sexual identity because of the bounds established by **gender-role stereotypes,** or generalizations about how men and women should express themselves and the characteristics each possesses. Our traditional sex roles are an example of gender-role stereotyping. Men, on the one hand, are traditionally expected to be independent, aggressive, logical, and always in control of their emotions. Women, on the other hand, are traditionally expected to be passive, nurturing, intuitive, sensitive, and emotional. **Androgyny** refers to the combination of traditional masculine and feminine traits in a single person. Androgynous people do not always follow traditional sex roles but instead choose behaviors based on a given situation.

By now you can see that defining sexual identity is not a simple matter. It is a lifelong process of growing and learning. Your sexual identity is made up of the unique combination of your biology, gender identity, chosen gender roles, sexual orientation, and personal experiences. It is up to you to take every opportunity to get to know and like yourself so that you may enjoy your life to the fullest.

gonads   The reproductive organs in a man (testes) or woman (ovaries).

puberty   The period of sexual maturation.

pituitary gland   The endocrine gland controlling the release of hormones from the gonads.

secondary sex characteristics   Characteristics associated with sex but not directly related to reproduction, such as vocal pitch, degree of body hair, and location of fat deposits.

gender   The psychological condition of being feminine or masculine as defined by the society in which one lives.

socialization   Process by which a society communicates behavioral expectations to its individual members.

gender roles   Expression of maleness or femaleness in everyday life.

gender identity   Personal sense or awareness of being masculine or feminine, a male or a female.

transgendered   When one's gender identity does not match one's biological sex.

transsexual   A person who is psychologically of one sex but physically of the other.

gender-role stereotypes   Generalizations concerning how men and women should express themselves and the characteristics each possesses.

androgyny   Combination of traditional masculine and feminine traits in a single person.

what do you THINK?

How often do you challenge existing gender-role stereotypes? ■ What is the outcome? ■ Do you think men and women have the same degree of freedom in gender-role expression?

Sexual Orientation

Sexual orientation refers to a person's enduring emotional, romantic, sexual, or affectionate attraction to other persons. You may be primarily attracted to members of the other sex (**heterosexual**), your same sex (**homosexual**), or both sexes (**bisexual**).

Many homosexuals prefer the terms **gay** and **lesbian** to describe their sexual orientations, because these terms go beyond the exclusively sexual connotation of the term *homosexual*. *Gay* can apply to both men and women, but *lesbian* refers specifically to women.

Gay, lesbian, and bisexual persons are repeatedly the targets of **sexual prejudice.** Sexual prejudice refers to negative attitudes and hostile actions directed at a social group and its members.[34] Hate crimes, discrimination, and hostility targeting sexual minorities are evidence of ongoing sexual prejudice. Recent data from the Department of Justice indicated that bias regarding sexual orientation was the motivation for over 15 percent of all hate crimes reported.[35]

Most researchers today agree that sexual orientation is best understood using a multifactorial model, which incorporates biological, psychological, and socioenvironmental factors. Biological explanations focus on research into genetics, hormones, and differences in brain anatomy, whereas psychological and socioenvironmental explanations examine

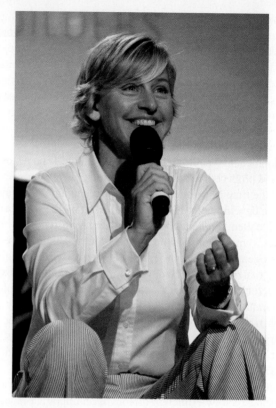

The presence of gay and lesbian celebrities in the media contributes to the increasing acceptance of gay relationships in everyday life. Ellen DeGeneres, now the host of her own daily talk show, is an openly gay comedian whose character in the 1990s sitcom *Ellen* famously came out as a lesbian on network television.

parent–child interactions, sex roles, and early sexual and interpersonal interactions. Collectively, this growing body of research suggests that the origins of homosexuality, like heterosexuality, are complex. To diminish the complexity of sexual orientation to "a choice" is a clear misrepresentation of current research. Homosexuals do not "choose" their sexual orientation any more than heterosexuals do.

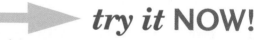 *try it* NOW!

Sexual orientation is often viewed as a simple concept based entirely on whom one has sex with, but this is an inaccurate and overly simplistic idea. Researcher F. Klein developed a questionnaire that not only looks at who you are sexually attracted to, fantasize about, and actually have sex with, but also considers factors such as who you feel more close to emotionally, like to socialize with, and in which "community" you feel most comfortable. Complete the worksheet in **Table 5.3**. You may realize that there are not just two (homosexual, heterosexual) or three (homosexual, heterosexual, bisexual) orientations, but indeed a whole range of complex, interacting, and fluid factors influencing our sexuality over time.

sexual orientation   A person's enduring emotional, romantic, sexual, or affectionate attraction to other persons.

heterosexual   Experiencing primary attraction to and preference for sexual activity with people of the other sex.

homosexual   Experiencing primary attraction to and preference for sexual activity with people of the same sex.

bisexual   Experiencing attraction to and preference for sexual activity with people of both sexes.

gay   Sexual orientation involving primary attraction to people of the same sex; usually but not always applies to men attracted to men.

lesbian   Sexual orientation involving attraction of women to other women.

sexual prejudice   Negative attitudes and hostile actions directed at social groups.

TABLE 5.3 Analyzing Sexual Preferences

To complete this worksheet, use the scales provided below and choose a number for each of the three aspects of your life: your past, your present, and your ideal. Remember that there are no right or wrong answers.

Variable	Past (your entire life up until one year ago)	Present (the last 12 months)	Ideal (if you could order your life any way you wanted)
A. SEXUAL ATTRACTION: To whom are you sexually attracted?	_____	_____	_____
B. SEXUAL BEHAVIOR: With whom do you have sex?	_____	_____	_____
C. SEXUAL FANTASIES: Who do you fantasize about?	_____	_____	_____
D. EMOTIONAL PREFERENCE: Who do you feel more drawn to or close to emotionally?	_____	_____	_____
E. SOCIAL PREFERENCE: With whom do you spend most of your social life?	_____	_____	_____
F. LIFESTYLE PREFERENCE: In which community (gay, straight, mixed) do you prefer to spend your time or feel most comfortable?	_____	_____	_____
G. SELF-IDENTIFICATION: How do you label or identify yourself?	_____	_____	_____

SCALE FOR A–E
0 = other sex only
1 = other sex mostly
2 = other sex somewhat more
3 = both sexes equally
4 = same sex somewhat more
5 = same sex mostly
6 = same sex only

SCALE FOR F AND G
0 = heterosexual only
1 = heterosexual mostly
2 = heterosexual somewhat more
3 = equally heterosexual and homosexual
4 = homosexual somewhat more
5 = homosexual mostly
6 = homosexual only

Source: From F. Klein, *The Bisexual Option.* Copyright © 1978 The Haworth Press, Inc. Used with permission.

Sexual Anatomy and Physiology

An understanding of the functions of the male and female reproductive systems will help you derive pleasure and satisfaction from your sexual relationships, be sensitive to your partner's wants and needs, and make responsible choices regarding your own sexual health.

Female Sexual Anatomy and Physiology

The female reproductive system includes two major groups of structures: the external genitals (**Figure 5.4**) and the internal genitals. The **external female genitals,** also referred to as the **vulva,** include all structures that are outwardly visible. Specifically, the external genitalia include the mons pubis, the labia minora and majora, the clitoris, the urethral and vaginal openings, and the vestibule of the vagina and its glands. The **mons pubis** is a pad of fatty tissue covering the pubic bone. The mons protects the pubic bone, and after onset of puberty it becomes covered with coarse hair. The **labia minora** are

inner lips, or folds, of mucous membrane, and the **labia majora** are folds of skin and erectile tissue that enclose the urethral and vaginal openings. The labia minora are found just inside the labia majora.

The **clitoris** is the female sexual organ whose only known function is sexual pleasure. It is located at the upper end of

external female genitals   The mons pubis, labia majora and minora, clitoris, urethral and vaginal openings, and the vestibule of the vagina and its glands.

vulva   Region that encloses the female's external genitalia.

mons pubis   Fatty tissue covering the pubic bone in females; in physically mature women, the mons is covered with coarse hair.

labia minora   "Inner lips," or folds of tissue just inside the labia majora.

labia majora   "Outer lips," or folds of tissue covering the female sexual organs.

clitoris   A pea-sized nodule of tissue located at the top of the labia minora; central to sexual arousal in women.

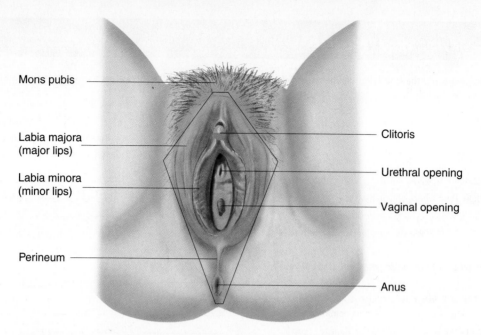

FIGURE 5.4 External Female Genital Structures

Source: From R. McAnulty and M. Burnette, *Exploring Human Sexuality: Making Healthy Decisions,* 2nd ed. (Boston: Allyn & Bacon, 2004). Copyright © 2004 by Pearson Education. Reprinted by permission of the publisher.

the labia minora and beneath the mons pubis. Directly below the clitoris is the **urethral opening,** through which urine is expelled from the body. Below the urethral opening is the vaginal opening. In some women, the vaginal opening is

urethral opening   The opening through which urine is expelled.

hymen   Thin tissue covering the vaginal opening in some women.

perineum   Tissue that forms the "floor" of the pelvic region; it covers a kite-shaped region including the external genitalia and anus.

internal female genitals   The vagina, uterus, fallopian tubes, and ovaries.

vagina   The passage in females leading from the vulva into the uterus.

uterus (womb)   Hollow, pear-shaped muscular organ whose function is to contain the developing fetus.

endometrium   Soft, spongy matter that makes up the uterine lining.

cervix   Lower end of the uterus that opens into the vagina.

ovaries   Almond-sized organs that house developing eggs and produce hormones.

fallopian tubes   Tubes that extend from near the ovaries to the uterus; site of fertilization and passageway for fertilized eggs.

covered by a thin membrane called the **hymen.** It is a myth that an intact hymen is proof of virginity. The **perineum** is the area of smooth tissue found between the vulva and the anus. Although not technically part of the external genitalia, the tissue in this area has many nerve endings and is sensitive to touch; it can play a part in sexual excitement.

The **internal female genitals** of the reproductive system include the vagina, uterus, fallopian tubes, and ovaries **(Figure 5.5).** The **vagina** is a tubular organ that serves as a passageway from the uterus to the outside of a woman's body. This passageway allows menstrual flow to exit from the uterus during a woman's monthly cycle, receives the penis during intercourse, and serves as the birth canal. The **uterus** (or **womb**) is a hollow, muscular, pear-shaped organ. Hormones acting on the soft, spongy matter that makes up the inner lining of the uterus, called the **endometrium,** either prepare the uterus for implantation and development of a fertilized egg or signal that no fertilization has taken place, in which case the endometrium deteriorates and becomes menstrual flow.

The lower end of the uterus, the **cervix,** extends down into the vagina. The **ovaries,** almond-sized organs suspended on either side of the uterus, produce the hormones estrogen and progesterone and are also the reservoir for immature eggs. All the eggs a woman will ever have are present in her ovaries at birth. Eggs mature and are released from the ovaries in response to hormone levels. Extending from the upper end of the uterus are two thin, flexible tubes called the **fallopian tubes.** The fallopian tubes, which do not actually touch the ovaries, capture eggs as they are released from the

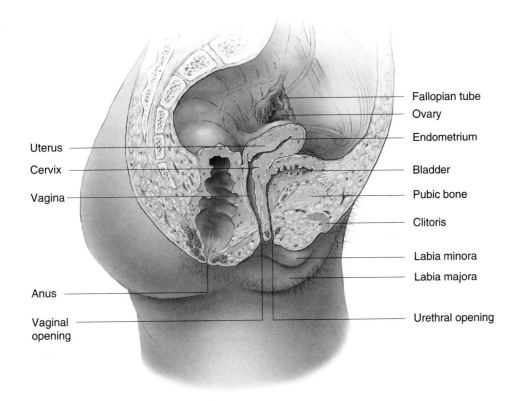

Uterus

Cervix

Vagina

Anus

Vaginal opening

Fallopian tube

Ovary

Endometrium

Bladder

Pubic bone

Clitoris

Labia minora

Labia majora

Urethral opening

FIGURE 5.5 Side View of the Female Reproductive Organs

ovaries during ovulation, and they are the site where sperm and egg meet and fertilization takes place. The fallopian tubes then serve as the passageway to the uterus, where the fertilized egg becomes implanted and development continues.

The Onset of Puberty and the Menstrual Cycle
With the onset of puberty, the female reproductive system matures, and the development of secondary sex characteristics transforms young girls into young women. The first sign of puberty is the development of breast buds, which generally occurs around age 11. The pituitary gland, **hypothalamus,** and ovaries all secrete hormones that act as chemical messengers among them. Working in a feedback system, hormonal levels in the bloodstream act as the trigger mechanism for release of more or different hormones.

Around age $9\frac{1}{2}$ to $11\frac{1}{2}$, the hypothalamus receives the message to begin secreting **gonadotropin-releasing hormone (GnRH).** The release of GnRH in turn signals the pituitary gland to release hormones called *gonadotropins.* Two gonadotropins, **follicle-stimulating hormone (FSH)** and **luteinizing hormone (LH),** signal the ovaries to start producing **estrogens** and **progesterone.** Estrogens regulate the menstrual cycle, and increased estrogen levels assist in the development of female secondary sex characteristics. Progesterone helps keep the endometrium developing to nourish a fertilized egg and helps maintain pregnancy.

The normal age range for the onset of the first menstrual period, termed **menarche,** is 9 to 17 years, with the average age being $11\frac{1}{2}$ to $13\frac{1}{2}$ years. Body fat heavily influences the onset of puberty, and increasing rates of obesity in children

hypothalamus An area of the brain located near the pituitary gland; works in conjunction with the pituitary gland to control reproductive functions.

gonadotropin-releasing hormone (GnRH) Hormone that signals the pituitary gland to release gonadotropins.

follicle-stimulating hormone (FSH) Hormone that signals the ovaries to prepare to release eggs and to begin producing estrogens.

luteinizing hormone (LH) Hormone that signals the ovaries to release an egg and to begin producing progesterone.

estrogens Hormones secreted by the ovaries that control the menstrual cycle.

progesterone Hormone secreted by the ovaries; helps keep the endometrium developing in order to nourish a fertilized egg; also helps maintain pregnancy.

menarche The first menstrual period.

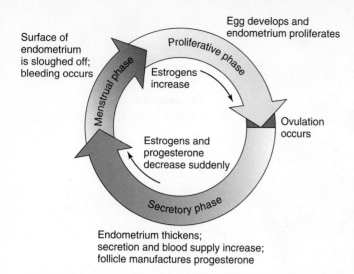

Surface of endometrium is sloughed off; bleeding occurs

Menstrual phase

Egg develops and endometrium proliferates

Proliferative phase

Estrogens increase

Ovulation occurs

Estrogens and progesterone decrease suddenly

Secretory phase

Endometrium thickens; secretion and blood supply increase; follicle manufactures progesterone

FIGURE 5.6 The Three Phases of the Menstrual Cycle

Source: From Spencer A. Rathus, Jeffrey S. Nevid, et al., *Human Sexuality in a World of Diversity,* 7/e. Published by Allyn and Bacon, Boston, MA. Copyright © 2008 by Pearson Education. Reprinted by permission of the publisher.

may account for the fact that girls here and in other countries seem to be reaching puberty much earlier than they used to.[36]

The average menstrual cycle is 28 days long and consists of three phases: the proliferative phase, the secretory phase, and the menstrual phase (**Figures 5.6 and 5.7**). The **proliferative phase** begins with the end of menstruation. During this time, the endometrium develops, or "proliferates." How does this process work? By the end of menstrua-

proliferative phase   First phase of the menstrual cycle.

ovarian follicles   Areas within the ovary in which individual eggs develop.

graafian follicle   Mature ovarian follicle that contains a fully developed ovum, or egg.

ovum   A single mature egg cell.

ovulation   The point of the menstrual cycle at which a mature egg ruptures through the ovarian wall.

secretory phase   Second phase of the menstrual cycle, during which the endometrium continues to prepare for a fertilized egg.

human chorionic gonadotropin (HCG)   Hormone that calls for increased levels of estrogen and progesterone secretion if fertilization has taken place.

menstrual phase   Final phase of the menstrual cycle, in which the endometrium sloughs off, and estrogen and progesterone levels decline in response to no fertilization having taken place.

menopause   The permanent cessation of menstruation, generally between the ages of 40 and 60.

tion, the hypothalamus senses very low levels of estrogen and progesterone in the blood. In response to these low levels, the hypothalamus increases its secretions of GnRH, which in turn triggers the pituitary gland to release FSH. When FSH reaches the ovaries, it signals several **ovarian follicles** (the part of the ovary where eggs develop) to begin to mature. Normally, only one of the follicles, called the **graafian follicle,** reaches full maturity in the days preceding ovulation. While the follicles mature, they begin to produce estrogen, which in turn signals the endometrium to proliferate. If fertilization occurs, the endometrial tissue will become a nesting place for the developing embryo. High estrogen levels signal the pituitary to slow down FSH production and increase release of LH. Under the influence of LH, the graafian follicle ruptures and releases a mature **ovum** (plural: *ova*) a single mature egg cell, near a fallopian tube (around day 14). This is the process of **ovulation.** The other ripening follicles degenerate and are reabsorbed by the body. Occasionally, two ova mature and are released during ovulation. If both are fertilized, fraternal (nonidentical) twins develop. Identical twins develop when one fertilized ovum divides into two separate egg cells.

The phase following ovulation is called the **secretory phase.** The ruptured graafian follicle, which has remained in the ovary, is transformed into the corpus luteum and begins to secrete large amounts of estrogen and progesterone. These hormone secretions peak around days 20 or 21 of the average cycle and cause the endometrium to thicken and continue to prepare for a potential fertilized ovum. If fertilization and implantation take place, cells surrounding the developing embryo release a hormone called **human chorionic gonadotropin (HCG),** increasing estrogen and progesterone secretions, which maintain the endometrium and signal the pituitary not to start a new menstrual cycle. If no implantation occurs, the hypothalamus responds to peak levels of progesterone in the blood by signaling the pituitary to stop producing FSH and LH. As levels of FSH and LH quickly fall, the corpus luteum begins to decompose. The decomposition of the corpus luteum leads to rapid declines in estrogen and progesterone levels. These hormones are needed to sustain the lining of the uterus, the endometrium. Without them, the endometrium is sloughed off in the menstrual flow, and this begins the **menstrual phase.** The low estrogen levels of the menstrual phase signal the hypothalamus to release GnRH, which acts on the pituitary to secrete FSH, and the cyclical process begins again.

Menopause   Just as menarche signals the beginning of a woman's reproductive years, **menopause**—the permanent cessation of menstruation—signals the end. Generally occurring between the ages of 40 and 60, and at age 51 on average in the United States, menopause results in decreased estrogen levels, which may produce troublesome symptoms in some women. Decreased vaginal lubrication, hot flashes,

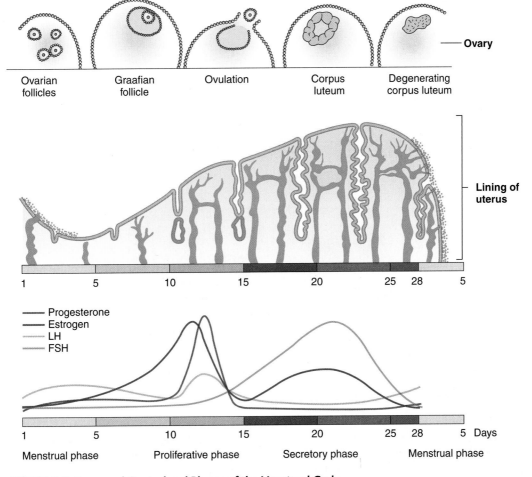

FIGURE 5.7 Hormonal Control and Phases of the Menstrual Cycle

headaches, dizziness, and joint pain all have been associated with the onset of menopause.

Hormones, such as estrogen and progesterone, have long been prescribed as **hormone replacement therapy** to relieve menopausal symptoms and reduce the risk of heart disease and osteoporosis. (The National Institutes of Health prefers the term **menopausal hormone therapy,** because this hormone treatment is not a replacement and does not restore the physiology of youth.) However, recent studies, including results from the Women's Health Initiative (WHI), suggest that hormone therapy may actually do more harm than good. In fact, the WHI terminated this research ahead of schedule because of concerns about participants' increased risk of breast cancer, heart attack, stroke, blood clots, and other health problems.[37] All women need to discuss the risks and benefits of menopausal hormone therapy with their health care provider and come to an informed decision. It is crucial to find a doctor who specializes in women's health and keeps up to date with the latest research findings. Certainly a healthy lifestyle, such as regular exercise, a balanced diet, and adequate calcium intake, can also help protect postmenopausal women from heart disease and osteoporosis.

Male Sexual Anatomy and Physiology

The structures of the male reproductive system may be divided into external and internal genitals **(Figure 5.8).** The penis and the scrotum make up the **external male genitals.** The **internal male genitals** include the testes, epididymides, vasa deferentia, ejaculatory ducts, urethra, and three other structures—the seminal vesicles, the prostate gland, and the Cowper's glands—which secrete components that, with sperm, make up semen. These three structures are sometimes referred to as the **accessory glands.**

hormone replacement therapy, menopausal hormone therapy   Use of synthetic or animal estrogens and progesterone to compensate for decreases in estrogens in a woman's body during menopause.

external male genitals   The penis and scrotum.

internal male genitals   The testes, epididymides, vasa deferentia, ejaculatory ducts, urethra, and accessory glands.

accessory glands   The seminal vesicles, prostate gland, and Cowper's glands.

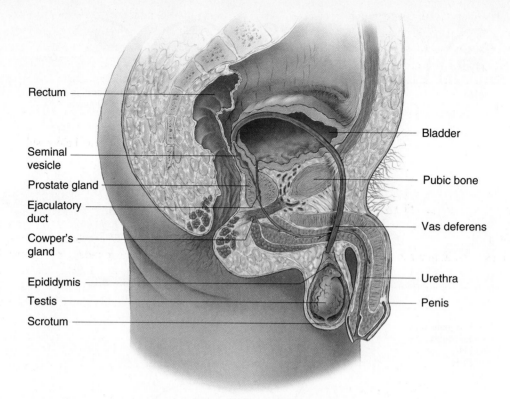

FIGURE 5.8 Side View of the Male Reproductive Organs

The **penis** is the organ that deposits sperm in the vagina during intercourse. The urethra, which passes through the center of the penis, acts as the passageway for both semen and urine to exit the body. During sexual arousal, the spongy tissue in the penis becomes filled with blood, making the organ stiff (erect). Further sexual excitement leads to **ejaculation,** a series of rapid, spasmodic contractions that propel semen out of the penis.

Situated behind the penis and also outside the body is a sac called the **scrotum.** The scrotum protects the testes and also helps control the temperature within the testes, which is vital to proper sperm production. The **testes** (singular: *testis*) manufacture sperm and **testosterone,** the hormone responsible for the development of male secondary sex characteristics.

The development of sperm is referred to as **spermatogenesis.** Like the maturation of eggs in the female, this process is governed by the pituitary gland. Follicle-stimulating hormone (FSH) is secreted into the bloodstream to stimulate the testes to manufacture sperm. Immature sperm are released into a comma-shaped structure on the back of each testis called the **epididymis** (plural: *epididymides*), where they ripen and reach full maturity.

Each epididymis contains coiled tubules that gradually "unwind" and straighten out to become the **vas deferens.** The two vasa deferentia, as they are called in the plural, make up the tubular transportation system whose sole function is to store and move sperm. Along the way, the **seminal vesicles** provide sperm with nutrients and other fluids that compose **semen.**

The vasa deferentia eventually connect each epididymis to the ejaculatory ducts, which pass through the prostate gland

penis   Male sexual organ that releases sperm into the vagina.

ejaculation   The propulsion of semen from the penis.

scrotum   Sac of tissue that encloses the testes.

testes   Two organs, located in the scrotum, that manufacture sperm and produce hormones.

testosterone   The male sex hormone manufactured in the testes.

spermatogenesis   The development of sperm.

epididymis   A comma-shaped structure atop the testis, where sperm mature.

vas deferens   A tube that stores and transports sperm toward the penis.

seminal vesicles   Storage areas for sperm where nutrient fluids are added to them.

semen   Fluid containing sperm and nutrient fluids that increase sperm viability and neutralize vaginal acid.

and empty into the urethra. The **prostate gland** contributes more fluids to the semen, including chemicals that help the sperm fertilize an ovum and neutralize the acidic environment of the vagina to make it more conducive to sperm motility (ability to move) and potency (potential for fertilizing an ovum).

Just below the prostate gland are two pea-shaped nodules called the **Cowper's glands.** The Cowper's glands secrete a fluid that lubricates the urethra and neutralizes any acid that may remain in the urethra after urination. Urine and semen do not come into contact with each other. During ejaculation of semen, a small valve closes off the tube to the urinary bladder.

Debate continues over the practice of *circumcision*, the surgical removal of a fold of skin covering the end of the penis known as the *foreskin.* Most circumcisions are performed for religious or cultural reasons or because of hygiene concerns. However, recent research supports the claim that circumcision yields medical benefits, including decreased risk of urinary tract infections in the first year, decreased risk of penile cancer (although cancer of the penis is very rare), and decreased risk of sexual transmission of human papillomavirus (HPV) and human immunodeficiency virus (HIV).[38]

Human Sexual Response

Psychological traits greatly influence sexual response and sexual desire. Thus, you may find a relationship with one partner vastly different from experiences with other partners.

Sexual response is a physiological process that generally follows a pattern. Sexual responses in both men and women are somewhat arbitrarily divided into four stages: excitement/ arousal, plateau, orgasm, and resolution. Researchers agree that each individual has a personal response pattern that may or may not conform to these phases. Regardless of the type of sexual activity (stimulation by a partner or self-stimulation), the response stages are the same.

During the first stage, *excitement/arousal*, **vasocongestion** (increased blood flow that causes swelling in the genitals) stimulates male and female genital responses. The vagina begins to lubricate in preparation for penile penetration, and the penis becomes partially erect. Both sexes may exhibit a "sex flush," or light blush all over their bodies. Excitement/ arousal can be generated through fantasy or by touching parts of the body, kissing, viewing films or videos, or reading erotic literature.

During the *plateau phase,* the initial responses intensify. Voluntary and involuntary muscle tensions increase. The woman's nipples and the man's penis become erect. The penis secretes a few drops of preejaculatory fluid, which may contain sperm.

During the *orgasmic phase,* vasocongestion and muscle tensions reach their peak, and rhythmic contractions occur through the genital regions. In women, these contractions are centered in the uterus, outer vagina, and anal sphincter.

In men, the contractions occur in two stages. First, contractions within the prostate gland begin propelling semen through the urethra. In the second stage, the muscles of the pelvic floor, urethra, and anal sphincter contract. Semen usually, but not always, is ejaculated from the penis. In both sexes, spasms in other major muscle groups also occur, particularly in the buttocks and abdomen. Feet and hands may also contract, and facial features often contort.

Muscle tension and congested blood subside in the *resolution phase,* as the genital organs return to their pre-arousal states. Both sexes usually experience deep feelings of well-being and profound relaxation. Following orgasm and resolution, many women can become aroused again and experience additional orgasms. However, some men experience a refractory period, during which their systems are incapable of subsequent arousal. This refractory period may last from a few minutes to several hours and tends to lengthen with age.

Men and women experience the same stages in the sexual response cycle; however, the length of time spent in any one stage varies. Thus, one partner may be in the plateau phase while the other is in the excitement or orgasmic phase. Such variations in response rates are entirely normal. Some couples believe that simultaneous orgasm is desirable for sexual satisfaction. Although simultaneous orgasm is pleasant, so are orgasms achieved at different times.

Sexual pleasure and satisfaction are also possible without orgasm or even intercourse. Expressing sexual feelings for another person involves many pleasurable activities, of which intercourse and orgasm may be only a part.

 what do you THINK?

Why do we place so much importance on orgasm? ■ Can sexual pleasure and satisfaction be achieved without orgasm? ■ What is the role of desire in sexual response?

Expressing Your Sexuality

Finding healthy ways to express your sexuality is an important part of developing sexual maturity. Many avenues of sexual expression are available.

prostate gland   Gland that secretes nutrients and neutralizing fluids into the semen.

Cowper's glands   Glands that secrete a fluid that lubricates the urethra and neutralizes any acid remaining in the urethra after urination.

vasocongestion   The engorgement of the genital organs with blood.

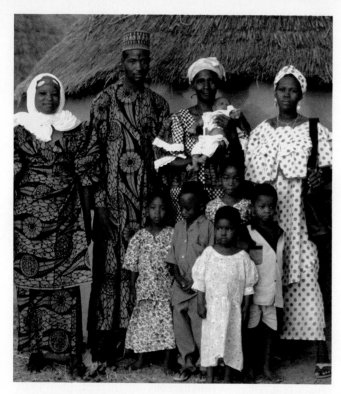
Our Western standard of monogamous heterosexual relationships may not be perceived as normal in other cultures. For example, this African family consists of one husband, several wives, and their children.

Sexual Behavior: What Is "Normal"?

Most of us want to fit in and be identified as normal, but how do we know which sexual behaviors are considered normal? What or whose criteria should we use? These are not easy questions.

What is "normal" sexual behavior?

Every society sets standards and attempts to regulate sexual behavior. Boundaries arise that distinguish good from bad, acceptable from unacceptable, and they result in criteria used to establish what is viewed as normal or abnormal. Some of the sociocultural standards for sexual behavior commonly held in Western culture today include the following:[39]

- *The coital standard.* Penile-vaginal intercourse (coitus) is viewed as the ultimate sex act.
- *The orgasmic standard.* Sexual interaction should lead to orgasm.

---

celibacy State of not being involved in a sexual relationship.

autoerotic behaviors Sexual self-stimulation.

sexual fantasies Sexually arousing thoughts and dreams.

- *The two-person standard.* Sex is an activity to be experienced by two.
- *The romantic standard.* Sex should be related to love.
- *The safer sex standard.* If we choose to be sexually active, we should act to prevent unintended pregnancy or disease transmission.

These are not laws or rules, but rather social scripts that have been adopted over time. Sexual standards often shift through the years, and many people choose not to follow them. We are a pluralistic nation, and that pluralism extends to our sexual practices. Rather than making blanket judgments about normal versus abnormal, we might ask the following questions:[40]

- Is a sexual behavior healthy and fulfilling for a particular person?
- Is it safe?
- Does it lead to the exploitation of others?
- Does it take place between responsible, consenting adults?

In this way, we can view behavior along a continuum that takes into account many individual factors. As you read about the options for sexual expression in the pages ahead, use these questions to explore your feelings about what is normal for you.

Options for Sexual Expression

The range of human sexual expression is virtually infinite. What you find enjoyable may not be an option for someone else. The ways you choose to meet your sexual needs today may be very different from what they were two weeks ago, or will be two years from now. Accepting yourself as a sexual person with individual desires and preferences is the first step in achieving sexual satisfaction. Curious about your college peers' sexual behavior? See Did You Know, and check out the **Spotlight on Your Health** box on page 144—you may be surprised by what it says!

Celibacy **Celibacy** is avoidance of or abstention from sexual activities with others. Some individuals choose celibacy for religious or moral reasons. Others may be celibate for a period of time because of illness, the breakup of a long-term relationship, or lack of an acceptable partner. For some, celibacy is a lonely, agonizing state, but others find it an opportunity for introspection, values assessment, and personal growth.

Autoerotic Behaviors **Autoerotic behaviors** involve sexual self-stimulation. The two most common are sexual fantasy and masturbation.

Sexual fantasies are sexually arousing thoughts and dreams. Fantasies may reflect real-life experiences, forbidden desires, or the opportunity to practice new or anticipated sexual experiences. The fact that you may fantasize about a particular sexual experience does not mean that you want to, or have to, act that experience out. Sexual fantasies are just that—fantasy.

Masturbation is self-stimulation of the genitals. Although many people feel uncomfortable discussing masturbation, it is a common sexual practice across the life span. Masturbation is a natural pleasure-seeking behavior in infants and children. It is a valuable and important means for adolescents, as well as adults, to explore sexual feelings and responsiveness.

Kissing and Erotic Touching

Kissing and erotic touching are two very common forms of nonverbal sexual communication. Both men and women have **erogenous zones,** areas of the body that when touched lead to sexual arousal. Erogenous zones may include genital as well as nongenital areas, such as the earlobes, mouth, breasts, and inner thighs. Almost any area of the body can be conditioned to respond erotically to touch. Spending time with your partner to explore and learn about his or her erogenous areas is another pleasurable, safe, and satisfying means of sexual expression.

Manual Stimulation

Both men and women can be sexually aroused and achieve orgasm through manual stimulation of the genitals by a partner. For many women, orgasm is more likely to be achieved through manual stimulation than through intercourse. *Sex toys* include a wide variety of objects that can be used for sexual stimulation alone or with a partner. Vibrators and dildos are two common types of toys and can be found in a variety of shapes, styles, and sizes. Sex toys can add zest to sexual experiences and, for women who may not reach orgasm by intercourse, may provide another option for satisfaction. Toys must be cleaned after each use.

Oral–Genital Stimulation

Cunnilingus refers to oral stimulation of a woman's genitals, and **fellatio** to oral stimulation of a man's genitals. Many partners find oral–genital stimulation intensely pleasurable. In one study, 45 percent of college students reported having oral sex in the past month.[41] For some people, oral sex is not an option because of moral or religious beliefs. Remember, HIV (human immunodeficiency virus) and other sexually transmitted infections (STIs) can be transmitted via unprotected oral–genital sex, just as they can through intercourse. Use of an appropriate barrier device is strongly recommended if either partner's health status is in question.

Vaginal Intercourse

The term *intercourse* generally refers to **vaginal intercourse** (*coitus,* or insertion of the penis into the vagina), which is the most often practiced form of sexual expression. Coitus can involve a variety of positions, including the missionary position (man on top facing the woman), woman on top, side by side, or man behind (rear entry). Many partners enjoy experimenting with different positions. Knowledge of yourself and your body, along with your ability to communicate effectively, will play a large part in determining the enjoyment or meaning of intercourse for you and your partner. Whatever your circumstance, you should practice safer sex to avoid disease and unwanted pregnancy.

Anal Intercourse

The anal area is highly sensitive to touch, and some couples find pleasure in the stimulation of this area. **Anal intercourse** is insertion of the penis into the anus. Research indicates that over 26 percent of college-aged men and women have had anal sex.[42] Stimulation of the anus by mouth or with the fingers also is practiced. As with all forms of sexual expression, anal stimulation or intercourse is not for everyone. If you do enjoy this form of sexual expression, remember to use condoms to avoid transmitting disease. Also, anything inserted into the anus should not be then directly inserted into the vagina, because bacteria commonly found in the anus can cause vaginal infections.

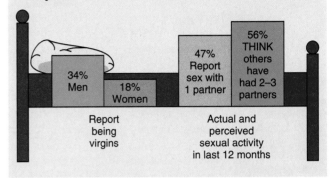

DID you KNOW?

According to a recent survey, American college students believe their peers are more sexually active than they really are.

34% Men / 18% Women — Report being virgins

47% Report sex with 1 partner

56% THINK others have had 2–3 partners

Actual and perceived sexual activity in last 12 months

Sources: "Smarter Sex Survey: Sexual Attitudes and Behaviors of U.S. Students Aged 18–24," www.smartersex.org *American College Health Association–National College Health Assessment*: Reference Group Data Report Spring 2006.

masturbation Self-stimulation of genitals.

erogenous zones Areas of the body of both men and women that, when touched, lead to sexual arousal.

cunnilingus Oral stimulation of a woman's genitals.

fellatio Oral stimulation of a man's genitals.

vaginal intercourse The insertion of the penis into the vagina.

anal intercourse The insertion of the penis into the anus.

ANALYZING STUDENT MISPERCEPTIONS OF SEX ON CAMPUS

College students often think everyone is having more sex than they are and with numerous partners. These perceptions may cause them to feel self-conscious about their own lack of sexual activity or encourage promiscuity so that they "measure up." In reality, college students' opinions about sex, relationships, contraception, and sexual activity vary greatly. Results from a survey answered by college students nationwide might help you sort through some of these misperceptions.

How much sex do my peers have?

- Within the previous school year approximately 76 percent of college students reported having had no sexual partner or only one sexual partner (oral, anal, or vaginal). However, when those same college students were asked how many sexual partners they perceived the typical student at their school had sex with in the previous year, over 82 percent thought the typical student had two or more partners.
- In the previous 30 days, 45 percent of students reported having had oral sex one or more times, but 93 percent thought the typical student had oral sex one or more times in the previous 30 days.
- In the previous 30 days, 49 percent of students reported having vaginal intercourse one or more times, yet 94 percent thought the typical student had vaginal intercourse one or more times in the previous 30 days.
- In the previous 30 days, 5 percent of students reported having anal intercourse one or more times, whereas 58 percent thought the typical student had anal sex one or more times in the previous 30 days.

- 2.1 percent of college students who had had vaginal intercourse within the previous school year reported experiencing an unintentional pregnancy.
- Approximately 28 percent of students reported having ever been tested for HIV.
- The most common methods of birth control used by sexually active students or their partners to prevent pregnancy the last time they had vaginal intercourse were the birth control pill (38 percent) and condoms (37 percent).

Source: American College Health Association. *American College Health Association—National College Health Assessment: Reference Group Data Report Spring 2006.* Baltimore: American College Health Association, 2006.

Variant Sexual Behavior

Although attitudes toward sexuality have changed radically since the Victorian era, some people still believe that any sexual behavior other than heterosexual intercourse is abnormal or perverted. People who study sexuality prefer the neutral term **variant sexual behavior** to describe sexual activities that most people do not engage in, for example:

- *Group sex.* Sexual activity involving more than two people. Participants in group sex run a higher risk of exposure to HIV and other STIs.
- *Transvestism.* Wearing the clothing of the opposite sex. Most transvestites are male, heterosexual, and married.
- *Fetishism.* Sexual arousal achieved by looking at or touching inanimate objects, such as underclothing or shoes.

variant sexual behavior A sexual behavior that most people do not engage in.

Some variant sexual behaviors can be harmful to the individual, to others, or to both. Many of the following activities are illegal in at least some states.

- *Exhibitionism.* Exposing one's genitals to strangers in public places. Most exhibitionists are seeking a reaction of shock or fear from their victims. Exhibitionism is a minor felony in most states.
- *Voyeurism.* Observing other people for sexual gratification. Most voyeurs are men who attempt to watch women undressing or bathing. Voyeurism is an invasion of privacy and is illegal in most states.
- *Sadomasochism.* Sexual activities in which gratification is received by inflicting pain (verbal or physical abuse) on a partner or by being the object of such infliction. A sadist is a person who enjoys inflicting pain, and a masochist is a person who enjoys experiencing it.
- *Pedophilia.* Sexual activity or attraction between an adult and a child. Any sexual activity involving a minor, including possession of child pornography, is illegal.
- *Autoerotic asphyxiation.* The practice of reducing or eliminating oxygen to the brain, usually by tying a cord around one's neck, while masturbating to orgasm. Tragically, some individuals accidentally strangle themselves.

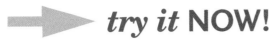

try it NOW!

How do you communicate with your partner about sex? Sex can be a difficult subject to talk about, even with someone you trust. Right now, take a moment to think about a sexual problem or desire you'd like to discuss with your partner, and brainstorm ways you can approach the subject.

Difficulties That Can Hinder Sexual Functioning

Research indicates that **sexual dysfunction,** the term used to describe problems that can hinder sexual functioning, is quite common. Don't feel embarrassed if you experience sexual dysfunction at some point in your life. The sexual part of you does not come with a lifetime warranty. You can have breakdowns involving your sexual function just as in any other body system. Sexual dysfunction can be divided into five major classes: disorders of sexual desire, sexual arousal, orgasm, sexual performance, and sexual pain. All of them can be treated successfully.

Sexual Desire Disorders

The most frequent reason why people seek out a sex therapist is **ISD, or inhibited sexual desire.**[43] ISD is the lack of a sexual appetite or simply a lack of interest and pleasure in sexual activity. In some instances, it can result from stress or boredom. **Sexual aversion disorder,** another type of desire dysfunction, is characterized by sexual phobias (unreasonable fears) and anxiety about sexual contact. The psychological stress of a punitive upbringing, a rigid religious background, or a history of physical or sexual abuse may be sources of these desire disorders.

Sexual Arousal Disorders

The most common sexual arousal disorder is **erectile dysfunction (ED)**—difficulty in achieving or maintaining a penile erection sufficient for intercourse. At some time in his life, every man experiences erectile dysfunction. Causes are varied and include underlying diseases, such as diabetes or prostate problems; reactions to some medications (for example, drugs for high blood pressure); depression; fatigue; stress; alcohol; performance anxiety; and guilt over real or imaginary problems (such as when a man compares himself to his partner's past lovers).

Some 30 million men in the United States, half of them under age 65, suffer from ED. The condition generally becomes more of a problem as men age, affecting one in four men over age 65.[44] The Food and Drug Administration (FDA) has approved several drugs such as Viagra (sildenafil citrate), Levitra (vardenafil hydrochloride), and Cialis (tadalafil) to treat ED. Additional oral medicines are being tested for safety and effectiveness.

Viagra, Levitra, and Cialis all belong to a class of drugs called phosphodiesterase (PDE) inhibitors. Taken an hour before sexual activity, these drugs work by enhancing the effects of nitric oxide, a chemical that relaxes smooth muscles in the penis during sexual stimulation and allows increased blood flow.

These medications are not, however, without risk. The most commonly reported side effects include headache, flushing, stomachache, urinary tract infection, diarrhea, rashes, and dizziness. In addition, among users of these medications there have been several instances of sudden vision loss due to blocked blood flow to the optic nerve. This side effect has prompted more caution in prescribing such drugs to patients with known cardiovascular disease, diabetes, high blood pressure, or high cholesterol.[45]

Orgasmic Disorders

Premature ejaculation—ejaculation that occurs prior to or very soon after the insertion of the penis into the vagina—affects up to 50 percent of men at some time in their lives. Treatment for premature ejaculation first involves a physical examination to rule out organic causes. If the cause of the problem is not physiological, therapy is available to help a man learn how to control the timing of his ejaculation. Fatigue, stress, performance pressure, and alcohol use can all contribute to orgasm disorders in men.

In a woman, the inability to achieve orgasm is termed **female orgasmic disorder.** A woman with this disorder often blames herself and learns to fake orgasm to avoid embarrassment or preserve her partner's ego. Contributing to this response are the messages women have historically been given about sex as a duty rather than a pleasurable act. As with men who experience orgasmic disorders, the first step in treatment is a physical exam to rule out organic causes. However, the problem is often solved by simple self-exploration to learn

---

sexual dysfunction   Problems associated with achieving sexual satisfaction.

inhibited sexual desire (ISD)   Lack of sexual appetite or simply a lack of interest and pleasure in sexual activity.

sexual aversion disorder   Type of desire dysfunction characterized by sexual phobias and anxiety about sexual contact.

erectile dysfunction (ED)   Difficulty in achieving or maintaining a penile erection sufficient for intercourse.

premature ejaculation   Ejaculation that occurs prior to or almost immediately following penile penetration of the vagina.

female orgasmic disorder   A woman's inability to achieve orgasm.

more about what forms of stimulation are arousing enough to produce orgasm. Through masturbation, a woman can learn how her body responds sexually to various types of touch. Once she has become orgasmic through masturbation, she learns to communicate her needs to her partner.

Sexual Performance Disorders

Both men and women can experience **sexual performance anxiety** when they anticipate some sort of problem in the sex act. A man may become anxious and unable to maintain an erection, or he may experience premature ejaculation. A woman may be unable to achieve orgasm or to allow penetration because of the involuntary contraction of vaginal muscles. Both can overcome performance anxiety by learning to focus on immediate sensations and pleasures rather than on orgasm.

Sexual Pain Disorders

Two common sexual pain disorders are dyspareunia and vaginismus. **Dyspareunia** is pain experienced by a woman during intercourse. This pain may be caused by diseases such as endometriosis, uterine tumors, chlamydia, gonorrhea, or urinary tract infections. Damage to tissues during childbirth and insufficient lubrication during intercourse may also cause discomfort. Dyspareunia can also be psychological in origin. As with other sexual problems, dyspareunia can be treated with good results.

Vaginismus is the involuntary contraction of vaginal muscles, making penile insertion painful or impossible. Most cases of vaginismus are related to fear of intercourse or to unresolved sexual conflicts. Treatment involves teaching a woman to achieve orgasm through nonvaginal stimulation.

Seeking Help for Sexual Dysfunction

Many theories and treatment models can help people with sexual dysfunction. A first important step is choosing a qualified sex therapist or counselor. A national organization,

---

sexual performance anxiety A condition of sexual difficulties caused by anticipating some sort of problem with the sex act.

dyspareunia Pain experienced by women during intercourse.

vaginismus A state in which the vaginal muscles contract so forcefully that penetration cannot be accomplished.

---

the American Association of Sex Educators, Counselors, and Therapists (AASECT), has been at the forefront of establishing criteria for certifying sex therapists. These criteria include appropriate degree(s) in the helping professions, specialized coursework in human sexuality, and sufficient hours of practical therapy work under the direct supervision of a certified sex therapist. Lists of certified counselors and sex therapists, as well as clinics that treat sexual dysfunctions, can be obtained by contacting AASECT or the Sexuality Information and Education Council of the United States (SIECUS).

Drugs and Sex

Because psychoactive drugs affect the body's entire physiological functioning, it is only logical that they affect sexual behavior. Promises of increased pleasure make drugs very tempting to people seeking greater sexual satisfaction. Too often, however, drugs become central to sexual activities and damage the relationship. Drug use can also lead to undesired sexual activity.

Alcohol is notorious for reducing inhibitions and promoting feelings of well-being and desirability. At the same time, alcohol inhibits sexual response; thus, the mind may be willing, but not the body.

Perhaps the greatest danger associated with use of drugs during sex is the tendency to blame the drug for negative behavior. "I can't help what I did last night because I was drunk" is a statement that demonstrates sexual immaturity. A sexually mature person carefully examines risks and benefits and makes decisions accordingly. If drugs are necessary to increase erotic feelings, it is likely that the partners are being dishonest about their feelings for each other. Good sex should not depend on chemical substances.

"Date Rape" Drugs
"Date rape" drugs have been a growing concern in recent years. They have become prevalent on college campuses, where they are often used in combination with alcohol. Rohypnol ("roofies," "rope," "forget pill"), GHB (gamma-hydroxybutyrate, or "liquid X," "Grievous Bodily Harm," "easy lay," "Mickey Finn"), and ketamine ("K," "Special K," "cat valium") have been used to facilitate rape. GHB and Rohypnol are difficult-to-detect drugs that depress the central nervous system. Ketamine can cause dreamlike states, hallucinations, delirium, amnesia, and impaired motor function. These drugs are often introduced to unsuspecting women through alcoholic drinks to render them unconscious and vulnerable to rape. This problem is so serious that the U.S. Congress passed the Drug-Induced Rape Prevention and Punishment Act of 1996 to increase federal penalties for using drugs to facilitate sexual assault. The dangers of these drugs are discussed in more detail in Chapter 4 (see the Spotlight on Your Health box on page 107) and in Chapter 7.

TAKING charge

Summary

- Characteristics of intimate relationships include behavioral interdependence, need fulfillment, emotional attachment, and emotional availability. These characteristics influence how we interact with others and the types of intimate relationships we form. Family, friends, and partners or lovers provide the most common opportunities for intimacy. Each relationship may include healthy and unhealthy characteristics that affect daily functioning.

- Gender differences in communication include conversation styles as well as differences in sharing feelings and disclosing personal facts and fears. These differences explain why men and women may relate differently in intimate relationships. Understanding these differences and learning how to deal with them are important aspects of healthy relationships.

- Barriers to intimacy often involve barriers to communication, which could result from a difference in background or the effects of alcohol and drugs. Other barriers may include the differences in the emotional needs of each partner, jealousy, and emotional wounds that could result from having been raised in a dysfunctional family.

- For most people, commitment is an important ingredient in successful relationships. The major types of committed relationships include marriage, cohabitation, and gay and lesbian partnerships.

- Success in committed relationships requires understanding the roles of partnering scripts, the importance of self-nurturance, and the elements of a good relationship.

- Life decisions such as whether to marry or whether to have children require serious consideration. Remaining single is more common than ever. Most single people lead healthy, happy, and well-adjusted lives. Those who decide to have or not to have children also can lead rewarding, productive lives as long as they have given this decision the utmost thought and weighed the pros and cons of each alternative in the context of their lifestyle.

- Today's family structure may look different from that of previous generations, but love, trust, and commitment to a child's welfare continue to be the cornerstones of successful child rearing.

- Before relationships fail, often many warning signs appear. By recognizing these signs and taking action to change behaviors, partners may save and enhance their relationships.

- Sexual identity is determined by a complex interaction of genetic, physiological, and environmental factors. Biological sex, gender identity, gender roles, and sexual orientation all are blended into our sexual identity.

- Sexual orientation refers to a person's enduring emotional, romantic, sexual, or affectionate attraction to other persons. Gay, lesbian and bisexual persons are repeatedly the targets of sexual prejudice. Sexual prejudice refers to negative attitudes and hostile actions directed at a social group and its members.

- The major components of the female sexual anatomy include the mons pubis, labia minora and majora, clitoris, urethral and vaginal openings, vagina, cervix, fallopian tubes, and ovaries. The major components of the male sexual anatomy are the penis, scrotum, testes, epididymides, vasa deferentia, ejaculatory ducts, and urethra.

- Physiologically, men and women experience the same four phases of sexual response: excitement/arousal, plateau, orgasm, and resolution.

- People can express their sexual selves in a variety of ways, including celibacy, autoerotic behaviors, kissing and erotic touch, manual stimulation, oral–genital stimulation, vaginal intercourse, and anal intercourse.

- Sexual dysfunctions can be classified into disorders of sexual desire, sexual arousal, orgasm, sexual performance, and sexual pain. Drug use also can also lead to sexual dysfunction.

Chapter Review

1. Intimate relationships fulfill our psychological need for someone to listen to our worries and concerns. This is known as our need for
   a. dependence.
   b. social integration.
   c. enjoyment.
   d. spontaneity.

2. Lovers tend to pay attention to the other person even when they should be involved in other activities. This is called
   a. inclusion.
   b. exclusivity.
   c. fascination.
   d. authentic intimacy.

3. Intense feelings of elation, sexual desire, and ecstasy in being with a partner are characteristic of
   a. companionate love.
   b. mature love.
   c. passionate love.
   d. intimacy.

4. According to anthropologist Helen Fisher, attraction and falling in love follow a pattern based on
   a. lust, attraction, and attachment.
   b. intimacy, passion, and commitment.
   c. imprinting, attraction, attachment, and the production of a cuddle chemical.
   d. fascination, exclusiveness, sexual desire, giving the utmost, and being a champion.

5. Who coined the term *genderlect*?
   a. Helen Fisher
   b. Robert Sternberg
   c. Deborah Tannen
   d. Carol Gilligan

6. Terms such as *behavioral interdependence, need fulfillment*, and *emotional availability* describe which type of relationship?
   a. dysfunctional relationship
   b. sexual relationship
   c. intimate relationship
   d. behavioral relationship

7. Predictability, dependability, and faith are three fundamental elements of
   a. trust.
   b. friendship.
   c. attraction.
   d. attachment.

8. One important factor in choosing a partner is *proximity*, which refers to
   a. mutual regard.
   b. attitudes and values.
   c. physical attraction.
   d. being in the same place at the same time.

9. Individuals who are sexually attracted to both sexes are identified as
   a. heterosexual.
   b. bisexual.
   c. homosexual.
   d. intersexual.

10. What is the role of testosterone in the male reproductive system?
    a. It is used to produce sperm for reproduction.
    b. It is the hormone that stimulates development of secondary male sex characteristics.
    c. It allows the penis to harden during sexual arousal.
    d. It secretes the seminal fluid preceding ejaculation.

Answers to these questions can be found on page A-1.

Questions for Discussion and Reflection

1. What are the characteristics of intimate relationships? What are behavioral interdependence, need fulfillment, emotional attachment, and emotional availability, and why is each important in relationship development?
2. Why are relationships with family important? Explain how your family unit was similar to or different from the traditional family unit in early America. Who made up your family of origin?
3. What problems can form barriers to intimacy? What actions can you take to reduce or remove these barriers?
4. What are the common elements of good relationships? What are some common warning signs of trouble?

What actions can you take to improve your own interpersonal relationships?
5. How have gender roles changed over your lifetime? Do you view the changes as positive for both men and women?
6. What is "normal" sexual behavior? What criteria should we use to determine healthful sexual practices?
7. If scientists ever establish the combination of factors that interact to produce homosexual, heterosexual, or bisexual orientation, will that put an end to antigay prejudice? Why or why not?

Accessing Your Health on the Internet

The following websites explore further topics and issues related to personal health. For links to the websites below, visit the Companion Website for *Health: The Basics*, Eighth Edition at www.aw-bc.com/donatelle.

1. *American Association of Sex Educators, Counselors, and Therapists (AASECT).* Professional organization providing standards of practice for treating sexual issues and disorders. www.aasect.org
2. *Bacchus and Gamma Peer Education Network.* Student-friendly source of information about sexual and other health issues. www.bacchusgamma.org

3. *Go Ask Alice.* An interactive question-and-answer resource from the Columbia University Health Services. "Alice" is available to answer questions about any health-related issues, including relationships, nutrition and diet, exercise, drugs, sex, alcohol, and stress. www.goaskalice.columbia.edu

4. *Sexuality Information and Education Council of the United States (SIECUS).* Information, guidelines, and materials for advancement of healthy and proper sex education. www.siecus.org

5. *Advocates for Youth.* Current news, policy updates, research, and other resources about the sexual health of and choices particular to high-school and college-aged students. www.advocatesforyouth.org

Further Reading

Caron, S. L. *Sex Matters for College Students: Sex FAQ's in Human Sexuality.* Englewood Cliffs, NJ: Prentice Hall, 2002.

  This is a brief, easy-to-read, and affordable paperback designed specifically to answer the basic sexual questions of today's young adults in a friendly and age-appropriate way.

Caster, W., R. Bussel, and J. May, *The Lesbian Sex Book: A Guide for Women Who Love Women,* 2nd ed. Los Angeles: Alyson Publications, 2003.

  A handbook for lesbian sexual practices and health.

Goldstone, S. *The Ins and Outs of Gay Sex: A Medical Handbook for Men.* New York: Dell, 1999.

  A comprehensive guide to the sexual and medical concerns of gay men.

Men's Health Books, ed. *The Complete Book of Men's Health: The Definitive, Illustrated Guide to Healthy Living, Exercise, and Sex.* Emmaus, PA: Rodale Press, 2000.

  A comprehensive and lushly illustrated guide to information on healthy lifestyles for men.

SIECUS (Sexuality Information and Education Council of the United States) Report. 130 West 42nd Street, New York, NY 10036.

  Highly acclaimed and readable bimonthly journal. Includes timely and thought-provoking articles on human sexuality, sexuality education, and AIDS.

Wingood, G. M., and R. DiClemente, eds. *Handbook of Women's Sexual and Reproductive Health.* Boston: Plenum Publishing, 2002.

  Medical researchers, including those in behavioral sciences and health education, summarize in depth the epidemiology, social and behavioral factors, policies, and effective intervention and prevention strategies related to women's sexual and reproductive health.

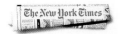

e-themes from *The New York Times*

For up-to-date articles about current health issues, visit www.aw-bc.com/donatelle, select *Health: The Basics*, Eighth Edition, Chapter 5, and click on "e-themes."

References

1. MayoClinic.com, "Nurture Relationships: A Healthy Habit for Healthy Aging," 2003, Mayo Foundation for Medical Education and Research (MFMER), www.mayohealth.org; K. Uberg et al., "Supportive Relationships as a Moderator of the Effects of Peer Drinking on Adolescents," *Journal of Research on Adolescents* 15, no.1 (2005): 1–20.

2. E. Weinstein and E. Rosen, *Teaching about Human Sexuality and Family: A Skills-Based Approach* (Belmont, CA: Thomson Higher Education, 2006).

3. Ibid.

4. L. Lefton and L. Brannon, *Psychology,* 9th ed. (Boston: Allyn & Bacon, 2005), 474.

5. Ibid.

6. H. Fisher, *Why We Love: The Nature and Chemistry of Romantic Love* (New York: Henry Holt, 2004).

7. E. Hatfield and R. L. Rapson, *Love, Sex, and Intimacy: Their Psychology, Biology, and History* (New York: Harper Collins, 1993).

8. R. Sternberg, "Construct Validation of a Triangular Love Scale," *European Journal of Social Psychology* 27 (1997): 313–35.

9. H. Fisher, *Why We Love;* H. Fisher, A. Aron, D. Mashek, H. Li, and L. L. Brown, "Defining the Brain System of Lust, Romantic Attraction, and Attachment," *Archives of Sexual Behavior,* 31, no. 5 (2002): 413–19.

10. A. Toufexis and P. Gray, "What Is Love? The Right Chemistry," *Time,* February 15, 1993, 47–52.

11. G. Kelly, *Sexuality Today: The Human Perspective,* 8th ed. (New York: McGraw-Hill, 2006).

12. Fisher et al., "Defining the Brain System," 413–19.

13. B. L. Seaward, *Managing Stress: Principles and Practices for Health and Well-Being,* 4th ed. (Boston: Jones & Bartlett, 2004), 100.

14. D. Tannen, *You Just Don't Understand: Women and Men in Conversation* (New York: William Morrow, 1990).

15. S. Michaud and R. Warner, "Gender Differences in Self Reported Response in Troubles Talk," *Sex Roles* 37 (1997): 528–40; K. Pasley, J. Kerpelman, and D. Guilbert, "Gender Conflict; Identity Disruption and Marital Instability: Expanding Gottman's Model," *Journal of Social and Personal Relationships* 18, no. 1 (2001): 1107–14; L. C. Gallo and T. W. Smith, "Attachment Style in Marriage: Adjustments and Responses to Interaction," *Journal of Social and Personal Relationships* 18, no. 2 (2001): 263–89; V. Manusov and J. Harvey, eds., *Attribution, Communication Behavior, and Close Relationships* (New York: Cambridge University Press, 2001).

16. S. A. Rathus, J. Nevid, and L. Fichner-Rathus, *Human Sexuality in a World of Diversity*, 6th ed. (Boston: Allyn & Bacon, 2005).

17. C. Morris and A. Maisto, *Psychology: An Introduction,* 12th ed. (Upper Saddle River, NJ: Prentice Hall, 2005).

18. Ibid.

19. S. Brehm et al., *Intimate Relationships,* 3rd ed. (New York: McGraw-Hill, 2002), 263.

20. B. Strong et al., *Human Sexuality: Diversity in Contemporary America,* 5th ed. (New York: McGraw-Hill, 2005).

21. The National Marriage Project, Rutgers, the State University of New Jersey, "The State of Our Unions," 2006, http://marriage.rutgers.edu.

22. U.S. Census Bureau, "Estimated Median Age at First Marriage, by Sex: 1890 to Present," March 27, 2007, www.census.gov/population/www/socdemo/hh-fam.html.

23. Mayo Clinic Staff, "Healthy Marriage: Why Love Is Good For You," Mayo Foundation for Medical Education and Research (MFMER), February 6, 2006, www.mayoclinic.com/print/healthy-marriage/MH00108.

24. C. A. Schoenborn, "Marital Status and Health:United States, 1999–2002," December 15, 2004, Advance Data from Vital and Health Statistics, Centers for Disease Control and Prevention.

25. Ibid.

26. Ibid.

27. National Gay and Lesbian Task Force, "Relationship Recognition of Same-Sex Couples in the U.S.," May 2007, www.theTaskForce.org.

28. U.S. Census Bureau, "March Current Population Survey," 2004, www.census.gov/population/www/socdemo/hh-fam.html.

29. U.S. Census Bureau, "Marital Status of People 15 Years and Older, March 2002," June 2003, www.census.gov/population/www/socdemo/hh-fam.html; Centers for Disease Control and Prevention, "Advance Data, First Marriage Dissolution, Divorce, and Remarriage: United States," 2001, www.cdc.gov/nchs/data/ad/ad323.pdf.

30. Ibid.

31. D. Hurley, "Divorce Rate: It's Not as High as You Think," *New York Times*, April 19, 2005.

32. The National Marriage Project, Rutgers, "The State of Our Unions."

33. Kelly, *Sexuality Today*, 271–72.

34. G. M. Herek, "The Psychology of Sexual Prejudice," *Current Directions in Psychological Science*, 9 (2000): 12–22.

35. H. Lerner, *The Dance of Intimacy* (New York: Perennial, 1990).

36. A. H. Slyper, "Childhood Obesity, Adipose Tissue Distribution, and the Pediatric Practitioner," *Pediatrics* 102 (1998): 4.

37. Writing Group for the Women's Health Initiative Investigators, "Risk and Benefits of Estrogen Plus Progestin in Healthy Postmenopausal Women: Principal Results from the Women's Health Initiative Randomized Controlled Trial," *Journal of the American Medical Association* 288, no. 3 (2002): 321–33.

38. N. Siegfried et al., "HIV and Male Circumcision—A Systematic Review with the Assessment of Quality of Studies," *The Lancet—Infectious Diseases* 5, no. 3 (2005): 165–73; A. Bertran et al., "Randomized, Controlled Intervention Trial of Male Circumcision for Reduction of HIV Transmission Risk: The ANRS 1265 Trial," *PLoS Medicine* 2, no. 11 (2005): 1112–22; B. G. Williams et al., "The Potential Impact of Male Circumcision on HIV in Sub-Saharan Africa," *PLoS Medicine* 3, no. 7 (2006): e 262; B. P. Homeier, "Circumcision," KidsHealth for Parents, Nemours Foundation, January 2005, http://kidshealth.org/parent/system/surgical/circumcision.html; Mayo Clinic Staff, "Circumcision: Weighing the Pros and Cons," MayoClinic.com, March 2006, www.mayoclinic.com/health/circumcision/PR00040.

39. Kelly, "Sexual Individuality and Sexual Values," in *Sexuality Today*.

40. Ibid.

41. American College Health Association. "American College Health Association–National College Health Assessment (ACHA-NCHA) Web Summary," April 2006, www.acha.org/projects_programs/ncha_sampledata.cfm.

42. Ibid.

43. Kelly, "Sexual Individuality and Sexual Values."

44. National Kidney and Urological Diseases Information Clearinghouse, "Erectile Dysfunction," 2005, http://kidney.niddk.nih.gov/kudiseases/pubs/impotence/index.htm.

45. U.S Food and Drug Administration. FDA "Updates Labeling for Viagra, Cialis and Levitra for Rare Post-Marketing Reports of Eye Problems," July 8, 2005, www.fda.gov/bbs/topics/NEWS/2005/NEW01201.html.

6

Birth Control, Pregnancy, and Childbirth

MANAGING YOUR FERTILITY

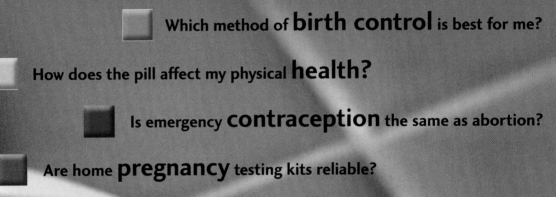

Which method of **birth control** is best for me?

How does the pill affect my physical **health?**

Is emergency **contraception** the same as abortion?

Are home **pregnancy** testing kits reliable?

What causes **infertility?**

OBJECTIVES

- Compare the different types of contraceptive methods and their effectiveness in preventing pregnancy and sexually transmitted infections.
- Summarize the legal decisions surrounding abortion and the various types of abortion procedures.
- Discuss key issues to consider when planning a pregnancy.
- Explain the importance of prenatal care and the physical and emotional aspects of pregnancy.
- Describe the basic stages of childbirth and complications that can arise during labor and delivery.
- Explain primary causes of and possible solutions to infertility.

oday we not only understand the intimate details of reproduction, but also possess technologies that control or enhance our **fertility,** our ability to reproduce. Along with information and technological advances comes choice, and choice goes hand in hand with responsibility. Choosing whether and when to have children is one of our greatest responsibilities. A woman and her partner have much to consider before planning or risking a pregnancy. Children transform people's lives. They require a lifelong personal commitment of love and nurturing. Are you physically, emotionally, and financially prepared to care for another human being?

One measure of maturity is the ability to discuss reproduction and birth control with one's sexual partner before engaging in sexual activity. Men often assume that their partners are taking care of birth control. Women often feel that bringing up the subject implies they are promiscuous. Both may feel that this discussion interferes with romance and spontaneity. You will find discussion easier and less embarrassing if you understand human reproduction and contraception and honestly consider your attitudes toward these matters.

Methods of Fertility Management

Conception refers to the fertilization of an ovum by a sperm. The following conditions are necessary for conception:

1. A viable egg
2. A viable sperm
3. Access to the egg by the sperm

---

fertility   A person's ability to reproduce.

conception   The fertilization of an ovum by a sperm.

contraception (birth control)   Methods of preventing conception.

sexually transmitted infections (STIs)   A variety of infections that can be acquired through sexual contact.

barrier methods   Contraceptive methods that block the meeting of egg and sperm by means of a physical barrier (such as condom, diaphragm, or cervical cap), a chemical barrier (such as spermicide), or both.

hormonal methods   Contraceptive method that introduces synthetic hormones into the woman's system to prevent ovulation, thicken cervical mucus, or prevent a fertilized egg from implanting.

male condom   A single-use sheath of thin latex or other material designed to fit over an erect penis and to catch semen on ejaculation.

The term **contraception** (sometimes called **birth control**) refers to methods of preventing conception. These methods offer varying degrees of control over when and whether pregnancies occur. Society has searched for a simple, infallible, and risk-free way to prevent pregnancy since people first associated sexual activity with pregnancy. We have not yet found one.

To evaluate the effectiveness of a particular contraceptive method, you must be familiar with two concepts: perfect failure rate and typical use failure rate. *Perfect failure rate* refers to the number of pregnancies that are likely to occur in the first year of use (per 100 uses of the method during sexual intercourse) if the method is used absolutely perfectly, that is, without any error. The *typical use failure rate* refers to the number of pregnancies that are likely to occur during the first year of use with typical use—that is, with the normal number of errors, memory lapses, and incorrect or incomplete use. The typical-use information is much more practical in helping people make informed decisions about contraceptive methods. We'll discuss various contraceptive methods in this chapter.

Some contraceptive methods can also protect, to some degree, against **sexually transmitted infections (STIs),** which you'll learn more about in Chapter 13. This is an important factor to consider in choosing a contraceptive.

Choosing a Method of Contraception

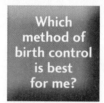

Which method of birth control is best for me?

Present methods of contraception fall into several categories. **Barrier methods** block the egg and sperm from joining. **Hormonal methods** introduce synthetic hormones into the woman's system that prevent ovulation, thicken cervical mucus, or prevent a fertilized egg from implanting. Surgical methods can prevent pregnancy permanently. Other methods may involve temporary or permanent abstinence or planning intercourse in accordance with fertility patterns.

There are many factors to consider when choosing a method of contraception. Issues to think about range from cost to comfort level to convenience and health risks associated with a particular method. **Table 6.1** summarizes the effectiveness and costs of various methods. The **Assess Yourself** box on page 154 will help you to determine which method is best for you and your partner.

Barrier Methods

The Male Condom   The **male condom** is a thin sheath designed to cover the erect penis and catch semen before it enters the vagina. The majority of male condoms are made of latex, although condoms made of polyurethane or lambskin are now available. The condom is the only temporary means of birth control available for men, and latex and polyurethane condoms are the only barriers that effectively

(Text continues on page 156.)

TABLE 6.1 Contraceptive Effectiveness, STI Prevention, and Costs

Method	Number of Unintended Pregnancies per 100 Women during the First Year of Use		Cost
	Typical Use	Perfect Use	
Continuous abstinence*	0	0	None
Female sterilization	0.5	0.5	$1,500–$6,000 for interview, counseling, examination, operation, and follow-up.
Male sterilization	0.15	0.1	$350–$1,000 for interview, counseling, examination, operation, and follow-up sperm count.
Implanon	0.05	0.05	Implanon was approved for use in the United States in July 2006. It is not yet known how much it will cost to have Implanon inserted or removed.
IUD (intrauterine device)			
ParaGard (copper T)	0.8	0.6	$175–$500 for exam, insertion, and follow-up visit.
Mirena (LNG-IUS)	0.2	0.2	$175–$500 for exam, insertion, and follow-up visit.
Depo-Provera	3	0.3	$30–$75 for 3-month injection; $35–$175 for initial exam; $20–$40 for further visits to clinician for shots.
Oral contraceptives (combined pill and progestin-only pill)	8	0.3	$15–$35 monthly pill pack at drugstores; often less at clinics; $35–$175 for initial exam.
Ortho Evra patch	8	0.3	$30–$40 per month at drugstores, often less at clinics; $35–$175 for initial exam.
NuvaRing	8	0.3	$30–$35 per month at drugstores, often less at clinics, $35–$175 for initial exam.
Male condom† (without Spermicides)	15	2	$0.50 and up per condom—some family planning centers give them away or charge very little. Available in drugstores, in family planning clinics, in some supermarkets, and from vending machines.
Diaphragm† (with Spermicidal Cream or Jelly)	16	6	$15–$75 for diaphragms, caps, and shields; $50–$200 for initial exam; $8–$17 for supplies of spermicide jelly or cream.
Sponge			$7.50–$9 for a package of 3 sponges. Available at family planning centers, in drugstores, online, and in some supermarkets.
Women who have never given birth	16	9	
Women who have given birth	32	20	
Female condom† (without Spermicides)	21	5	$2.50 per condom. Available at family planning centers, in drugstores, and in some supermarkets.
Fertility awareness methods	25	12	$10–$12 for temperature kits. Charts and classes often free in health centers and churches.
Withdrawal	27	4	None
Spermicides† (foams, creams, gels, vaginal suppositories, and vaginal film)	29	18	$8–$17 for applicator kits of foam and gel ($4–$8 for refills). Film and suppositories are priced similarly. Available at family planning clinics, in drugstores, and in some supermarkets.
No method	85	85	None
Emergency contraceptive pill			Treatment initiated within 72 hours after unprotected intercourse reduces the risk of pregnancy by 75–89% (with no protection against STIs). Costs depend on what services are needed: $10 to $45 for Plan B, available without a prescription to women 18 and older; $20–$50 for one pack of combination pills; $50–$70 for two packs of progestin-only pills; $35–$150 for visit with health care provider; $10–$20 for pregnancy test.

*Indicates complete protection from STIs.

†Indicates limited protection from STIs.

Note: "Typical Use" refers to failure rates for men and women whose use is not consistent or always correct. "Perfect Use" refers to failure rates for those whose use is consistent and always correct.

Note: Some family planning clinics charge for services and supplies on a sliding scale according to income.

Source: R. Hatcher et al., *Contraceptive Technology*, 19th rev. ed. Copyright © 2007 Contraceptive Technology Communications, Inc. Used with permission.

ASSESS yourself

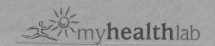

CONTRACEPTIVE COMFORT AND CONFIDENCE SCALE

Fill out this assessment online at www.aw-bc.com/MyHealthLab or www.aw-bc.com/donatelle.

These questions will help you assess whether the method of contraception you or your partner are using now—or may consider using in the future—will be effective for you. Answering yes to any of these questions predicts potential problems. Most individuals will have a few yes answers. If you have more than a few yes responses, however, you may want to talk to a health care provider, counselor, partner, or friend to decide whether to use this method or how to use it so that it will really be effective. In general, the more yes answers you have, the less likely you are to use this method consistently and correctly with every act of intercourse.

Method of contraception you use now or are considering: _____

Length of time you used this method in the past: _____

Answer yes or no to the following questions:

	Yes	No
1. Have I ever had problems using this method?	❑	❑
2. Have I or my partner ever become pregnant while using this method?	❑	❑
3. Am I afraid of using this method?	❑	❑
4. Would I really rather not use this method?	❑	❑
5. Will I have trouble remembering to use this method?	❑	❑
6. Will I have trouble using this method correctly?	❑	❑
7. Do I still have unanswered questions about this method?	❑	❑
8. Does this method make menstrual periods longer or more painful for me or my partner?	❑	❑
9. Does this method cost more than I can afford?	❑	❑
10. Could this method cause serious complications?	❑	❑
11. Am I opposed to this method because of any religious or moral beliefs?	❑	❑
12. Is my partner opposed to this method?	❑	❑
13. Am I using this method without my partner's knowledge?	❑	❑
14. Will using this method embarrass my partner?	❑	❑
15. Will using this method embarrass me?	❑	❑
16. Will I enjoy intercourse less because of this method?	❑	❑
17. If this method interrupts lovemaking, will I avoid using it?	❑	❑
18. Has a nurse or doctor ever told me not to use this method?	❑	❑
19. Is there anything about my personality that could lead me to use this method incorrectly?	❑	❑
20. Am I at risk of being exposed to HIV (the human immunodeficiency virus) or other sexually transmitted infections (STIs) if I use this method?	❑	❑

Total number of yes answers: _____

Source: From R. A. Hatcher et al., *Contraceptive Technology,* 19th rev. ed. Copyright © 2007 Contraceptive Technology Communications, Inc. Used with permission.

MAKE it happen!

ASSESSMENT: The Assess Yourself activity gave you the chance to assess your comfort and confidence with the contraceptive method you are using now or may use in the future. Depending on the results of the assessment, you may consider making a change in your birth control method.

MAKING A CHANGE: To change your behavior, you need to develop a plan. Follow these steps and complete your Behavior Change Contract to take action.

1. Evaluate your behavior, and identify patterns. What can you change now? What can you change in the near future?

2. Select one pattern of behavior that you want to change.

3. Fill out the Behavior Change Contract found at the front of your book. It should include your long-term goal for change, your short-term goals, the rewards you'll give yourself for reaching these goals, potential obstacles along the way, and strategies for overcoming these obstacles. For each goal, list the small steps and specific actions that you will take.

4. Chart your progress in a journal. At the end of a week, consider how successful you were in following your plan. What helped you be successful? What made change more difficult? What will you do differently next week?

5. Revise your plan as needed: Are the short-term goals attainable? Are the rewards satisfying?

EXAMPLE: Marissa had been using a diaphragm as her form of birth control. When she completed the self-assessment, she discovered that there were several aspects of it that made her uncomfortable. The questions to which she answered yes showed that she sometimes forgot to bring her diaphragm when she planned to see her boyfriend, Ben, and she disliked using it because it interrupted her sexual activity. She also was embarrassed to use it because she didn't like inserting it in front of Ben. She decided she should investigate other birth control options and discuss them with her boyfriend. Her first step was to visit her student health center and, based on her likes and dislikes, to choose one or two alternatives to the diaphragm. Among the options suggested to her were the contraceptive patch (Ortho Evra) and the vaginal ring (NuvaRing), both of which she would not have to remember to use and would not interrupt sexual activity. Marissa's next step was to talk to her boyfriend about his likes and dislikes and then to make a final decision based on her confidence in the method, its convenience, and its cost.

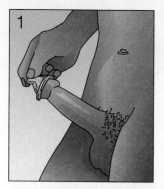
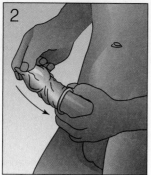
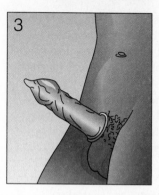
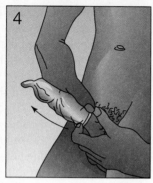

FIGURE 6.1 How to Use a Condom
The condom should be rolled over the erect penis before any penetration occurs. A small space (about 1/2 inch) should be left at the end of the condom to collect the semen after ejaculation (1). Hold the tip of the condom, and unroll it all the way to the base of the penis (2, 3). Hold the base of the condom before withdrawal to avoid spilling any semen (4).

prevent the spread of some STIs and HIV (human immuno-deficiency virus). ("Skin" condoms, made from lamb intestines, are not effective against STIs.)

Condoms come in a wide variety of styles. All may be purchased with or without spermicide in pharmacies, supermarkets, public bathrooms, and many health clinics. A new condom must be used for each act of vaginal, oral, or anal intercourse.

A condom must be rolled onto the penis before the penis touches the vagina and held in place when removing the penis from the vagina after ejaculation **(Figure 6.1)**. Condoms come with or without spermicide and with or without lubrication. Spermicides can cause irritation for some users, and there is no evidence that using a spermicide with condoms reduces the risk of pregnancy. If desired, users can lubricate their own condoms with contraceptive foams, creams, and jellies or other water-based lubricants (e.g., K-Y jelly, ForPlay Lubricants, Astroglide, or Wet or Aqua Lube). Never use products such as baby oil, cold cream, petroleum jelly, vaginal yeast infection medications, or hand or body lotion

spermicides   Substances designed to kill sperm.

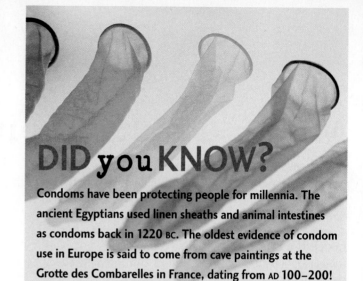

with a condom. These products contain mineral oil and will cause the latex to begin to disintegrate within 60 seconds.

Condoms are less effective and more likely to break during intercourse if they are old or poorly stored. To maintain effectiveness, store them in a cool place (not in a wallet or hip pocket), and inspect them for small tears before use. Discard all condoms that have passed their expiration date.

For some people, a condom ruins the spontaneity of sex because stopping to put it on may break the mood for them. Others report that the condom decreases sensation. These inconveniences and perceptions contribute to improper use or avoiding condoms altogether. Partners who put a condom on as part of foreplay are generally more successful with this form of birth control.

Jellies, Creams, Foams, Suppositories, and Film

Like condoms, some other barrier methods—jellies, creams, foam, suppositories, and film—do not require a prescription. They are referred to as **spermicides**—substances designed to kill sperm.

Jellies and creams are packaged in tubes, and foams are available in aerosol cans. All have tubes designed for insertion into the vagina. They must be inserted far enough to cover the cervix, thus providing both a chemical barrier that kills sperm and a physical barrier that stops sperm from continuing toward an egg **(Figure 6.2)**.

Suppositories are waxy capsules that are inserted deep in the vagina, where they melt. They must be inserted 10 to 20 minutes before intercourse to have time to melt, but no longer than one hour prior to intercourse, or they lose their effectiveness. Additional contraceptive chemicals must be applied for each subsequent act of intercourse.

Vaginal contraceptive film is another method of spermicide delivery. A thin film infused with spermicidal gel is inserted into the vagina, so that it covers the cervix. The

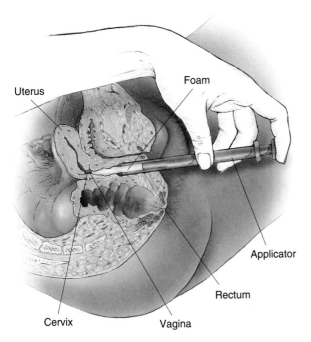

FIGURE 6.2 **The Proper Method of Applying Spermicide within the Vagina**

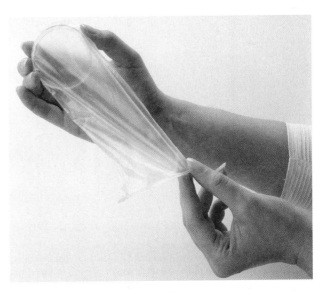

The female condom.

film dissolves into a spermicidal gel that is effective for up to 3 hours. As with other spermicides, a new film must be inserted for each act of intercourse.

Recent studies indicate that spermicides containing nonoxynol 9 (N-9) are not effective in preventing some STIs, such as gonorrhea, chlamydia, and HIV. In fact, frequent use of spermicides containing nonoxynol 9 has been shown to cause irritation and breaks in the mucous layer or skin of the genital tract, creating a point of entry for viruses and bacteria that cause disease. Spermicides containing nonoxynol 9 have also been associated with increased risk of urinary tract infection.[1] Although they are not recommended as the primary form of contraception, spermicides are often recommended for use with other methods and are most effective when used in conjunction with a condom.

The Female Condom

The **female condom** (brand name: Reality Condom) is a single-use, soft, loose-fitting polyurethane sheath meant for internal use. It is designed as one unit with two flexible rings. One ring, which lies inside the sheath, serves as an insertion mechanism and internal anchor. The other ring, which remains outside the vagina once the device is inserted, protects the labia and the base of the penis from infection. Many women like the female condom because it gives them more control over reproduction than the male condom. When used correctly, the female condom provides protection against HIV and STIs comparable to that of a latex male condom. Because the polyurethane is thin and pliable, there is less loss of sensation than with the latex male condom. Some disadvantages of the female condom are similar to those associated with the male condom: they interfere with

spontaneity and are slightly awkward to use. The female condom can also can be used by either gender for anal intercourse.

The Diaphragm with Spermicidal Jelly or Cream

Invented in the mid-nineteenth century, the **diaphragm** was the first widely used birth control method for women. This device is a soft, shallow cup made of thin latex rubber. Its flexible, rubber-coated ring is designed to fit snugly behind the pubic bone in front of the cervix and over the back of the cervix on the other side so it blocks access to the uterus. Diaphragms are manufactured in different sizes and must be fitted to the woman by a trained practitioner. The practitioner also should be certain that the user knows how to insert her diaphragm correctly before she leaves the practitioner's office.

Diaphragms must be used with spermicidal cream or jelly, which is applied to the inside of the diaphragm before it is inserted. A diaphragm can be inserted up to 6 hours before intercourse. The diaphragm holds the spermicide in place, creating a physical and chemical barrier against sperm. Additional spermicide must be applied before each subsequent act of intercourse; the diaphragm must be left in place for 6 to 8 hours after intercourse to allow the chemical to kill any sperm remaining in the vagina. When used with spermicidal jelly or cream, the diaphragm offers significant protection against gonorrhea and, possibly, chlamydia and human papilloma virus (HPV), but not HIV (**Figure 6.3**).

> **female condom** A single-use polyurethane sheath for internal use during vaginal or anal intercourse to catch semen on ejaculation.
>
> **diaphragm** A latex, cup-shaped device designed to cover the cervix and block access to the uterus; should always be used with spermicide.

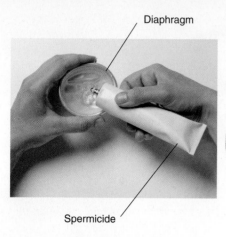

Diaphragm

Spermicide

(a) Place spermicide inside and around the rim of the diaphragm.

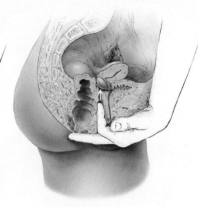

(b) Insertion: squeeze rim together; insert with spermicide-side up.

(c) Check placement, making certain cervix is covered.

FIGURE 6.3 The Proper Use and Placement of a Diaphragm

Using the diaphragm during the menstrual period or leaving it in place longer than 24 hours slightly increases the user's risk of **toxic shock syndrome (TSS).** This condition results from the multiplication of bacteria that spread to the bloodstream and cause sudden high fever, rash, nausea, vomiting, diarrhea, and a rapid drop in blood pressure. If not treated, TSS can be fatal. The diaphragm (as well as a tampon left too long in place) creates conditions conducive to the growth of these bacteria. To reduce the risk of TSS, women should wash their hands carefully with soap and water before inserting or removing a diaphragm.

Another problem with the diaphragm is that it can put undue pressure on the urethra, blocking urinary flow and predisposing the user to bladder infections. Inserting the device also can be awkward, especially if the woman is rushed. Diaphragms are much less effective when inserted incorrectly.

The Cervical Cap with Spermicidal Jelly or Cream
One of the oldest methods used to prevent pregnancy, early **cervical caps** were made from beeswax, silver, or copper. The Prentif cervical cap, a small cup made of latex, is no longer produced by the manufacturer, but many are still in use. The "new" cervical cap, the FemCap, is a clear silicone cup that fits snugly over the entire cervix. It comes in three sizes and must be fitted by a practitioner. The FemCap is designed for use with spermicidal jelly or cream. It is somewhat more difficult to insert than a diaphragm because of its smaller size.

The cap works by blocking sperm from the uterus. It is held in place by suction created during application. It may be inserted up to 6 hours prior to intercourse, and the device must be left in place for 6 to 8 hours after intercourse. If removed and cleaned, it can be reinserted immediately. Like the diaphragm, the cervical cap used with spermicide may offer protection against some STIs, but not HIV.

Some women report unpleasant vaginal odors after use. Because the device can become dislodged during intercourse, placement must be checked frequently. The cap cannot be used during the menstrual period or for longer than 48 hours because of the risk of TSS.

Lea's Shield is a one-size-fits-all silicon rubber device that covers the cervix. The device can be inserted anytime prior to

toxic shock syndrome (TSS) A potentially life-threatening disease that occurs when specific bacterial toxins multiply and spread to the bloodstream, most commonly through improper use of tampons or diaphragms.

cervical cap A small cup made of latex that is designed to fit snugly over the entire cervix.

Lea's Shield A one-size-fits-all silicon rubber contraceptive device that covers the cervix and is available by prescription.

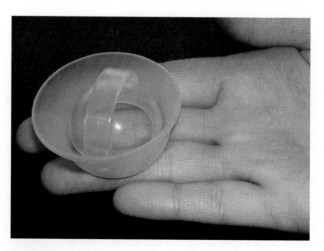

FemCap.

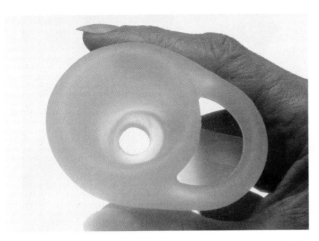
Lea's Shield.

intercourse, but it must remain in place for 8 hours after intercourse; it can remain in place for a maximum of 48 hours. The shield is outfitted with a small loop that aids in both insertion and removal. It must be used with spermicidal jelly or cream, as with the diaphragm or cervical cap. Approved by the FDA in 2002, it is available by prescription. Because the shield is made of silicon rubber, not latex, it is a suitable alternative for people allergic to latex. Other benefits and disadvantages are similar to those of the diaphragm and cervical cap.

The Sponge
The original version of the sponge, the **Today sponge,** was available in the United States from 1983 to 1995, at which time the manufacturer shut down production rather than bring its facility up to FDA standards. In 2005 the Today sponge, now produced by a different company, was approved by the FDA and was made available for purchase in retail stores.

The sponge is made of polyurethane foam and contains nonoxynol 9. It fits over the cervix and creates a barrier against sperm. A main advantage is convenience, because it

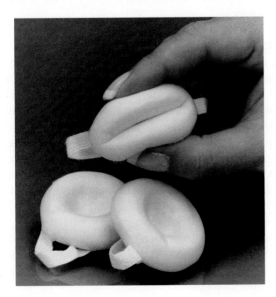
The contraceptive sponge.

does not require a trip to the doctor for fitting. Protection begins right away on insertion and lasts for up to 24 hours. There is no need to reapply spermicide or insert a new sponge for any subsequent acts of intercourse within the same 24-hour period; it must be left in place for at least 6 hours after the last intercourse. Disadvantages of the sponge are limited protection from STIs and only moderate protection against pregnancy. Allergic reactions, such as irritations of the vagina, are more common with sponge. Should the vaginal lining become irritated, the risk of yeast infections and other STIs may increase. Some cases of toxic shock syndrome have been reported in women using the sponge. The same precautions should be taken as with the diaphragm and cervical cap.

Hormonal Methods

Oral Contraceptives
Oral contraceptive pills were first marketed in the United States in 1960. Their convenience quickly made them the most widely used reversible method of fertility control. Most modern pills are up to 99% effective at preventing pregnancy with perfect use. Today, oral contraceptives are the most commonly used contraceptive among college-aged women **(Figure 6.4).**

Much of the pill's popularity comes from its convenience and discreetness. Users like that it does not interrupt or interfere with lovemaking. In addition to protecting against pregnancy, the pill may lessen menstrual difficulties, such as cramps and premenstrual syndrome. Oral contraceptives also lower the risk of several health conditions, including endometrial and ovarian cancers, noncancerous breast disease, osteoporosis, ovarian cysts, pelvic inflammatory disease (PID), and iron-deficiency anemia.[2]

Most oral contraceptives work through the combined effects of synthetic estrogen and progesterone *(combination pills)*. Estrogen in the pill prevents ovulation by inhibiting the production of follicle-stimulating hormone (FSH; Chapter 5). Progesterone in the pill prevents proper growth of the uterine lining and thickens the cervical mucus, thus forming a barrier against sperm.

Combination pills are taken in a cycle. At the end of each 3-week cycle, the user discontinues the drug or takes placebo pills for 1 week. The resultant drop in hormones causes the uterine lining to disintegrate, and the user will have a menstrual period, usually within 1 to 3 days. Menstrual flow is generally lighter than it is for women who don't use the pill because the hormones in the pill prevent thick endometrial buildup.

Today sponge   A contraceptive device, made of polyurethane foam and containing nonoxynol 9, that fits over the cervix to create a barrier against sperm.

oral contraceptives   Pills taken daily for 3 weeks of the menstrual cycle that prevent ovulation by regulating hormones.

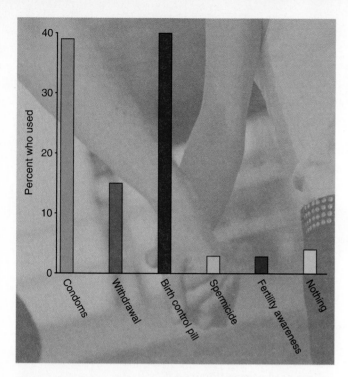

FIGURE 6.4 **Types of Contraception Sexually Active College Students Have Used in the Past 30 Days**

Source: From *American College Health Association–National College Health Assessment* (ACHA–NCHA) Web Summary, updated April 2006. www.acha-ncha.org/data_highlights.html.

A newer type of pill available since 2003 is **Seasonale,** a 91-day (extended-cycle) oral contraceptive. A woman using this type of regimen takes active pills for 12 weeks, followed by 1 week of placebos. Under this cycle, women can expect to have a menstrual period every 3 months. Data indicate that women do have an increased occurrence of spotting or bleeding in the first few cycles.[3] Side effects and risks are similar to those of 28-day cycle pills.

How does the pill affect my physical health?

Because the chemicals in oral contraceptives change the way the body metabolizes certain nutrients, all women using the pill should check with their practitioners to see whether dietary supplements are advisable. A nutritious diet that includes whole grains, fresh fruits and vegetables, lean meats, fish and poultry, and non-fat dairy products is important.

Oral contraceptives can interact negatively with other drugs. For example, some antibiotics diminish the pill's effectiveness and may require an adjustment in the antibiotic dosage. Women in doubt should check with their practitioners or pharmacists.

Seasonale An extended-cycle oral contraceptive that causes a woman to menstruate only once every 3 months.

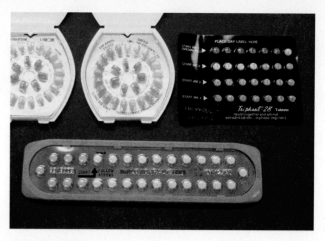

Oral contraceptives.

Return of fertility may be delayed after a woman discontinues the pill, but the pill is not known to cause infertility. Women who had irregular menstrual cycles before going on the pill are more likely to have problems conceiving, regardless of pill use.

Possible serious health problems associated with the pill include blood clots, which can lead to strokes or heart attacks, and an increased risk for high blood pressure **(Figure 6.5).** The risk is low for most healthy women under 35 who do not smoke; it increases with age and especially with cigarette smoking.

Apart from these risk factors and certain side effects associated with the pill, its greatest disadvantage is that it must be taken every day. If a woman misses one pill, she should use an alternative form of contraception for the remainder of that cycle. Another drawback is that the pill does not protect against STIs. Cost also may be a problem for some women. Some teenagers report that the requirement to have a complete gynecological examination to get a prescription for the pill is a huge obstacle. Educating young women about what goes on in a gynecological exam certainly would help ease their anxiety.

Progestin-Only Pills Progestin-only pills (or mini-pills) contain small doses of progesterone and no estrogen. Women who feel uncertain about using estrogen pills, who suffer from side effects related to estrogen, or who are nursing may choose these medications rather than combination pills. There is still some question about how progestin-only pills work. Current thought is that they change the composition of the cervical mucus, thus impeding sperm travel. They also may inhibit ovulation in some women. The effectiveness rate of progestin-only pills is 96 percent, slightly lower than that of estrogen-containing pills. Also, their use usually leads to irregular menstrual bleeding. As with all oral contraceptives, the user has no protection against STIs. Progestin-only pills share some of the risks and benefits associated with combination pills, though they are without estrogen-related risks.

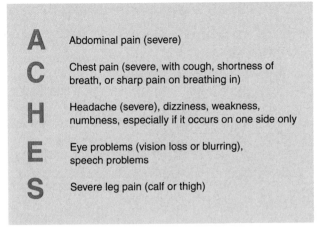

A	Abdominal pain (severe)
C	Chest pain (severe, with cough, shortness of breath, or sharp pain on breathing in)
H	Headache (severe), dizziness, weakness, numbness, especially if it occurs on one side only
E	Eye problems (vision loss or blurring), speech problems
S	Severe leg pain (calf or thigh)

FIGURE 6.5 Early Warning Signs of Medical Complications for Users of the Birth Control Pill

Source: R. A. Hatcher et al., *Contraceptive Technology,* 19th rev. ed. Copyright © 2007 Contraceptive Technology Communications, Inc. Used with permission.

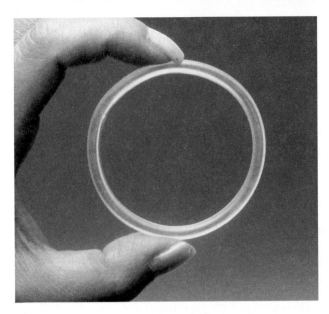

NuvaRing (actual size).

Ortho Evra (The Patch)

Ortho Evra is a square patch, as thin as a plastic strip bandage, that is worn for 1 week and replaced on the same day of the week for 3 consecutive weeks; the fourth week is patch-free. Ortho Evra is 99 percent effective and works by delivering continuous levels of estrogen and progestin through the skin and into the bloodstream. The patch can be worn on one of four areas of the body: buttocks, abdomen, upper torso (front and back, excluding the breasts), or upper outer arm.

In 2005, amidst evidence that the patch may increase a woman's risk for life-threatening blood clots, the FDA mandated an additional warning label explaining that the patch exposes women to about 60 percent more total estrogen than a typical combination birth control pill. Although studies on this health concern continue, the FDA will monitor the safety of Ortho Evra, and women should discuss these risks with

their health care provider when determining whether the patch is right for them.[4]

NuvaRing

NuvaRing is a hormonal contraceptive that offers protection 4 weeks at a time when used as prescribed. It is a soft, flexible ring about 2 inches in diameter. The user inserts the ring into her vagina, leaves it in place for 3 weeks, and removes it for 1 week for her menstrual period. Once the ring is inserted, it continuously releases a steady flow of estrogen and progestin. When used properly, the ring is 99 percent effective.

Advantages to NuvaRing include protection against pregnancy for 1 month; no pill to take daily; no need to be fitted by a clinician; no requirement to use spermicide; and rapid return of the ability to become pregnant after use is stopped. Possible side effects include increased vaginal discharge and vaginal irritation or infection. Oil-based vaginal medicines to treat yeast infections cannot be used when the ring is in place, and a diaphragm or cervical cap cannot be used as a backup method for contraception.

Depo-Provera and Other Injections

Depo-Provera is a long-acting synthetic progesterone that is injected intramuscularly every 3 months by a health care provider. Researchers believe that the drug prevents

Ortho Evra   A patch that releases hormones similar to those in oral contraceptives; each patch is worn for 1 week.

NuvaRing   A soft, flexible ring inserted into the vagina that releases hormones, preventing pregnancy.

Depo-Provera   An injectable method of birth control that lasts for 3 months.

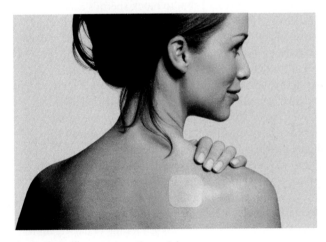

Ortho Evra, the contraceptive patch.

ovulation. There are fewer health problems associated with Depo-Provera than with estrogen-containing pills. However, use of this contraceptive comes with a warning that prolonged use of the drug is linked with loss of bone density. The main disadvantage is irregular bleeding, which can be troublesome at first, but within a year most women are amenorrheic (i.e., they have no menstrual periods). Weight gain (an average of 5 pounds in the first year) is common. Other possible side effects include dizziness, nervousness, and headache. Some women feel Depo-Provera encourages sexual spontaneity because they do not have to remember to take a pill or insert a device.

However, unlike other methods of contraception, Depo-Provera cannot be stopped immediately if problems arise. Also, women who wish to become pregnant may find that it takes up to a year after their last injection to succeed.

Implanon and Other Implants A new single-rod implantable contraceptive, Implanon, has been approved for use by the FDA. Implanon is a small (about the size of a matchstick), soft capsule that is inserted just beneath the skin on the inner side of a woman's upper underarm by a health care provider. After insertion, Implanon is generally not visible, making it a discreet method of birth control. Implanon continually releases a low, steady dose of progestin for up to 3 years, suppressing ovulation during that time. Implanon does not protect against HIV and other sexually transmitted infections. As with other progestin-only contraceptives, users of Implanon can experience irregular bleeding. Jadelle, a two-rod implant, is currently waiting approval by the FDA to enter the market in the United States.

what do you THINK?

Who do you think is responsible for deciding which method of contraception should be used in a sexual relationship? ■ What are some examples of good opportunities for you and your partner to have a discussion about contraceptives? ■ What do you think are the biggest barriers in our society to the use of condoms?

Surgical Methods

Sterilization has become the second leading method of contraception for women of all ages in the United States, and the leading method of contraception among married women in the United States.[5] Because sterilization is

sterilization Permanent fertility control achieved through surgical procedures.

tubal ligation Sterilization of the woman that involves cutting and tying off or cauterizing the fallopian tubes.

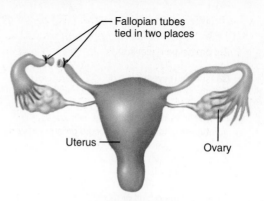

(a) Tubal ligation

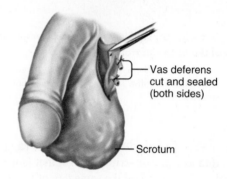

(b) Vasectomy

FIGURE 6.6 Sterilization
(a) In a tubal ligation, the fallopian tubes are tied or sealed shut.
(b) In a vasectomy, the surgeon makes an incision in the scrotum, then locates the vas deferens, and either seals or ties them shut.
Source: M. Johnson, *Human Biology: Concepts and Current Issues,* 4th ed. Copyright © 2008 Benjamin Cummings. Reprinted by permission of Pearson Education.

permanent, anyone considering it should think through possibilities, such as divorce and remarriage or a future improvement in financial status, that might make a pregnancy realistic or desirable.

Female Sterilization One method of sterilization for women is **tubal ligation,** a surgical procedure in which the fallopian tubes are sealed shut to block sperm's access to released eggs (**Figure 6.6a**). The operation usually is done laparoscopically in a hospital on an outpatient basis, under some form of anesthesia. The procedure itself usually takes less than an hour, and the patient is generally allowed to return home within a short time.

A tubal ligation does not affect ovarian and uterine function. The woman's menstrual cycle continues, and released eggs simply disintegrate and are absorbed by the lymphatic system. As soon as her incisions heals, the woman may resume sexual intercourse with no fear of pregnancy.

As with any surgery, there are risks. Although rare, the possible complications of a tubal ligation include infection, pulmonary embolism, hemorrhage, anesthesia complication, and ectopic pregnancy. Women considering a tubal ligation should thoroughly discuss all the risks with their physician before the operation.

A new sterilization procedure, **Essure,** involves the placement of small microcoils into the fallopian tubes via the vagina by a physician. Once in place, the microcoils expand to the shape of the fallopian tubes. The coils promote the growth of scar tissue around the device and cause the fallopian tubes to become blocked. Like traditional forms of tubal ligation, Essure is permanent.

A potential advantage of the Essure procedure is that it does not require an incision. The entire procedure takes only 35 minutes and can be performed in the doctor's office. It is recommended for women who definitely do not want more children and especially for those who cannot have a tubal ligation because of chronic health conditions, such as obesity or heart disease. Essure is a relatively new technique, and as a result the long-term risks are unknown.

A **hysterectomy,** or removal of the uterus, is a method of sterilization requiring major surgery. It is usually done only when the patient's uterus is diseased or damaged.

Male Sterilization

Sterilization in men is less complicated than it is in women. A **vasectomy** is frequently done on an outpatient basis, using a local anesthetic (Figure 6.6b).

In a small percentage of cases, serious complications occur, such as formation of a blood clot in the scrotum (which usually disappears without medical treatment), infection, or inflammatory reactions. Because sperm are stored in other areas of the reproductive system besides the vasa deferentia, couples must use alternative methods of birth control for at least 1 month after the vasectomy. The man must check with his physician (who will do a semen analysis) to determine when unprotected intercourse can take place. The pregnancy rate after 1 year in women whose partners have had vasectomies is 0.15 percent.[6]

Many men are reluctant to consider sterilization because they fear it will affect sexual performance. However, a vasectomy in no way affects sexual response. Because sperm constitute only a small percentage of semen, the amount of ejaculate does not change significantly. The testes continue to produce sperm, but the sperm can no longer enter the ejaculatory duct. After a time, sperm production may diminish. Any sperm that are manufactured disintegrate and are absorbed into the lymphatic system.

Although a vasectomy should be considered permanent, surgical reversal sometimes can restore fertility. Recent improvements in microsurgery techniques have resulted in annual pregnancy rates of 40 to 60 percent for women whose partners have had reversals. The two major factors influencing the success rate of reversal are the doctor's expertise and the time elapsed since the vasectomy.

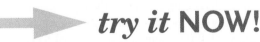

try it NOW!

Be prepared. Any method of contraception can fail. Take steps to protect yourself from unintended pregnancy and STIs at all times. Whether you are on the pill or rely on condoms or other barrier methods, always have a backup plan in mind and supplies available in case the condom tears or you forget to take a pill. An extra pack of condoms and spermicidal jelly, foam, or film are good items to have on hand.

Other Methods of Contraception

Intrauterine Devices

Women have been using **intrauterine devices (IUDs)** since 1909, and they are currently the most popular form of reversible contraception throughout the world. However, in the United States, the number of users of IUDs is relatively small. The IUD is a safe and highly effective method of birth control, but it does not protect against STIs. The exact mode of operation is not clearly understood, but researchers believe IUDs work by affecting the way the sperm and egg move, thereby preventing fertilization and/or affecting the lining of the uterus to prevent a fertilized ovum from implanting.

Two IUDs are currently available in the United States. *ParaGard* is a T-shaped plastic device with copper wrapped around the shaft. It does not contain any hormones and can be left in place for 10 years before replacement. A newer IUD, *Mirena,* is effective for 5 years and releases small amounts of the progestin levonorgestrel.

A physician must fit and insert an IUD. For insertion, the device is folded and placed into a long, thin plastic applicator. The practitioner measures the depth of the uterus with a special instrument and then uses these measurements to place the IUD accurately so the arms of the T open out across the top of the uterus. One or two strings extend from the IUD into the vagina so the user can check to make sure that her IUD is in place. The device is removed by a practitioner when desired.

Disadvantages of IUDs include possible discomfort, cost of insertion, and potential complications. The device can cause heavy menstrual flow and severe cramps. Women using IUDs have a higher risk of uterine perforation, ectopic pregnancy, pelvic inflammatory disease, infertility, and tubal infections. If a pregnancy occurs while the IUD is in place, the device should be removed as soon as possible, because the chance of miscarriage is 25 to 50 percent. Doctors often offer therapeutic abortion to women who become pregnant while using an IUD because of the

Essure A nonsurgical female sterilization procedure in which a physician places small microcoils into the fallopian tubes to block them.

hysterectomy The surgical removal of the uterus.

vasectomy Sterilization of the man that involves cutting and either sealing or tying off both vasa deferentia.

intrauterine device (IUD) A T-shaped device that is implanted in the uterus to prevent pregnancy.

serious risks (including premature delivery, infection, and congenital abnormalities) associated with continuing the pregnancy.

Withdrawal

Withdrawal, also called *coitus interruptus,* involves removing the penis from the vagina just prior to ejaculation. Because there can be up to 500,000 sperm in the drop of fluid at the tip of the penis before ejaculation, this method is unreliable. Timing withdrawal is also difficult, and men concentrating on accurate timing may not be able to relax and enjoy intercourse. In the 2006 American College Health Association–National College Health Assessment, approximately 14 percent of respondents reported that withdrawal was their method of birth control the last time they had sexual intercourse. This statistic is startlingly high, considering the very high risk of pregnancy or contracting an STI associated with this method of birth control.[7]

Emergency Contraception

Emergency contraception is the use of contraception to prevent unintended pregnancy after unprotected intercourse, a sexual assault, or the failure of another form of contraception. Combination estrogen-progestin pills and progestin-only pills are two common types of **emergency contraception pills (ECPs).** The copper-bearing intrauterine device (IUD) has also been used as emergency contraception for years.

There are 6.4 million pregnancies every year in the United States. Half of these pregnancies are unintended, and ECPs have the potential to reduce this number by at least half. Researchers estimate that widespread use of ECPs could prevent 1.7 million unintended pregnancies and 800,000 abortions each year in the United States.[8] In a nationwide survey of colleges and universities, 62 percent of all college health centers provide emergency contraception. On campuses that provide ECPs, 22 percent are open for at least part of the weekend.[9] Public colleges and universities are much more likely to provide ECPs; only slightly more than half of private college health centers offer ECPs. A recent study revealed that approximately 12 percent of sexually active college women reported that they used emergency contraception in the last school year.[10]

Pills used for emergency contraception are sometimes referred to as "morning-after pills." They are not the same as the "abortion pill," RU-486, though the two are often confused. Emergency contraception is taken after unprotected

Is emergency contraception the same as abortion?

intercourse, but before a woman misses her period. A woman taking ECP does so to prevent pregnancy; it will not work if she is already pregnant. Mifeprex or mifepristone, which is the early abortion pill, is taken after a woman is sure she is pregnant, having already taken a pregnancy test with a positive result. This and other methods of abortion are discussed in more detail later in the chapter.

ECPs prevent pregnancy in the same way as other hormonal contraceptives: they delay or inhibit ovulation, inhibit fertilization, or block implantation of a fertilized egg, depending on a women's phase in her menstrual cycle. Although ECPs use the same hormones as birth control pills, not all brands of birth control pills can be used for emergency contraception. When taken within 24 hours, ECP is up to 95 percent effective; when taken 2 to 5 days later, ECP lowers a woman's risk of becoming pregnant by 75 to 88 percent.[11]

In August 2006, the FDA approved the sale of one brand of emergency contraceptive pills, Plan B, without a prescription in the United States to women aged 18 and older. For women under 18, a prescription still is required. As of June 2007, nine states (Washington, California, New Mexico, Alaska, Hawaii, Maine, New Hampshire, Massachusetts, and Vermont) had enacted laws that permit a pharmacist to provide emergency contraception to customers of any age. However, the pharmicist in these states is required to act within a colloborative agreement with a physician or under state-approved protocols.[12]

Plan B is a progestin-only pill whose first dose should be taken as soon as possible (but not later than 120 hours, or 5 days) after unprotected intercourse. A second pill follows 12 hours after the first pill. Overall, Plan B reduces pregnancy risk by about as much as do other ECPs that require a prescription from a health care provider.

Abstinence and "Outercourse"

Strictly defined, *abstinence* means deliberately avoiding intercourse. This strict definition would allow one to engage in such forms of sexual intimacy as massage, kissing, and solitary masturbation. But many people today have broadened the definition of abstinence to include all forms of sexual contact, even those that do not culminate in sexual intercourse. Abstinence is the only method of avoiding pregnancy that is 100 percent effective.

Couples who go a step further than massage and kissing and engage in activities such as oral–genital sex and mutual masturbation are sometimes said to be engaging in "outercourse." Like abstinence, outercourse can be 100 percent effective for birth control, as long as the male does not ejaculate near the vaginal opening. Unlike abstinence, however, outercourse is not 100 percent effective against STIs. Oral–genital contact can transmit disease, although the practice can be made safer by using a condom on the penis or a dental dam on the vaginal opening.

withdrawal A method of contraception that involves withdrawing the penis from the vagina before ejaculation; also called *coitus interruptus*.

emergency contraceptive pills (ECPs) Drugs taken within 3 days after intercourse to prevent fertilization or implantation.

EMERGENCY CONTRACEPTIVE PILLS: FACTS AND CONTROVERSY

The findings from American College Health Association's National College Health Assessment (ACHA–NCHA) indicate that in 2006 approximately 71 percent of students reported having at least one sexual partner in the last school year and that approximately 2 percent of female students reported experiencing an unintentional pregnancy.

Clinicians have been prescribing emergency contraception for decades, and it first appeared as specific product in the United States in 1998, becoming available over-the-counter in 2006. In spite of its increase in availability, there is still confusion over whether it is the same as abortion. It is not. Rather, emergency contraceptive pills (ECPs) can be an effective method for preventing unintended pregnancies, including those on college campuses. According to the NCHA findings, approximately 11 percent of sexually active college students reported using (or reported that their partner had used) emergency contraception within the last school year. In fact, the Alan Guttmacher Institute estimates that ECP use prevented 51,000 abortions in 2000 alone. Though ECPs are no substitute for taking proper precautions before having sex (such as using latex condoms), their potential for reducing the rate of unintended pregnancy and, ultimately, abortion is very strong.

However, emergency contraception is available at only 67 percent of college or university student health centers nationwide. Opponents fear that easy access to emergency contraception will encourage irresponsible sexual activity among young people. Research indicates otherwise: a recent study of women aged 15 to 20 revealed that providing increased access to ECPs does not increase the likelihood of unprotected sex. Some opposition also identifies ECP use with abortion, arguing that preventing fertilization of an egg or its implantation into a woman's uterus is the equivalent to aborting a growing fetus. Proponents of ECP do not consider the prevention of implantation or fertilization equivalent to abortion. One thing is clear: the proliferation of emergency contraceptive pills has opened up a new debate across America as to when pregnancy begins.

Sources: American College Health Association, "American College Health Association–National College Health Assessment (ACHA–NCHA) Web Summary," April 2006, www.acha.org/projects_programs/ncha_sampledata.cfm; R. G. Sawyer and E. Thompson, "Knowledge and Attitudes about Emergency Contraception in University Students," College Student Journal 4 (December 2003): 523–31; Alan Guttmacher Institute, "Emergency Contraception Has Tremendous Potential In the Fight to Reduce Unintended Pregnancy," May 2005, www.agi-usa.org. L. Miller and R. Sawyer, "Emergency Contraceptive Pills: A 10 Year Follow-Up Survey of Use and Experiences at Colleges Health Centers in the Mid-Atlantic United States," American Journal of College Health, March/April 2006: 249–59.

Fertility Awareness Methods

Methods of fertility control that rely on altering sexual behavior are called **fertility awareness methods (FAMs).** These techniques require observing female fertile periods and abstaining from sexual intercourse (penis–vagina contact) during fertile times.

Two decades ago, the rhythm method was ridiculed because of its low effectiveness rates. However, it was the only method of birth control available to women belonging to religious denominations that forbid the use of oral contraceptives, barrier methods, and sterilization. Our present reproductive knowledge enables women and their partners to use natural methods of birth control with less risk of pregnancy, although these methods remain far less effective than others.

Fertility awareness methods rely on a knowledge of basic physiology **(Figure 6.7).** A released ovum can survive for up to 48 hours after ovulation. Sperm can live for as long as 5 days in the vagina. Natural methods of birth control teach women to recognize their fertile times. Changes in cervical mucus prior to and during ovulation and a rise in basal body temperature are two frequently used indicators. Another method involves charting a woman's menstrual cycle and ovulation times on a calendar. Women may use any combination of these methods to determine their fertile times more accurately.

Cervical Mucus Method The **cervical mucus method** requires women to examine the consistency and color of their normal vaginal secretions. Prior to ovulation, vaginal mucus becomes gelatinous and stretchy, and normal vaginal secretions may increase. To avoid pregnancy, partners must avoid sexual activity involving penis–vagina

fertility awareness methods (FAMs) Several types of birth control that require alteration of sexual behavior rather than chemical or physical intervention in the reproductive process.

cervical mucus method A birth control method that relies on observation of changes in cervical mucus to determine when the woman is fertile so the couple can abstain from penis–vagina contact during those times.

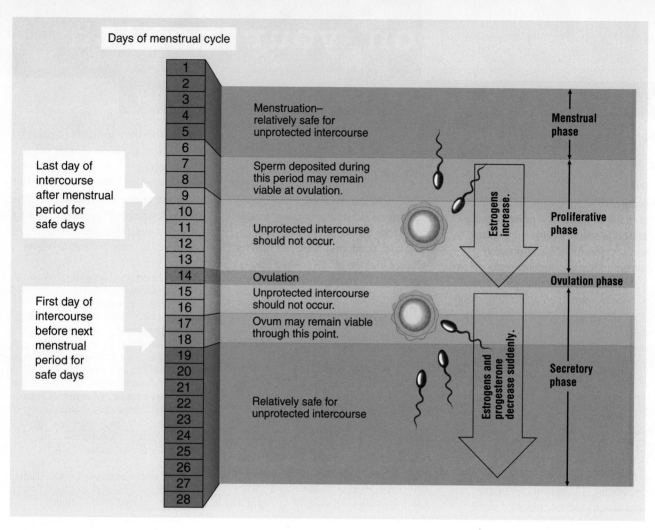

Days of menstrual cycle

Day	
1–6	Menstruation– relatively safe for unprotected intercourse
7–9	Sperm deposited during this period may remain viable at ovulation.
10–13	Unprotected intercourse should not occur.
14	Ovulation
15–16	Unprotected intercourse should not occur.
17–18	Ovum may remain viable through this point.
19–28	Relatively safe for unprotected intercourse

Last day of intercourse after menstrual period for safe days

First day of intercourse before next menstrual period for safe days

Menstrual phase

Estrogens increase.

Proliferative phase

Ovulation phase

Estrogens and progesterone decrease suddenly.

Secretory phase

FIGURE 6.7 The Fertility Cycle
Fertility awareness methods, or FAMs, can combine the use of a calendar, the cervical mucus method, and body temperature measurements to identify the fertile period. It is important to remember that most women do not have a consistent 28-day cycle.

contact while this mucus is present and for several days afterward.

Body Temperature Method
The **body temperature method** relies on the fact that the woman's basal body temperature rises between 0.4 and 0.8 degrees after ovulation has occurred. For this method to be effective, the woman must chart her temperature for several months to learn to recognize her body's temperature fluctuations. To avoid pregnancy, the partners must abstain from penis–vagina contact preceding the temperature rise until several days after the temperature rise was first noted.

Calendar Method
The **calendar method** requires the woman to record the exact number of days in her menstrual cycle. Because few women menstruate with complete regularity, this method involves keeping a record of the menstrual cycle for 12 months, during which time some other method of birth control must be used. This method assumes that ovulation occurs during the midpoint of the cycle. To avoid pregnancy, the couple must abstain from penis–vagina contact during the fertile time.

Women interested in fertility awareness methods are advised to take classes in their use. Women who are untrained in these techniques run a high risk of unintended pregnancy.

body temperature method A birth control method in which a woman monitors her body temperature for the rise that signals ovulation, so that the couple can abstain from penis–vagina contact around this time.

calendar method A birth control method in which a woman's menstrual cycle is mapped on a calendar to determine presumed fertile times, so that the couple can abstain from penis–vagina contact during those times.

Abortion

In 1973, the landmark U.S. Supreme Court decision in *Roe v. Wade* stated that the "right to privacy . . . founded on the Fourteenth Amendment's concept of personal liberty . . . is broad enough to encompass a woman's decision whether or not to terminate her pregnancy."[13] The decision maintained that during the first trimester of pregnancy, a woman and her practitioner have the right to terminate the pregnancy through **abortion** without legal restrictions. It allowed individual states to set conditions for second-trimester abortions. Third-trimester abortions were ruled illegal unless the mother's life or health was in danger.

Prior to the legalization of first- and second-trimester abortions, women wishing to terminate a pregnancy had to travel to a country where the procedure was legal, consult an illegal abortionist, or perform their own abortions. These procedures sometimes led to death from hemorrhage or infection or to infertility from internal scarring. Today, nearly half of all pregnancies that occur each year are unintended, and 50 percent of these pregnancies are terminated by abortion. The U.S. abortion rate has declined in recent years but is still higher than that of many of the other industrialized nations. There are several possible factors that influence this difference. Many other nations have fewer unintended pregnancies, strongly emphasize early sex education, and have made contraception easier and cheaper to obtain.[14]

Opponents of abortion believe that the embryo or fetus is a human being with rights that must be protected. The political debate continues as opponents of abortion pressure state and local governments to pass laws prohibiting the use of public funds for abortion and abortion counseling. In recent years, new legislation has given states the right to impose certain restrictions on abortions. Abortions cannot be performed in publicly funded clinics in some states, and other states have laws requiring parental notification before a teenager can obtain an abortion. In 2005 alone, states enacted 98 new sexual and reproductive health laws, over half of which were aimed at restricting abortion access. However, 17 states currently do appropriate public funds to women in poverty who seek an abortion.[15]

On the federal level, the U.S. Congress has banned access to abortion for virtually all women who receive health care through the federal government. This affects Medicaid recipients, women in the military, military dependents stationed overseas, women in federal prison, Native Americans, federal employees, and even Peace Corps volunteers. Since the Federal Abortion Ban was signed by President George W. Bush in 2003, it has been challenged by the American Civil Liberties Union (ACLU), the National Abortion Federation, Planned Parenthood, and the Center for Reproductive Rights in federal courts across the country on the grounds that it is unconstitutional. The two main reasons for challenging the ban are that the broad language could ban abortion as early as the 12th week in pregnancy and that it does not include exceptions to protect women's health.[16] The U.S. Supreme Court struck down an identical law as unconstitutional in 2000, and the

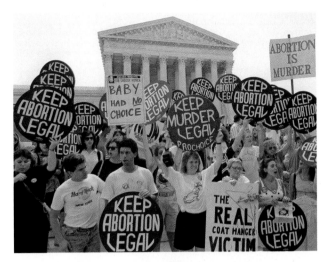

Abortion continues to be a controversial and emotional issue in the United States.

2003 law has been declared unconstitutional by all the federal courts of appeals that have heard challenges to it. However, on April 18, 2007, the U.S. Supreme Court handed down a decision to uphold the Federal Abortion Ban. *Roe v. Wade* has not been overturned, but it faces many future challenges.

Although many opponents work through the courts and the political process, attacks on abortion clinics and on doctors who perform abortions are not uncommon. Nearly all clinics have faced some form of threats or acts of violence. Legal protection, such as the Freedom of Access to Clinic Entrance Act (FACE), offers some relief from the harassment and violence directed at abortion clinics. However, because of such harassment, the biggest threat to a woman's access to an abortion now is finding a clinic rather than legal restrictions.

The best birth control methods can fail. Women can be raped. Pregnancies can occur despite every possible precaution. When an unintended pregnancy does occur, a woman must decide whether to terminate it, carry to term and keep the baby, or carry to term and give the baby away. This is a personal decision that each woman must make, based on her personal beliefs, values, and resources, after carefully considering all alternatives.

Methods of Abortion

The choice of abortion procedure is determined by how many weeks the woman has been pregnant. Length of pregnancy is calculated from the first day of her last menstrual period.

Surgical Abortions
If performed during the first trimester of pregnancy, abortion presents a relatively low risk to the woman. The most commonly used method of

---

abortion The expulsion or removal of an embryo or fetus from the uterus.

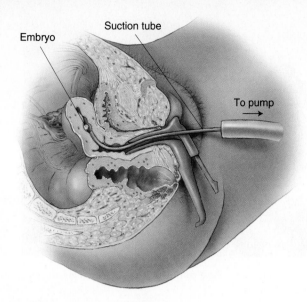

Embryo Suction tube

To pump →

FIGURE 6.8 Vacuum Aspiration Abortion

first-trimester abortion is **vacuum aspiration (Figure 6.8).** The procedure is usually performed under a local anesthetic. The cervix is dilated with instruments or by placing laminaria, a sterile seaweed product, in the cervical canal. The laminaria is left in place for a few hours or overnight and slowly dilates the cervix. After it is removed, a long tube is inserted into the uterus through the cervix, and gentle suction removes fetal tissue from the uterine walls.

Pregnancies that progress into the second trimester can be terminated through **dilation and evacuation (D&E).** For this procedure, the cervix is dilated for 1 to 2 days, and a combination of instruments and vacuum aspiration is used to empty the uterus. Second-trimester abortions may be done under general anesthetic. The D&E can be performed on an outpatient basis (usually in the physician's office), with or

---

vacuum aspiration An abortion technique that uses gentle suction to remove fetal tissue from the uterus.

dilation and evacuation (D&E) An abortion technique that uses a combination of instruments and vacuum aspiration; fetal tissue is both sucked and scraped out of the uterus.

induction abortion Abortion technique in which chemicals are injected into the uterus through the uterine wall; labor begins, and the woman delivers a dead fetus.

hysterotomy The surgical removal of the fetus from the uterus.

intact dilation and extraction (D&X) A late-term abortion procedure in which the body of the fetus is extracted up to the head and then the contents of the cranium are aspirated.

mifepristone A steroid hormone that induces abortion by blocking the action of progesterone.

---

without pain medication. Generally, however, the woman is given a mild tranquilizer to help her relax. This procedure may cause moderate to severe uterine cramping and blood loss. After a D&E a return visit to the clinician is an important follow-up procedure.

Two other methods used in second-trimester abortions, though less common than the D&E, are prostaglandin or saline **induction abortions.** Prostaglandin hormones or saline solution are injected into the uterus, which kills the fetus and initiates labor contractions. After 24 to 48 hours, the fetus and placenta are expelled from the uterus.

The **hysterotomy,** or surgical removal of the fetus from the uterus, may be used during emergencies, when the mother's life is in danger, or when other types of abortions are deemed too dangerous.

The risks associated with surgical abortion include infection, incomplete abortion (when parts of the placenta remain in the uterus), excessive bleeding, and cervical and uterine trauma. Follow-up and attention to danger signs decrease the chances of long-term problems.

The mortality rate for women undergoing first-trimester abortions averages 1 death per every 500,000 procedures at 8 or fewer weeks. The risk of death increases with the length of pregnancy. At 16 to 20 weeks, the mortality is 1 per 27,000, and at 21 weeks or more it increases to 1 per 8,000.[17] This higher rate later in the pregnancy is due to the increased risks of uterine perforation, bleeding, infection, and incomplete abortion, which in turn are due to the fact that the uterine wall becomes thinner as the pregnancy progresses.

One surgical method of performing abortion that has been the target of abortion opponents is **intact dilation and extraction (D&X),** sometimes referred to by the nonmedical term *partial-birth abortion.* This procedure is rarely performed, but it is considered when other abortion methods could injure the mother and when there are severe fetal abnormalities. The dilation and extraction procedure is used after 21 weeks' gestation. Two days before the procedure, laminaria is inserted vaginally to dilate the cervix. The water should break on the third day, at which time the woman should return to the clinic. The fetus is rotated to a breech (feet first) position, and forceps are used to pull the legs, shoulders, and arms through the birth canal. The head is collapsed to allow it to pass through the cervix. Then the fetus is completely removed.

Medical Abortions Unlike surgical abortions, medical abortions are performed without entering the uterus. **Mifepristone,** formerly known as RU-486 and currently sold in the U.S. under the brand name Mifeprex, is a steroid hormone that induces abortion by blocking the action of progesterone, a hormone produced by the ovaries and placenta that maintains the lining of the uterus. As a result, the uterine lining and the embryo are expelled from the uterus, terminating the pregnancy.

Mifepristone's nickname, the "abortion pill," may imply an easy process. However, this treatment actually involves more steps than a surgical abortion, which takes approximately 15 minutes followed by a physical recovery of about

CONTRACEPTIVE USE HELPS REDUCE THE INCIDENCE OF ABORTION WORLDWIDE

Nearly 80 million pregnancies occur worldwide every year. More than half of these pregnancies end in abortion, often in countries where abortion is illegal and access to contraception is limited. Access to voluntary family planning services, including contraception, is essential in helping to reduce the number of unintended pregnancies and, consequently, the incidence of abortion.

- The primary cause of abortion is unplanned pregnancy. When modern contraceptives are unavailable, women often turn to abortion to end unwanted pregnancy.
- Whether abortion is legal or not has little to do with its overall incidence.

In many countries where abortion is illegal or severely restricted (e.g., many Latin American and African countries), abortion rates are higher than in countries where it is legal (e.g., countries in Western Europe).

- Increased use of contraception has been accompanied by significant declines in abortion rates in a number of countries, including Bangladesh, Bulgaria, Chile, Estonia, Hungary, Latvia, Romania, Russia, and Turkey.
- Contraceptive use increased in Russia by 74 percent, while abortion rates decreased by 61 percent, between 1988 and 2001.
- Abortion rates declined in the 1990s in tandem with a rise in the use of modern

contraception in the republics of Kazakhstan, Uzbekistan, and Kyrgyzstan. In Kazakhstan, contraception prevalence increased by 50 percent in the 1990s, and abortion rates decreased by nearly the same amount.

Sources: Adapted from the Population Action International Fact Sheet, August 2005, www.populationaction.org/Publications/Fact_Sheets/Index. Alan Guttmacher Institute, "Issues in Brief: The Role of Contraception in Reducing Abortion," 2005, www.agi-usa.org/pubs/ib19.html; C. Marston and J. Cleland, *The Effects of Contraception on Obstetric Outcomes* (Geneva, Switzerland: World Health Organization, 2004); M. Reynolds, "Abortion Rate Drops to Lowest Level Ever," *The Prague Post*, July 27, 2005, www.praguepost.com/P03/2005/Art/0728/news4.php.

---

1 day. With mifepristone, a first visit to the clinic involves a physical exam and a dose of three tablets, which may cause minor side effects such as nausea, headaches, weakness, and fatigue. The patient returns 2 days later for a dose of prostaglandins (misoprostol; brand name: Cytotec), which cause uterine contractions that expel the fertilized egg. The patient is required to stay under observation at the clinic for 4 hours and to make a follow-up visit 12 days later.[18]

Ninety-six percent of women who take mifepristone and prostaglandins during the first 9 weeks of pregnancy will experience a complete abortion. The side effects of this treatment are similar to those reported during heavy menstruation and include cramping, minor pain, and nausea. Approximately 1 in 1,000 women requires a blood transfusion because of severe bleeding. The procedure does not require hospitalization; women may be treated on an outpatient basis.

Another drug that has been used to induce early-term medical abortions is methotrexate, although it is not approved by the FDA for this purpose. Typically a woman receives an injection from her clinician and, during an office visit 3 to 7 days later, receives a prostaglandin dose. The pregnancy usually ends within 4 hours.

Emotional Aspects of Abortion

The emotional aftereffects of abortion have been the subject of much interest. Do women who have had abortions suffer symptoms similar to those of post-traumatic stress disorder? Are they forever haunted by the experience?

Although a variety of feelings, such as regret, guilt, sadness, relief, and happiness, are normal, no evidence has shown that an abortion causes long-term psychological trauma for a woman. In a longitudinal study of over 5,000 women who had had abortions, researchers found that the best predictor of a woman's emotional well-being following an abortion was her emotional well-being prior to the procedure. Even factors such as marital status or affiliation with a religion that strongly opposes abortion were found to have no effect on a woman's later sense of self-esteem and well-being.[19]

A small percentage of women who undergo abortions experience depressive symptoms similar to postpartum blues, but the vast majority express no regrets about their decision and state they would make the choice again if they found themselves in similar circumstances. Certainly the presence of a support network and the assistance of mental health professionals is helpful to any woman who is struggling with the emotional aspects of the abortion decision in her own life.

what do you THINK?

If you or your partner unexpectedly became pregnant, would you choose to terminate the pregnancy? ■ How might an abortion affect your relationship? ■ What factors would you consider in making your decision? Why?

Planning a Pregnancy

The many methods available to control fertility give you choices that did not exist when your parents—and even you—were born. If you are in the process of deciding whether to have children, take the time to evaluate your emotions, finances, and physical health.

Emotional Health

First and foremost, consider why you want to have a child: To fulfill an inner need to carry on the family? To escape loneliness? Other reasons? Are you ready to make all the sacrifices necessary to bear and raise a child? Can you care for this new human being in a loving and nurturing manner?

If you feel that you are ready to be a parent, the next step is preparation. You can prepare for this change in your life in several ways: read about parenthood, take classes, talk to parents of children of all ages, and join a support group. If you choose to adopt, you will find many support groups available as well.

Maternal Health

Before becoming pregnant, a woman should have a thorough medical examination. **Preconception care** should include assessment of potential complications that could occur during pregnancy. Medical problems such as diabetes and high blood pressure should be discussed, as well as any genetic disorders that run in the family. Additional suggestions for a healthy pregnancy include the following:

- If you smoke or drink alcohol, stop; reduce or eliminate caffeine intake.
- Avoid X rays and environmental chemicals, such as lawn and garden chemicals.
- Maintain a normal weight; lose weight if necessary.
- Take prenatal vitamins, which are especially important in providing adequate folic acid.

Paternal Health

It is common wisdom that mothers-to-be should steer clear of toxic chemicals that can cause birth defects, should eat a healthy diet, and should stop smoking and drinking alcohol. Now, similar precautions are recommended for fathers-to-be. New research suggests that a man's exposure to chemicals influences not only his ability to father a child, but also the future health of his child.

Fathers-to-be have been overlooked in past preconception and prenatal studies for several reasons. Researchers assumed that the genetic damage leading to birth defects and other health problems occurred while a child was in the mother's womb or were caused by random errors of nature. However, it now appears that some disorders can be traced to sperm damaged by chemicals. Sperm are naturally vulnerable to toxic assault and genetic damage. Many drugs and ingested chemicals can readily invade the testes from the bloodstream; others ambush sperm after they leave the testes and pass through the epididymides, where they mature and are stored. By one route or another, half of 100 chemicals studied so far (including by-products of cigarette smoke) apparently harm sperm.

Financial Evaluation

Finances are another important consideration. Are you prepared to go out to dinner less often, forego a new pair of shoes, or drive an older car? These are important questions to ask yourself when considering the financial aspects of being a parent. Can you afford to give your child the life you would like him or her to enjoy?

First, check your medical insurance: Does it provide pregnancy benefits? If not, you can expect to pay on average $7,000 for a normal delivery, and up to $11,450 for a C-section. These costs don't include prenatal medical care, and complications can also increase the average cost substantially. Both partners should investigate their employers' policies concerning parental leave, including length of leave available and conditions for returning to work.

The U.S. Department of Agriculture estimates that it can cost as much as $260,000 for a middle-class married couple to raise a child to the age of 17. (Housing costs and food are the two largest expenditures.)[20] That figure does not include college, which can now run over $40,000 per year with room and board at a private institution. Also consider the cost and availability of quality child care. How much family assistance can you realistically expect with a new baby, and is non-family child care available? How much does full-time child care cost? Costs vary by region and type of care. According to statistics gathered in the last U.S. census, families with young children spent 10 percent of their total income on child care in 2002.[21]

Although you may be aware of the federal tax credit available for child care, you may not realize how little assistance it actually provides. For example, a family with an income of over $28,000 can expect to receive a maximum yearly credit of $480 for one child. A second child doubles the credit, but no further assistance is provided for a third child or more children.

Contingency Planning

A final consideration is how to provide for the child should something happen to you and your partner. If both of you were to die while the child is young, do you have relatives or close friends who would raise the child? If you have more than one child, would they have to be split up, or could they

---

preconception care Medical care received prior to becoming pregnant that helps a woman assess and address potential maternal health issues.

be kept together? Though unpleasant to think about, this sort of contingency planning is crucial. Children who lose their parents are heartbroken and confused. A prearranged plan of action will smooth their transition into new families.

 what do you THINK?

Which factors will you consider in deciding whether or when to have children? ▪ Is there a certain age at which you feel you will be ready to be a parent? ▪ What goals do you hope to achieve first? ▪ What are your biggest concerns about parenthood?

Pregnancy

Pregnancy is an important event in a woman's life. The actions taken before a pregnancy begins, as well as behaviors during pregnancy, can have a significant effect on the health of both infant and mother.

Prenatal Care

A successful pregnancy depends on a mother who takes good care of herself and the fetus. Good nutrition; exercise; avoiding drugs, alcohol, and other harmful substances; and regular medical checkups beginning early in the pregnancy are essential. Early detection of fetal abnormalities, identification of high-risk mothers and infants, and a complication-free pregnancy are the major purposes of prenatal care.

Women should also consider their confidence in their own ability to give birth and the availability of a support system (spouse or partner, family, friends, community groups) willing to give her and her child love and emotional support during and after her pregnancy.

Choosing a Practitioner and Receiving Medical Care
A woman should carefully choose a practitioner to oversee her pregnancy and delivery. If possible, she should make this choice before she becomes pregnant. Recommendations from friends and from one's family physician are a good starting point. Also consider a practitioner's philosophy about pain management during labor, experience handling complications, and willingness to accommodate your personal beliefs on these issues.

Two types of physicians can attend pregnancies and deliveries. The *obstetrician-gynecologist (OB-Gyn)* is a medical doctor (MD) who specializes in obstetrics (pregnancy and birth) and gynecology (care of women's reproductive organs). These practitioners are trained to handle all types of pregnancy-related and delivery-related emergencies. A *family practitioner* is a licensed MD who provides comprehensive care for people of all ages. Most family practitioners have obstetrical experience but will refer a patient to a specialist

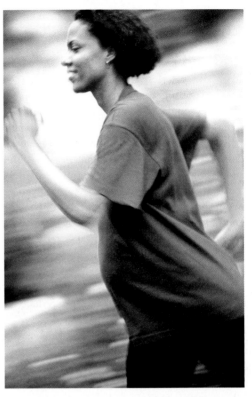

A doctor-approved exercise program during pregnancy can help control weight, make delivery easier, and have a healthy effect on the fetus.

if necessary. Unlike the OB-Gyn, the family practitioner can serve as the baby's physician after attending the birth.

Midwives are also experienced practitioners who can assist with both pregnancies and deliveries. *Certified nurse-midwives* are registered nurses with specialized training in pregnancy and delivery. Most midwives work in private practice or in conjunction with physicians. Those who work with physicians have access to traditional medical facilities to which they can turn in an emergency. *Lay midwives* may or may not have extensive training in handling an emergency. They may be self-taught or trained through formal certification procedures. Women should carefully evaluate the credentials of a prospective midwife and make sure access to medical care is available in case it is needed.

Regular check-ups to measure weight gain and blood pressure and to monitor the size and position of the fetus should continue throughout the pregnancy. Ideally, a woman should begin medical checkups as soon as possible after becoming pregnant (within the first 3 months). This early care reduces infant mortality and low birth weight. The American College of Obstetricians and Gynecologists recommends seven or eight prenatal visits for women with low-risk pregnancies. Unfortunately, prenatal care is not available to everyone.

midwives Experienced practitioners who assist with pregnancy and delivery.

Native American and African American women have the lowest rates of prenatal care in the United States.[22]

Nutrition and Exercise Pregnant women need additional protein, calories, vitamins, and minerals, so their diets should be carefully monitored by a qualified practitioner. Special attention should be paid to getting enough folic acid (found in dark leafy greens), iron (found in dried fruits, meats, legumes, liver, and egg yolks), calcium (found in nonfat or low-fat dairy products and some canned fish), and fluids.

Vitamin supplements can correct some deficiencies, but there is no substitute for a well-balanced diet. Babies born to poorly nourished mothers run high risks of substandard mental and physical development. Folic acid, when consumed before and during early pregnancy, reduces the risk of spina bifida, a disabling birth condition that results from failure of the spinal column to close. Manufacturers of breads, pastas, rice, and other grain products now are required to add folic acid to their products to reduce neural tube defects in newborns.

Weight gain during pregnancy helps nourish a growing baby. For a woman of normal weight before pregnancy, the recommended weight gain during pregnancy is 25 to 35 pounds. For obese or overweight women, weight gain of 15 to 25 pounds is recommended. Underweight women can gain 28 to 40 pounds, and women carrying twins should gain about 35 to 45 pounds. Gaining too much or too little weight can lead to complications. With higher weight gains, women may develop gestational diabetes, hypertension, or increased risk for delivery complications. Gaining too little weight increases the chance of a low–birth weight baby.

Of the total number of pounds gained during pregnancy, about 6 to 8 are the baby. The baby's birth weight is important because low weight can mean health problems during labor and the baby's first few months. Pregnancy is not the time to think about losing weight—doing so may endanger the fetus.

As in all other stages of life, exercise is an important factor in weight control during pregnancy and in overall maternal health. Pregnant women should consult their physicians before starting any exercise program.

Drugs and Alcohol A woman should avoid all types of drugs during pregnancy. Even common over-the-counter medications, such as aspirin, and some beverages, such as coffee and tea, can damage a developing fetus.

During the first 3 months of pregnancy, the fetus is especially subject to the **teratogenic** (birth defect–causing) effects of drugs, environmental chemicals, X rays, or diseases. The fetus also can develop an addiction to or tolerance for drugs that the mother is using. Of particular concern to medical professionals is the use of tobacco and alcohol during pregnancy.

Consumption of alcohol is detrimental to a growing fetus. Symptoms of **fetal alcohol syndrome (FAS)** include mental retardation, slowed nerve reflexes, and small head size. The exact amount of alcohol necessary to cause FAS is not known, but researchers doubt that it is safe to consume any alcohol. Therefore, they recommend total abstinence from alcohol during pregnancy.

Smoking Tobacco use, in particular smoking, harms every phase of reproduction. Women who smoke have more difficulty becoming pregnant and a higher risk of being infertile. Women who smoke during pregnancy have a greater chance of complications, premature births, low–birth weight infants, stillbirth, and infant mortality.[23] In fetuses, tobacco use by the mother appears to be a significant factor in the development of cleft lip and palate.

Studies are now revealing that secondhand smoke is also detrimental. The exposed fetus is likely to experience low birth weight, increased susceptibility to childhood diseases, and sudden infant death syndrome.[24] Smoking clearly has an influence throughout the pregnancy cycle.

Other Factors A pregnant woman should avoid exposure to X rays, toxic chemicals, heavy metals, pesticides, gases, and other hazardous compounds. She should not clean cat-litter boxes, because cat feces can contain organisms that cause a disease called **toxoplasmosis.** If a pregnant woman contracts this disease, her baby may be stillborn or suffer mental retardation or other birth defects.

If she has never had rubella (German measles), a woman should be immunized for it prior to becoming pregnant. A rubella infection can kill the fetus or cause blindness or hearing disorders in the infant. Sexually transmitted infections such as genital herpes or HIV are also risk factors. A woman should inform her physician of any infectious condition so proper precautions and treatment options can be taken.

A Woman's Reproductive Years

About half of the average American woman's life span is spent between menarche (first menses) and menopause (last menses), a period of approximately 40 years. Deciding whether and when to have children, as well as how to prevent pregnancy when necessary, is a long-term concern.

Today, a woman over 35 who is pregnant has plenty of company. There are some advantages to having a baby later in life. In fact, many doctors note that older mothers tend to be more conscientious about following medical advice during pregnancy and are more psychologically mature and ready to include an infant in their family than are some younger women.

teratogenic Causing birth defects; may refer to drugs, environmental chemicals, X rays, or diseases.

fetal alcohol syndrome (FAS) A collection of symptoms, including mental retardation, that can appear in infants of women who drink alcohol during pregnancy.

toxoplasmosis A disease caused by an organism found in cat feces that, when contracted by a pregnant woman, may result in stillbirth or an infant with mental retardation or birth defects.

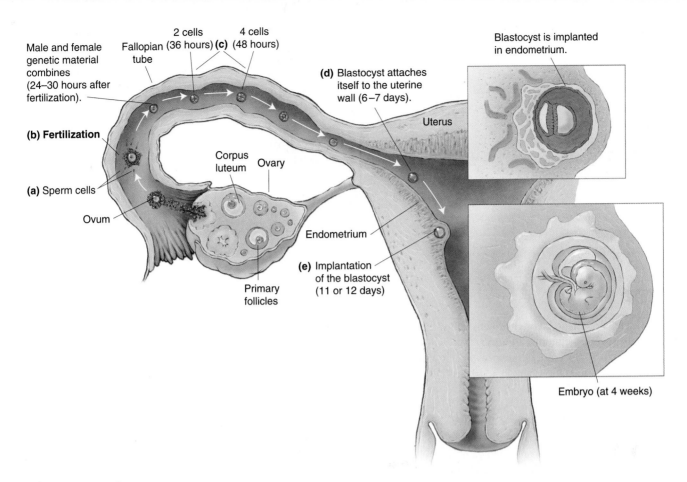

FIGURE 6.9 Fertilization

(a) The efforts of hundreds of sperm may allow one sperm to penetrate the ovum's *corona radiata,* an outer layer of cells, and then the *zona pellucida,* a thick inner membrane. (b) The sperm nucleus fuses with the egg nucleus at fertilization, producing a *zygote.* (c) The zygote divides first into two cells, then four cells, and so on. (d) The *blastocyst* attaches itself to the uterine wall. (e) The blastocyst implants itself in the endometrium.

Statistically, the chances of having a baby with birth defects do increase after age 35. For example, the incidence of **Down syndrome,** a genetic disorder characterized by mild to severe mental retardation and a variety of physical abnormalities, increases with maternal age.[25] Women who delay motherhood also worry about their physical ability to carry and deliver their babies. A comprehensive exercise program will assist in a healthy pregnancy and delivery.

Pregnancy Testing

A woman may suspect she is pregnant before she takes any pregnancy tests. A pregnancy test scheduled in a medical office or birth control clinic will confirm the pregnancy. Women who wish to know immediately can purchase home pregnancy test kits sold over the counter in drugstores. A positive test is based on the secretion of **human chorionic gonadotropin (HCG),** which is found in the woman's urine (HCG is also detectable in blood).

Home pregnancy test kits are about 85 to 95 percent reliable. Instructions must be followed carefully. If the test is done too early in the pregnancy, it may show a false nega-

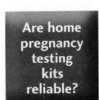

Are home pregnancy testing kits reliable?

tive. Other causes of false negatives are unclean test tubes, ingestion of certain drugs, and vaginal or urinary tract infections. Accuracy also depends on the quality of the test itself and the user's ability to perform it and interpret the results. Blood tests administered and analyzed by a medical laboratory are more accurate.

The Process of Pregnancy

The process of pregnancy begins the moment a sperm fertilizes an ovum in the fallopian tubes **(Figure 6.9).** From there, the single fertilized cell, now called a *zygote,* multiplies and

Down syndrome A genetic disorder characterized by mental retardation and a variety of physical abnormalities.

human chorionic gonadotropin (HCG) Hormone detectable in blood or urine samples of a mother within the first few weeks of pregnancy.

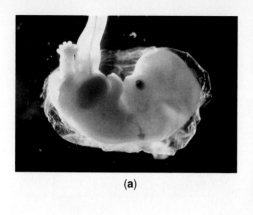

(a)

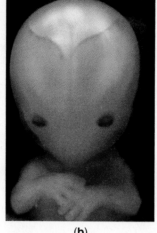

(b)

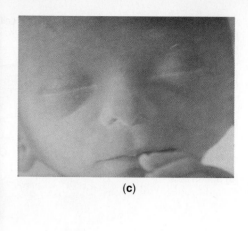

(c)

This series of fetoscopic photographs shows the development of the fetus in the (a) first, (b) second, and (c) third trimesters of pregnancy.

becomes a sphere-shaped cluster of cells called a *blastocyst,* as it travels toward the uterus, a journey that may take 3 to 4 days. On arrival, the embryo burrows into the thick, spongy endometrium (implantation) and is nourished from this carefully prepared lining.

Early Signs of Pregnancy

The first sign of pregnancy is usually a missed menstrual period (although some women "spot" in early pregnancy, which may be mistaken for a period). Other signs include breast tenderness, emotional upset, extreme fatigue, nausea, sleeplessness, and vomiting (especially in the morning).

Pregnancy typically lasts 40 weeks. The due date is calculated from the expectant mother's last menstrual period. Pregnancy is typically divided into three phases, or **trimesters,** of approximately 3 months each.

The First Trimester

During the first trimester, few noticeable changes occur in the mother's body. She may urinate more frequently and experience morning sickness, swollen breasts, or undue fatigue. These symptoms may not be frequent or severe, so she may not even realize she is pregnant unless she has a pregnancy test.

During the first 2 months after conception, the **embryo** differentiates and develops its various organ systems, beginning with the nervous and circulatory systems. At the start of the third month, the embryo is called a **fetus,** which indicates that all organ systems are in place. For the rest of the pregnancy, growth and refinement occur in each major body system so that they can function independently, yet in coordination, at birth. The photos above illustrate physical changes during fetal development.

The Second Trimester

At the beginning of the second trimester, physical changes in the mother become more visible. During this time, the fetus makes greater demands on the mother's body. In particular, the **placenta,** the network of blood vessels connected to the umbilical cord that carry nutrients and oxygen to the fetus and fetal waste products to the mother, becomes well established.

The Third Trimester

From the end of the sixth month through the ninth is considered the third trimester. This is the period of greatest fetal growth, when the fetus gains most of its weight. During the third trimester, the fetus must get large amounts of calcium, iron, and nitrogen from the food the mother eats.

Although the fetus may live if it is born during the seventh month, it needs the layer of fat it acquires during the eighth month and time for the organs (especially the respiratory and digestive organs) to develop to their full potential. Babies born prematurely usually require intensive medical care.

Emotional Changes

Of course, the process of pregnancy involves much more than the changes in a woman's body and the developing fetus. Many important emotional changes occur from the time a woman learns she is pregnant through the "**fourth trimester**" (the first 6 weeks of an infant's life outside the uterus). Throughout pregnancy,

trimester   A 3-month segment of pregnancy; used to describe specific developmental changes that occur in the embryo or fetus.

embryo   The fertilized egg from conception until the end of 2 months' development.

fetus   The term for a developing baby from the third month of pregnancy until birth.

placenta   The network of blood vessels connected to the umbilical cord that carries nutrients, oxygen, and wastes between the developing infant and the mother.

"fourth trimester"   The first 6 weeks of an infant's life outside the uterus.

women may experience fear of pregnancy complications, anxiety over becoming a parent, and wonder and excitement over the developing baby.

Prenatal Testing and Screening

Modern technology enables medical practitioners to detect health defects in a fetus as early as the 14th to 18th weeks of pregnancy. One common test is *ultrasound*, which uses high-frequency sound waves to create a *sonogram*, or visual image of the fetus in the uterus. The sonogram is used to determine the size and position of the fetus. Knowing the position of the fetus helps health care providers perform other tests and deliver the infant. Sonograms can also detect birth defects in the central nervous system and digestive system. New three-dimensional ultrasound techniques clarify images and improve doctors' efforts to detect and treat defects prenatally. Ultrasound does not provide any genetic information about the fetus.

The **triple marker screen (TMS)** is a maternal blood test that is used to identify certain birth defects and genetic abnormalities in growing fetuses (e.g., neural tube defects, Down syndrome). Optimally the test is conducted during the 16th and 18th week of pregnancy. A blood sample is taken and sent to a lab for analysis. The lab analyzes the levels of alpha-fetoprotein (AFP), human chorionic gona-dotropin (HCG), and unconjugated estriol (uE3) in the blood and determines whether they fall in a "normal" range for this stage of the pregnancy, based on the mother's age, weight, race, and other factors (such as having diabetes). TMS is a screening test, not a diagnostic test; it can detect susceptibility for a birth defect or genetic abnormality, but is not meant to confirm a diagnosis of any condition. In the case of abnormal TMS results, parents may choose to have further testing such as ultrasound or aminocentesis.

Amniocentesis is a common testing procedure that is strongly recommended for women over 35. This procedure involves inserting a long needle through the mother's abdominal and uterine walls into the **amniotic sac,** the protective pouch surrounding the fetus. The needle draws out 3 to 4 teaspoons of fluid, which is analyzed for genetic information about the baby. This test can reveal the presence of 40 genetic abnormalities, including Down syndrome, Tay-Sachs disease (a fatal disorder of the central nervous system common among Jewish people of Eastern European descent), and sickle cell disease (a debilitating blood disorder found primarily among African Americans). Amniocentesis can also reveal sex, a fact some parents may choose not to know until after birth. Although widely used, amniocentesis is not without risk. The chance of miscarriage as a result of testing is 1 in 200 or less.

Another procedure, *chorionic villus sampling (CVS),* involves snipping tissue from the developing fetal sac. CVS can be used at 10 to 12 weeks of pregnancy, and the test results are available in 12 to 48 hours. CVS is an attractive option for couples who are at high risk for having a baby with Down syndrome or a debilitating hereditary disease.

Fetoscopy involves making a small incision in the abdominal and uterine walls and inserting an optical viewer into the uterus to view the fetus directly. This device is used with ultrasound to determine fetal age and location of the placenta. This method is still experimental and involves some risk. It causes miscarriage in approximately 5 percent of cases.

If any of these tests reveals a serious birth defect, parents are advised to undergo genetic counseling. In the case of a chromosomal abnormality such as Down syndrome, the parents are usually offered the option of a therapeutic abortion. Some parents choose this option; others research the disability and decide to go ahead with the birth.

? *what do you* THINK?

As you look at your current lifestyle, what behaviors (e.g., nutritional choices, fitness) would you cease or begin to promote a healthy pregnancy? ▪ What would you look for in selecting a health care provider during your own or your partner's pregnancy? ▪ Would you want to know whether you or your partner were carrying a child with a genetic defect or other abnormality? Why or why not?

Childbirth

Prospective parents need to make a number of key decisions long before the baby is born. These include where to have the baby, whether to use drugs during labor and delivery, which childbirth method to choose, and whether to breast-feed or bottle-feed. Answering these questions will ensure a smoother passage into parenthood.

Choosing Where to Have Your Baby

Prospective mothers have many delivery options, ranging from traditional hospital birth to home birth. Parental values are important. Many couples, for instance, feel that the modern medical establishment has dehumanized the birth process. Thus, they choose to deliver at home or at a *birthing center,* a homelike setting outside a hospital where

triple marker screen (TMS)   A maternal blood test that can be used to help identify fetuses with certain birth defects and genetic abnormalities.

amniocentesis   A medical test in which a small amount of fluid is drawn from the amniotic sac to test for Down syndrome and other genetic abnormalities.

amniotic sac   The protective pouch surrounding the baby.

women can give birth and receive postdelivery care by a team of professional practitioners that includes physicians and registered nurses.

However, hospitals have responded to the desire for a more relaxed, less medically oriented birthing process. Many hospitals now offer labor–delivery–postpartum birthing rooms, which allow patients with noncomplicated deliveries to spend the entire process in one room. "Rooming-in," or keeping the baby in the same room with the mother at all times, is encouraged to facilitate bonding and breast-feeding. Partners are generally encouraged to room-in with mother and baby as well.

Labor and Delivery

During the few weeks preceding delivery, the baby normally shifts to a head-down position, and the cervix begins to dilate (widen). The junction of the pubic bones loosens to permit expansion of the pelvic girdle during birth. The exact mechanisms that initiate labor are unknown. Contractions in the abdomen and lower back usually signal the beginning of labor. Another common early signal of labor is the breaking of the amniotic sac, which causes a rush of fluid from the vagina (commonly referred to as "water breaking").

The birth process has three stages, described in **Figure 6.10**, which can last from several hours to more than a day. In some cases, the attending practitioner may perform an **episiotomy**, a straight incision in the mother's perineum (the area between the vulva and the anus), toward the end of the second stage to prevent the baby's head from tearing vaginal tissues and to speed the baby's exit from the vagina. Upon exit, the baby takes its first breath, which is generally accompanied by a loud wail.

After delivery, the attending practitioner assesses the baby's overall condition, cleans the baby's mucus-filled breathing passages, and ties and severs the umbilical cord. Most mothers prefer to have their new infants next to them following the birth. Together with their spouse or partner, they feel a need to share this time of bonding with their infant.

Managing Labor: Medical and Nonmedical Approaches

Painkilling drugs given to the mother during labor can cause sluggish responses in the newborn and other complications. For this reason, many women choose drug-free labor and delivery—but it is important to keep a flexible attitude about pain relief, because each labor is different. Working in partnership with a health care provider to make the best decision for mother and baby is optimal. Use of painkilling medication during a delivery is not a sign of weakness. One person is not a "success" for delivering without medication and another a "failure" for using medical measures. Remember, pain is to be expected. In fact, many experts say that the pain of labor is the most difficult in the human experience. There is no one right answer for managing that pain.

The Lamaze method is the most popular birth alternative in the United States. It discourages the use of drugs; prelabor classes teach the mother to control her pain through special breathing patterns, focusing exercises, and relaxation. Lamaze births usually take place in a hospital or birthing center with a physician or midwife in attendance. The partner (or labor coach) assists by giving emotional support, physical comfort, and coaching for proper breath control during contractions.

Other methods prospective parents can research include the Harris method, Childbirth without Fear, the Leboyer method, the Bradley method, and water birth. These vary in their philosophies regarding painkillers, partner participation, and other issues.

The Postpartum Period

The postpartum period typically lasts 4 to 6 weeks after delivery. During this period, many women experience fluctuating emotions. For many new mothers, the physical stress of labor, dehydration and blood loss, and other stresses challenge their stamina. About 50 to 80 percent of new mothers experience what is called the "baby blues," characterized by periods of sadness, anxiety, headache, sleep disturbances, and irritability. For most women, these symptoms disappear after a short while. About 10 percent of new mothers experience **postpartum depression,** a more disabling syndrome characterized by mood swings, lack of energy, crying, guilt, and depression. It can happen anytime within the first year after childbirth. Mothers experiencing postpartum depression should be encouraged to seek professional treatment. Counseling and in some cases medication are two of the most common types of treatment.[26]

Breast-Feeding

Although the new mother's milk will not begin to flow for 2 or more days, her breasts secrete a thick yellow substance called *colostrum*. Because this fluid contains vital antibodies to help fight infection, the newborn baby should be allowed to suckle.

The American Academy of Pediatrics strongly recommends that infants be breast-fed for at least 6 months and ideally for 12 months. Scientific findings indicate there are many advantages to breastfeeding. Breast-fed babies have

episiotomy   A straight incision in the mother's perineum in the area between the vulva and the anus, sometimes performed toward the end of the second stage of labor to prevent the tearing of vaginal tissues and to speed delivery.

postpartum depression   Energy depletion, anxiety, mood swings, and depression that women may feel during the postpartum period.

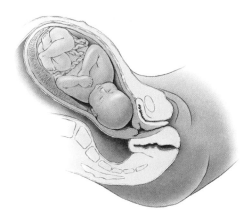

Stage I: Dilation of the cervix

Contractions in the abdomen and lower back push the baby downward, putting pressure on the cervix and dilating it. The first stage of labor may last from a couple of hours to more than a day for a first birth, but it is usually much shorter during subsequent births.

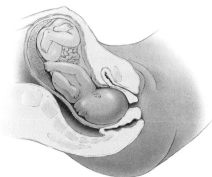

End of Stage I: Transition

The cervix becomes fully dilated, and the baby's head begins to move into the vagina (birth canal). Contractions usually come quickly during transition, which generally lasts 30 minutes or less.

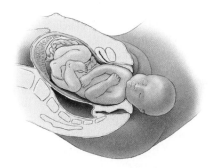

Stage II: Expulsion

Once the cervix has become fully dilated, contractions become rhythmic, strong, and more painful as the uterus pushes the baby headfirst through the birth canal. The expulsion stage lasts 1 to 4 hours and concludes when the infant is finally pushed out of the mother's body.

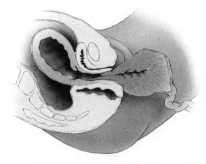

Stage III: Delivery of the placenta

In the third stage, the placenta detaches from the uterus and is expelled through the birth canal. This stage is usually completed within 30 minutes after delivery.

FIGURE 6.10 The Birth Process

fewer illnesses and a much lower hospitalization rate, because breast milk contains maternal antibodies and immunological cells that stimulate the infant's immune system. When breast-fed babies do get sick, they recover more quickly. They are also less likely to be obese than babies fed on formulas, and they have fewer allergies. They may even be more intelligent: a recent study found that the longer a baby was breast-fed, the higher the IQ in adulthood. Researchers theorize that breast milk contains substances that enhance brain development.[27] Another study found that women who were able to breast-feed successfully for longer periods of time generally viewed breast-feeding as more positive, had more knowledge about the process, and had higher self-efficacy in their ability to breast-feed.[28]

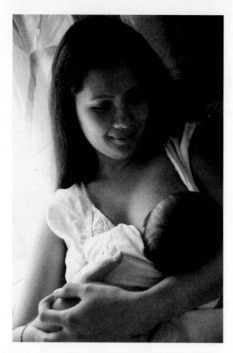
Breast-feeding enhances the development of intimate bonds between mother and child.

Some women are unable or unwilling to breast-feed. Prepared formulas can provide nourishment that allows a baby to grow and thrive. When deciding whether to breast- or bottle-feed, mothers need to consider their own desires and preferences, too. Both feeding methods can supply the physical and emotional closeness essential to the parent-child relationship.

Complications

Problems can occur during labor and delivery, even following a successful pregnancy. The possibilities should be discussed prior to labor.

Preeclampsia and Eclampsia
Preeclampsia is a condition that is characterized by high blood pressure, protein in the urine, and edema (fluid retention), which usually causes swelling of the hands and face. This condition complicates approximately 10 percent of pregnancies and is responsible for 18 percent of U.S. maternal deaths each year. Symptoms may include sudden weight gain, headache, nausea or vomiting, changes in vision, racing pulse, mental confusion, and stomach or right shoulder pain. If preeclampsia is not treated, it can cause strokes and seizures, a condition called **eclampsia.** Potential problems can include liver and kidney damage, internal bleeding, stroke, poor fetal growth, and fetal and maternal death.

This condition tends to occur in the late second or third trimesters. The cause is not known; however, the incidence of preeclampsia is higher in first-time mothers, women over 40 or under 18 years of age, women carrying multiple fetuses, and women with a history of chronic hypertension, diabetes, kidney disorder, or previous history of preeclampsia. Family history of preeclampsia is also a risk factor, whether the history is on the man's or woman's side. Treatment for preeclampsia ranges from bed rest and monitoring for women with mild cases, to hospitalization and close monitoring for more severe cases, which have the potential to be life-threatening for the woman and her fetus.

Cesarean Section
If labor lasts too long or if a baby is in physiological distress or is about to exit the uterus any way but head first, a **cesarean section (C-section)** may be necessary. This surgical procedure involves making an incision across the mother's abdomen and through the uterus to remove the baby. This operation also is performed if labor is extremely difficult, maternal blood pressure falls rapidly, the placenta separates from the uterus too soon, the mother has diabetes, or other problems occur.

The rate of delivery by C-section in the United States has increased from 5 percent in the mid-1960s to 29 percent in 2004.[29] Although necessary in certain cases, some physicians and critics, including the Centers for Disease Control and Prevention (CDC), feel that C-sections are performed too frequently in the United States.

Miscarriage
One in ten pregnancies does not end in delivery. Loss of the fetus before it is viable is called a **miscarriage** (also referred to as *spontaneous abortion*). An estimated 70 to 90 percent of women who miscarry eventually become pregnant again.

Reasons for miscarriage vary. In some cases, the fertilized egg has failed to divide correctly. In others, genetic abnormalities, maternal illness, or infections are responsible. Maternal hormonal imbalance also may cause a miscarriage, as may a weak cervix, toxic chemicals in the environment, or physical trauma to the mother. In most cases, the cause is not known.

Rh Factor
Rh is a blood protein. Problems with **Rh factors** occur when the mother is Rh-negative and the fetus is Rh-positive. During a first birth, some of the baby's blood passes into the mother's bloodstream. An Rh-negative mother

preeclampsia A complication in pregnancy characterized by high blood pressure, protein in the urine, and edema.

eclampsia Potentially fatal complication resulting from untreated preeclampsia; involves maternal strokes and seizures.

cesarean section (C-section) A surgical birthing procedure in which a baby is removed through an incision made in the mother's abdominal and uterine walls.

miscarriage Loss of the fetus before it is viable; also called *spontaneous abortion.*

Rh factor A blood protein related to the production of antibodies. If an Rh-negative mother is pregnant with an Rh-positive fetus, the mother will manufacture antibodies that can harm the fetus.

may manufacture antibodies to destroy the Rh-positive blood introduced into her bloodstream at the time of birth. Her first baby will be unaffected. However, subsequent babies with positive Rh factor will be at risk for a severe anemia called *hemolytic disease,* because the mother's Rh antibodies will attack the fetus's red blood cells.

Prevention is preferable to treatment. All women with Rh-negative blood should be injected with a medication called RhoGAM within 72 hours of any birth, miscarriage, or abortion. This injection will prevent them from developing the Rh antibodies.

Ectopic Pregnancy
The implantation of a fertilized egg outside the uterus, usually in the fallopian tube or occasionally in the pelvic cavity, is called an **ectopic pregnancy.** Because these structures are not capable of expanding and nourishing a developing fetus, the pregnancy must be terminated surgically, or a miscarriage will occur. Ectopic pregnancy generally is accompanied by pain in the lower abdomen or aching in the shoulders as the blood flows up toward the diaphragm. If bleeding is significant, blood pressure drops, and the woman can go into shock. If an ectopic pregnancy goes undiagnosed and untreated, the fallopian tube will rupture, putting the woman at great risk of hemorrhage, peritonitis (infection in the abdomen), and even death.

Over the past 12 years, the incidence of ectopic pregnancy has tripled, and no one really understands why. We do know that ectopic pregnancy is a potential side effect of pelvic inflammatory disease, which has become increasingly common in recent years. The scarring or blockage of the fallopian tubes that is characteristic of this disease prevents the fertilized egg from passing to the uterus.

Stillbirth
One of the most traumatic events a couple can face is a **stillbirth.** A stillborn baby is born dead, often for no apparent reason. The grief experienced following a stillbirth is devastating. Nine months of happy anticipation have been thwarted. Family, friends, and other children may be in a state of shock and need comfort as well. The mother's breasts produce milk, and there is no infant to be fed. A room with a crib and toys is left empty.

Some communities have groups called the Compassionate Friends to help parents and other family members through this grieving process. This nonprofit organization is for parents who have lost a child of any age for any reason.

Sudden Infant Death Syndrome
The unexpected death of a child under 1 year of age, for no apparent reason, is called **sudden infant death syndrome (SIDS).** Though SIDS is the leading cause of death for children aged 1 month to 1 year and affects about 1 in 1,000 infants in the United States each year, it is not a specific disease. Rather, it is ruled the cause of death after all other possibilities are ruled out. A SIDS death is sudden and silent; death occurs quickly, often during sleep, with no signs of suffering.

Doctors do not know what causes SIDS. However, research done in countries including England, New Zealand, Australia, and Norway has shown that placing children on their backs or sides to sleep cuts the rate of SIDS by as much as half. The American Academy of Pediatrics advises parents to lay infants on their backs and sponsors the Back to Sleep educational campaign urging parents to do so. Additional precautions against SIDS include having a firm surface for the infant's bed, not allowing the infant to become too warm, maintaining a smoke-free environment, having regular pediatric visits, breast-feeding, and seeking prenatal care. The use of a pacifier is also recommended and should be offered to an infant up to 1 year old during daytime naps and during the night. Research has shown that this practice does reduce the risk of SIDS.[30]

what do you THINK?

What are your thoughts on medical versus natural management of labor and delivery? ▪ Do you have strong preferences for how you'd like to manage your own birthing process? If so, what are they? ▪ What might be the advantages and disadvantages of breast-feeding?

Infertility

For the couple desperately wishing to conceive, the road to parenthood may be frustrating. An estimated one in six American couples experiences **infertility,** or difficulties in conceiving. Reasons include the trend toward delaying childbirth (as a woman gets older, she is less likely to conceive), endometriosis, pelvic inflammatory disease, and low sperm count.

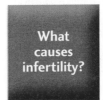

What causes infertility?

Causes of Infertility in Women

Endometriosis is the leading cause of infertility in women in the United States. With this very painful disorder, parts of the endometrial lining of the uterus implant themselves

---

ectopic pregnancy Implantation of a fertilized egg outside the uterus, usually in a fallopian tube; a medical emergency that can end in death from hemorrhage or peritonitis.

stillbirth The birth of a dead baby.

sudden infant death syndrome (SIDS) The sudden death of an infant under 1 year of age for no apparent reason.

infertility Difficulties in conceiving.

endometriosis A disorder in which uterine lining tissue establishes itself outside the uterus; the leading cause of infertility in women in the United States.

outside the uterus and block the fallopian tubes. The disorder can be treated surgically or with hormonal therapy. Success rates vary.

Another cause of infertility is **pelvic inflammatory disease (PID),** a serious infection that scars the fallopian tubes and blocks sperm migration. PID often results from chlamydia or gonorrheal infections that spread to the fallopian tubes or ovaries. (See Chapter 13 for more on PID.) The past 30 years have brought a tremendous increase in the annual number of PID cases, from 17,800 to about 1 million per year. One episode of PID causes sterility in 10 to 15 percent of women, and 50 to 75 percent become sterile after three or four infections.[31]

Causes of Infertility in Men

Among men, the single largest fertility problem is **low sperm count.** Although only one viable sperm is needed for fertilization, research has shown that all the other sperm in the ejaculate aid in the fertilization process. There are normally 60 to 80 million sperm per milliliter of semen. When the count drops below 20 million, fertility declines.

Low sperm count may be attributable to environmental factors (such as exposure of the scrotum to intense heat or cold, radiation, or altitude) or even to wearing excessively tight underwear or outerwear. However, other factors, such as the mumps virus, can damage the cells that make sperm. Varicose veins above one or both testicles also can render men infertile. Male infertility problems account for about 40 percent of infertility cases.

---

pelvic inflammatory disease (PID)   An infection that scars the fallopian tubes and consequently blocks sperm migration, causing infertility.

low sperm count   A sperm count below 20 million sperm per milliliter of semen; the leading cause of infertility in men.

fertility drugs   Hormones that stimulate ovulation in women who are not ovulating; often responsible for multiple births.

alternative insemination   Fertilization accomplished by depositing a partner's or a donor's semen into a woman's vagina via a thin tube; almost always done in a doctor's office.

in vitro fertilization (IVF)   Fertilization of an egg in a nutrient medium and subsequent transfer back to the mother's body.

gamete intrafallopian transfer (GIFT)   Procedure in which an egg harvested from the woman's ovary is placed with the man's sperm in her fallopian tube, where it is fertilized and then migrates to the uterus for implantation.

Infertility Treatments

Medical treatment can identify the cause of infertility in about 90 percent of cases. The chances of becoming pregnant range from 30 to 70 percent, depending on the reason for infertility. The countless tests and the invasion of privacy that characterize some couples' efforts to conceive can put stress on an otherwise strong, healthy relationship. A good physician or fertility team will take the time to ascertain the couple's level of motivation.

Workups to determine the cause of infertility can be expensive, and the costs are not usually covered by insurance companies. Fertility workups for men include a sperm count, a test for sperm motility, and analysis of any disease processes present. Women are thoroughly examined by an obstetrician-gynecologist for the composition of cervical mucus and evidence of problems such as tubal scarring or endometriosis.

Fertility Drugs   **Fertility drugs** stimulate ovulation in women who are not ovulating. Ninety percent of women who use these drugs will begin to ovulate, and half will conceive. Fertility drugs can have many side effects, including headaches, irritability, restlessness, depression, fatigue, edema (fluid retention), abnormal uterine bleeding, breast tenderness, vasomotor flushes (hot flashes), and visual difficulties. Women using fertility drugs are also at increased risk of developing multiple ovarian cysts (fluid-filled growths) and liver damage. The drugs sometimes trigger the release of more than one egg—a woman treated with one of these drugs has a one in ten chance of having multiple births. Most such births are twins, but triplets and even quadruplets are not uncommon.

Alternative Insemination   Another treatment option is **alternative insemination** of a woman with her partner's sperm. This technique has led to an estimated 250,000 births in the United States, primarily for couples in which the man is infertile. The couple may also choose insemination by an anonymous donor through a sperm bank. The sperm are medically screened, classified according to the physical characteristics of the donor (for example, blond hair, blue eyes), and then frozen for future use. In the last few years, concern has been expressed about the possibility of transmitting the AIDS virus through alternative insemination. As a result, donors are routinely screened for the disease.

In Vitro Fertilization   Often referred to as *test tube fertilization,* **in vitro fertilization (IVF)** involves collecting a viable ovum from the prospective mother and transferring it to a nutrient medium in a laboratory, where it is fertilized with sperm from the woman's partner or a donor. After a few days, the embryo is transplanted into the mother's uterus, where, it is hoped, it will develop normally. Since 1984, the in vitro process has been responsible for an estimated 60,000 babies.

Gamete Intrafallopian Transfer   In **gamete intrafallopian transfer (GIFT),** the egg is harvested from the woman's ovary and placed in the fallopian tube with the man's sperm. Less expensive and time consuming than in vitro fertilization, GIFT mimics nature by allowing the egg to be fertilized in the fallopian tube and migrate to the uterus according to the normal timetable.

Intracytoplasmic Sperm Injection

In **intracytoplasmic sperm injection (ICSI),** a sperm cell is injected into an egg. First performed successfully in 1992, this procedure required researchers to learn how to manipulate both egg and sperm without damaging them. ICSI can help men with low sperm counts or motility, and even those who cannot ejaculate or have no live sperm in their semen as a result of vasectomy, chemotherapy, or a medical disorder. However, recent studies have found that infants conceived with the use of ICSI or in vitro fertilization have twice the risk of a major birth defect as do those conceived naturally.[32]

Nonsurgical Embryo Transfer and Other Techniques

In **nonsurgical embryo transfer,** a donor egg is fertilized by the man's sperm and implanted in the woman's uterus. This procedure may also be used to transfer an already fertilized ovum into the uterus of another woman. In **embryo transfer,** an ovum from a donor is artificially inseminated by the man's sperm, allowed to stay in the donor's body for a time, and then transplanted into the woman's body.

Infertile couples have another alternative—**embryo adoption programs.** The adopting couple can experience pregnancy and control prenatal care. The cost is approximately $4,000 for the embryos to be thawed and transferred to an infertile woman's uterus or uterine tubes.

The ethical and moral questions surrounding experimental infertility treatments are staggering. Before moving forward with any of these treatments, individuals need to ask themselves a few important questions. Has infertility been absolutely confirmed? Are reputable infertility counseling services accessible? Have they explored all possible alternatives and considered potential risks? Have all parties examined their attitudes, values, and beliefs about conceiving a child in this manner? Finally, they need to consider what and how they will tell the child about their method of conception.

Surrogate Motherhood

Sixty to 70 percent of infertile couples are able to conceive after treatment. The rest decide to live without children, to adopt, or to attempt surrogate motherhood. In this option, the couple hires a woman to be alternatively inseminated by the male partner. The surrogate then carries the baby to term and surrenders it to the couple at birth. Surrogate mothers are reportedly paid about $10,000 for their services and are reimbursed for medical expenses. Legal and medical expenses can run as high as $30,000 for the infertile couple.

Couples considering surrogate motherhood are advised to consult a lawyer regarding contracts. Most of these legal documents stipulate that the surrogate mother undergo amniocentesis and that if the fetus is defective, she must consent to an abortion. In that case, or if the surrogate miscarries, she is reimbursed for her time and expenses. The prospective parents must also agree to take the baby if it is carried to term, even if it is unhealthy or has physical abnormalities.

Adoption

For couples who have decided that biological childbirth is not an option, adoption provides an alternative. About 50,000 children are available for adoption in the United States every year. This is far fewer than the number of couples seeking adoptions. By some estimates, only 1 in 30 couples receives the child they want. On average, couples spend 2 years and $100,000 on the adoption process.

Increasingly, couples are choosing to adopt children from other countries. In 2006, U.S. families adopted over 20,679 foreign-born children.[33] The cost of intercountry adoption varies from approximately $10,000 to more than $30,000, including agency fees, dossier and immigration processing fees, and court costs. However, it may be a good alternative for many couples, especially those who want to adopt an infant rather than an older child.

what do you THINK?

If you or your partner had infertility problems, how much time and money would you be willing to invest in treatment? ■ Do you think that single women and lesbians should have equal access to alternative methods of insemination? Why or why not? ■ Do you think single women, single men, gay men, and lesbians should have equal opportunities to adopt? ■ How do you think society views these types of adoptions?

intracytoplasmic sperm injection (ICSI) Fertilization accomplished by injecting a sperm cell directly into an egg.

nonsurgical embryo transfer In vitro fertilization of a donor egg by the male partner's (or donor's) sperm and subsequent transfer to the female partner's or another woman's uterus.

embryo transfer Artificial insemination of a donor with the male partner's sperm; after a time, the embryo is transferred from the donor to the female partner's uterus.

embryo adoption programs A procedure whereby an infertile couple is able to purchase frozen embryos donated by another couple.

TAKING charge

Summary

- Latex male condoms and the female condom, when used correctly for oral sex or intercourse, provide the most effective protection in preventing sexually transmitted infections (STIs). Other contraceptive methods include abstinence, outercourse, oral contraceptives, foams, jellies, implants, suppositories, creams, film, the diaphragm, the cervical cap, Lea's shield, FemCap, the Today Sponge, Ortho Evra, NuvaRing, intrauterine devices, Depo-Provera, and withdrawal. Fertility awareness methods rely on altering sexual practices to avoid pregnancy. Whereas all these methods of contraception are reversible, sterilization is permanent.
- Abortion is legal in the United States through the second trimester. Abortion methods include vacuum aspiration, dilation and evacuation (D&E), dilation and curettage (D&C), intact dilation and extraction (D&X), hysterectomy, induction abortion, mifepristone, and methotrexate.
- Parenting is a demanding job that requires careful planning. Prospective parents need to take into account emotional health, maternal and paternal health, financial plans, and contingency planning.

- Prenatal care includes a complete physical exam within the first trimester and avoidance of all substances that could have teratogenic effects on the fetus, such as alcohol and drugs, smoking, X rays, and harmful chemicals. Full-term pregnancy covers three trimesters.
- Childbirth occurs in three stages. Partners should jointly choose a labor method early in the pregnancy to be better prepared for labor when it occurs. Possible complications of pregnancy and childbirth include preeclampsia and eclampsia, miscarriage, Rh factor problems, ectopic pregnancy, stillbirth, and the need for a C-section.
- Infertility in women may be caused by pelvic inflammatory disease (PID) or endometriosis. In men, it may be caused by low sperm count. Treatments may include alternative insemination, in vitro fertilization, gamete intrafallopian transfer (GIFT), intracytoplasmic sperm injection (ICSI), nonsurgical embryo transfer, embryo transfer, and embryo adoption programs. Surrogate motherhood involves hiring a fertile woman to be alternatively inseminated by the male partner. Adoption, including international adoptions, can be a viable option.

Chapter Review

1. What type of contraceptive method involves long-acting synthetic progesterone injected intramuscularly every 3 months?
   a. Seasonale
   b. Ortho Evra
   c. Depo-Provera
   d. Lea's Shield

2. Which of the following is *not* a barrier contraceptive?
   a. cervical cap
   b. condom
   c. diaphragm
   d. contraceptive patch

3. What is the most commonly used method of first-trimester abortion?
   a. vacuum aspiration
   b. dilation and evacuation (D&E)
   c. dilation and curettage (D&C)
   d. induction abortions

4. What is meant by the *failure rate* of contraceptive use?
   a. the number of times a woman fails to get pregnant when she wanted to
   b. the number of times a woman gets pregnant when she did not want to
   c. the number of pregnancies that occur for women using a particular method of birth control
   d. the reliability of alternative methods of birth control that do not use condoms

5. Toxic chemicals, pesticides, X rays, and other hazardous compounds that cause birth defects are referred to as
   a. carcinogens.
   b. teratogens.
   c. mutants.
   d. environmental assaults.

6. In an ectopic pregnancy, the fertilized egg grows into the fetus in the woman's
   a. fallopian tube.
   b. uterus.
   c. vagina.
   d. ovaries.

7. For a woman of normal weight before pregnancy, what is the recommended weight gain during pregnancy?
   a. 15 to 20 pounds
   b. 20 to 30 pounds
   c. 25 to 35 pounds
   d. 30 to 45 pounds

8. What prenatal test involves snipping tissue from the developing fetal sac?
   a. fetoscopy
   b. ultrasound
   c. amniocentesis
   d. chorionic villus sampling

9. Rh factor problems occurs when the mother is _____ and the fetus is _____
   a. Rh positive; Rh positive
   b. Rh positive; Rh negative
   c. Rh negative; Rh positive
   d. Rh negative; Rh negative

10. The number of American couples who experience infertility is
   a. 1 in 6.
   b. 1 in 24.
   c. 1 in 60.
   d. 1 in 100.

Answers to these questions can be found on page A-1.

Questions for Discussion and Reflection

1. List the most effective contraceptive methods. What are their drawbacks? What medical conditions would keep a person from using each one? What are the characteristics of the methods that you think would be most effective for you? Why do you consider them most effective for you personally?
2. What are the various methods of abortion? What are the two opposing viewpoints concerning abortion? What is *Roe v. Wade,* and what impact did it have on the abortion debate?
3. What are the most important considerations in deciding whether the time is right to become a parent? If you choose to have children, what factors will you consider regarding the number of children to have?
4. Discuss the growth of the fetus through the three trimesters. What medical checkups or tests should be done during each trimester?
5. Discuss the emotional aspects of pregnancy. What types of emotional reactions are common in each trimester and the postpartum period (the "fourth trimester")?
6. If you and your partner are unable to have children, what alternative methods of conception would you consider? Is adoption an option you would consider?

Accessing Your Health on the Internet

The following websites explore further topics and issues related to personal health. For links to the websites below, visit the Companion Website for *Health: The Basics,* Eighth Edition at www.aw-bc.com/donatelle.

1. *The Alan Guttmacher Institute (AGI).* AGI is a nonprofit organization focused on sexual and reproductive health research, policy analysis, and public education. www.agi-usa.org
2. *Go Ask Alice.* This website enables you to ask health questions anonymously. It is designed to help visitors make informed decisions about all aspects of their health by providing nonjudgmental, science-based responses to their questions. www.goaskalice.columbia.edu
3. *The American Pregnancy Association.* A national organization offering a wealth of resources to promote reproductive and pregnancy wellness. The website includes educational materials and information on the latest in research. www.americanpregnancy.org
4. *Dr. Drew.* Provides answers and advice on sex, relationships, and many other topics of interest for college students. www.drdrew.com
5. *Planned Parenthood.* This site offers a range of up-to-date information on sexual health issues, such as birth control, deciding when and whether to have a child, sexually transmitted infections, and safer sex. www.plannedparenthood.org
6. *Sexuality Information and Education Council of the United States.* Information, guidelines, and materials for the advancement of sexuality education. The site advocates the right of individuals to make responsible sexual choices. www.siecus.org

Further Reading

Boston Women's Health Collective. *Our Bodies, Ourselves: A New Edition for a New Era*. New York: Simon and Schuster, 2005.

> *Like its earlier editions, this volume contains information about women's health from a decidedly feminist angle. Every aspect of health is covered, including nutrition, emotional health, fitness, relationships, reproduction, contraception, and pregnancy.*

Feldt, G. *The War on Choice*. New York: Bantam, 2004.

> *A history and analysis of threats to women's reproductive rights. Feldt describes political efforts to outlaw abortion and argues that women should mobilize to support pro-choice causes.*

Hatcher, R. A., et al. *Contraceptive Technology*, 19th rev. ed. New York: Ardent Media, 2007.

> *Perhaps the best primary reference concerning birth control for physicians, family planning centers, student health services, and educators. Contributors include staff members from the Centers for Disease Control and Prevention.*

Hatcher, R. A., et al. *Safely Sexual*, 2nd ed. New York: Ardent Media, 2005.

> *Provides practical recommendations for unplanned pregnancy, as well as for preventing STIs and HIV infection.*

Strong, B., et al. *Human Sexuality: Diversity in Contemporary America*, 6th ed. New York: McGraw-Hill, 2006.

> *A comprehensive introduction into human sexuality.*

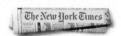

e-themes from *The New York Times*

For up-to-date articles about current health issues, visit www.aw-bc.com/donatelle, select *Health: The Basics*, Eighth Edition, Chapter 6, and click on "e-themes."

References

1. World Health Organization, "Nonoxynol-9 Ineffective in Preventing HIV Infection," June 8, 2006, www.who.int/mediacentre/notes/release55/en.
2. R. A. Hatcher et al., *Contraceptive Technology*, 19th rev. ed. (New York: Ardent Media, 2007); R. Burkman et al., "Safety Concerns and Health Benefits Associated with Oral Contraception," *American Journal of Obstetrics and Gynecology* 190, 4 Suppl. S (2004): S5–S22.
3. U.S. Department of Health and Human Services, "FDA Approves Seasonale Oral Contraceptive," FDA Talk Paper TO3–65, September 5, 2003, www.fda.gov.
4. U.S. Food and Drug Administration, "FDA Updates Labeling for Ortho Evra Contraceptive Patch," *FDA News*, November 10, 2005, www.fda.gov/bbs/topics/news/2005/NEW01262.html.
5. D. Bensyl et al., "Contraceptive Use—United States and Territories, Behavioral Risk Factor Surveillance System, 2002," *Morbidity and Mortality Weekly Report* 54, SS6 (November 18, 2005): 1–72.
6. Ibid; Hatcher et al., *Contraceptive Technology*.
7. American College Health Association, "American College Health Association–National College Health Assessment (ACHA–NCHA) Web Summary," April 2006, www.acha.org/projects_programs/ncha_sampledata.cfm.
8. S. J. Ventura, J. C. Abma, W. D. Mosher, and S. Henshaw, "Estimated Pregnancy Rates for the United States, 1990–2000: An Update," *National Vital Statistic Reports* 52 (2004): 1–2; H. Boonstra, "Emergency Contraception: The Need to Increase Public Awareness," *Guttmacher Report on Public Policy* 5(2002): 3–6; Planned Parenthood Federation of America, "Emergency Contraception," 2007, www.plannedparenthood.org/birth-control-pregnancy/emergency-contraception-4363%20.htm.
9. American College Health Association, "Access to Emergency Contraception on College and University Campuses: American College Health Association–National College Health Assessment (ACHA–NCHA) Spring 2006 Reference Group Data Report (Abridged)," *Journal of American College Health* 55, no. 4 (January 2007), 195–206.
10. Ibid.
11. Ibid.
12. National Conference of State Legislatures, "50 State Summary of Emergency Contraception Laws," June 2007, www.ncsl.org/programs/health/ecleg.htm.
13. Boston Women's Health Collective, *Our Bodies, Ourselves: A New Edition for a New Era* (New York: Simon and Schuster, 2005).
14. Ibid.
15. The Alan Guttmacher Institute, "State Policies in Brief: An Overview of Abortion Laws," April 1, 2007, www.agi-usa.org; The Alan Guttmacher Institute, "Sexual and Reproductive Health Issues in the States: Major Trends in 2005," www.agi-usa.org.
16. NARAL and Pro Choice America, "Federal Abortion Ban Update," May 27, 2007, www.prochoiceamerica.org/issues/abortion/abortion-bans/fab-update.html.
17. The Alan Guttmacher Institute, "Facts in Brief: Induced Abortion in the United States," 2005, www.agi-usa.org.
18. Planned Parenthood, "The Difference between Emergency Contraception Pills and Medication Abortion," July 9, 2005, www.plannedparenthood.org.
19. N. F. Russo and A. J. Dabul, "The Relationship of Abortion to Well-Being: Do Race and Religion Make a Difference?" *Professional Psychology: Research and Practice* 28, no. 1 (2000): 23–31.
20. Center for Policy and Promotion, "Expenditures on Children by Families, 2006," April 2007, www.cnpp.usda.gov/Publications/CRC/crc2006.pdf.
21. J. Overturf-Johnson, "Who's Minding the Kids? Child Care Arrangements: Winter 2002," *Current Population Reports*, Pub. no. 70–101 (Washington, DC: U.S. Census Bureau, 2005).

22. National Center for Health Statistics, *Health, United States, 2006 with Chartbook on Trends in the Health of Americans* (Hyattsville, MD: U.S. Government Printing Office, 2006).

23. National Center for Chronic Disease Prevention and Health Promotion, "Maternal and Infant Health: Smoking During Pregnancy," 2006, www.cdc.gov/reproductivehealth/MaternalInfantHealth/related/SmokingPregnancy.htm.

24. M. Kharrazi et al., "Environmental Tobacco Smoke and Pregnancy Outcome," *Epidemiology* 15, no. 6 (November 2006), 660–70.

25. National Institute of Child Health and Human Development, "Facts about Down's Syndrome," 2005, www.nichd.nih.gov/publications/downsyndrome.

26. National Institute of Mental Health, "Frequently Asked Questions: Depression During and After Pregnancy," April 2005, www.4woman.gov.

27. E. de Lisser, "Breast Feeding Boosts Adult I.Q., Research Suggests," *Wall Street Journal*, May 2, 2002, D2.

28. American Pregnancy Association, "What's in Breast Milk?" June 9, 2006, www.americanpregnancy.org.

29. J. A. Martin et al., *Preliminary Births for 2004: Infant and Maternal Health* (Hyattsville, MD: National Center for Health Statistics, 2006).

30. F. R. Hawk et al., "Do Pacifiers Reduce the Risk of Sudden Infant Death Syndrome? A Meta-Analysis," *Pediatrics,* October 10, 2005, 716–23.

31. Centers for Disease Control and Prevention, "Pelvic Inflammatory Disease—Fact Sheet," 2006, www.cdc.gov/std/pid.

32. K. Powell, "Fertility Treatments: Seeds of Doubt," *Nature* 422 (2003): 656–658.

33. Bureau of Consular Affairs, "Immigrant Visas Issued to Orphans Coming to the U.S.," 2006, http://travel.state.gov/family/adoption/stats/stats_451.html.

7

Addictive Behaviors, Licit and Illicit Drugs

USE, MISUSE, AND ABUSE

How can I recognize the signs of **addiction** in a loved one or even myself?

Is my roommate's **obsessive** gambling an addiction?

Should I be concerned about the **safety** of prescription drugs?

Are there any **negative** long-term effects from marijuana use?

OBJECTIVES

- Identify the signs of addiction and discuss types of addictions, including compulsive behaviors such as gambling and shopping.
- Discuss the six categories of drugs and their routes of administration.
- Compare choices in prescription and over-the-counter drugs, and understand how to use them safely and how hazardous drug interactions can occur.
- Profile illicit drug use in the United States, including who uses illicit drugs, financial impact, and impact on college campuses and the workplace.
- Discuss the use and abuse of controlled substances, including cocaine, amphetamines, marijuana, opiates, hallucinogens, designer drugs, inhalants, and steroids.

I t isn't difficult these days to find high-profile cases of compulsive and destructive behavior. Stories of celebrities and politicians struggling with addictions to alcohol, drugs, and sex are splashed in the headlines and profiled on television news programs. But millions of "everyday" people throughout the world are staging their own battles with addiction as well. Addictions can be perplexing, because many potentially addictive activities may actually enhance the lives of those who engage in them moderately. In addition to alcohol and drugs, commonly recognized objects of addiction include gambling, shopping, and borrowing money.

Defining Addiction

Addiction is continued involvement with a substance or activity despite ongoing negative consequences. Addictive behaviors initially provide a sense of pleasure or stability that is beyond the addict's power to achieve in other ways. Eventually, the addicted person needs to be involved in the behavior to feel normal.

In this chapter, *addiction* is used interchangeably with *physiological addiction.* However, **physiological dependence,** the adaptive state that occurs with regular addictive behavior and results in withdrawal symptoms, is only one indicator of addiction. Psychological dynamics play an important role, which explains why behaviors not related to the use of chemicals—gambling, for example—may also be addictive. A person who possesses a strong desire to continue engaging in a particular activity is said to have developed a psychological dependence. In fact, psychological and physiological dependence are so intertwined that it is not really possible to separate the two. For every psychological state, there is a corresponding physiological state. In other words, everything you feel is tied to a chemical process occurring in your body.[1] Thus, addictions once thought to be entirely psychological in nature are now understood to have physiological components.

To be addictive, a substance or behavior must have the potential to produce a positive mood change. Chemicals are responsible for the most profound addictions, not only because they produce dramatic mood changes, but also because they cause cellular changes to which the body adapts so well that it eventually requires the chemical to function normally. Yet other behaviors, such as gambling, spending money, working, and sex, also create changes at the cellular level along with positive mood changes. Although the mechanism is not well understood, all forms of addiction probably reflect dysfunction of certain biochemical systems in the brain.[2]

Traditionally, diagnosis of an addiction was limited to drug addiction and was based on four criteria as defined by the American Psychological Association:

1. Use for the purpose of relieving **withdrawal** symptoms— a series of temporary physical and psychological symptoms that occurs when the addicted person abruptly stops using the drug.

2. Continued use of the substance despite knowledge of the harm it causes oneself and others (deterioration in work performance, relationships, and social interaction).

3. Unsuccessful efforts to cut down or cease using the drug, including **relapse,** the tendency to return to the addictive behavior after a period of abstinence.

4. **Tolerance** or an acquired reaction to a drug in which continued intake of the same dose has diminished effects. In response to tolerance, drug users must increase the dose to achieve the desired effect.

Until recently, health professionals were unwilling to diagnose an addiction until medical symptoms appeared in the patient. Now we know that although withdrawal, pathological behavior, relapse, and tolerance are valid indicators of addiction, they do not characterize all addictive behavior.

Signs of Addiction

How can I recognize the signs of addiction in a loved one or even myself?

Studies show that all animals share the same basic pleasure and reward circuits in the brain that turn on when they engage in something pleasurable. We all engage in potentially addictive behaviors to some extent because some are essential to our survival and are highly reinforcing, such as eating, drinking, and sex. At some point along the continuum, however, some individuals are not able to engage in these behaviors moderately, and they become addicted.

Addictions are characterized by four common symptoms: (1) **compulsion,** or excessive preoccupation with the behavior

addiction Continued involvement with a substance or activity despite ongoing negative consequences.

physiological dependence The adaptive state that occurs with regular addictive behavior and results in withdrawal symptoms.

withdrawal A series of temporary physical and biopsychosocial symptoms that occur when an addict abruptly abstains from an addictive chemical or behavior.

relapse The tendency to return to an addictive behavior after a period of abstinence.

tolerance Phenomenon in which progressively larger doses of a drug or more intense involvement in a behavior are needed to produce the desired effects.

compulsion Preoccupation with a behavior and an overwhelming need to perform it.

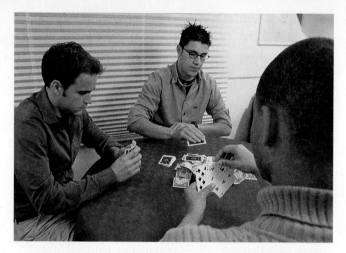

As a result of the growing popularity of poker games, betting on sports events, and online gambling, college students have a problem gambling rate two or three times that of the general population.

and an overwhelming need to perform it; (2) **loss of control,** or the inability to predict reliably whether any isolated occurrence of the behavior will be healthy or damaging; (3) **negative consequences,** such as physical damage, legal trouble, financial problems, academic failure, or family dissolution, which do not occur with healthy involvement in any behavior; and (4) **denial,** the inability to perceive that the behavior is self-destructive. These four components are present in all addictions, whether chemical or behavioral.

Addictive Behaviors

Clearly, tobacco, alcohol, and other drugs are addictive, and addictions to these drugs create multiple problems for addicted individuals as well as their families and society. Later in this chapter, and in other chapters in this book, we will discuss specific substance-related addictions. But first, we will examine two behaviors known to be addictive because they are mood-altering: compulsive gambling and shopping.

loss of control Inability to predict reliably whether a particular instance of involvement with an addictive substance or behavior will be healthy or damaging.

negative consequences Physical damage, legal trouble, financial ruin, academic failure, family dissolution, and other severe problems associated with addiction.

denial Inability to perceive or accurately interpret the self-destructive effects of an addictive behavior.

compulsive (pathological) gambler A person addicted to gambling.

Compulsive or Pathological Gambling

Gambling is a form of recreation and entertainment for millions of Americans. Most people who gamble do so casually and moderately to experience the excitement of anticipating a win.

Is my roommate's obsessive gambling an addiction?

However, over 3 million Americans are **compulsive,** or **pathological, gamblers** (addicted to gambling), and 15 million more are considered to be at risk for developing a gambling addiction.[3] The American Psychiatric Association (APA) recognizes pathological gambling as a mental disorder and lists ten characteristic behaviors, including preoccupation with gambling, unsuccessful efforts to cut back or quit, using gambling to escape problems, and lying to family members to conceal the extent of involvement with gambling.

Gamblers and drug addicts describe many similar cravings and highs. A recent study supports what many experts believe to be true: that compulsive gambling is like drug addiction. Compulsive gamblers in this study were found to have decreased blood flow to a key section of the brain's reward system. Much as with people who abuse drugs, it is thought that compulsive gamblers compensate for this deficiency in their brain's reward system by overdoing it and getting hooked.[4] Most compulsive gamblers state that they seek excitement even more than money. They place increasingly larger bets to obtain the desired level of excitement.

Who is at risk for getting hooked to the rush of gambling? Men are more likely to have gambling problems than women are. Gambling prevalence is also higher among lower-income individuals, those who are divorced, African Americans, older adults, and individuals residing within 50 miles of a casino. Residents in southern states, where opportunities to gamble have increased significantly over the past 20 years, also have higher gambling rates.[5]

Gambling among college students appears to be on the rise across the nation. In a 2005 telephone poll conducted by University of Pennsylvania's Annenburg Public Policy Center, 15.5 percent of college students reported gambling once a week, up from 8.3 percent in 2002, an 87 percent increase. Men dominated the gambling scene, with 26 percent reporting gambling each week, whereas 5.5 percent of women reported gambling weekly.[6]

What accounts for this trend? College students have easier access to gambling opportunities than ever before with the advent of online gambling, a growing number of casinos, scratch tickets, lotteries, and sports betting networks. In particular, the largest boost has come from the increasing popularity of poker. Access to poker on the Internet and televised poker tournaments have revived the game, causing many young people to spend an unhealthy amount of time and money participating in online poker tournaments.

On campus, it is more common for men to gamble than women. Other characteristics associated with gambling among college students include spending more time watching TV, using computers for nonacademic purposes, spending less time studying, earning lower grades, participating in intercollegiate athletics, and engaging in heavy, episodic drinking and using illicit drugs in the past year.[7]

Whereas casual gamblers can stop anytime they wish and are capable of seeing the necessity to do so, compulsive gamblers are unable to control the urge to gamble even in the face of devastating consequences: high debt, legal problems, and the loss of everything meaningful, including homes, families, jobs, health, and even their lives. Gambling can also have a detrimental affect on health: cardiovascular problems affect 38 percent of compulsive gamblers, and their suicide rate is 20 times higher than that of the general population.

Compulsive Shopping and Borrowing

Although compulsive spending has been a pervasive problem in the United States for some time, a more insidious form of the addiction lurks in the new "plastic generation." Credit card companies entice you with fantasies of having it all, right now—whether or not you can afford it.

The credit card companies seem to be succeeding. There are 400 million MasterCards and Visas out there. Add to that cable shopping stations, catalog shopping, and shopping over the Internet, and the opportunity to overspend is greater than ever before. The resulting debt from all this spending is phenomenal. After bankruptcies, formerly a last resort, reached a record high in 2005, new laws came into effect in 2006 reducing the number of bankruptcy filings by 70 percent to 618,000 for 2006. But consumer debt remains high, and it is expected that the number of bankruptcies filed will soon increase again.[8] On average, compulsive spenders are $23,000 in debt, usually in the form of credit card debt or mortgages against their homes.[9]

Although most people can manage debt with careful planning, some spend money to meet emotional needs they can't fulfill elsewhere. Anxiety, self-doubt, and anger all lead to spending as a way of coping with daily stressors. College students may be particularly vulnerable to spending problems because advertisers and credit card companies heavily target them.

Compulsive gambling and shopping can frequently lead to compulsive borrowing to help support the addiction. Irresponsible investments and purchases lead to debts that the addict tries to repay by borrowing more. Compulsive debtors borrow money repeatedly from family, friends, or institutions in spite of the problems this causes. Whereas most people incur overwhelming debt through a combination of hardship and ignorance about financial management, compulsive debtors incur debt primarily as a result of buying or gambling behaviors in which they have engaged to relieve painful feelings.

How Addiction Affects Family and Friends

The family and friends of an addicted person also suffer many negative consequences. Often they struggle with **codependence,** a self-defeating relationship pattern in which a person is "addicted to the addict." It is the primary outcome of dysfunctional relationships or families.

Codependence is not accurately defined by isolated incidents, but rather by a pattern of behavior. Codependents find it hard to set healthy boundaries and often live in the chaotic, crisis-oriented mode that naturally occurs around addicts. They assume responsibility for meeting others' needs to the point that they subordinate or even cease being aware of their own needs. They may be unable to perceive their needs because they have repeatedly been taught that their needs are inappropriate or less important than someone else's. Their behavior goes far beyond performing kind services for another person. Codependents feel less than human if they fail to respond to the needs of someone else, even when their help was not requested. Although the term *codependent* is used less frequently today, treatment professionals still recognize the importance of helping addicts see how their behavior affects those around them and of working with family and friends to establish healthier relationships and boundaries.

Family and friends can play an important role in getting an addict to seek treatment. They are most helpful when they refuse to be enablers. **Enablers** are people who knowingly or unknowingly protect addicts from the natural consequences of their behavior. If they don't have to deal with the consequences, addicts cannot see the self-destructive nature of their behavior and will therefore continue it. Codependents are the primary enablers of their addicted loved ones, although anyone who has contact with an addict can be an enabler and thus contribute (perhaps powerfully) to continuation of the addictive behavior. Enablers are generally unaware that their behavior has this effect. In fact, enabling is rarely conscious and certainly not intentional.

---

codependence A self-defeating relationship pattern in which a person is "addicted to the addict."

enablers People who knowingly or unknowingly protect addicts from the natural consequences of their behavior.

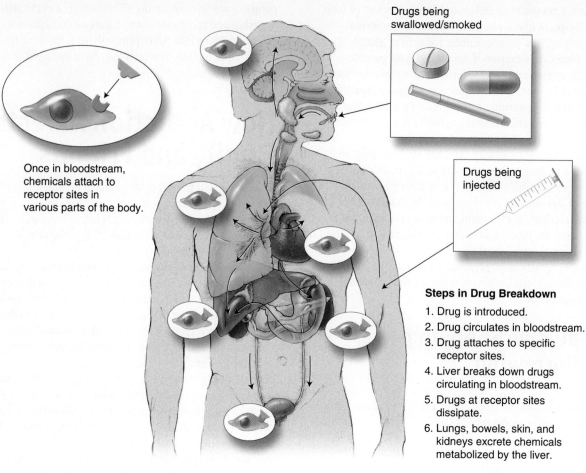

Drugs being swallowed/smoked

Once in bloodstream, chemicals attach to receptor sites in various parts of the body.

Drugs being injected

Steps in Drug Breakdown

1. Drug is introduced.
2. Drug circulates in bloodstream.
3. Drug attaches to specific receptor sites.
4. Liver breaks down drugs circulating in bloodstream.
5. Drugs at receptor sites dissipate.
6. Lungs, bowels, skin, and kidneys excrete chemicals metabolized by the liver.

FIGURE 7.1 **How the Body Metabolizes Drugs**

 what do you THINK?

Why do we tend to protect others from the natural consequences of their destructive behaviors? ■ Have you ever confronted someone you were concerned about? If so, was the confrontation successful?
■ What tips would you give someone who wants to confront a loved one about an addiction?

Drug Dynamics

Drug misuse and abuse are problems of staggering proportions in our society. Each year, drug and alcohol abuse contributes to the destruction of families and jobs and to the deaths of more than 120,000 Americans. Drug abuse costs taxpayers more than $294 billion in preventable health care costs, extra law enforcement, vehicle crashes, crime, and lost productivity.[10] It's impossible to put a dollar amount on the pain, suffering, and dysfunction that drugs cause in our everyday lives.

receptor sites Specialized locations on cell membranes to which drugs can attach themselves.

Although overall use of drugs in the United States has fallen by 50 percent in the last 20 years, the past 10 years have shown an increase in the use of certain drugs by adolescents.[11] It is important to understand how drugs work and why people use them. Humans appear to have a need to alter their consciousness, or mental state. We like to feel good or escape the normal. Consciousness can be altered in many ways: children spinning until they become dizzy and adults enjoying the rush of thrilling extreme sports are examples. To change our awareness, many of us listen to music, skydive, ski, read, daydream, meditate, pray, or have sexual relations. Others turn to drugs to alter consciousness.

Drugs work because they physically resemble the chemicals produced naturally within the body (**Figure 7.1**). Most bodily processes result from chemical reactions or from changes in electrical charge. Because drugs possess an electrical charge and chemical structure similar to those of chemicals that occur naturally in the body, they can affect physical functions in many different ways. For example, many painkillers resemble the endorphins (meaning "morphine within") that are manufactured in the body.

A current explanation of how drugs work is the receptor site theory, which states that drugs bind to specific **receptor sites** in the body. These sites are locations on the membranes of some cells to which, because of their size, shape, electrical charge, and chemical properties, drugs can attach themselves. Most drugs attach to multiple receptor sites on cells located throughout the body in places such as the heart and circulatory system, the lungs, liver, kidneys, brain, and gonads (testicles or ovaries).

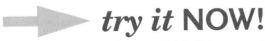

try it NOW!

Achieve a drug-free and "natural high." Many people become addicted to drugs because of the positive, short-term effects they can exert on mood. Right now, you can take a walk in a beautiful and sense-stimulating location, lose yourself in a favorite song, or visit an amusement park and ride the roller coaster to satisfy a craving for an endorphin rush or simply to lift your spirits.

Types of Drugs

Scientists divide drugs into six categories: prescription, over-the-counter, recreational, herbal, illicit, and commercial drugs. These classifications are based primarily on drug action, although some are based on the source of the chemical in question. Each category includes some drugs that stimulate body functions and some that depress body functions. Each category also includes **psychoactive drugs,** which have the potential to alter a person's mood or behavior.

- **Prescription drugs** can be obtained only with the written prescription of a licensed physician or other health care provider with prescription rights. More than 10,000 types of prescription drugs are sold in the United States, at an annual cost of over $200 billion to consumers.[12]
- **Over-the-counter (OTC) drugs** can be purchased without a prescription. Each year, Americans spend more than $20 billion on OTC products, and the market is increasing at the rate of 20 percent annually. More than 300,000 OTC products are available, and an estimated three out of four people routinely self-medicate with them.
- **Recreational drugs** belong to a somewhat vague category whose boundaries depend on how the term *recreation* is defined. Generally, these drugs contain chemicals used to help people relax or socialize. Most of them are legally sanctioned even though they are psychoactive. Alcohol, tobacco, coffee, tea, and chocolate products are usually included in this category.
- **Herbal preparations** form another vague category. Included among these approximately 750 substances are herbal teas and other products of botanical (plant) origin that are believed to have medicinal properties. (See Chapter 17 for more on herbal preparations.)
- **Illicit (illegal) drugs** are the most notorious type of drug. Although laws governing their use, possession, cultivation, manufacture, and sale differ from state to state, illicit drugs generally are recognized as harmful. All of them are psychoactive.
- **Commercial preparations** are the most universally used yet least commonly recognized chemical substances. More than 1,000 of these substances exist, including seemingly

benign items such as perfumes, cosmetics, household cleansers, paints, glues, inks, dyes, gardening chemicals, pesticides, and industrial by-products.

Routes of Administration of Drugs

Route of administration refers to the way in which a given drug is taken into the body. The most common methods include **oral ingestion** (by mouth), **inhalation** (administration of drugs through the mouth or nostrils via sniffing or smoking), and **injection** into the muscles (intramuscular) bloodstream (intravenous), or just under the skin (subcutaneous). **Intravenous injection,** which involves the insertion of a hypodermic syringe directly into a vein, is the most common method of injection for drug misusers because the drug's effect is felt rapidly. It is also the most dangerous method of administration because of the risk of contracting HIV and/or hepatitis B and damage to blood vessels. Drugs can also be absorbed through the skin or tissue linings (**inunction**)—the nicotine patch is a common example of a drug that is administered in this manner—or

psychoactive drugs Drugs that have the potential to alter mood or behavior.

prescription drugs Medications that can be obtained only with the written prescription of a licensed physician.

over-the-counter (OTC) drugs Medications that can be purchased without a physician's prescription.

recreational drugs Drugs that contain chemicals that help people relax or socialize; most, but not all, drugs in this category are legal.

herbal preparations Substances of plant origin that are believed to have medicinal properties.

illicit (illegal) drugs Drugs whose use, possession, cultivation, manufacture, and/or sale are against the law because they generally are recognized as harmful.

commercial preparations Commonly used chemical substances including cosmetics, household cleaning products, and industrial by-products.

route of administration The manner in which a drug is taken into the body.

oral ingestion Intake of drugs through the mouth and into the digestive tract.

inhalation The introduction of drugs through the nostrils or mouth and into the lung.

injection The introduction of drugs into the body via a hypodermic needle.

intravenous injection The introduction of drugs directly into a vein.

inunction The introduction of drugs by absorption through the skin.

through the vagina or anus in the form of **suppositories.** Suppositories are typically mixed with a waxy medium that melts at body temperature so the drug can be released into the bloodstream. However the drug enters the system, most drugs remain active in the body for several hours.

Using, Misusing, and Abusing Drugs

Although drug abuse usually is referred to in connection with illicit psychoactive drugs, many people abuse and misuse prescription and OTC medications. **Drug misuse** involves the use of a drug for a purpose for which it was not intended. For example, taking a friend's high-powered prescription painkiller for your headache is a misuse of that drug. This is not too far removed from **drug abuse,** the excessive use of any drug, and may result in serious harm.

The misuse and abuse of any drug may lead to addiction. Both risks and benefits are involved in the use of any chemical substance. Intelligent decision making requires a clearheaded evaluation of these risks and benefits.

 what do you THINK?

What are some situations in which students misuse drugs? ▪ Other than alcohol, which drugs (prescription or OTC) do students tend to abuse while they are in college?

Prescription Drugs

Even though prescription drugs are administered under medical supervision, the wise consumer still takes precautions. Hazards and complications arising from the use of prescription drugs are common.

suppositories Mixtures of drugs and a waxy medium designed to melt at body temperature that are inserted into the anus or vagina.

drug misuse The use of a drug for a purpose for which it was not intended.

drug abuse Excessive use of a drug.

antibiotics Prescription drugs designed to fight bacterial infection.

central nervous system depressants Sedative or hypnotic medications commonly used to treat anxiety.

benzodiazepines Central nervous system depressants that relieve anxiety, relax the body, and induce sleep.

antidepressants Prescription drugs used to treat clinically diagnosed depression.

Today, consumers have a variety of resources available to them for determining risks of various prescription medicines and can make educated decisions about whether or not to take a certain drug. One of the best resources is the U.S. Food and Drug Administration (FDA) Center for Drug Evaluation and Research website (www.fda.gov/cder). This special consumer section of the FDA provides current information on risks and benefits of prescription drugs. Being knowledgeable about what you are taking or thinking about taking is a sound strategy to ensure safety. (See the **Consumer Health** box for more on prescription drug safety issues.)

Types of Prescription Drugs

Antibiotics are drugs used to fight bacterial infection. Bacterial infections continue to be among the most common serious diseases throughout the world, but the vast majority can be cured with antibiotics. There are close to 100 different antibiotics, which may be dispensed by intramuscular injection or in tablet or capsule form. Some, called *broad-spectrum antibiotics,* are designed to control disease caused by a number of bacterial species. These medications may also kill off helpful bacteria in the body, thus triggering secondary infections. For example, some vaginal infections are related to long-term use of antibiotics. It is important to follow your health care provider's directions when taking antibiotics and to use them only when you have a bacterial infection. The misuse of antibiotics has led to a dangerous increase in drug-resistant bacteria in recent years.

Central nervous system depressants are sedative or hypnotic medications commonly used to treat anxiety. The two main types of drugs in this group are **benzodiazepines** (such as Valium, Ativan, and Xanax), and *barbiturates* (including Amytal and Seconal). The benzodiazepines are the most widely used drug in this category, most commonly prescribed for tension, muscular strain, sleep problems, anxiety, panic attacks, and alcohol withdrawal. They differ widely in their mechanism of action, absorption rate, and metabolism, but all produce similar intoxication and withdrawal symptoms. Benzodiazepine sleeping pills have largely replaced barbiturates, which were used medically in the past for relieving tension and inducing relaxation and sleep.

All sedative or hypnotic drugs can produce physical and psychological dependence in several weeks. A complication specific to sedatives is cross-tolerance, which occurs when users develop tolerance for one sedative or become dependent on it and develop tolerance for others as well. Withdrawal from sedative or hypnotic drugs may range from mild discomfort to severe symptoms, depending on the degree of dependence. A major public health issue is whether or not persons using benzodiazepines have an increased risk of cognitive decline and dementia. Ongoing research is investigating this possible link.[13]

Antidepressants are medications typically used to treat major depression, although occasionally they are used for other forms of depression that resist conventional therapy. There are several groups of antidepressant medications

IMPROVING THE SAFETY OF PRESCRIPTION AND OVER-THE-COUNTER DRUGS

In 1993, the Food and Drug Administration (FDA) changed its policies to speed the approval process of new drugs. These changes were made for humanitarian reasons, in response to activists seeking rapid approval of experimental drugs that offered at least a ray of hope to AIDS patients who otherwise faced certain death. The "accelerated development/review" process was seen as a way to offer drugs that might be a significant improvement over existing treatments or that could benefit people with life-threatening illnesses for which no treatment currently exists.

Should I be concerned about the safety of prescription drugs?

Hundreds of new drugs have been approved since then. Of that number, a handful have been withdrawn after reports of deaths and severe side effects. Two examples are the prescription drugs Bextra and Lotronex. Bextra, a drug widely used for treating arthritis pain, was taken off the market after a large-scale study revealed a series of cardiovascular risks associated with it, including heart attack and stroke, and an increased risk for a potentially fatal skin reaction. Lotronex, a drug for treating irritable bowel syndrome, was pulled from the market after being linked to five deaths, the removal of one patient's colon, and other bowel complications.

In response to these events and others, the Food and Drug Administration has launched a new drug safety initiative. It established the Drug Safety Oversight Board to oversee safety issues, consult with medical experts and consumer groups, and provide new information on medication risks and benefits to consumers and health care providers. The FDA has also developed new and improved communication channels to the general public on drug safety information.

New communication channels include the following:

- *The Drug Watch Web Page.* This page includes emerging information, for both previously and newly approved drugs, about possible serious side effects or other safety risks and how risks can be avoided. The agency will enhance access to this information and call for assistance in prioritizing and further evaluating potential adverse health concerns.

- *Healthcare Professional Information Sheets.* These information sheets for health care professionals contain the most important new information for safe use, including known and potential safety issues based on reports of adverse events, new information that may affect prescribing of the drug, and its approved indications and benefits.

- *Patient Information Sheets.* These are one-page information sheets for patients in a consumer-friendly format for all products on Drug Watch. Information includes new safety information as well as basic information about how to use the drug.

Sources: U.S. Food and Drug Administration, "The FDA Speeds Medical Treatment for Serious Diseases," March-April 2006, www.fda.gov/cder; U.S. Food and Drug Administration, "Accelerated Development Review," 2006. www.fda.gov/cder/handbook; U.S. Department of Health and Human Services, "News Release: Reforms Will Improve Oversight and Openness at FDA," February 15, 2005, www.fda.gov/cder/drugsafety.htm.

---

approved for use in the United States. Prozac, Zoloft, and Paxil are well-known examples. Over the past decade, the use of antidepressant drugs in the United States has increased by 48 percent overall, and by 124 percent in children.[14]

Generic Drugs

Generic drugs, medications sold under a chemical name rather than under a brand name, have gained popularity in recent years. They contain the same active ingredients as brand-name drugs but are less expensive. If your doctor prescribes a drug, always ask whether a generic equivalent exists and whether it would be safe and effective for you to try. Not all drugs are available as generics.

Be aware, though, that there is some controversy about the effectiveness of generic drugs because substitutions sometimes are made in minor ingredients that can affect the way the drug is absorbed, potentially causing discomfort or even allergic reactions in some users. Always note any reactions you have to medications, and tell your doctor about them.

Over-the-Counter Drugs

Over-the-counter (OTC) drugs are nonprescription substances used in the course of self-diagnosis and self-medication. More than one-third of the time, people treat their routine health problems with OTC medications. In fact, American consumers spend billions of dollars yearly on OTC preparations for relief of everything from runny noses to ingrown toenails. There are 40,000 OTC drugs and more than 300,000 brand names for them.

generic drugs Medications marketed by chemical name rather than brand name.

"PHARMING" PARTIES: THE NEW DRUG ABUSE VENUE

Several teens are sitting at the kitchen table listening to one describe how she obtained OxyContin from the medicine chest at home. "It was left over," she says, "from my sister's wisdom teeth surgery." Says another, "I'll give you some of this Ritalin for some of that painkiller."

This is not an ordinary party—it's a pharming party, a get-together arranged so young adults can barter for their favorite prescription drugs. Pharming parties represent a growing trend among teenaged drug abusers and college students. According to a report by the National Center on Addiction and Substance Abuse (CASA) at Columbia University, the use of illegal substances such as cocaine, heroin, and other illegal drugs on college campuses had increased by 52 percent in 2005 over 1993 rates. (Marijuana use was not included in the study.) CASA findings during this time also show that the proportion of students abusing prescription drugs had significantly increased:

- 343 percent for opiods such as Percocet, Vicodin and OxyContin
- 93 percent for abuse of stimulants such as Ritalin and Adderall
- 450 percent for tranquilizers such as Xanax and Valium

- 225 percent for sedatives such as Nembutal and Seconal

Unfortunately, prescription drugs are often easier to obtain than illegal ones. Some teenagers and college students come by them legitimately (such as those who have a prescription for an amphetamine-based prescription medication) but trade them for others, such as painkillers, that hold more appeal because of their potent high. Others order from shady Internet pharmacies where prescriptions are not always required. Some students may fake or exaggerate symptoms to persuade physicians to write prescriptions.

Studies also find that many who are abusing prescription medications are also abusing illegal drugs at the same time. According to another study, a national survey on drug use called "Monitoring the Future," students who obtained prescription painkillers from peers reported higher levels of binge drinking and marijuana abuse than nonabusers or those who received painkillers from family. This poses another set of problems, because alcohol in combination with any one of these medications can make a dangerous cocktail.

Because abuse of prescription medicines is a growing and not highly recognized problem, many people do not realize the dangers. "My friend told me to save the painkillers for when I'm drinking or getting high," says a 17-year-old with a chuckle. She doesn't think of herself as an addict, but she recognizes the signs of addiction among her friends: "I know a lot of people who live by pills. Pills can dictate your life—I have seen it." Painkillers such as OxyContin, Percocet, Percodan, Vicodin, and others are highly addictive if taken for prolonged periods of time. OxyContin, in particular, can be a very addictive and dangerous narcotic when abused. Users may take the pill orally, snort it, or dissolve it in a solution they can inject. The "rush" is similar to that of heroin. Chronic use can also result in increasing tolerance, and more of the drug is needed to achieve the desired effect. Occasional pharming parties can quickly spiral into an out-of-control addiction.

Sources: Excerpt from C. Banta, "Trading for a High," *Time,* August 1, 2005; L. D Johnston et al., *Monitoring the Future: National Survey Results on Drug Use, 1975–2004: Volume II, College Students and Adults,* NIH publication no. 05-5727 (Bethesda, MD: National Institute on Drug Abuse, 2005); L. Whitten, "Studies Identify Factors Surrounding Rise in Abuse of Prescription Drugs by College Students," *NIDA Notes* 20, no. 4, 2006; The National Center on Addiction and Substance Abuse at Columbia University, "Wasting the Best and the Brightest," March 2007, www.casacolumbia.org/supportcasa/item.asp?cID=12&PID=155.

Most OTC drugs are manufactured from a basic group of 1,000 chemicals. The many different products available to us are produced by combining as few as two and as many as ten substances.

How Prescription Drugs Become Over-the-Counter Drugs

The FDA regularly reviews prescription drugs to evaluate how suitable they would be as OTC products. For a drug to be switched from prescription to OTC status, it must meet the following criteria.

1. The drug has been marketed as a prescription medication for at least 3 years.

2. The use of the drug has been relatively high during the time it was available as a prescription drug.

3. Adverse drug reactions are not alarming, and the frequency of side effects has not increased during the time it was available to the public.

Since this policy has been in effect, the FDA has moved hundreds of drugs to OTC status. Some examples are ibuprofen, Claritin, and Prilosec. Many more prescription drugs are currently being considered for OTC status.

Types of Over-the-Counter Drugs

The FDA has categorized 26 types of OTC preparations. Those most commonly used are analgesics; cold, cough, allergy, and asthma relievers; stimulants; sleeping aids and relaxants; and dieting aids.

Analgesics
More than 50 million Americans experience chronic pain. Is it any wonder that we spend more than $2 billion annually on **analgesics** (pain relievers), the largest sales category of OTC drugs in the United States? These pain relievers come in several forms. Aspirin, acetaminophen (Tylenol, Pamprin, Panadol), ibuprofen (Advil, Motrin, Nuprin), and ibuprofen-like drugs such as naproxen (Aleve) and ketoprofen (Orudis) are the most common.

Most pain relievers work at receptor sites by interrupting pain signals. Some are categorized as *NSAIDs* (non-steroidal anti-inflammatory drugs), also called **prostaglandin inhibitors.** Prostaglandins are chemicals released by the body in response to pain. Prostaglandin inhibitors restrain the release of prostaglandins and thus reduce the pain. Common NSAIDs include ibuprofen, naproxen, and aspirin.

Besides relieving pain, aspirin lowers fever by increasing the flow of blood to the skin surface, which causes sweating and cools the body. Aspirin long has been used to reduce the inflammation and swelling associated with arthritis. It is widely accepted that a low dose of aspirin has anticoagulant effects (that is, it interferes with blood clotting) and can reduce the risk of heart attack and stroke.

Possible side effects for many NSAIDs include allergic reactions, ringing in the ears, stomach bleeding, and ulcers. Combining aspirin with alcohol can compound aspirin's gastric irritant properties. As with all drugs, read the labels. Some analgesic labels caution against driving or operating heavy machinery when using the drug, and most warn that analgesics should not be taken with alcohol.

Research has also linked aspirin to a potentially fatal condition called Reye's syndrome. Children, teenagers, and young adults (up to age 19) who are treated with aspirin while recovering from the flu or chickenpox are at risk for developing this syndrome. Aspirin substitutes are recommended for people in these age groups.

Acetaminophen is an aspirin substitute found in Tylenol and related medications. Like aspirin, acetaminophen is an effective analgesic and antipyretic (fever-reducing drug). However, it does not relieve inflamed or swollen joints. The side effects associated with acetaminophen generally are minimal, though overdose can cause liver damage. Both aspirin and acetaminophen are on the government's lists of medications that are **Generally Recognized as Safe (GRAS)** and **Generally Recognized as Effective (GRAE).**

TABLE 7.1 Types of Over-the-Counter Cold, Cough, and Allergy Relievers

- **Expectorants.** These drugs loosen phlegm, which allows the user to cough it up and clear congested respiratory passages. GRAS and GRAE reviewers question the effectiveness of many expectorants. When combined with other medications, particularly among those used by frail or very ill individuals, safety issues may arise.

- **Antitussives.** These OTC drugs calm or curtail the cough reflex. They are most effective when the cough is dry (does not produce phlegm). Oral codeine, dextromethorphan, and diphenhydramine are the most common antitussives that are on both the GRAE and GRAS lists.

- **Antihistamines.** These central nervous system depressants dry runny noses, clear postnasal drip, clear sinus congestion, and reduce tears.

- **Decongestants.** These remedies reduce nasal stuffiness due to colds.

- **Anticholinergics.** These substances often are added to cold preparations to reduce nasal secretions and tears. None of the preparations tested have been found to be GRAE or GRAS. Some cold compounds contain alcohol in concentrations that may exceed 40 percent.

Cold, Cough, Allergy, and Asthma Relievers
Most cold, cough, allergy, and asthma relievers are designed to alleviate the discomforting symptoms associated with maladies of the upper respiratory tract. The operative word in this category is *reliever;* unfortunately, no drugs exist to cure the actual diseases. The drugs available provide only temporary relief until the sufferer's immune system prevails over the disease. **Table 7.1** describes the basic types of OTC cold, cough, and allergy relievers.

Sleeping Aids and Relaxants
A study by the World Health Organization, conducted in 15 health centers around the globe, found that 27 percent of patients reported difficulties with sleeping.[15] Many people routinely treat their insomnia with OTC sleep aids (such as Nytol, Sleep-Eze, and

---

analgesics Pain relievers.

prostaglandin inhibitors Drugs that inhibit the production and release of prostaglandins, hormone-like substances often associated with arthritis or menstrual pain. Also called *non-steroidal anti-inflammatory drugs (NSAIDs).*

Generally Recognized as Safe (GRAS) A list of drugs generally recognized as safe, which seldom cause side effects when used properly.

Generally Recognized as Effective (GRAE) A list of drugs generally recognized as effective, which work for their intended purpose when used properly.

Sominex) that are advertised as providing "safe and restful" sleep. These drugs induce the drowsy feelings that precede sleep. The principal ingredient in OTC sleeping aids is an antihistamine called pyrilamine maleate. Chronic reliance on sleeping aids may lead to addiction; people accustomed to using these products may eventually find it impossible to sleep without them.

Dieting Aids
In the United States, there is a $200 million market for dieting aids. Some of these drugs (e.g., Acutrim, Dexatrim) are advertised as "appetite suppressants." The FDA has pulled several appetite suppressants off the market because their active ingredient was phenylpropanolamine (PPA), which has been linked to increased risk of stroke.[16] More recently, the FDA has also prohibited the sale of ephedra, a naturally occurring substance often billed as a diet aid or sports and energy enhancement drug. Ephedra use has been linked to heart attack, stroke, and death.[17]

Estimates show that when taken as recommended, even the best OTC dieting aids significantly reduce appetite in fewer than 30 percent of users, and tolerance occurs in only 1 to 3 days of use. Manufacturers of appetite suppressants often include a written 1,200-calorie diet to complement their drug. However, most people who limit themselves to 1,200 calories per day will lose weight—without any help from appetite suppressants. Clearly, these products have no real value in treating obesity.

Some people rely on **laxatives** and **diuretics** ("water pills") to lose weight. Frequent use of laxatives disrupts the body's natural elimination patterns and may cause constipation or even *obstipation* (inability to have a bowel movement). The use of laxatives to produce weight loss has unspectacular results and robs the body of needed fluids, salts, and minerals.

Taking diuretics to lose weight is also dangerous. Not only will the user gain the weight back upon drinking fluids, but diuretic use also may contribute to dangerous chemical imbalances. The potassium and sodium eliminated by diuretics play important roles in maintaining electrolyte balance. Depletion of these vital minerals can cause weakness, dizziness, fatigue, and sometimes death.

---

laxatives Medications used to soften stool and relieve constipation.

diuretics Drugs that increase the excretion of urine from the body.

polydrug use Use of multiple medications or illicit drugs simultaneously.

synergism Interaction of two or more drugs that produces more profound effects than would be expected if the drugs were taken separately. Also known as *potentiation*.

Rules for Proper Use of Over-the-Counter Drugs

Despite a common belief that OTC products are safe and effective, indiscriminate use and abuse can occur with these drugs as with all others. For example, people who frequently drop medication into their eyes to "get the red out" or pop antacids after every meal are likely to become addicted. Many people also experience adverse side effects because they ignore the warnings on the labels or simply do not read them.

The FDA has developed a standard label that appears on most OTC products (**Figure 7.2**). It provides directions for use, warnings, and other useful information. (Diet supplements, which are regulated as food products, have their own label that includes a Supplement Facts panel.)

OTC medications are far more powerful than ever before, and the science behind them is stronger as well. Therefore, as with any type of medication, do your homework. Observe the following rules when taking nonprescription drugs.

1. Always know what you are taking. Identify the active ingredients in the product.

2. Know the effects, both desired and undesired, of each active ingredient.

3. Read the warnings and cautions.

4. Don't use anything for more than 1 or 2 weeks.

5. Be particularly cautious if you are also taking prescription drugs because the drugs may interact.

6. If you have questions, ask your pharmacist.

7. *If you don't need it, don't take it!*

Drug Interactions

Sharing medications, using expired prescriptions, taking higher doses than recommended, or using medications as a substitute for dealing with personal problems may result in serious health consequences. **Polydrug use,** taking several medications (including vitamins) or illegal drugs simultaneously, also can lead to dangerous health problems associated with drug interactions. The most hazardous interactions are synergism, antagonism, inhibition, intolerance, and cross-tolerance. Hazardous interactions may also occur between drugs and foods and beverages. Talk with your doctor about possible interactions before taking any medicines.

Synergism, also known as *potentiation,* is an interaction of two or more drugs in which the effects of the individual drugs are multiplied beyond what normally would be expected if they were taken alone. You might think of synergism as $2 + 2 = 10$.

A synergistic reaction can be very dangerous. Prescription and OTC medications carry labels warning the user not to combine them with certain other drugs or with alcohol. You should always verify any possible drug interactions before

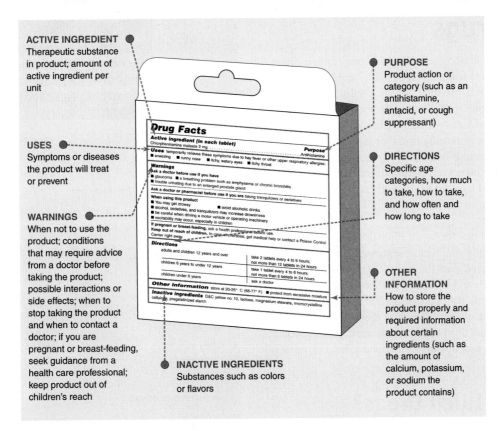

ACTIVE INGREDIENT
Therapeutic substance in product; amount of active ingredient per unit

USES
Symptoms or diseases the product will treat or prevent

WARNINGS
When not to use the product; conditions that may require advice from a doctor before taking the product; possible interactions or side effects; when to stop taking the product and when to contact a doctor; if you are pregnant or breast-feeding, seek guidance from a health care professional; keep product out of children's reach

INACTIVE INGREDIENTS
Substances such as colors or flavors

PURPOSE
Product action or category (such as an antihistamine, antacid, or cough suppressant)

DIRECTIONS
Specific age categories, how much to take, how to take, and how often and how long to take

OTHER INFORMATION
How to store the product properly and required information about certain ingredients (such as the amount of calcium, potassium, or sodium the product contains)

Drug Facts

Active ingredient (in each tablet)
Chlorpheniramine maleate 2 mg .... **Purpose**
.... Antihistamine

Uses temporarily relieves these symptoms due to hay fever or other upper respiratory allergies:
■ sneezing ■ runny nose ■ itchy, watery eyes ■ itchy throat

Warnings
Ask a doctor before use if you have
■ glaucoma ■ a breathing problem such as emphysema or chronic bronchitis
■ trouble urinating due to an enlarged prostate gland
Ask a doctor or pharmacist before use if you are taking tranquilizers or sedatives
When using this product
■ You may get drowsy ■ avoid alcoholic drinks
■ alcohol, sedatives, and tranquilizers may increase drowsiness
■ be careful when driving a motor vehicle or operating machinery
■ excitability may occur, especially in children
If pregnant or breast-feeding, ask a health professional before use.
Keep out of reach of children. In case of overdose, get medical help or contact a Poison Control Center right away.

Directions

adults and children 12 years and over	take 2 tablets every 4 to 6 hours; not more than 12 tablets in 24 hours
children 6 years to under 12 years	take 1 tablet every 4 to 6 hours; not more than 6 tablets in 24 hours
children under 6 years	ask a doctor

Other information store at 20-25° C (68-77° F) ■ protect from excessive moisture
Inactive ingredients D&C yellow no. 10, lactose, magnesium stearate, microcrystalline cellulose, pregelatinized starch

FIGURE 7.2 The Over-the-Counter Drug Label

Source: From "The New Over-the-Counter Medicine Label," 2002. © 2002 Consumer Health Care Products. Reprinted by permission.

using a prescribed or OTC drug. Pharmacists, physicians, drug information centers, or community drug education centers can answer your questions. Even if one of the drugs in question is illegal, you still should attempt to determine the dangers involved in combining it with other drugs. Health care professionals are legally bound to maintain confidentiality even when they know that a client is using illegal substances.

Antagonism, although usually less serious than synergism, can also produce unwanted and unpleasant effects. In an antagonistic reaction, drugs work at the same receptor site so that one blocks the action of the other. The blocking drug occupies the receptor site and prevents the other substance from attaching, thus altering its absorption and action.

With **inhibition,** the effects of one drug are eliminated or reduced by the presence of another drug at the receptor site. One common inhibitory reaction occurs between antacid tablets and aspirin. The antacid inhibits the absorption of aspirin and makes it less effective as a pain reliever. Other inhibitory reactions occur between alcohol and antibiotics and between antibiotics and contraceptive pills.

Intolerance occurs when drugs combine in the body to produce extremely uncomfortable reactions. The drug Antabuse, used to help alcoholics give up alcohol, works by

producing this type of interaction. It binds liver enzymes (the chemicals the liver produces to break down alcohol), making it impossible for the body to metabolize alcohol. As a result, an Antabuse user who drinks alcohol experiences nausea, vomiting, and, occasionally, fever.

Cross-tolerance occurs when a person develops a physiological tolerance to one drug and shows a similar tolerance to selected other drugs as a result. Taking one drug may actually increase the body's tolerance to another substance. For example, cross-tolerance can develop between alcohol and barbiturates, two depressant drugs.

antagonism A type of drug interaction in which two or more drugs work at the same receptor site, so that one blocks the action of the other.

inhibition A type of drug interaction in which the effects of one drug are eliminated or reduced by the presence of another drug at the receptor site.

intolerance A type of drug interaction in which two or more drugs produce extremely uncomfortable symptoms.

cross-tolerance Development of a tolerance to one drug that reduces the effects of another, similar drug.

Illicit Drugs

Whereas some people become addicted to prescription drugs and painkillers, others use illicit drugs. The problem of illicit drug use touches us all. We may use illicit substances ourselves, watch someone we love struggle with drug abuse, or become the victim of a drug-related crime. At the very least, we are forced to pay increasing taxes for law enforcement and drug rehabilitation. When our co-workers use drugs, the effectiveness of our own work is diminished. If the car we drive was assembled by drug-using workers at the plant, we are in danger. A drug-using bus driver, train engineer, or pilot jeopardizes our safety.

The good news is that the use of illicit drugs has declined significantly in recent years in most segments of society. Use of most drugs increased from the early 1970s to the late 1970s, peaked between 1979 and 1986, and declined until 1992, from which point it has not changed. In 2003, an estimated 19.2 million Americans were illicit drug users, about three-quarters the 1979 peak level of 25 million users. Among youth, however, illicit drug use, notably of marijuana, has been rising in recent years.[18]

Who Uses Illicit Drugs?

Many of us have stereotypes in our minds of who uses illicit drugs, but it is difficult to generalize. Illicit drug users span all age groups, ethnicities, occupations, and socioeconomic groups. No matter the group, illicit drug use has a devastating effect on users and their families in the United States and many other countries.

After more than a decade of declining use on American college campuses, illicit drugs have reappeared. In 2004, the number of college students nationwide who had tried any drug stood at almost 52 percent; over a third had smoked pot in the past year, and 20 percent had done so in the past month. Daily use of marijuana was at its highest point since 1989.[19] Cocaine use is down sharply, but LSD use has more than doubled. These figures vary from school to school.

Patterns of drug use vary only slightly by age. For example, a nationwide study of college campuses reported that approximately 33.3 percent of students had tried marijuana during the previous year (**Table 7.2**), and that percentage is nearly the same as the percentage of all Americans under the age of 45 who used marijuana during that time: 33.7 percent. Approximately 5.7 percent of college students surveyed reported using cocaine in the past year, whereas 8.5 percent of all Americans under age 45 said they had used cocaine during the previous year.[20]

Most antidrug programs have not been effective because they have focused on only one aspect of drug abuse, rather than examining all factors that contribute to the problem. The pressures to take drugs are often tremendous, and the reasons for using them are complex. People who develop drug problems generally begin with the belief that they can control their drug use. Initially, they often view taking drugs as a fun and manageable pastime. Peer influence is a strong motivator, espe-

cially among adolescents, who greatly fear not being accepted as part of the group. Other people use drugs to cope with feelings of worthlessness and despair or to battle depression and anxiety. Because most illegal drugs produce physical and psychological dependence, it is unrealistic to think that a person can use them regularly without becoming addicted. Consider whether you are controlled by drugs or a drug user by answering the questions in the **Assess Yourself** box on page 202.

TABLE 7.2	Annual Prevalence of Use for Various Types of Drugs, 2005: Full-Time College Students versus Respondents 1–4 Years beyond High School

	Full-Time College (%)	Others (%)
Any illicit drug	36.6	39.6
Any illicit drug other than marijuana	18.5	23.4
Marijuana	33.3	34.6
Inhalants	1.8	1.8
Hallucinogens	5.0	7.3
LSD	0.7	2.1
Cocaine	5.7	9.0
Crack	0.8	2.9
MDMA (Ecstasy)	2.9	4.9
Heroin	0.3	1.1
Other narcotics	8.4	12.7
OxyContin	2.1	6.2
Vicodin	9.6	14.0
Amphetamines, adjusted	6.7	7.2
Ritalin	4.2	4.3
Methamphetamine	1.7	4.9
Ice	1.4	3.1
Sedatives (barbiturates)	3.9	6.9
Tranquilizers	6.4	9.3
Rohypnol	0.1	0.6
GHB	0.4	0.6
Ketamine	0.5	1.5
Alcohol	83.0	76.9
Cigarettes	36.0	45.2
Approximate weighted N=	*1,360*	*850*

Source: L. D. Johnston et al., *Monitoring the Future: National Survey Results on Drug Use, 1975–2005: Volume II, College Students and Adults* (Bethesda, MD: National Institute on Drug Abuse, 2006), 233.

what do you THINK?

What factors do you believe influence illicit drug use in the United States? ■ What is the attitude toward drug use on your campus? ■ Are some substances considered more acceptable than others? ■ Is drug use considered more acceptable at certain times or occasions?

Controlled Substances

Drugs are classified into five schedules (categories) based on their potential for abuse, their medical uses, and accepted standards of safe use **(Table 7.3)**. Schedule I drugs, those with the highest potential for abuse, are considered to have no valid medical uses. Although Schedule II, III, IV, and V drugs have known and accepted medical applications, many of them present serious threats to health when abused or misused. Penalties for illegal use are tied to the drugs' schedule level.

Hundreds of illegal drugs exist. For general purposes, they can be divided into seven representative categories: *stimulants, depressants, hallucinogens/psychedelics, designer drugs, inhalants,* and *steroids.*

Stimulants

Cocaine A white crystalline powder derived from the leaves of the South American coca shrub (not related to cocoa plants), **cocaine** ("coke") has been described as one of the most powerful naturally occurring stimulants.

Methods of Cocaine Use Cocaine can be taken in several ways. The powdered form of the drug is "snorted" through the nose. When cocaine is snorted, it can damage mucous membranes in the nose and cause sinusitis. It can destroy the user's sense of smell, and occasionally it even eats a hole through the septum.

Smoking (known as freebasing) and intravenous injections are even more dangerous means of taking cocaine. Freebasing has become more popular than injecting in recent years because people fear contracting diseases such as AIDS and hepatitis by sharing contaminated needles. But freebasing involves other dangers. Because the volatile mixes it requires are very explosive, some people have been killed or seriously burned. Smoking cocaine can also cause lung and liver damage.

Many cocaine users still occasionally "shoot up," a method that introduces large amounts into the body rapidly. Within seconds, a sense of euphoria sets in. This intense high lasts for 15 to 20 minutes, and then the user heads into a "crash." To prevent the unpleasant effects of the crash, users must shoot up frequently, which can severely damage veins. Injecting users place themselves at risk not only for AIDS and hepatitis, but also for skin infections, inflamed arteries, and infection of the lining of the heart.

Physical Effects of Cocaine The effects of cocaine are felt rapidly. Snorted cocaine enters the bloodstream through the lungs in less than 1 minute and reaches the brain in less than 3 minutes. When cocaine binds at its receptor sites in the central nervous system, it produces intense pleasure. The euphoria quickly abates, however, and the desire to regain the pleasurable feelings makes the user want more cocaine **(Figure 7.3)**.

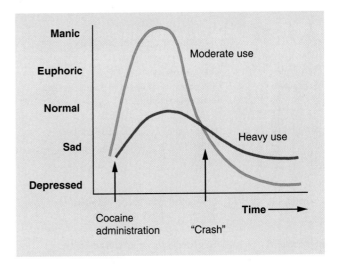

FIGURE 7.3 Ups and Downs of a Typical Dose of Cocaine

Source: From Charles F. Levinthal, *Drugs, Behavior, and Modern Society,* 5th ed. Published by Allyn & Bacon, Boston, MA. Copyright © 2007 by Pearson Education. Reprinted by permission of the publisher.

Cocaine is both an anesthetic and a central nervous system stimulant. In tiny doses, it can slow heart rate. In larger doses, the physical effects are dramatic: increased heart rate and blood pressure, loss of appetite that can lead to dramatic weight loss, convulsions, muscle twitching, irregular heartbeat, and even eventual death due to overdose. Other effects of cocaine include temporary relief of depression, decreased fatigue, talkativeness, increased alertness, and heightened self-confidence. However, as the dose increases, users become irritable and apprehensive, and their behavior may turn paranoid or violent.

Types of Cocaine **Freebase** is a form of cocaine that is more powerful and costly than powder or crack (see next section) and is taken by smoking. Street cocaine (cocaine hydrochloride) is converted to pure base by using ether to remove the hydrochloride salt and many of the "cutting agents" used to dilute the drug. This volatile chemical mixture is very dangerous and can cause severe burns. (The use of ether, which is flammable, adds to the danger.) The end product, freebase, is smoked through a water pipe.

Freebase cocaine reaches the brain within seconds and produces a quick, intense high that disappears quickly, leaving an intense craving for more. Freebasers typically increase the amount and frequency of the dose, often become severely addicted, and experience serious health problems.

cocaine A powerful stimulant drug made from the leaves of the South American coca shrub.

freebase The most powerful distillate of cocaine.

TABLE 7.3   How Drugs are Scheduled

Schedule	Characteristics	Examples
Schedule I	High potential for abuse and addiction; no accepted medical use	Heroin LSD Marijuana
Schedule II	High potential for abuse and addiction; restricted medical use	Cocaine Amphetamine (DMA, STP) Methadone OxyContin Ritalin
Schedule III	Some potential for abuse and addiction; currently accepted medical use	Anabolic steroids Nalorphine Vicodin
Schedule IV	Low potential for abuse and addiction; currently accepted medical use	Xanax Minor tranquilizers
Schedule V	Lowest potential for abuse; accepted medical use	Robitussin AC OTC preparations

Source: National Institute on Drug Abuse, "Commonly Abused Drugs," 2007, www.drugabuse.gov/DrugPages/DrugsofAbuse.html.

Side effects of freebasing cocaine include weight loss, increased heart rate and blood pressure, depression, paranoia, and hallucinations. Freebase is an extremely dangerous drug and is responsible for a large number of cocaine-related hospital emergency-room visits and deaths.

The street name **crack** is given to freebase cocaine processed from cocaine hydrochloride by using ammonia or sodium bicarbonate (baking soda), water, and heat to remove the hydrochloride. The mixture (90 percent pure cocaine) is then dried. The soapy-looking substance that results can be broken into "rocks" and smoked. These rocks are approximately five times as strong as cocaine. Crack gets its name from the popping noises it makes when burned. A recent study found that 2 percent of college students reported using crack during their lives.[21]

Because crack is such a pure drug, it takes much less time to achieve the desired high. One puff of a pebble-sized rock produces an intense high that lasts for approximately 20 minutes. The user can usually get three or four hits off a rock before it is used up. Crack is typically sold in small vials, folding papers, or heavy tinfoil containing two or three rocks.

A crack user can become addicted quickly. Addiction is accelerated by the speed at which crack is absorbed through the lungs (it hits the brain within seconds) and by the intensity of the high.

Cocaine-Affected Babies Because cocaine rapidly crosses the placenta (as virtually all drugs do), the fetus is vulnerable when a pregnant woman uses cocaine. It is estimated that 2.4 to 3.5 percent of pregnant women between the ages of 12 and 34 abuse cocaine. It is difficult to gauge how many newborns have been exposed to cocaine because pregnant users are reluctant to discuss their drug habit with health care providers for fear of prosecution. The most threatening problem during pregnancy is the increased risk of a miscarriage.

crack   A distillate of powdered cocaine that comes in small, hard "chips" or "rocks"; not the same as rock cocaine.

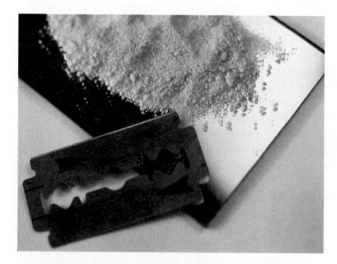

Although cocaine abuse has declined from its peak in the 1980s, it continues to be a commonly abused illicit drug today.

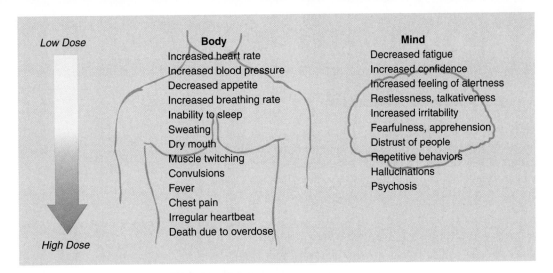

FIGURE 7.4 Effects of Amphetamines on the Body and Mind

Fetuses exposed to cocaine in the womb are more likely to have a small head, premature delivery, reduced birth weight, increased irritability, and subtle learning and cognitive deficits. Research suggests that a significant number of these children develop problems with learning and language skills that require remedial attention.[22] It is critical to identify these children early so they can receive immediate intervention. For both financial and humane reasons, prenatal care and education programs for mothers at risk should be considered a priority for state and local government.

Cocaine Addiction and Society Cocaine addicts often suffer both physiological damage and serious disruption in lifestyle, including loss of employment and self-esteem. It is estimated that the annual cost of cocaine addiction in the United States exceeds $3.8 billion. However, there is no way to measure the cost in wasted lives. In 2005, 33.7 million Americans aged 12 and over reported lifetime use of cocaine, and 7.9 million reported using crack. About 5.5 million reported annual use of cocaine, and 1.4 million reported using crack. An estimated 2.4 million Americans reported current use of cocaine, 682,000 of whom reported using crack. There were an estimated 872,000 new users of cocaine in 2005 (approximately 2,400 per day), and most were aged 18 or older, although the average age of first use was approximately 20 years.[23]

Cocaine has been called unpredictable by drug experts, deadly by coroners, dangerous by former users, and disastrous by the media. Yet to date, there has been no successful weapon to combat its use in the United States. Apparently, the risks do not override users' desire to experience its effects.

Because cocaine is illegal, a complex underground network has developed to manufacture and sell the drug. Buyers may not always get the product they think they are purchasing. Cocaine marketed for snorting may be only 60 percent pure. Usually, it is mixed, or "cut," with other white, powdery substances such as mannitol or sugar, though occasionally it is cut with arsenic or other cocaine-like powders that may themselves be highly dangerous.

Amphetamines The **amphetamines** include a large and varied group of synthetic agents that stimulate the central nervous system. Small doses of amphetamines improve alertness, lessen fatigue, and generally elevate mood. With repeated use, however, physical and psychological dependence develops. Sleep patterns are affected (insomnia); heart rate, breathing rate, and blood pressure increase; and restlessness, anxiety, appetite suppression, and vision problems are common **(Figure 7.4).** High doses over long time periods can produce hallucinations, delusions, and disorganized behavior.

Certain types of amphetamines are used for medicinal purposes. Drugs such as Ritalin and Adderall are used to treat children with attention deficit hyperactivity disorder. However, in recent years these drugs have taken the place of caffeine on college campuses, and many students misuse them to stay awake for all-night cramming sessions. In fact, Ritalin is on the Drug Enforcement Agency's top ten list of most often stolen prescription drugs. There is a false perception that these drugs improve academic performance. According to a recent national survey, over 4 percent of college students had used Ritalin in the past year.[24]

Methamphetamine An increasingly common form of amphetamine, **methamphetamine** (commonly called simply "meth") is a potent, long-acting, addictive drug that strongly

amphetamines A large and varied group of synthetic agents that stimulate the central nervous system.

methamphetamine (meth) A powerfully addictive drug that strongly activates certain areas of the brain and affects the central nervous system.

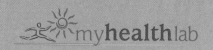
RECOGNIZING A DRUG PROBLEM

Fill out this assessment online at
www.aw-bc.com/myhealthlab or
www.aw-bc.com/donatelle.

ARE YOU CONTROLLED BY DRUGS?

How do you know whether you are chemically dependent? A dependent person can't stop using drugs. This abuse hurts the user and everyone around him or her. Take the following assessment; the more often you check yes, the more likely you have a problem.

	Yes	No
1. Do you use drugs to handle stress or escape from life's problems?	❑	❑
2. Have you unsuccessfully tried to cut down on or quit using your drug?	❑	❑
3. Have you ever been in trouble with the law or been arrested because of your drug use?	❑	❑
4. Do you think a party or social gathering isn't fun unless drugs are available?	❑	❑
5. Do you avoid people or places that do not support your usage?	❑	❑
6. Do you neglect your responsibilities because you'd rather use your drug?	❑	❑
7. Have your friends, family, or employer expressed concern about your drug use?	❑	❑
8. Do you do things under the influence of drugs that you would not normally do?	❑	❑
9. Have you seriously thought that you might have a chemical dependency problem?	❑	❑

ARE YOU CONTROLLED BY A DRUG USER?

Is your life controlled by a chemical abuser? Your love and care (codependence) may actually be enabling the person to continue the abuse, hurting you and others. Try this assessment; the more often you check yes, the more likely there's a problem.

	Yes	No
1. Do you often have to lie or cover up for the chemical abuser?	❑	❑
2. Do you spend time counseling the person about the problem?	❑	❑
3. Have you taken on additional financial or family responsibilities?	❑	❑
4. Do you feel that you have to control the chemical abuser's behavior?	❑	❑
5. At the office, have you done work or attended meetings for the abuser?	❑	❑
6. Do you often put your own needs and desires after the user's?	❑	❑
7. Do you spend time each day worrying about your situation?	❑	❑
8. Do you analyze your behavior to find clues to how it might affect the chemical abuser?	❑	❑
9. Do you feel powerless and at your wit's end about the abuser's problem?	❑	❑

Source: Reprinted by permission of Krames Communications, 1100 Grundy Lane, San Bruno, CA 94066-3030, www.krames.com.

activates the brain's reward center by producing a sense of euphoria. Meth can cause brain damage that impairs motor skills and cognitive functions, leads to psychosis, and increases risk for heart attack and stroke.

Methods of Methamphetamine Use Methamphetamine can be snorted, smoked, injected, or orally ingested. Depending on the method of use, the drug will affect the user in different ways. Users often experience tolerance immediately, making meth a highly addictive drug from the very first time it is used. When snorted, the effects can be felt in 3 to 5 minutes; if orally ingested, the user will experience effects within 15 to 20 minutes. The pleasurable effects of meth are typically an intense rush lasting only a few minutes when snorted; in contrast, smoking the drug can produce a high lasting over 8 hours.

MAKE it happen!

ASSESSMENT: The Assess Yourself activity describes signs of being controlled by drugs or by a drug user. Depending on your results, you may need to change certain behaviors that may be detrimental to your health.

MAKING A CHANGE: To change your behavior, you need to develop a plan. Follow these steps below and complete your Behavior Change Contract to take action.

1. Evaluate your behavior, and identify patterns and specific things you are doing. What can you change now? What can you change in the near future?

2. Select one pattern of behavior that you want to change.

3. Fill out the Behavior Change Contract found at the front of your book. It should include your long-term goals for change, your short-term goals, the rewards you'll give yourself for reaching these goals, potential obstacles along the way, and strategies for overcoming these obstacles. For each goal, list the small steps and specific actions that you will take.

4. Chart your progress in a journal. At the end of a week, consider how successful you were in following your plan. What helped you be successful? What made change more difficult? What will you do differently next week?

5. Revise your plan as needed. Are the short-term goals attainable? Are the rewards satisfying?

EXAMPLE: Tranh was surprised to find he had several yes answers to the self-assessment section about being controlled by a drug user. He realized that his girlfriend Kim's drug use was hurting their relationship and negatively affecting him. Kim smoked marijuana almost every day and took club drugs at least twice a month. Tranh often had to lie to Kim's employer if she was too incapacitated to go to work. Recently, she had been in a car accident after smoking pot for several hours, which damaged Tranh's car and increased his insurance rate. And whenever she went out for an evening, he worried that she was taking Ecstasy and would find herself in a compromising situation.

These worries, financial consequences, and pressure to lie all made Tranh resolve to take steps to make a change in his responses to Kim's behavior. His first step was to plan what he wanted to say to Kim about her drug use and how it affected both of them. He also started investigating drug counseling resources at school and in the community, both for Kim and for himself to help him cope with the issues raised by Kim's drug use. Finally, he began talking to Kim's friends, who, it turned out, also were concerned about her behavior. They worked together to develop strategies to help Kim and provide alternatives to her drug use; Tranh also felt less alone and more supported as soon as he started reaching out to his peers.

Physical Effects of Methamphetamine

As shown in Figure 7.4, smaller doses of methamphetamine increase physical activity and alertness and decrease appetite. However, the drug's effects quickly wear off, and the user seeks more. Long-term use of meth can cause severe dependence, psychosis, paranoia, aggression, weight loss, and stroke. Abusers often do not sleep or eat for days, as they continually inject up to 1 gram of the drug every 2 to 3 hours. A high state of irritability and agitation has been associated with violent behavior among some users.

Abuse of methamphetamine is an increasingly serious problem, especially in more rural areas of the United States, Hawaii, and the West Coast. In 2005, 4.5 percent of high school seniors reported using methamphetamine in their lifetime. Rates among adults are difficult to determine, but it is believed that over 12 million Americans have tried meth.[25] A possible contributing factor to the increasing rate of methamphetamine use that it is relatively easy to make. Methamphetamine is produced by "cookers" using

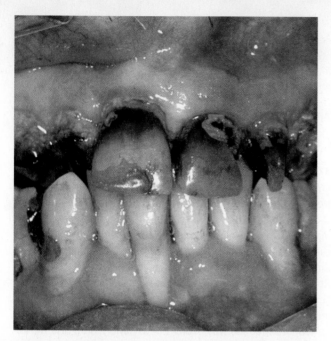

Methamphetamine users often damage their teeth beyond repair because of the toxic chemicals the substance. This condition is commonly referred to as "meth mouth."

recipes that often include common over-the-counter ingredients such as ephedrine and pseudoephedrine, which are found in cold and allergy medications. Many states have taken action by moving all cold and allergy medications behind the pharmacist's counter, so high-volume buyers can be carefully monitored. Additionally, laws have strengthened the penalties associated with manufacturing methamphetamine.

Ice is a potent form of methamphetamine that is imported primarily from Asia, particularly from South Korea and Taiwan. It is purer and more crystalline than the version manufactured in many large U.S. cities, and is odorless when smoked. Ice is usually smoked, like crack cocaine, and its effects can last for more than 12 hours.

Like other methamphetamines, the "down" side of this drug is devastating. Prolonged use can cause fatal lung and kidney damage as well as long-lasting psychological damage. In some instances, major psychological dysfunction can persist as long as 2½ years after last use.

ice   A potent, inexpensive form of methamphetamine that has long-lasting effects.

marijuana   Chopped leaves and flowers of the *Cannabis indica* or *Cannabis sativa* plants (hemp); a psychoactive stimulant that intensifies reactions to environmental stimuli.

tetrahydrocannabinol (THC)   The chemical name for the active ingredient in marijuana.

hashish   The sticky resin of the cannabis plant; it is high in THC.

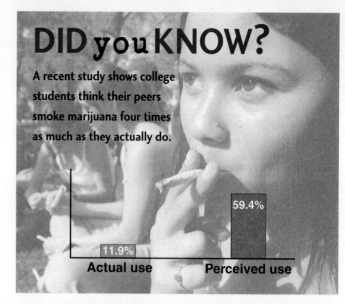
Marijuana

Although archaeological evidence documents the use of **marijuana** ("grass," "weed," "pot") as far back as 6,000 years, the drug did not become popular in the United States until the 1960s. Today marijuana is the most commonly used illicit drug in the United States. Nearly one of every three Americans over the age of 12 has tried marijuana at least once. Some 12 million Americans have used it; more than 1 million cannot control their use of it. Its use is also on the rise on college campuses, following the trend of increased use set by the general population.[26] However, students do not use marijuana as much as is sometimes perceived (see Did You Know?).

Physical Effects of Marijuana   Marijuana is derived from either the *Cannabis sativa* or *Cannabis indica* (hemp) plants. Current American-grown marijuana is a turbocharged version of the hippie weed of the late 1960s. **Tetrahydrocannabinol (THC)** is the psychoactive substance in marijuana and the key to determining how powerful a high it will produce. Today, most marijuana contains 5 percent THC; more potent forms of the drug can contain up to 27 percent THC but average 12 percent.[27]

Hashish, a potent cannabis preparation derived mainly from the thick, sticky resin of the plant, contains high concentrations of THC. Hash oil, a tarlike liquid produced by percolating a solvent such as ether through dried marijuana to extract the THC, may contain up to 300 mg of THC in a dose, or an average of 10 percent.[28]

Most of the time, marijuana is rolled into cigarettes (joints) or smoked in a pipe or water pipe (bong). Effects are generally felt within 10 to 30 minutes and usually wear off within 3 hours.

The most noticeable effect of THC is dilation of the blood vessels of the eyes, which produces the characteristic bloodshot eyes. Smokers of the drug also exhibit coughing, dry mouth and throat ("cotton mouth"), increased thirst and appetite, lowered blood pressure, and mild muscular weakness, primarily exhibited in drooping eyelids. Users can also experience severe anxiety, panic, paranoia, and psychosis.

Users of marijuana may have intensified reactions to various stimuli; colors, sounds, and the speed at which things move may seem altered. High doses of hashish may produce vivid visual hallucinations.

Effects of Chronic Marijuana Use

Because

> Are there any negative long-term effects from marijuana use?

marijuana is illegal in most parts of the United States and has been widely used only since the 1960s, long-term studies of its effects have been difficult to conduct. Also, studies conducted in the 1960s involved marijuana with THC levels constituting only a fraction of today's plant levels, so their results may not apply to the stronger forms available today.

Most current information about chronic marijuana use comes from countries such as Jamaica and Costa Rica, where the drug is not illegal. These studies of long-term users (for 10 or more years) indicate that marijuana causes lung damage comparable to that caused by tobacco smoking. Indeed, smoking a single joint may be as bad for the lungs as smoking three tobacco cigarettes. Inhaling marijuana transfers carbon monoxide to the bloodstream. Because the blood has a greater affinity for carbon monoxide than it does for oxygen, this action diminishes the oxygen-carrying capacity of the blood. The heart must work harder to pump the vital element to oxygen-starved tissues. Furthermore, the cannabis tar contains higher levels of carcinogens than does tobacco smoke. Smoking marijuana results in three times as much tar inhalation and retention in the respiratory tract than tobacco use.

Other risks associated with marijuana include suppression of the immune system, blood pressure changes, and impaired memory function. Recent studies suggest that pregnant women who smoke marijuana are at a higher risk for stillbirth or miscarriage and for delivering low–birth weight babies and babies with abnormalities of the nervous system. Babies born to marijuana smokers are five times more likely to have features similar to those exhibited by children with fetal alcohol syndrome.

Debates concerning the effects of marijuana on the reproductive system have yet to be resolved. Studies conducted in the mid-1970s suggested that marijuana inhibited testosterone (and thus sperm) production in men and caused chromosomal breakage in both ova and sperm. Subsequent research in these areas is inconclusive. The question of whether the high-level THC plants currently available will increase the risks associated with this drug is, as yet, unanswered.[29]

Marijuana and Medicine

Although recognized as a dangerous drug by the U.S. government, marijuana has several medical purposes. It helps control such side effects as the severe nausea and vomiting produced by chemotherapy, the chemical treatment for cancer. It improves appetite and forestalls the loss of lean muscle mass associated with AIDS-wasting syndrome. Marijuana reduces the muscle pain and spasticity caused by diseases such as multiple sclerosis. It also temporarily relieves the eye pressure of glaucoma, although it is unclear whether it is more effective than legal glaucoma drugs.[30] Marijuana's legal status for medicinal purposes continues to be hotly debated.

Marijuana and Driving

Marijuana use presents clear hazards for drivers of motor vehicles as well as others on the road. The drug substantially reduces a driver's ability to react and make quick decisions. In a study by the National Highway Traffic Safety Administration, a moderate dose of marijuana alone was shown to impair driving performance; however, the effects of even a low dose of marijuana combined with alcohol were markedly greater than for either drug alone. Studies show that approximately 6 to 11 percent of fatal accident victims test positive for THC.[31] In many of these cases, alcohol is detected as well. Perceptual and other performance deficits resulting from marijuana use may persist for some time after the high subsides. Users who attempt to drive, fly, or operate heavy machinery often fail to recognize their impairment.

what do you THINK?

Why do you think that marijuana is the most popular illicit drug on college campuses? ▪ How widespread is marijuana use at your school?

Opiates

Opiates cause drowsiness, relieve pain, and induce euphoria. Also called *narcotics,* they are derived from the parent drug **opium,** a dark, resinous substance made from the milky juice of the opium poppy seed pod. Opiates include morphine, codeine, heroin, and black tar heroin.

The word *narcotic* comes from the Greek word for "stupor" and generally is used to describe sleep-inducing substances. Until the early twentieth century, many patent medicines contained opiates and were advertised as cures for everything from menstrual cramps to teething pains. More powerful than opium, **morphine** (named after Morpheus,

> **opiates** Drugs that induce sleep and relieve pain; includes derivatives of opium and synthetics with similar chemical properties. Also called *narcotics.*
>
> **opium** The parent drug of the opiates; made from the seed pod resin of the opium poppy.
>
> **morphine** A derivative of opium; sometimes used by medical practitioners to relieve pain.

the Greek god of sleep) was widely used as a painkiller during the Civil War. **Codeine,** a less powerful analgesic (pain reliever) derived from morphine, also became popular.

As opiates became more common, physicians noted that patients tended to become dependent on them. Growing concern about addiction led to government controls of narcotic use. The Harrison Act of 1914 prohibited the production, dispensation, and sale of opiate products unless prescribed by a physician. Subsequent legislation required physicians prescribing opiates to keep careful records. Physicians are still subject to audits of their prescriptions.

Some opiates are still used today for medical purposes. Morphine is sometimes prescribed for severe pain, and codeine is found in prescription cough syrups and other painkillers. Several prescription drugs, including Percodan, Vicodin, and Dilaudid, contain synthetic opiates. Although all opiate use is strictly regulated, illicit use of OxyContin, another powerful opiate, has increased dramatically in recent years.

Physical Effects of Opiates
Opiates are powerful depressants of the central nervous system. In addition to relieving pain, these drugs lower heart rate, respiration, and blood pressure. Side effects include weakness, dizziness, nausea, vomiting, euphoria, decreased sex drive, visual disturbances, and lack of coordination. Of all the opiates, heroin has the greatest notoriety as an addictive drug. The following section discusses the progression of heroin addiction; addiction to any opiate follows a similar path.

Heroin Addiction
Heroin is a white powder derived from morphine. **Black tar heroin** is a sticky, dark brown, foul-smelling form of heroin that is relatively pure and inexpensive. Once considered a cure for morphine dependence, heroin was later discovered to be even more addictive and potent than morphine. Today, heroin has no medical use.

An estimated 3.7 million people have used heroin at one time in their lives. The highest number of users are young adults aged 26 or older.[32] Heroin can be snorted, injected, or smoked. Injection remains the most common route of administration; however, the contemporary version of heroin is so potent that users can get high by snorting or smoking the drug. This has attracted a more affluent group of users who may not want to inject, for reasons such as the increased risk of contracting diseases such as HIV.

Heroin is a depressant that produces drowsiness and a dreamy, mentally slow feeling. It can cause drastic mood swings, with euphoric highs followed by depressive lows. Heroin slows respiration and urinary output and constricts the pupils of the eyes. Symptoms of tolerance and withdrawal can appear within 3 weeks of first use.

The most common route of administration for heroin addicts is "mainlining"—intravenous injection of powdered heroin mixed in a solution. Many users describe the "rush" they feel when injecting themselves as intensely pleasurable, whereas others report unpredictable and unpleasant side effects. The temporary nature of the rush contributes to the drug's high potential for addiction—many addicts shoot up four or five times a day. Mainlining can cause veins to scar and eventually collapse. Once a vein has collapsed, it can no longer be used to introduce heroin into the bloodstream. Addicts become expert at locating new veins to use: in the feet, the legs, the temples, under the tongue, or in the groin.

The physiology of the human body could be said to encourage opiate addiction. Opiate-like substances called **endorphins** are manufactured in the body and have multiple receptor sites, particularly in the central nervous system. When endorphins attach at these points, they create feelings of painless well-being. Medical researchers refer to them as "the body's own opiates." When endorphin levels are high, people feel euphoric. The same euphoria occurs when opiates or related chemicals are active at the endorphin receptor sites.

Treatment for Opiate Addiction
Programs to help heroin addicts and people addicted to other opiates kick the habit have not been very successful. Some addicts resume drug use even after years of drug-free living because the craving for the injection rush is very strong. It takes a great deal of discipline to seek alternative nondrug highs.

Heroin addicts experience a distinct pattern of withdrawal. Symptoms of withdrawal include intense desire for the drug, sleep disturbance, dilated pupils, loss of appetite, irritability, goose bumps, and muscle tremors. The most difficult time in the withdrawal process occurs 24 to 72 hours following last use. All of the preceding symptoms continue, along with nausea, abdominal cramps, restlessness, insomnia, vomiting, diarrhea, extreme anxiety, hot and cold flashes, elevated blood pressure, and rapid heartbeat and respiration. Once the peak of withdrawal has passed, all these symptoms begin to subside. Still, the recovering addict has many hurdles to jump.

Methadone maintenance is one treatment available for people addicted to heroin or other opiates. Methadone is a synthetic narcotic that blocks the effects of opiate withdrawal. It is chemically similar enough to the opiates to control the tremors, chills, vomiting, diarrhea, and severe abdominal pains of withdrawal. Methadone dosage is

codeine A drug derived from morphine; used in cough syrups and certain painkillers.

heroin An illegally manufactured derivative of morphine, usually injected into the bloodstream.

black tar heroin A dark brown, sticky form of heroin.

endorphins Opiate-like hormones that are manufactured in the human body and contribute to natural feelings of well-being.

methadone maintenance A treatment for people addicted to opiates that substitutes methadone, a synthetic narcotic, for the opiate of addiction.

decreased over a period of time until the addict is weaned off the drug.

Methadone maintenance is controversial because of the drug's own potential for addiction. Critics contend that the program merely substitutes one addiction for another. Proponents argue that people on methadone maintenance are less likely to engage in criminal activities to support their habits than heroin addicts are. For this reason, many methadone maintenance programs are financed by state or federal government and are available free of charge or at reduced cost.

A number of new drug therapies for opiate dependence are emerging. Naltrexone (Trexan), an opiate antagonist, has been approved as a treatment. While on naltrexone, recovering addicts do not have the compulsion to use heroin, and if they do use it, they don't get high, so there is no point in using the drug. More recently, researchers have reported promising results with Temgesic (buprenorphine) a mild, nonaddicting synthetic opiate, which, like heroin and methadone, bonds to certain receptors in the brain, blocks pain messages, and persuades the brain that its cravings for heroin have been satisfied. Addicts report that while they are taking buprenorphine, they do not crave heroin anymore.

Hallucinogens (Psychedelics)

Hallucinogens are substances that are capable of creating auditory or visual hallucinations. These drugs are also known as **psychedelics,** a term adapted from the Greek phrase meaning "mind-manifesting." Hallucinogens alter a user's feelings, perceptions, and thoughts. The major receptor sites for most of these drugs are located in the brain region that is responsible for interpreting outside stimuli before these signals travel to other parts of the brain. This area, the **reticular formation,** lies in the brainstem at the upper end of the spinal cord **(Figure 7.5).** When a hallucinogen is present at a reticular formation site, messages become scrambled, and the user may see wavy walls instead of straight ones or may "smell" colors and "hear" tastes. This mixing of sensory messages is known as **synesthesia.** Users may also become less inhibited or recall events long buried in the subconscious mind.

The most widely recognized hallucinogens are LSD, mescaline, psilocybin, and PCP. All are illegal and carry severe penalties for manufacture, possession, transportation, or sale.

LSD Of all the psychedelics, **lysergic acid diethylamide (LSD)** is the most notorious. First synthesized in the late 1930s by Swiss chemist Albert Hoffman, LSD resulted from experiments to derive medically useful drugs from the ergot fungus found on rye and other cereal grains. Because LSD seemed capable of unlocking the secrets of the mind, psychiatrists initially felt it could be beneficial to patients unable to remember suppressed traumas. From 1950 through 1968, the drug was used for such purposes.

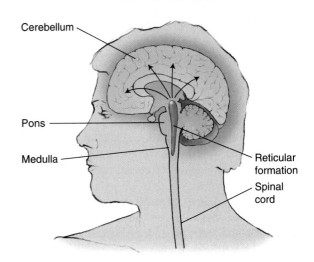

FIGURE 7.5 Reticular Formation

Media attention focused on LSD in the 1960s. Young people used the drug to "turn on" and "tune out" the world that gave them the war in Vietnam, race riots, and political assassinations. In 1970, federal authorities, under intense pressure from the public, placed LSD on the list of controlled substances (Schedule I). LSD's popularity peaked in 1972 then tapered off, primarily because of users' inability to control dosages accurately.

Because of the recent wave of nostalgia for the 1960s, this dangerous psychedelic drug, known on the street as "acid," has been making a comeback. Over 11 million Americans, most of them under age 35, have tried LSD at least once. LSD especially attracts younger users. A national survey of college students showed that 1.2 percent had used the drug in the past year.[33]

The most common and most popular form of LSD is blotter acid—small squares of blotterlike paper that have been impregnated with a liquid LSD mixture. The blotter is swallowed or chewed briefly. LSD also comes in tiny thin squares of gelatin called windowpane and in tablets called microdots,

hallucinogens Substances capable of creating auditory or visual distortions and heightened states.

psychedelics Drugs that distort the processing of sensory information in the brain.

reticular formation An area in the brainstem that is responsible for relaying messages from the senses to other areas in the brain.

synesthesia A drug-created effect in which sensory messages are incorrectly assigned—for example, the user "hears" a taste or "smells" a sound.

lysergic acid diethylamide (LSD) Psychedelic drug causing sensory disruptions; also called "acid."

which are less than an eighth of an inch across (it would take 10 or more to add up to the size of an aspirin tablet). As with any illegal drug, purchasers run the risk of buying an impure product.

One of the most powerful drugs known to science, LSD can produce strong effects in doses as low as 20 micrograms. (To give you an idea of how small a dose this is, the average postage stamp weighs approximately 60,000 micrograms.) The potency of the typical dose currently ranges from 20 to 80 micrograms, compared to 150 to 300 micrograms commonly used in the 1960s.

Despite its reputation as primarily a psychedelic, LSD produces a number of physical effects, including increased heart rate, elevated blood pressure and temperature, goose flesh (roughened skin), increased reflex speeds, muscle tremors and twitches, perspiration, increased salivation, chills, headaches, and mild nausea. The drug also stimulates uterine muscle contractions, so it can lead to premature labor and miscarriage in pregnant women. Research into long-term effects has been inconclusive.

The psychological effects of LSD vary. Euphoria is the common psychological state produced by the drug, but *dysphoria* (a sense of evil and foreboding) may also be experienced. The drug also shortens attention span, causing the mind to wander. Thoughts may be interposed and juxtaposed, so the user experiences several different thoughts simultaneously. Users become introspective, and suppressed memories may surface, often taking on bizarre symbolism. Many more effects are possible, including decreased aggressiveness and enhanced sensory experiences.

LSD causes distortions of ordinary perceptions, such as the movement of stationary objects. "Bad trips," the most publicized risk of LSD, are commonly related to the user's mood. The person, for example, may interpret increased heart rate as a heart attack (a "bad body trip"). Often bad trips result when a user confronts a suppressed emotional experience or memory (a "bad head trip").

Although there is no evidence that LSD creates physical dependence, it may well create psychological dependence. Many LSD users become depressed for 1 or 2 days following a trip and turn to the drug to relieve this depression. The result is a cycle of LSD use to relieve post-LSD depression, which often leads to psychological addiction.

---

mescaline A hallucinogenic drug derived from the peyote cactus.

peyote A cactus with small "buttons" that, when ingested, produce hallucinogenic effects.

psilocybin The active chemical found in psilocybe mushrooms; it produces hallucinations.

phencyclidine (PCP) A hallucinogen, commonly called "angel dust," that causes hallucinations, delusions, and delirium.

what do you THINK?

Are people today using LSD for the same reasons they did in the 1960s? ■ What are the perceived attractions and the real dangers of LSD?

Mescaline **Mescaline** is one of hundreds of chemicals derived from the **peyote** cactus, a small cactus that grows in the southwestern United States and parts of Latin America. Natives of these regions have long used dried peyote "buttons" for religious purposes. In fact, members of the Native American Church (a religion practiced by thousands of North American native tribes) have been granted special legal permission to use the drug during religious ceremonies in some states.

Users typically swallow 10 to 12 buttons. They taste bitter and generally induce immediate nausea or vomiting. Long-time users claim that the nausea becomes less noticeable with frequent use. Those who are able to keep the drug down begin to feel the effects within 30 to 90 minutes, when mescaline reaches maximum concentration in the brain. (It may persist for up to 9 or 10 hours.) Mescaline is both a powerful hallucinogen and a central nervous system stimulant.

Products sold on the street as mescaline are likely to be synthetic chemical relatives of the true drug. Street names of these products include DOM, STP, TMA, and MMDA. Any of these can be toxic in small quantities.

Psilocybin **Psilocybin** and *psilocin* are the active chemicals in a group of mushrooms sometimes called "magic mushrooms." Psilocybe mushrooms, which grow throughout the world, can be cultivated from spores or harvested wild. Because many mushrooms resemble the psilocybe variety, people who harvest wild mushrooms for any purpose should be certain of what they are doing. Mushroom varieties can be easily misidentified, and mistakes can be fatal. Psilocybin is similar to LSD in its physical effects, which generally wear off in 4 to 6 hours.

PCP **Phencyclidine,** or **PCP,** is a synthetic substance that became a black-market drug in the early 1970s. PCP was originally developed as a dissociative anesthetic, which means that patients receiving this drug could keep their eyes open and apparently remain conscious but feel no pain during a medical procedure. Afterward, patients would experience amnesia for the time the drug was in their system. Such a drug had obvious advantages as an anesthetic, but its unpredictability and drastic effects (postoperative delirium, confusion, and agitation) made doctors abandon it, and it was withdrawn from the legal market.

On the illegal market, PCP is a white, crystalline powder that users often sprinkle onto marijuana cigarettes. It is dangerous and unpredictable regardless of the method of administration. Common street names for PCP are "angel dust" for the crystalline powdered form and "peace pill" and "horse tranquilizer" for the tablet form.

The effects of PCP depend on the dose. A dose as small as 5 mg will produce effects similar to those of strong central nervous system depressants—slurred speech, impaired coordination, reduced sensitivity to pain, and reduced heart and respiratory rate. Doses between 5 and 10 mg cause fever, salivation, nausea, vomiting, and total loss of sensitivity to pain. Doses greater than 10 mg result in a drastic drop in blood pressure, coma, muscular rigidity, violent outbursts, and possible convulsions and death.

Psychologically, PCP may produce either euphoria or dysphoria. It also is known to produce hallucinations as well as delusions and overall delirium. Some users experience a prolonged state of "nothingness." The long-term effects of PCP use are unknown.

Designer Drugs (Club Drugs)

Designer drugs are synthetic drugs that produce effects similar to existing illegal drugs. They are manufactured in chemical laboratories and homes and are sold illegally. These drugs are easy to produce from available raw materials. The drugs themselves were once technically legal because the law had to specify the exact chemical structure of an illicit substance. However, a law is now in place that bans all chemical cousins of illegal drugs.

Collectively known as **club drugs,** these dangerous substances include Ecstasy, gamma-hydroxybutyrate (GHB), ketamine (Special K), and Rohypnol. Although users may think them harmless, research has shown that club drugs can produce a range of unwanted effects, including hallucinations, paranoia, amnesia, and, in some cases, death. Some club drugs work on the same brain mechanisms as alcohol and can dangerously boost the effects of both substances. Because the drugs are odorless and tasteless, people can easily slip them into drinks. Some of them have been associated with sexual assault and for that reason are referred to as "date rape drugs" (see the Spotlight on Your Health box in Chapter 4, as well as the discussion of drugs and sex on page 146 of Chapter 5).

Ecstasy (methylene dioxymethamphetamine, or MDMA) use has been reported by almost one of every four students at some universities. Ecstasy creates feelings of openness and warmth, combined with the mind-expanding characteristics of hallucinogens. Effects begin within 30 minutes and can last for 4 to 6 hours. Young people may use Ecstasy initially to improve mood or get energized so they can keep dancing; it also increases heart rate and blood pressure and may raise body temperature to the point of kidney and/or cardiovascular failure. Chronic use appears to damage the brain's ability to think and to regulate emotion, memory, sleep, and pain. Combined with alcohol, Ecstasy can be extremely dangerous and sometimes fatal. Recent studies indicate that Ecstasy may cause long-lasting neurotoxic effects by damaging brain cells that produce serotonin.[34]

Rohypnol is a potent tranquilizer similar in nature to Valium, but many times stronger. The drug produces a sedative effect, amnesia, muscle relaxation, and slowed psychomotor

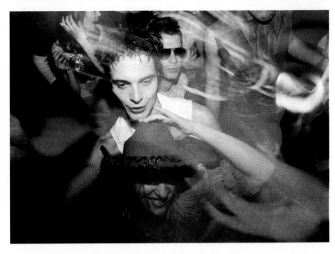

Ecstasy is popular in various nightclub, rave, and trance music scenes for its combination of stimulant and psychedelic effects.

responses. The most publicized "date rape" drug, Rohypnol has gained notoriety as a problem on college campuses. The drug has been added to punch and other drinks at parties, where it is reportedly given to women in hopes of lowering their inhibitions and facilitating potential sexual conquests. The manufacturer changed the formula to give the drug a bright blue color that would make it easy to detect in most drinks, so would-be perpetrators are turning to blue tropical drinks and punches to disguise the drug.

GHB (gamma-hydroxybutyrate) is a central nervous system depressant known to have euphoric, sedative, and anabolic (body-building) effects. It was originally sold over the counter to body builders as an aid to reduce fat and build muscle. Concerns about GHB led the FDA to ban over-the-counter sales in 1992, and GHB is now a Schedule I controlled substance.[35] GHB is an odorless, tasteless fluid that can be made easily at home or in a chemistry lab. Like Rohypnol, GHB has been slipped into drinks without being detected, resulting in loss of memory, unconsciousness, amnesia, and even death. Other dangerous side effects include nausea, vomiting, seizures, memory loss, hallucinations, coma, and respiratory distress.

designer drugs (club drugs) Synthetic analogs (drugs that produce similar effects) of existing illicit drugs.

Ecstasy (MDMA) A club drug that creates feelings of openness and warmth but also raises heart rate and blood pressure.

Rohypnol A powerful sedative, commonly known as the "date rape" drug for its ability to cause semiconsciousness and facilitate unwanted sexual encounters.

gamma-hydroxybutyrate (GHB) A central nervous system depressant alleged to have body-building properties that has been used as a "date rape" drug.

Ketamine is used as an anesthetic in many hospital and veterinary clinics. It is called Special K on the street, where it is most often diverted in liquid form from veterinary offices or medical suppliers. Dealers dry the liquid (usually by cooking it) and grind the residue into powder. Special K causes hallucinations as it inhibits the relay of sensory input; the brain fills the resulting void with visions, dreams, memories, and sensory distortions. The effects of Special K are less severe than those of Ecstasy, so it has grown in popularity among people who have to go to work or school after a night of partying.

Inhalants

Inhalants are chemicals that produce vapors that, when inhaled, can cause hallucinations and create intoxicating and euphoric effects. Not commonly recognized as drugs, inhalants are legal to purchase and universally available but dangerous when used incorrectly. They generally appeal to young people who can't afford or obtain illicit substances. Some products often misused as inhalants include rubber cement, model glue, paint thinner, lighter fluid, varnish, wax, spot removers, and gasoline. Most of these substances are sniffed or "huffed" by users in search of a quick, cheap high.

Because they are inhaled, the volatile chemicals in these products reach the bloodstream within seconds. An inhaled substance is not diluted or buffered by stomach acids or other body fluids and thus is more potent than it would be if swallowed. This characteristic, along with the fact that dosages are extremely difficult to control because everyone has unique lung and breathing capacities, makes inhalants particularly dangerous.

The effects of inhalants usually last fewer than 15 minutes and resemble those of central nervous system depressants. Combining inhalants with alcohol produces a synergistic effect and can cause severe liver damage that can be fatal. Users may experience dizziness, disorientation, impaired coordination, reduced judgment, and slowed reaction times.

An overdose of fumes from inhalants can cause unconsciousness. If the user's oxygen intake is reduced during the inhaling process, death can result within 5 minutes. Whether a user is a first-time or chronic user, sudden sniffing death (SSD) syndrome can be a fatal consequence. This syndrome can occur if a user inhales deeply and then participates in physical activity or is startled.

Amyl Nitrite Sometimes called "poppers" or "rush," **amyl nitrite** is packaged in small, cloth-covered glass capsules that can be crushed to release the active chemical. The drug is often prescribed to alleviate chest pain in heart disease patients because it dilates small blood vessels and reduces blood pressure. Dilation of blood vessels in the genital area is thought to enhance sensations or perceptions of orgasm. It also produces fainting, dizziness, warmth, and skin flushing.

Nitrous Oxide **Nitrous oxide** is sometimes used as an adjunct to dental anesthesia or minor surgical anesthesia. It is also a propellant chemical in aerosol products such as whipped toppings. Users who inhale nitrous oxide experience a state of euphoria, floating sensations, and illusions. Effects also include pain relief and a silly feeling demonstrated by laughing and giggling (hence its nickname, "laughing gas"). Regulating dosages of this drug can be difficult. Sustained inhalation can lead to unconsciousness, coma, and death.

Anabolic Steroids

Public awareness of **anabolic steroids** recently has been heightened by media stories about their use by amateur and professional athletes, especially in major league baseball. Anabolic steroids are artificial forms of the male hormone testosterone that promote muscle growth and strength. These **ergogenic drugs** are used primarily by people who believe the drugs will increase their strength, power, bulk (weight), speed, and athletic performance.

Most steroids are obtained through the black market. It was once estimated that approximately 17 to 20 percent of college athletes used them. Now that stricter drug-testing policies have been instituted by the National Collegiate Athletic Association (NCAA), reported use of anabolic steroids among intercollegiate athletes has dropped to 1.1 percent. However, a recent survey among high school students found a significant increase in the use of anabolic steroids since 1991. Few data exist on the extent of steroid abuse by adults. It has been estimated that hundreds of thousands of people aged 18 and older abuse anabolic steroids at least once a year. Among both adolescents and adults, steroid abuse is higher among men than women. However, steroid abuse is growing most rapidly among young women.[36]

Steroids are available in two forms: injectable solutions and pills. Anabolic steroids produce a state of euphoria, diminished fatigue, and increased bulk and power in both sexes. These qualities give steroids an addictive quality. When users stop, they can experience psychological withdrawal and

ketamine (Special K) An anesthetic used primarily in veterinary settings that has gained popularity as a club drug with potentially dangerous hallucinogenic effects.

inhalants Products that are sniffed or inhaled to produce highs.

amyl nitrite A drug that dilates blood vessels and is properly used to relieve chest pain.

nitrous oxide The chemical name for "laughing gas," a substance properly used for surgical or dental anesthesia.

anabolic steroids Artificial forms of the hormone testosterone that promote muscle growth and strength.

ergogenic drugs Substances believed to enhance athletic performance.

sometimes severe depression, in some cases leading to suicide attempts. If untreated, depression associated with steroid withdrawal has been known to last for a year or more after steroid use stops.

Men and women who use steroids experience a variety of adverse effects. These drugs cause mood swings (aggression and violence), sometimes known as "'roid rage"; acne; liver tumors; elevated cholesterol levels; hypertension; kidney disease; and immune system disturbances. There is also a danger of transmitting AIDS and hepatitis (a serious liver disease) through shared needles. In women, large doses of anabolic steroids may trigger the development of masculine attributes such as lowered voice, increased facial and body hair, and male-pattern baldness; they may also result in an enlarged clitoris, smaller breasts, and changes in or absence of menstruation. When taken by healthy men, anabolic steroids shut down the body's production of testosterone, causing men's breasts to grow and testicles to atrophy.

To combat the growing problem of steroid use, the U.S. Congress passed the Anabolic Steroids Control Act (ASCA) of 1990. This law makes it a crime to possess, prescribe, or distribute anabolic steroids for any use other than the treatment of specific diseases. Anabolic steroids are now classified as a Schedule III drug. Penalties for their illegal use include up to 5 years' imprisonment and a $250,000 fine for the first offense and up to 10 years' imprisonment and a $500,000 fine for subsequent offenses.

A new and alarming trend is the use of other drugs to achieve the effects of steroids. The two most common steroid alternatives are gamma-hydroxybutyrate (GHB) and clenbuterol. GHB (also discussed earlier) is a deadly, illegal drug that is a primary ingredient in many "performance-enhancing" formulas. GHB does not produce a high. It does, however, cause headaches, nausea, vomiting, diarrhea, seizures, and other central nervous system disorders, and possibly death. Clenbuterol is used in some countries for veterinary treatments but is not approved for any use—in animals or humans—in the United States.

New attention was drawn to the issue of steroids and related substances when former St. Louis Cardinals slugger Mark McGwire admitted to using a supplement containing androstenedione (andro), an adrenal hormone that is produced naturally in both men and women. Andro raises levels of testosterone, which helps build lean muscle mass and promotes quicker recovery after injury. McGwire had done nothing illegal, because the supplement could be purchased over the counter (with sales estimated at $800 million a year), and its use was legal in baseball at that time. However, the supplement had been banned by the NFL, NCAA, and International Olympic Committee. A recent study found that when men take 100 milligrams of andro three times daily, it increases estrogen levels by up to 80 percent, enlarges the prostate gland, and increases heart disease risk by 10 to 15 percent. Major league baseball banned its use in 2004.

Visits to the locker rooms of many sports teams would disclose large containers of other alleged muscle-building supplements, such as creatine. Although they are legal, questions remain whether enough research has been done

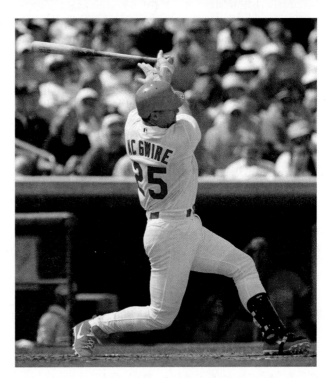

In March 2005, Mark McGwire and other major league baseball players were subpoenaed to testify before Congress on the use of steroids in the sport. McGwire has admitted to the use of andro, a hormonal supplement, in the past.

concerning the safety of these supplements. Some experts worry that they may bring consequences similar to those of steroids, such as liver damage and heart problems.

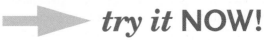

try it NOW!

Take steps against drug misuse. Drug misuse can eventually lead to addiction and hurt your chances of achieving lifelong goals. On a piece of paper, identify one long-term goal you would like to achieve, such as becoming a lawyer. Be sure your goal is specific. Next, write down three steps you need to take to reach this goal (e.g., an internship with the district attorney, getting into the law school of your choice, passing the bar exam). Finally, think about drug misuse, its consequences, and how these factors will make your goal difficult to achieve or prevent you from reaching it at all.

Illegal Drug Use in the United States

Stories of people who have tried illegal drugs, enjoyed them, and suffered no consequences may tempt you to try them yourself. You may tell yourself it's "just this once," convincing yourself that one-time use is harmless. Given the dangers surrounding these substances, however, you should think twice. The risks associated with drug use extend beyond the personal. The decision to try any illicit substance encourages illicit drug manufacture and transport, thus contributing to the national drug problem. The financial burden of illegal drug use on the U.S. economy is staggering, with an estimated economic cost of around $180.9 billion per year.[37] This estimate includes costs associated with substance abuse treatment and prevention, health care, reduced job productivity and lost earnings, and social consequences such as crime and social welfare.

In addition, roughly half of all expenditures to combat crime are related to illegal drugs. The burden of these costs is absorbed primarily by the government (46 percent), followed by people who abuse drugs and members of their households (44 percent). One study found that Americans spend $64 billion on illicit drugs annually. These numbers break down as follows: $35 billion on cocaine, $10 billion each on marijuana and heroin, and $5 billion on methamphetamines. This is eight times what the federal government spends on research on HIV/AIDS, cancer, and heart disease put together.[38]

Solutions to the Problem

Americans are alarmed by the increasing use of illegal drugs. Respondents in public opinion polls feel that the most important strategy for fighting drug abuse is educating young people. They also endorse strategies such as stricter border surveillance to reduce drug trafficking, longer prison sentences for drug dealers, increased government spending on prevention, enforcing antidrug laws, and greater cooperation among government agencies, private groups, and individuals providing treatment assistance. All of these approaches will probably help up to a point, but they do not offer a total solution to the problem. Drug abuse has been a part of human behavior for thousands of years, and it is not likely to disappear in the near future. For this reason, it is necessary to educate ourselves and to develop the self-discipline necessary to avoid dangerous drug dependence.

For many years, the most popular antidrug strategies were total prohibition and "scare tactics." Both approaches proved ineffective. Prohibition of alcohol during the 1920s created more problems than it solved, as did prohibition of opiates in 1914. Outlawing other illicit drugs has neither eliminated them nor curtailed their traffic across U.S. borders.

In general, researchers in the field of drug education agree that a multimodal approach is best. Students should be taught the difference between drug use and abuse. Factual information that is free of scare tactics must be presented; lecturing and moralizing do not work. Emphasis should be placed on things that are important to young people. Telling adolescent boys that girls will find them disgusting if their breath stinks of cigarettes or pot will get their attention. Likewise, lecturing on the negative effects of drug use is a much less effective deterrent than teaching young people how to negotiate the social scene. One program intended to educate students, Drug Abuse Resistance Education (commonly called DARE), has been largely ineffective. Education efforts need to focus on achieving better outcomes for preventing drug use.

We must also study at-risk groups so we can better understand the circumstances that make them susceptible to drug use. Time, money, and effort by educators, parents, and policymakers are needed to ensure that today's youth receive the love and security essential for building productive and meaningful lives and rejecting drug abuse.

TAKING charge

Summary

- Addiction is the continued involvement with a substance or activity despite ongoing negative consequences. Some behaviors, such as compulsive gambling and shopping, are addictive because they are mood-altering. Codependents are "addicted to the addict."
- The six categories of drugs are prescription drugs, over-the-counter (OTC) drugs, recreational drugs, herbal preparations, illicit drugs, and commercial preparations. Administration routes include oral ingestion, injection (intravenous, intramuscular, and subcutaneous), inhalation, and inunction.
- Prescription drugs are administered under medical supervision. There are dozens of categories, including antibiotics, sedatives, tranquilizers, and antidepressants. Generic drugs often can be substituted for more expensive brand-name products.
- OTC drug categories include analgesics; cold, cough, allergy, and asthma relievers; stimulants; sleeping aids and relaxants; and dieting aids. Exercise personal responsibility by reading directions for OTC drugs and asking your pharmacist or doctor whether any special precautions are advised when taking these substances.

- People from all walks of life use illicit drugs, although college students report higher usage rates than do the general population. Drug use declined from the mid-1980s to the early 1990s but has remained steady since then. However, among young people, use of drugs has been rising in recent years.

- Controlled substances include cocaine and its derivatives, amphetamines, methamphetamine and ice, marijuana, opiates, hallucinogens/psychedelics, designer drugs (club drugs), inhalants, and steroids. Users tend to become addicted quickly to such drugs.
- The drug problem reaches everyone through crime and elevated health care costs.

Chapter Review

1. An individual who knowingly tries to protect an addict from natural consequences of his or her destructive behaviors is
   a. enabling.
   b. coddling.
   c. practicing intervention.
   d. controlling.

2. Chemical dependence *relapse* refers to
   a. a person who is experiencing a blackout memory loss.
   b. a gap in one's drinking or drugging patterns.
   c. a full return to addictive behavior.
   d. the failure to change one's behavior.

3. Taking excessive drugs on a continual basis, even when it is not necessary to, describes
   a. drug misuse.
   b. drug addiction.
   c. drug tolerance.
   d. drug abuse.

4. Cross-tolerance occurs when
   a. drugs work at the same receptor site so that one blocks the action of the other.
   b. the effects of one drug are eliminated or reduced by the presence of another drug at the receptor site.
   c. a person develops a physiological tolerance to one drug and shows a similar tolerance to selected other drugs as a result.
   d. two or more drugs interact and the effects of the individual drugs are multiplied beyond what normally would be expected if they were taken alone.

5. Rebecca takes a number of medications for various conditions, including Prinivil (an antihypertensive drug), insulin (a diabetic medication), and Claritin (an antihistamine). This is an example of
   a. synergism.
   b. illegal drug use.
   c. polydrug use.
   d. antagonism.

6. Prozac, Zoloft, and Paxil are among the most frequently prescribed
   a. antibiotics.
   b. sedatives.
   c. antidepressants.
   d. tranquilizers.

7. Drugs that are marketed by their chemical names rather than a brand name are called
   a. generic drugs.
   b. OTC drugs.
   c. recreational drugs.
   d. commercial drugs.

8. Which of the following is classified as a stimulant drug?
   a. amphetamines
   b. alcohol
   c. marijuana
   d. LSD

9. Freebasing is
   a. mixing cocaine with heroin.
   b. inhaling heroin fumes.
   c. injecting a drug into the veins.
   d. smoking the fumes of cocaine.

10. The psychoactive drug mescaline is found in what plant?
    a. mushrooms
    b. peyote cactus
    c. marijuana
    d. belladonna

Answers to these questions can be found on page A-1.

Questions for Discussion and Reflection

1. What is the current theory that explains how drugs work in the body? Explain how this theory works.
2. Explain the terms *synergism, antagonism,* and *inhibition.*
3. Why do you think many people today feel that marijuana use is not dangerous? What are the arguments in favor of legalizing marijuana? What are the arguments against legalization? How common is the use of marijuana on your campus?
4. What could you do to help a friend who is fighting a substance abuse problem? What resources on your campus could help you?
5. What types of programs do you think would be effective in preventing drug abuse among high school and college students? How would programs for high school students differ from those for college students?
6. Discuss how addiction affects family and friends. What role do family and friends play in helping the addict get help and maintain recovery?

Accessing Your Health on the Internet

The following websites explore further topics and issues related to personal health. For links to the websites below, visit the Companion Website for *Health: The Basics,* Eighth Edition at www.aw-bc.com/donatelle.

1. *Club Drugs.* A website that disseminates science-based information about club drugs. www.clubdrugs.org
2. *U.S. Food and Drug Administration (FDA).* The federal agency responsible for approving prescription and over-the-counter drugs, with information on product approvals, recalls, and more. www.fda.gov
3. *Join Together.* An excellent site for the most current information related to substance abuse. Also includes information on gun violence and provides advice on organizing and taking political action. www.jointogether.org

4. *National Institute on Drug Abuse (NIDA).* The home page of this U.S. government agency has information on the latest statistics and findings in drug research. www.nida.nih.gov
5. *Substance Abuse and Mental Health Services Administration (SAMHSA).* Outstanding resource for information about national surveys, ongoing research, and national drug interventions. www.samhsa.gov
6. *National Council on Problem Gambling.* Provides information and help for people with gambling problems and their families, including a searchable directory for counselors. www.ncpgambling.org

Further Reading

Elster, J., ed. *Addiction: Entries and Exits.* New York: Russell Sage Foundation, 2000.

> Addresses current addiction controversies from an international perspective, with authors from the United States and Norway. Topics include whether addicts have a choice in their behavior and current addiction theories.

Goldstein, A. *Addiction: From Biology to Drug Policy.* New York: Oxford University Press, 2001.

> Discusses how drugs affect the brain, how each drug causes addiction, and how addictive drugs impact society. The author explains what we know about drug addiction, how we know what we know, and what we can and cannot do about the drug problem.

Griffith, W. H., and S. Moore. *Complete Guide to Prescription and Nonprescription Drugs 2007.* New York: Perigee, 2006.

> This essential guide answers every conceivable question about prescription and nonprescription drugs and contains information about dosages, side effects, precautions,

> interactions, and more. More than 5,000 brand-name and 800 generic drugs are profiled in an easy-to-use format.

The National Center on Addiction and Substance Abuse. *Women Under the Influence: Alcohol Problems in Adolescents and Young Adults: Epidemiology, Neurobiology, Prevention and Treatment.* Baltimore: Johns Hopkins University Press, 2006.

> A scholarly analysis of substance abuse among American women. This lucidly written book provides a perceptive and compassionate discussion of the factors that contribute to abuse of a wide spectrum of substances and of the associated social and health consequences for women.

Physician's Desk Reference for Nonprescription Drugs, Dietary Supplements and Herbs: The Definitive Guide to OTC Medications. Montvale, NJ: Thomson PDR, 2006.

> Outlines proper uses, possible dangers, and effective ingredients of nonprescription medications.

Ray, O. S. and C. Ksir. *Drugs, Society and Human Behavior*, 12th ed. New York: McGraw-Hill, 2008.

> This book examines drugs and behavior from the behavioral, pharmacological, historical, social, legal, and clinical perspectives.

Shaw, B. *Addiction and Recovery for Dummies*. Wiley Publishing Co. 2005.

> This compassionate guide helps you identify the problem and work toward a healthy, realistic approach to recovery, explaining the latest clinical and self-help treatments for both adults and teens.

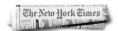

e-themes from *The New York Times*

For up-to-date articles about current health issues, visit www.aw-bc.com/donatelle, select *Health: The Basics*, Eighth Edition, Chapter 7, and click on "e-themes."

References

1. H. F. Doweiko, *Concepts of Chemical Dependency*, 6th ed. (Belmont, CA: Wadsworth, 2005), 11.
2. R. Goldberg, *Drugs across the Spectrum*, 5th ed. (Belmont, CA: Thomson/Brooks/Cole, 2006).
3. National Council on Problem Gambling. "Fact Sheets," September 1, 2004, www.ncpgambling.org.
4. "Gambling as Addiction," *Science* 307, no. 5708 (2005): 349, www.sciencemag.org/cgi/content/summary
5. J. W. Welte et al., "Gambling Participation and Pathology in the United States," *Addictive Behaviors* 29, no. 5 (2004): 983–989.
6. The Annenburg Public Policy Center, "Card Playing Trend in Young People Continutes," Press Release, September 28, 2005, www.annenbergpublicpolicycenter.org.
7. W. DeJong et. al., "Gambling: The New Addiction Crisis in Higher Education," *Prevention Profile* (March 2006): 11–13.
8. MSNBC, "Bankruptcy Filings Fell by 70 percent in 2006," April 17, 2007, www.msnbc.msn.com.
9. American Bankruptcy Institute, "Quarterly Non-business Filings by Year, 2005," www.abiworld.org; Women's Wall Street, "Conquer the Compulsive Shopping Blues." June 19, 2004.
10. Substance Abuse and Mental Health Services Administration, "Substance Abuse: A National Health Challenge," October 4, 2006, www.samhsa.gov/oas/oas.html.
11. Ibid.
12. P. Kittenger and D. Herron, "Patient Power: Over-the-Counter Drugs—Brief Analysis," National Center for Policy Analysis, 2005, www.ncpa.org/pub/ba/ba524.
13. H. Verdoux et al., "Is Benzodiazepine Use a Risk Factor for Cognitive Decline and Dementia?" *Psychological Medicine* 35 (2005): 307–15.
14. National Center for Health Statistics, "New Study Shows Critical Role for Primary Care Specialists. National Ambulatory Medical Care Survey: 2002 Summary," August 26, 2004, www.cdc.gov/nchs/pressroom/04facts/primarycare.htm.
15. J. Rowley et al., "Insomnia," June 17, 2004, www.emedicine.com/neuro/topic418.htm.
16. U.S. Food and Drug Administration, "Phenylpropanolamine (PPA) Information Page," 2002, www.fda.gov/cder/drug/infopage/ppa/default.htm.
17. U.S. Food and Drug Administration, "Sales of Supplements Containing Ephedrine Alkaloids Prohibited." April 12, 2004, www.fda.gov.
18. U.S. Department of Health and Human Services, *Marijuana: Facts for Teens*, NIH Publication no. 04-4037 (Bethesda, MD: National Institute on Drug Abuse, 2004).
19. L. D. Johnston et al., *Monitoring the Future: National Survey Results on Drug Use, 1975–2004: Volume II, College Students and Adults*, NIH Publication no. 05-5728 (Bethesda, MD: National Institute on Drug Abuse, 2005).
20. Ibid.
21. Ibid.
22. M. Fisherman and C. Johanson, "Cocaine," in *Pharmacological Aspects of Drug Dependence: Towards an Integrated Neurobehavior Approach, Handbook of Experimental Pharmacology*, C. Shuster and M. Kuhar, eds. (Hamburg, Germany: Springer Verlag, 1996): 159–95.
23. Substance Abuse and Mental Health Services Administration, *Results from the 2005 National Survey on Drug Use and Health: National Findings* (Rockville, MD: Office of Applied Studies, 2006).
24. L. D. Johnston et al., *Monitoring the Future: National Survey Results on Drug Use, 1975–2005: Volume I, Secondary School Students*, NIH Publication no. 06-5883 (Bethesda, MD: National Institute on Drug Abuse, 2006).
25. Ibid.
26. W. Compton et al., "Prevalence of Marijuana Use Disorders in the United States 2001–2002," *Journal of the American Medical Association* 291 (2004): 2114–21.
27. U.S. Department of Health and Human Services, *Marijuana*.
28. Ibid.
29. J. Burkman et al., "Marijuana Impacts Sperm Function both in In-Vivo and In-Vitro: Semen Analysis From Men Smoking Marijuana" (paper presented at a conference of the American Society of Reproduction Medicine, San Antonio, TX, October, 2003), 11–15.
30. American Academy of Ophthalmology, Medical Library, "The Use of Marijuana in the Treatment of Glaucoma," 2003, www.medem.com.
31. National Institute on Drug Abuse, *Marijuana Abuse*, NIH Publication no. 05-3859 (Bethesda, MD: National Institute on Drug Abuse, 2005).
32. National Institute on Drug Abuse, *Research Report Series on Heroin Abuse and Addiction* (NIH Publication no. 05-4165 (Bethesda, MD: National Institute on Drug Abuse, 2005).
33. Johnston, *Monitoring the Future, Volume I*.
34. National Institute on Drug Abuse, "NIDA InfoFacts: Club Drugs," 2006, www.drugabuse.gov/infofacts/clubdrugs.html.
35. Ibid.
36. National Institute on Drug Abuse, "Anabolic Steroids," *NIDA for Teens*, 2005, http://teens.drugabuse.gov/drnida/drnida_ster1.asp.
37. National Drug Intelligence Center, "National Drug Threat Assessment, 2006: The Impact of Drugs on Society," 2006, www.usdoj.gov/ndic/pubs11/18862/impact.htm.
38. Office of National Drug Control Strategy, "2002 National Drug Control Strategy," 2002, www.whitehousedrugpolicy.gov.

8

Alcohol, Tobacco, and Caffeine

DAILY PLEASURES, DAILY CHALLENGES

Aren't the majority of college students **heavy** drinkers?

Is there any cure for a **hangover?**

Is secondhand smoke a **risk** to my health?

Is **caffeine** really addictive?

OBJECTIVES

■ Discuss the alcohol use patterns of college students and overall trends in consumption.

■ Explain the physiological and behavioral effects of alcohol, including blood alcohol concentration, absorption, metabolism, and immediate and long-term effects of alcohol consumption.

■ Explain the symptoms and causes of alcoholism, its cost to society, effects on the family, and treatment options.

■ Discuss the social and political issues involved in tobacco use.

■ Discuss the health risks of smoking, spit (smokeless) tobacco, and environmental tobacco smoke, and describe how the chemicals in tobacco products affect the body.

■ Summarize the benefits, risks, and potential health consequences associated with caffeine use.

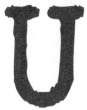

Usually the word *drug* conjures up images of people abusing illegal substances. We use the term to describe dangerous chemicals such as heroin or cocaine, without recognizing that socially accepted substances can be drugs, too—for example, alcohol, tobacco, and caffeine.

Alcohol: An Overview

Moderate use of alcohol can enhance celebrations and special times. Research shows that very low levels of use may actually decrease some health risks. However, always remember that alcohol is a chemical substance that affects your physical and mental behavior.

An estimated 65 percent of Americans consume alcoholic beverages regularly, though consumption patterns are unevenly distributed throughout the drinking population. Ten percent are heavy drinkers, and they account for half of all the alcohol consumed. The remaining 90 percent of the drinking population are infrequent, light, or moderate drinkers.

Alcohol and College Students

Alcohol is the most widely used (and abused) recreational drug in our society. It is also the most popular drug on college campuses, where approximately 70 percent of students report having consumed alcoholic beverages in the last 30 days.[1] Almost half of all college students engage in **heavy episodic (binge) drinking,** meaning that they consume five or more drinks in a row (men), or four or more in a row (women). Therefore, students who might go out and drink only once a week are considered heavy drinkers if they consume a great deal of alcohol during that occasion. In a new trend on college campuses, women's consumption of alcohol has come close to equaling men's.

College is a critical time to become aware of and responsible for drinking. There is little doubt that drinking is a part of campus culture and tradition. Many students are away from home, often for the first time, and are excited by their newfound independence. For some students, this independence and the rite of passage into the college culture are symbolized by the use of alcohol. It provides the answer to one of the most commonly heard statements on any college campus: "There is nothing to do." Additionally, many students say they drink to have fun. Having fun, which often means drinking simply to get drunk, may really be a way of coping with stress, boredom, anxiety, or pressures created by academic and social demands.

Statistics about college students' drinking may not always reflect actual consumption. Many college and universities are trying a social norms approach, sending a consistent message to students about actual drinking behavior on campus. There is growing research that college students' drinking behavior is strongly influenced by the incorrect perception of peer drinking norms. Many students misperceive that their peers drink more than they actually do. This misperception is true not only about the frequency and amount that students drink, but also about the actual consequences students experience as a result of their drinking. For example, at a large midwestern university, 42 percent of students reported not having had a hangover in the past 6 months. Yet the same group of surveyed students perceived that only 3 percent of their peers had not had a hangover in the past month.

Today, many campuses are working to change misperceptions of normal drinking behavior. As a result, heavy episodic alcohol consumption—"binge drinking"—has declined at campuses across the country **(Table 8.1).**

Binge Drinking and College Students

There are, however, some students who indulge in binge drinking. The stakes of binge drinking are high because it poses high risk for alcohol-related injuries and death. According to a recent study, 1,700 college students die each year because of alcohol-related, unintentional injuries, including car accidents. Binge drinking is the number-one cause of preventable death among undergraduate college students in the United States today.[2]

A study by the Harvard School of Public Health found that 44.4 percent of students were binge drinkers, and, of those, 22.8 percent were frequent bingers (people who binge drink three times or more in a 2-week period; **Table 8.2).**[3] Compared with nonbinge drinkers, frequent binge drinkers are 16 times more likely to miss class, 8 times more likely to get behind in their school work, and more apt to get into trouble with campus or local police.[4] Unfortunately, recent studies confirm what students have been experiencing for a long time—binge drinkers cause problems not only for themselves, but also for those around them.

Although everyone is at some risk for alcohol-related problems, college students seem to be particularly vulnerable for the following reasons:

- Alcohol exacerbates their already high risk for suicide, automobile crashes, and falls.
- Many college and university customs, norms, traditions, and mores encourage certain dangerous practices and patterns of alcohol use.
- University campuses are heavily targeted by advertising and promotions from the alcoholic beverage industry.

> **Aren't the majority of college students heavy drinkers?**

heavy episodic (binge) drinking   Drinking for the express purpose of becoming intoxicated; five drinks or more on a single occasion for men and four drinks or more for women.

THE FACTS ABOUT COLLEGE STUDENTS AND DRINKING

College administrators estimate that alcohol is involved with 29 percent of dropouts, 38 percent of academic failures, and 64 percent of violent behaviors.

Perhaps you've heard conflicting reports in the media about the prevalence and effects of drinking on campus. The statistic above is just one of many that detail the scope of the problem. Consider the following facts about students and alcohol consumption:

- Alcohol kills more people below age 21 than cocaine, marijuana, and heroin combined.
- Half a million students between ages 15 and 24 are unintentionally injured each year while intoxicated.
- Eight percent of students reported alcohol use as one of their top ten impediments to academic performance in the previous year.
- Of today's first-year college students, 159,000 will drop out of school next year for alcohol or other drug-related reasons.

- Over the past decade, there has been a threefold increase in the number of college women who report having been drunk on ten or more occasions in the previous month.
- Areas of a college campus offering cheap beer prices have more crime, including trouble between students and police or other campus authorities, arguments, physical fighting, property damage, false fire alarms, and sexual misconduct.
- Alcohol is involved in more than two-thirds of suicides among college students, 90 percent of campus rapes and sexual assaults, and 95 percent of violent crime on campus.
- Seventy-five percent of male students and 55 percent of female students involved in acquaintance rape had been drinking or using drugs at the time.
- Each year, more than 100,000 students between the ages of 18 and 24 report having been too intoxicated to know whether they consented to having sex.
- College students under the age of 21 are more prone to binge drinking and

pay less for their alcohol than their older classmates do. Though underage students drink less often, they consume more per occasion than students age 21 and older who are allowed to drink legally.

Source: Data were compiled from the numerous studies cited throughout this chapter and from M. Mohler-Kuo et al., "College Rapes Linked to Binge-Drinking Rates," *Journal of Studies on Alcohol* 65, no. 1 (2004); H. Weschler, "Watering Down the Drinks: The Moderating Effect of College Demographics on Alcohol Use in High Risk Groups," *American Journal of Public Health* 93, no. 11 (2003): 1929–33; T. F. Nelson et al., "Alcohol and Collegiate Sports Fans," *Addictive Behaviors* 28, no. 1 (2003): 1–11; R. W. Hingson et al., "Magnitude of Alcohol-Related Mortality and Morbidity among U.S. College Students Aged 18–24," *Journal of Studies on Alcohol* 63, no. 2 (2002): 136–44; American College Health Association, "American College Health Association–National College Health Assessment (ACHA–NCHA) Spring 2006 Reference Group Data Report," *Journal of American College Health* 55, no. 4 (2007): 195–206; Facts on Tap, "The College Experience: Alcohol and Student Life," 2006, www.factsontap.org.

TABLE 8.1	Reported Change in Alcohol Use as a Result of Social Norms Campaigns

The statistics below represent a small number of institutions using social norms campaigns to reduce alcohol consumption among college students, and their reported results.

University or College with a Social Norms Campaign	Reduction in Heavy Episodic Alcohol Consumption Due to Social Norms Campaign
Northern Illinois University	44% over 10 years
Hobart & William Smith Colleges	40% over 5 years
Rowan University	23% over 5 semesters
University of Missouri–Columbia	21% over 2 years
University of North Carolina	30% over 5 years
University of Arizona	29% over 3 years
Western Washington University	20% over 3 years
Florida State University	22% over 3 years
Michigan State University	26% over 3 years

Source: National Social Norms Resource Center, July 17, 2006, www.socialnorms.org.

College Students' Patterns of Alcohol Use, 2001

Category	Total (%)	Men (%)	Women (%)
Abstainer (past year)	19.3	20.1	18.7
Nonbinge drinker	36.3	31.3	40.4
Occasional binge drinker	21.6	23.4	20.0
Frequent binge drinker	22.8	25.2	20.9

Alcohol-Related Problems

Problem Reported	Nonbinge Drinkers (%)	Frequent Binge Drinkers (%)
Did something regrettable	18	62
Missed a class	9	63
Forgot where they were or what they did	10	54
Got behind in schoolwork	10	46
Argued with friends	10	43
Got hurt or injured	4	27
Damaged property	2	23
Engaged in unplanned sexual activities	8	42
Drove after drinking	19	57

Sources: H. Wechsler et al., "Trends in College Binge Drinking during a Period of Increased Prevention Efforts: Findings from Four Harvard School of Public Health College Study Surveys: 1993–2001," *Journal of American College Health* 50, no. 5 (2002): 207. Reprinted with permission of Helen Dwight Reid Educational Foundation. Published by Heldref Publications, 1319 18th St. NW, Washington DC 20036. Copyright 2002.

- It is more common for college students than their non-collegiate peers to drink recklessly and to engage in drinking games and other dangerous drinking practices.
- College students are particularly vulnerable to peer influence and have a strong need to be accepted by their peers.
- There is institutional denial by college administrators that alcohol problems exist on their campuses.

Binge drinking is especially dangerous because it often involves drinking a lot of alcohol in a very short period of time. This type of consumption can quickly lead to extreme intoxication, involving unconsciousness, alcohol poisoning, and even death. Often, drinking competitions or games and hazing rituals encourage this type of drinking. To see whether your alcohol consumption is a problem, complete the quiz in the **Assess Yourself** box on page 220.

There is also significant evidence that campus rape is linked to binge drinking. Women from colleges with medium to high binge drinking rates are 1.5 times more at risk of being raped than those from schools with a low binge drinking rate. Seventy-two percent of campus rapes occur when the victim is so intoxicated that she is unable to consent to or refuse sex.[5] For more on rape, see Chapter 4.

Binge drinking also affects students who do not participate in binge drinking behavior. One study indicated that over 696,000 students between the ages of 18 and 24 were assaulted by another student who had been drinking.[6] Other students report sleep and study disruptions, sexual abuse and other unwanted sexual advances, and vandalism of personal property.

To curb binge drinking and alcohol abuse, many schools are instituting strong policies against drinking. University presidents have formed a leadership group to help curb the problem of alcohol abuse. Many fraternities have elected to have "dry" houses. At the same time, schools are making more help available to students with drinking problems. Today, most campuses offer both individual and group counseling and are directing more attention toward preventing alcohol abuse. Student organizations such as BACCHUS (Boost Alcohol Consciousness Concerning the Health of University Students) promote responsible drinking and party hosting.

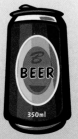

DID you KNOW?

College students consume an estimated 430 million gallons of beer, wine, and liquor per year. This is enough alcohol to fill more than 650 Olympic-sized swimming pools.

(Text continues on page 222.)

ASSESS yourself

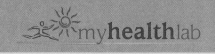

ALCOHOL ABUSE: EVALUATING YOUR RISK

Fill out this assessment online at
www.aw-bc.com/myhealthlab
or www.aw-bc.com/donatelle.

For each question, choose the answer that is correct for you.

1. How often do you have a drink containing alcohol?

| Never | Monthly or less | 2 to 4 times a month | 2 to 3 times a week | 4 or more times a week |

2. How many drinks containing alcohol do you have on a typical day when you are drinking?

| 1 or 2 | 3 or 4 | 5 or 6 | 7 to 9 | 10 or more |

3. How often do you have 6 drinks or more on one occasion?

| Never | Less than monthly | Monthly | Weekly | Daily or almost daily |

4. How often during the last year have you found that you were not able to stop drinking once you had started?

| Never | Less than monthly | Monthly | Weekly | Daily or almost daily |

5. How often during the last year have you failed to do what was normally expected from you because of drinking?

| Never | Less than monthly | Monthly | Weekly | Daily or almost daily |

6. How often during the last year have you needed a first drink in the morning to get yourself going after a heavy drinking session?

| Never | Less than monthly | Monthly | Weekly | Daily or almost daily |

7. How often during the last year have you had a feeling of guilt or remorse after drinking?

| Never | Less than monthly | Monthly | Weekly | Daily or almost daily |

8. How often during the last year have you been unable to remember what happened the night before because you had been drinking?

| Never | Less than monthly | Monthly | Weekly | Daily or almost daily |

9. Have you or someone else been injured as a result of your drinking?

| No | Yes, but not in the last year | Yes, during the last year |

10. Has a relative or friend or a doctor or other health worker been concerned about your drinking or suggested you cut down?

| No | Yes, but not in the last year | Yes, during the last year |

Analyzing Your Answers

Each question has its own set of scores. Assign yourself the correct number of points as indicated below, based on your answers.

Question 1: 0 = never; 1 = monthly or less; 2 = 2–4 times/ month; 3 = 2–3 times/week; 4 = 4 or more times/week

Question 2: 0 = 1–2 drinks; 1 = 3–4 drinks; 2 = 5–6 drinks; 3 = 7–9 drinks; 4 = 10 or more drinks

Questions 3–8: 0 = never; 1 = less than monthly; 2 = monthly; 3 = weekly; 4 = daily or almost daily

Questions 9 and 10: 0 = no; 1 = yes, but not in the last year; 2 = yes, during the last year

Scores below 6: Congratulations! You are in control of your drinking behaviors and do a good job of consuming alcohol responsibly and in moderation.

Scores between 6 and 8: Your alcohol consumption is possibly risky. Try to take steps to change your drinking behavior. It might be hard when you are surrounded by friends who participate in the same risky actions, but try to make some positive changes for your health and safety.

Scores above 8: Your drinking patterns are putting you at high risk for illness, unsafe sexual situations, or alcohol-related injuries, and they may even be affecting your academic performance. Look back at how you answered each question, and identify some changes you can make to reduce your risk.

Source: K. Bush et al., "The AUDIT Alcohol Consumption Questions (Audit-C)," *Archives of Internal Medicine* 158, no. 16 (1998): 1789–95; World Health Organization, Division of Mental Health and Prevention of Substance Abuse, "Alcohol Use Disorders Identification Text (AUDIT)," 2006, www.who.net.

MAKE it happen!

ASSESSMENT: The Assess Yourself activity gave you the chance to evaluate your alcohol consumption and determine whether it is harmful to you and those around you. If you were surprised by some of your answers, or couldn't be sure how to answer some of the questions, you may want to take steps to change your behavior.

MAKING A CHANGE: To change your behavior, you need to develop a plan. Follow these steps below and complete your Behavior Change Contract to take action.

1. Evaluate your behavior, and identify patterns and specific things you are doing. What can you change now? What can you change in the near future?

2. Select one pattern of behavior that you want to change.

3. Fill out the Behavior Change Contract found at the front of your book. It should include your long-term goals for change, your short-term goals, the rewards you'll give yourself for reaching these goals, potential obstacles along the way, and strategies for overcoming these obstacles. For each goal, list the small steps and specific actions that you will take.

4. Chart your progress in a journal. At the end of a week, consider how successful you were in following your plan. What helped you be successful? What made change more difficult? What will you do differently next week?

5. Revise your plan as needed: Are the short-term goals attainable? Are the rewards satisfying?

EXAMPLE: After completing the quiz in the Assess Yourself box, Mark was surprised to discover that he drank much more often than he had thought. In particular, he was surprised to realize that he was a heavy episodic drinker. During his 3 years in college, Mark had grown used to consuming 5 or more drinks once a week, and he had never seen this as a problem before he completed this questionnaire. He decided to address his concerns about his alcohol use in several steps.

First, Mark kept a log of his alcohol consumption over 2 weeks. He saw that he was drinking almost every night of the week, and drinking very heavily at least once a week. Mark decided he wanted to reduce his drinking and set two goals: taking a break from drinking altogether for 3 weeks and, after that, drinking only 3 drinks on Friday and Saturday nights for the rest of the semester. Mark explained to his friends that he was taking a break and invited them to go with him on hikes, to the movies, and to other alcohol-free environments. After successfully taking this break, Mark decided to set some goals and limits for himself on the alcohol he would consume in the future. He went to a fraternity party on a Friday night and drank 2 beers, his predetermined limit. He was happy to realize when he woke up the next morning that he felt refreshed, not hung over. When he went out for dinner with his friends Saturday night, they wanted to go barhopping afterwards. He volunteered to be the designated driver, and the bar gave him free sodas for the night. The next weekend, Mark found he had extra money that he hadn't spent on beer during the week and bought himself a new DVD.

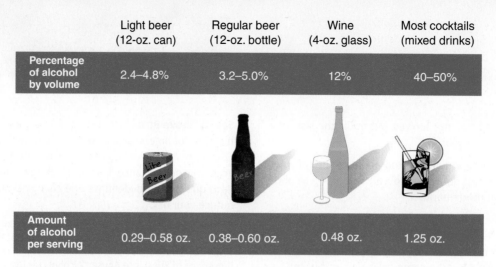

	Light beer (12-oz. can)	Regular beer (12-oz. bottle)	Wine (4-oz. glass)	Most cocktails (mixed drinks)
Percentage of alcohol by volume	2.4–4.8%	3.2–5.0%	12%	40–50%
Amount of alcohol per serving	0.29–0.58 oz.	0.38–0.60 oz.	0.48 oz.	1.25 oz.

FIGURE 8.1 Alcoholic Beverages and Their Alcohol Equivalencies

Trends in Consumption

In general, alcohol consumption levels among Americans have declined steadily since the late 1970s. In 2005, the estimated per capita consumption was the equivalent of 2.2 gallons of pure alcohol per person.[7] This represents a substantial decline from 2.64 gallons reported for 1977. (This measure indicates the amount of alcohol that a person would obtain by drinking approximately 50 gallons of beer, 20 gallons of wine, or more than 4 gallons of distilled spirits.)

This downward trend has been tied to a growing attention to weight, personal health, and physical activity. The alcohol industry has responded by introducing beer and wines with fewer calories and carbohydrates and with reduced alcohol content.

 what do you THINK?

Why do some college students drink excessive amounts of alcohol? ■ Are there particular traditions or norms related to when and why students drink on your campus? ■ Have you ever had your sleep or studies interrupted, or have you had to babysit a friend because he or she had been drinking?

ethyl alcohol (ethanol)   An addictive drug produced by fermentation and found in many beverages.

fermentation   The process whereby yeast organisms break down plant sugars to yield ethanol.

distillation   The process whereby mash is subjected to high temperatures to release alcohol vapors, which are then condensed and mixed with water to make the final product.

proof   A measure of the percentage of alcohol in a beverage.

The Chemical Makeup of Alcohol

The intoxicating substance found in beer, wine, liquor, and liqueurs is **ethyl alcohol,** or **ethanol.** It is produced during a process called **fermentation,** in which yeast organisms break down plant sugars, yielding ethanol and carbon dioxide. Fermentation continues until the solution of plant sugars (called mash) reaches a concentration of 14 percent alcohol. For beers, ales, and wines, the process ends with fermentation. Manufacturers then add other ingredients that dilute the alcohol content of the beverage.

Hard liquor is produced through further processing called **distillation,** during which alcohol vapors are released from the mash at high temperatures. The vapors are then condensed and mixed with water to make the final product.

The **proof** of an alcoholic drink is a measure of the percentage of alcohol in the beverage and therefore the strength of the drink. Alcohol percentage is half of the given proof. For example, 80 proof whiskey or scotch is 40 percent alcohol by volume, and 100 proof vodka is 50 percent alcohol by volume. Lower-proof drinks will produce fewer alcohol effects than the same amount of higher-proof drinks will produce. Most wines are between 12 and 15 percent alcohol, and most beers are between 2 and 8 percent, depending on state laws and type of beer (**Figure 8.1**).

Absorption and Metabolism

Unlike the molecules found in most foods and drugs, alcohol molecules are sufficiently small and fat soluble to be absorbed throughout the entire gastrointestinal system. A negligible amount of alcohol is absorbed through the lining of the mouth. Approximately 20 percent of ingested alcohol diffuses through the stomach lining into the bloodstream, and nearly 80 percent passes through the lining of the upper third of the small intestine. Absorption into the bloodstream is rapid and complete.

Several factors influence how quickly your body will absorb alcohol: the alcohol concentration in your drink, the amount of alcohol you consume, the amount of food in your stomach, pylorospasm (spasm of the pyloric valve in the digestive system), your metabolism, weight and body mass index, and your mood. The higher the concentration of alcohol in your drink, the more rapidly it will be absorbed in your digestive tract. As a rule, wine and beer are absorbed more slowly than distilled beverages. Carbonated alcoholic beverages—such as champagne and carbonated wines—are absorbed more rapidly than those containing no sparkling additives, or fizz. Carbonated beverages and drinks served with mixers cause the pyloric valve—the opening from the stomach into the small intestine—to relax, thereby emptying the contents of the stomach more rapidly into the small intestine. Because the small intestine is the site of the greatest absorption of alcohol, carbonated beverages increase the rate of absorption. In contrast, if your stomach is full, absorption slows because the surface area exposed to alcohol is smaller. A full stomach also retards the emptying of alcoholic beverages into the small intestine.

The more alcohol you consume, the longer absorption takes. Alcohol can irritate the digestive system, which causes pylorospasm. When the pyloric valve is closed, nothing can move from the stomach to the upper third of the small intestine, which slows absorption. If the irritation continues, it can cause vomiting.

Mood is another factor, because emotions affect how long it takes for the contents of the stomach to empty into the intestine. Powerful moods, such as stress and tension, are likely to cause the stomach to dump its contents into the small intestine. That is why alcohol is absorbed much more rapidly when people are tense than when they are relaxed.

Alcohol is metabolized in the liver, where it is converted to *acetaldehyde* by the enzyme *alcohol dehydrogenase*. It is then rapidly oxidized to *acetate,* converted to carbon dioxide and water, and eventually excreted from the body. Acetaldehyde is a toxic chemical that can cause immediate symptoms, such as nausea and vomiting, as well as long-term effects, such as liver damage. A very small portion of alcohol is excreted unchanged by the kidneys, lungs, and skin.

Alcohol contains 7 calories (kcal) per gram (you will learn more about calories in Chapter 9). This means that the average regular beer contains about 150 calories. Mixed drinks may contain more if they are combined with sugary soda or fruit juice. The body uses the calories in alcohol in the same manner it uses those found in carbohydrates: for immediate energy or for storage as fat if not immediately needed.

When compared to the variable breakdown rates of foods and other beverages, the breakdown of alcohol occurs at a fairly constant rate of 0.5 ounce per hour. This amount of alcohol is equivalent to 12 ounces of 5 percent beer, 5 ounces of 12 percent wine, or 1.5 ounces of 40 percent (80 proof) liquor. Unmetabolized alcohol circulates in the bloodstream until enough time passes for the body to break it down.[8]

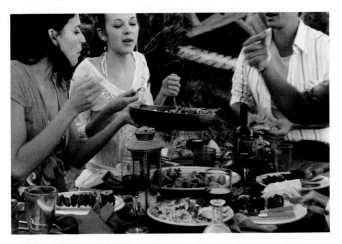

Many factors influence how rapidly your body absorbs alcohol. For example, eating while drinking slows down the absorption of alcohol into your bloodstream.

Blood Alcohol Concentration

Blood alcohol concentration (BAC) is the ratio of alcohol to total blood volume. It is the factor used to measure the physiological and behavioral effects of alcohol. Despite individual differences, alcohol produces some general behavioral effects, depending on BAC **(Table 8.3).** At a BAC of 0.02 percent, a person feels slightly relaxed and in a good mood. At 0.05, relaxation increases, there is some motor impairment, and a willingness to talk becomes apparent. At 0.08, the person feels euphoric, and there is further motor impairment. At 0.10, the depressant effects of alcohol become apparent, drowsiness sets in, and motor skills are further impaired, followed by a loss of judgment. Thus, a driver may not be able to estimate distance or speed, and some drinkers lose their ability to make value-related decisions and may do things they would not do when sober. As BAC increases, the drinker suffers increased physiological and psychological effects. All these changes are negative. Alcohol ingestion does not enhance any physical skills or mental functions.

A drinker's BAC depends on weight and body fat, the water content in body tissues, the concentration of alcohol in the beverage consumed, the rate of consumption, and the volume of alcohol consumed. Heavier people have larger body surfaces through which to diffuse alcohol; therefore, they have lower concentrations of alcohol in their blood than do thin people after drinking the same amount. Because alcohol does not diffuse as rapidly into body fat as into water, alcohol concentration is higher in a person with more body fat. Because a woman is likely to have more body fat and less water in her body tissues than a man of the same weight, she will be more intoxicated than a man after drinking the same amount of alcohol.

blood alcohol concentration (BAC) The ratio of alcohol to total blood volume; the factor used to measure the physiological and behavioral effects of alcohol.

Number of Drinks[†]	Blood Alcohol Concentration (%)	Psychological and Physical Effects
2	0.05–0.06	Feeling of relaxation, warmth; slight decrease in reaction time and in fine-muscle coordination
3	0.08–0.09	Balance, speech, vision, and hearing slightly impaired; feelings of euphoria, increased confidence; loss of motor coordination
3–4	0.08–0.10	Legal intoxication in most states; some have lower limits
4	0.11–0.12	Coordination and balance becoming difficult; distinct impairment of mental faculties, judgment
5	0.14–0.15	Major impairment of mental and physical control; slurred speech, blurred vision, lack of motor skills
7	0.20	Loss of motor control—must have assistance in moving about; mental confusion
>10	>0.30	Severe intoxication; minimal conscious control of mind and body
14	0.40	Unconsciousness, coma, death

*For each hour elapsed since the last drink, subtract 0.015 percent blood alcohol concentration, or approximately one drink.

†One drink = one beer (4% alcohol, 12 ounces), one highball (1 ounce whiskey), or one glass table wine (5 ounces).

Source: Modified from data given in Ohio State Police Driver Information Seminars and the National Clearinghouse for Alcohol and Alcoholism Information, Rockville, MD.

Both breath analysis (Breathalyzer tests) and urinalysis are used to determine whether an individual is legally intoxicated, but blood tests are more accurate measures of BAC. An increasing number of states are requiring blood tests for people suspected of driving under the influence of alcohol, but legal limits of BAC while driving do vary from one state to another. In some states, refusal to take the breath or urine test results in immediate revocation of the person's driver's license.

People can acquire physical and psychological tolerance to the effects of alcohol through regular use. The nervous system adapts over time, so greater amounts of alcohol are required to produce the same physiological and psychological effects. Though BAC may be quite high, the individual has learned to modify his behavior to appear sober. This ability is called **learned behavioral tolerance.**

Physiological and Behavioral Effects of Alcohol

Alcohol and Injuries

Alcohol use plays a significant role in the types of injuries people experience. Thirteen percent of emergency room visits by undergraduates are related to alcohol; of this total, 34 percent were the result of acute intoxication. A recent study

learned behavioral tolerance The ability of heavy drinkers to modify behavior so that they appear to be sober even when they have high BAC levels.

found that injured patients with a BAC of over 0.08 percent who were treated in emergency rooms were 3.2 times more likely to have a violent injury than an unintentional injury.[9] Most people admitted to emergency rooms are men 21 years or older, mostly as the result of accidents or fights where alcohol was involved.[10]

Alcohol Poisoning

Alcohol poisoning occurs much more frequently than people realize, and all too often it can be fatal. Drinking large amounts of alcohol in a short period of time can cause the blood alcohol level to reach the lethal range quickly. Alcohol, used either alone or in combination with other drugs, is responsible for more deaths due to toxic overdose than any other substance.

Death from alcohol poisoning can be caused by either central nervous system (CNS) and respiratory depression or the inhalation of vomit or fluid into the lungs. The amount of alcohol it takes for a person to become unconscious is dangerously close to the lethal dose. Signs of alcohol poisoning include inability to be roused; a weak, rapid pulse; an unusual or irregular breathing pattern; and cool (possibly damp), pale, or bluish skin. If you are with someone who has been drinking heavily and who exhibits these conditions or if you are unsure about the person's condition, call your local emergency number (911 in most areas) for immediate assistance. Don't wait for the individual to become unconscious; by then, the risk of death increases tenfold.

Alcohol and Sexual Decision Making

Alcohol has a clear influence on one's abilities to make good decisions about sex because it lowers inhibitions, and you may do things you might not do when sober. Seventy percent of college students admit to having engaged in sexual activity primarily as a result of being under the influence of alcohol. Students who are intoxicated are less likely to use safer sex practices and are more likely to engage in high-risk sexual activity. The risk of acquiring a sexually transmitted infection or an unplanned pregnancy also increases among students who drink more heavily compared to those who drink moderately or not at all.

Women and Alcohol

Body fat is not the only contributor to the differences in alcohol's effects on men and women. Compared to men, women have half as much *alcohol dehydrogenase*, the enzyme that breaks down alcohol in the stomach before it has a chance to reach the bloodstream and the brain. Therefore, if a man and a woman drink the same amount of alcohol, the woman's BAC will be approximately 30 percent higher than the man's BAC, leaving her more vulnerable to slurred speech, careless driving, and other drinking-related impairments.

Hormonal differences can also affect a woman's BAC. Certain times in the menstrual cycle and the use of oral contraceptives are likely to contribute to longer periods of intoxication. This prolonged peak appears to be related to estrogen levels.

Immediate Effects of Alcohol

The most dramatic effects produced by ethanol occur within the central nervous system. Alcohol depresses CNS functions, which decreases respiratory rate, pulse rate, and blood pressure. As CNS depression deepens, vital functions become noticeably affected. In extreme cases, coma and death can result.

Alcohol is a diuretic that causes increased urinary output. Although this effect might be expected to lead to automatic **dehydration** (loss of water), the body actually retains water, most of it in the muscles or in the cerebral tissues. The reason is that water is usually pulled out of the **cerebrospinal fluid** (fluid within the brain and spinal cord), leading to what is known as mitochondrial dehydration at the cellular level within the nervous system. Mitochondria are miniature *organelles* within cells that are responsible for cell respiration, and they rely heavily on fluid balance. When mitochondrial dehydration occurs, the mitochondria cannot carry out their normal functions. This results in symptoms that include the "morning-after" headaches some drinkers suffer.

Alcohol irritates the gastrointestinal system and may cause indigestion and heartburn if taken on an empty stomach. In addition, people who engage in brief drinking sprees during which they consume unusually high amounts of alcohol put themselves at risk for irregular heartbeat or even total loss of heart rhythm, which can disrupt blood flow and damage the heart muscle.

Is there any cure for a hangover?

Hangover A **hangover** is often experienced the morning after a drinking spree. The symptoms of a hangover are familiar to most people who drink:

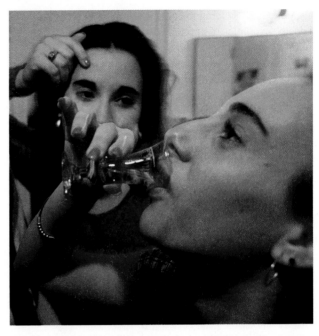

Increasing numbers of women on college campuses are trying to keep up with their male peers when binge drinking. The results can be dangerous; a woman's BAC will be higher than a man's after the same number of drinks.

headache, muscle aches, upset stomach, anxiety, depression, diarrhea, and thirst. **Congeners,** forms of alcohol that are metabolized more slowly than ethanol and are more toxic, are thought to play a role in the development of a hangover. The body metabolizes the congeners after the ethanol is gone from the system, and their toxic by-products may contribute to the hangover. Alcohol also upsets the water balance in the body, which results in excess urination, dehydration, and thirst the next day. Increased production of hydrochloric acid can irritate the stomach lining and cause nausea. It usually takes 12 hours to recover from a hangover. Bed rest, solid food, and aspirin may help relieve its discomforts, but the only cure for a hangover is abstaining from excessive alcohol use.

Drug Interactions When you use any drug (and alcohol is a drug), you need to be aware of its possible interactions with other drugs (Chapter 7), whether prescription or over-the-counter (OTC). Using alcohol while taking any other drug that causes CNS depression increases the effects of both of the

dehydration Loss of fluids from body tissues.

cerebrospinal fluid Fluid within and surrounding the brain and spinal cord tissues.

hangover The physiological reaction to excessive drinking, including symptoms such as headache, upset stomach, anxiety, depression, diarrhea, and thirst.

congeners Forms of alcohol that are metabolized more slowly than ethanol and produce toxic by-products.

drugs, potentially leading to coma, respiratory depression, and death. Examples of common drugs that can result in over-sedation when combined with alcohol include barbiturates, Valium-like drugs, codeine and other narcotics, and OTC antihistamines such as Benadryl. If you are taking any medication, ask your doctor of pharmacist whether it is safe for you to consume alcohol while taking the medication. Avoid using alcohol when taking antihistamines, antibiotics, analgesics, antidepressants, and anti-anxiety medications; the interactions between alcohol and these medications can be hazardous.

Long-Term Effects

Alcohol is distributed throughout most of the body and may affect many organs and tissues. Problems associated with long-term, habitual use of alcohol include diseases of the nervous system, cardiovascular system, and liver, as well as some cancers.

Effects on the Nervous System
The nervous system is especially sensitive to alcohol. Even people who drink moderately experience shrinkage in brain size and weight and a loss of some degree of intellectual ability.

New research suggests that developing brains in adolescents are much more prone to brain damage than was previously thought. Alcohol appears to damage the frontal areas of the adolescent brain, which are crucial for controlling impulses and thinking through consequences of intended actions.[11] In addition, researchers suggest that people who begin drinking at an early age face enormous risks of becoming alcoholics: 47 percent of people who begin drinking alcohol before age 14 become alcohol dependent at some time in their lives, compared with 9 percent of those who wait until at least age 21.[12]

Cardiovascular Effects
Alcohol affects the cardiovascular system in a number of ways. Numerous studies have associated light to moderate alcohol consumption (no more than 2 drinks a day) with a reduced risk of coronary artery disease. Several mechanisms have been proposed to explain how this might happen. The strongest evidence points to an increase in high-density lipoprotein (HDL) cholesterol, which is known as "good" cholesterol. Studies have shown that moderate drinkers have higher levels of HDL. Another factor that might help is an *antithrombotic effect*. Alcohol consumption is associated with a decrease in clotting factors that contribute to the development of atherosclerosis.

However, this does not mean that alcohol consumption is recommended as a preventive measure against heart disease—

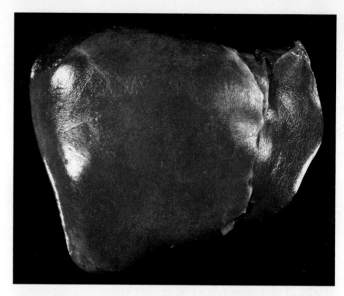

A normal liver

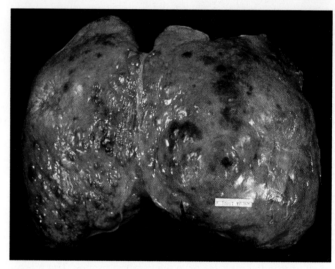

A liver with cirrhosis

it causes many more cardiovascular health hazards than benefits. Alcohol contributes to high blood pressure and slightly increased heart rate and cardiac output. People who report drinking 3 to 5 drinks a day, regardless of race or sex, have higher blood pressure than those who drink less.

Liver Disease
One of the most common diseases related to alcohol abuse is **cirrhosis** of the liver. It is among the top ten causes of death in the United States. One result of heavy drinking is that the liver begins to store fat—a condition known as *fatty liver.* If there is insufficient time between drinking episodes, this fat cannot be transported to storage sites, and the fat-filled liver cells stop functioning. Continued drinking can cause a further stage of liver deterioration called *fibrosis,* in which the damaged area of the liver develops fibrous scar tissue. Cell function can be partially restored at this stage with proper nutrition and abstinence from alcohol. If the person continues to drink, however, cirrhosis results. At this point, the liver cells die, and the damage becomes permanent.

cirrhosis The last stage of liver disease associated with chronic heavy use of alcohol, during which liver cells die and damage becomes permanent.

alcoholic hepatitis Condition resulting from prolonged use of alcohol, in which the liver is inflamed; can be fatal.

Alcoholic hepatitis is a serious condition resulting from prolonged use of alcohol. A chronic inflammation of the liver develops, which may be fatal in itself or progress to cirrhosis.

Cancer

Alcohol is considered a carcinogen. The repeated irritation caused by long-term use of alcohol has been linked to cancers of the esophagus, stomach, mouth, tongue, and liver. There is substantial evidence that women consuming high levels of alcohol (more than 3 drinks per day) have a higher risk of breast cancer compared with abstainers.[13] In one study, a team of scientists from the National Institute of Alcohol Abuse and Alcoholism discovered a possible link between acetaldehyde and DNA damage that could help to explain the connection between drinking and certain types of cancer.[14]

Other Effects

Alcohol abuse is a major cause of chronic inflammation of the pancreas, the organ that produces digestive enzymes and insulin. Chronic abuse of alcohol inhibits enzyme production, which further inhibits the absorption of nutrients. Drinking alcohol can block the absorption of calcium, a nutrient that strengthens bones. This should be of particular concern to women because of their risk for osteoporosis; bone thinning and calcium loss (see Chapter 14) increases with age. Heavy consumption of alcohol worsens this condition.

Evidence also suggests that alcohol impairs the body's ability to recognize and fight foreign bodies, such as bacteria and viruses. The relationship between alcohol and AIDS is unclear, especially because some of the populations at risk for AIDS are also at risk for alcohol abuse. But any stressor, including alcohol, with a known effect on the immune system would probably contribute to the development of the disease.

Alcohol and Pregnancy

Recall from Chapter 6 that *teratogenic* substances cause birth defects. Of the 30 known teratogens in the environment, alcohol is one of the most dangerous and common. More than 10 percent of all children have been exposed to high levels of alcohol in utero. All will suffer varying degrees of effects, ranging from mild learning disabilities to major physical, mental, and intellectual impairment. Alcohol consumed during the first trimester poses the greatest threat to organ development; exposure during the last trimester, when the brain is developing rapidly, is most likely to affect CNS development. A disorder called **fetal alcohol syndrome (FAS)** is associated with alcohol consumption during pregnancy. FAS is the third most common birth defect and the second leading cause of mental retardation in the United States, with an estimated incidence of 1 to 2 in every 1,000 live births. It is the most common preventable cause of mental impairment in the Western world.

If a woman ingests alcohol while pregnant, it will pass through the placenta and enter the growing fetus's bloodstream. It is recommended that women not consume any alcohol during pregnancy. Among the symptoms of FAS are mental retardation, small head, tremors, and abnormalities of the face, limbs, heart, and brain. Children with FAS may experience problems such as poor memory and impaired learning, reduced attention span, impulsive behavior, and poor problem-solving abilities, among others.[15]

Some children have fewer than the full physical or behavioral symptoms of FAS and can be categorized as having **fetal alcohol effects (FAE)**. FAE is estimated to occur three to four times more often than FAS, although it is much less recognized. The signs of FAE in newborns are low birth weight and irritability, and there may be permanent mental impairment. Infants whose mothers habitually consumed more than 3 ounces of alcohol (approximately 6 drinks) in a short time period when pregnant are at high risk for FAE. Risk levels for babies whose mothers consume smaller amounts are uncertain.

Drinking and Driving

Traffic accidents are the leading cause of death for all age groups from 5 to 45 years old (including college students). Approximately 39 percent of all traffic fatalities in 2005 were alcohol related.[16] It is estimated that three out of every ten Americans will be involved in an alcohol-related accident at some time in their lives.[17] Unfortunately, college students are overrepresented in alcohol-related crashes. Surveys report over 2.8 million college students, or 31.4 percent, have driven under the influence of alcohol.[18]

In 2005, there were 16,885 alcohol-related traffic fatalities (ARTFs), a 5 percent reduction from 1982.[19] Over the past 20 years, intoxication rates (BAC of 0.10 percent or greater) decreased for drivers of all age groups involved in fatal crashes **(Figure 8.2)**. This number represents an average of one alcohol-related fatality approximately every 30 minutes. Several factors probably contributed to these reductions in ARTFs: laws that raised the drinking age to 21; stricter law enforcement; increased emphasis on zero tolerance (laws prohibiting anyone under 21 from driving with any detectable BAC); and educational programs designed to discourage drinking and driving. The legal limit for BAC in all states is 0.08. Furthermore, many states do have zero tolerance laws, and the penalty usually is suspension of the driver's license.[20]

Laboratory and test-track research shows that the vast majority of drivers are impaired even at 0.08 BAC with regard to critical driving tasks. Braking, steering, lane changing, judgment, and divided attention, among other measures, are all affected significantly at 0.08 BAC. National groups such as MADD (Mothers Against Drunk Driving) and SADD

---

fetal alcohol syndrome (FAS) A disorder that may affect the fetus when the mother consumes alcohol during pregnancy. Among its effects are mental retardation, small head, tremors, and abnormalities of the face, limbs, heart, and brain.

fetal alcohol effects (FAE) A syndrome describing children with a history of prenatal alcohol exposure but without all the physical or behavioral symptoms of FAS. Among its symptoms are low birth weight, irritability, and possible permanent mental impairment.

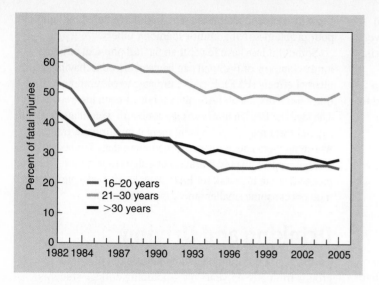

FIGURE 8.2 Percentage of Fatally Injured Passenger Vehicle Drivers with BACs > 0.08 Percent, by Driver Age
Source: Insurance Institute for Highway Safety, "Fatality Facts: Alcohol 2005," 2007, www.iihs.org.

(Students Against Destructive Decisions) try to educate their peers about the dangers of drinking and driving.

Despite all these measures, the risk of being involved in an alcohol-related automobile crash remains substantial. Researchers have shown a direct relationship between the amount of alcohol in a driver's bloodstream and the likelihood of a crash. A driver with a BAC level of 0.10 percent is approximately ten times more likely to be involved in a car accident than a driver who has not been drinking. At a BAC of 0.15 on weekend nights, the likelihood of dying in a single-vehicle crash is more than 380 times higher than for nondrinkers. Only 28 percent of fatally injured drivers involved in nighttime single-vehicle crashes had no alcohol in their blood.[21]

Alcohol-related fatal crashes occur more often at night than during the day; the hours between midnight and 3:00 AM are the most dangerous. The risk of being involved in an alcohol-related crash increases not only with the time of day, but also with the day of the week. In 2005, 24 percent of all fatal crashes during the week were alcohol related; among those taking place on weekends, 45 percent involved alcohol.[22]

 what do you THINK?

What do you think the legal BAC for drivers should be? ▪ What should the penalty be for people arrested for driving under the influence of alcohol (DUI) for the first offense? The second offense? The third offense?

alcohol abuse Use of alcohol that interferes with work, school, or personal relationships or that entails violations of the law.

alcoholism (alcohol dependence) Condition in which personal and health problems related to alcohol use are severe and stopping alcohol use results in withdrawal symptoms.

Alcohol Abuse and Alcoholism

Alcohol use becomes **alcohol abuse** when it interferes with work, school, or social and family relationships, or when it entails any violation of the law, including driving under the influence (DUI). **Alcoholism,** or **alcohol dependence,** results when personal and health problems related to alcohol use are severe, and stopping alcohol use results in withdrawal symptoms. Approximately 6 million Americans can be described as alcoholics.

Identifying a Problem Drinker

As with other drug addictions, tolerance, psychological dependence, and withdrawal symptoms must be present to qualify a drinker as an addict (see Chapter 7). Irresponsible and problem drinkers, such as people who get into fights or embarrass themselves or others when they drink, are not necessarily alcoholics. Also, most alcoholics are not found on skid row: 95 percent live in some type of extended family unit. Alcoholics can be found at all socioeconomic levels and in all professions, ethnic groups, geographical locations, religions, and races.

Studies suggest that the lifetime risk of alcoholism in the United States is about 10 percent for men and 3 percent for women. Moreover, almost 25 percent of the American population (50 million people) is affected by the alcoholism of a friend or family member.[23]

Recognizing and admitting the existence of an alcohol problem is often extremely difficult. Alcoholics themselves deny their problem, often making statements such as, "I can stop any time I want to. I just don't want to right now." Their families also tend to deny the problem, saying things like, "He really has been under a lot of stress lately. Besides, he only drinks beer." The fear of being labeled a "problem drinker" often prevents people from seeking help.

Alcoholics tend to have a number of symptoms in common (see the Assess Yourself box). People who recognize one or more of these behaviors in themselves may wish to seek professional help to determine whether alcohol has become a controlling factor in their lives.

Women are the fastest-growing population of alcohol abusers. They tend to become alcoholic at a later age and after fewer years of heavy drinking than do male alcoholics. Women at highest risk for alcohol-related problems are those who are unmarried but living with a partner, are in their twenties or early thirties, or have a husband or partner who drinks heavily.

College Students and Problem Drinking

One study has shown that 6 percent of college students meet the criteria for a diagnosis of alcohol dependence (also referred to as alcoholism), and 31 percent meet the criteria for alcohol abuse. Students who attend colleges with heavy drinking environments are more likely to be diagnosed with abuse or dependence. Despite the prevalence of alcohol disorders on campus, very few students seek treatment.[24]

The Causes of Alcohol Abuse and Alcoholism

We know that alcoholism is a disease with biological and social/environmental components, but we do not know what role each component plays in the disease.

Biological and Family Factors Research into the hereditary and environmental causes of alcoholism has found higher rates of alcoholism among children of alcoholics than in the general population. In fact, alcoholism is four to five times more common among children of alcoholics. These children may be strongly influenced by their parents' behavior.

Despite evidence of heredity's role in alcoholism, scientists do not yet understand the precise role of genes and increased risk for alcoholism, nor have they identified a specific "alcoholism" gene. Studies of identical twins (twins who share the same genes) and fraternal twins (who share about half of their genes, like other siblings) suggest that heredity, in both men and women, accounts for two-thirds of the risk for becoming alcoholic.

Social and Cultural Factors Social and cultural factors may trigger the affliction for many people who are not genetically predisposed to alcoholism. Some people begin drinking as a way to dull the pain of an acute loss or an emotional or social problem. For example, college students may drink to escape the stress of college life; disappointment over unfulfilled expectations; difficulties in forming relationships; or loss of the security of home, loved ones, and close friends. Involvement in a painful relationship, death of a family member, and other problems may trigger a search for an anesthetic. Unfortunately, the emotional discomfort that causes many people to turn to alcohol also ultimately causes them to become even more uncomfortable as the depressant

effect of the drug begins to take its toll. Thus, the person who is already depressed may become even more depressed, antagonizing friends and other social supports. Eventually, the drinker becomes physically dependent on the drug.

Family attitudes toward alcohol also seem to influence whether a person will develop a drinking problem. It has been clearly demonstrated that people who are raised in cultures in which drinking is a part of religious or ceremonial activities or in which alcohol is a traditional part of the family meal are less prone to alcohol dependence. In contrast, in societies in which alcohol purchase is carefully controlled and drinking is regarded as a rite of passage to adulthood, the tendency for abuse appears to be greater.

Apparently, then, some combination of heredity and environment plays a decisive role in the development of alcoholism. Certain ethnic and racial groups also have special alcohol abuse problems.

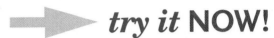

try it NOW!

Make a conscious effort to alter your drinking habits. Take these measures to be sure you do not become extremely intoxicated the next time you go out: switch to light beers or other beverages with a lower alcohol content; don't drink fast—be sure to space your drinks farther apart; and eat a meal if you plan on drinking to slow down the rate of alcohol absorption.

Effects of Alcoholism on the Family

Only recently have people begun to recognize that it is the alcoholic *and* the alcoholic's entire family that suffer. Although most research focuses on family effects during the late stages of alcoholism, the family unit actually begins to react early on as the person starts to show symptoms of the disease.

An estimated 77 million Americans (about 43 percent of the U.S. adult population) have been exposed to alcoholism in the family.[25] Twenty-two million members of alcoholic families are age 18 or older, and many have carried childhood emotional scars into adulthood. Approximately one in four children under age 18 lives in an atmosphere of anxiety, tension, confusion, and denial.[26]

In dysfunctional families, children learn certain rules from an early age: don't talk, don't trust, and don't feel. These unspoken rules allow the family to avoid dealing with real problems and issues as family members unconsciously adapt to the alcoholic's behavior by adjusting their own behavior. Unfortunately, these behaviors enable the alcoholic to keep drinking. Children in such dysfunctional families generally assume at least one of the following roles:

- *Family hero.* Tries to divert attention from the problem by being too good to be true.
- *Scapegoat.* Draws attention away from the family's primary problem through delinquency or misbehavior.

- *Lost child.* Becomes passive and quietly withdraws from upsetting situations.
- *Mascot.* Disrupts tense situations by providing comic relief.

For children in alcoholic homes, life is a struggle. They have to deal with constant stress, anxiety, and embarrassment. Because the alcoholic is the center of attention, the children's wants and needs are often ignored. It is not uncommon for these children to be victims of violence, abuse, neglect, or incest. As we have seen, when such children grow up, they are much more prone to alcoholic behaviors themselves than are children from nonalcoholic families.

In the past decade, we have come to recognize the unique problems of adult children of alcoholics whose difficulties in life stem from a lack of parental nurturing during childhood. Among these problems are difficulty in developing social attachments, a need to be in control of all emotions and situations, low self-esteem, and depression. Fortunately, not all individuals who have grown up in alcoholic families are doomed to have lifelong problems. As many of these people mature, they develop a resiliency in response to their families' problems. They thus enter adulthood armed with positive strengths and valuable career-oriented skills, such as the ability to assume responsibility, strong organizational skills, and realistic expectations of their jobs and others. (For more information on how addiction can impact families, see Chapter 7.)

Costs to Society

It is estimated that alcohol-related costs to society reach well over $184.6 billion when health insurance, criminal justice costs, treatment costs, and lost productivity are factored in. Reportedly, alcoholism is directly or indirectly responsible for over 25 percent of the nation's medical expenses and lost earnings.[27]

The Cost of Underage Drinking A recent study estimated that underage drinking costs society $61.9 billion annually. These costs take into consideration crashes, violence, property crime, suicide, burns, drowning, fetal alcohol syndrome, high-risk sex, poisoning, psychosis, and treatments for alcohol dependence. The largest costs were related to violence ($34.7 billion) and drunken driving accidents ($13.5 billion), followed by high-risk sex (nearly $5 billion), property crime ($3 billion), and addiction treatment programs (nearly $2 billion). By dividing the cost of underage drinking by the estimated number of underage drinkers, the study estimated that every underage drinker costs society an average of $4,680 a year.[28]

Women and Alcoholism

Studies indicate that there are now almost as many female as male alcoholics. Women get addicted faster with less alcohol use and then suffer the consequences more profoundly. Women alcoholics have death rates 50 to 100 percent higher than male alcoholics, including deaths from suicide, alcohol-related accidents, heart disease and stroke, and cirrhosis.[29]

Risk factors for drinking problems among *all women* include a family history of drinking problems, pressure to drink from a peer or spouse, depression, and stress.

Drinking patterns among different age groups also differ in these ways:[30]

- Younger women drink more overall, and they experience more alcohol-related problems, such as drinking and driving, assaults, suicide attempts, and difficulties at work.
- Middle-aged women are more likely to develop drinking problems in response to a traumatic or life-changing event, such as divorce, surgery, or death of a significant other.
- Older women are more likely than older men to have developed drinking problems within the past 10 years.

It is estimated that only 14 percent of women who need treatment get it. In one study, women cited the following reasons for not seeking treatment: potential loss of income, not wanting others to know they may have a problem, inability to pay for treatment, and fear that treatment would not be confidential.[31]

Alcohol and Ethnic or Racial Differences

Different ethnic and racial minority groups have their own patterns of alcohol consumption and abuse. Among Native American populations, alcohol is the most widely used drug; the rate of alcoholism in this population is two to three times higher than the national average, and the death rate from alcohol-related causes is eight times higher than the national average. Some possible factors for the alcoholism problem in the Native American population are poor economic conditions and the cultural belief that alcoholism is a spiritual problem, not an actual disease.

African American and Latino populations also exhibit distinct patterns of abuse. On average, African Americans drink less than white Americans; however, those who do drink tend to be heavy drinkers. Among Latinos, men have a higher-than-average rate of alcohol abuse and alcohol-related health problems. Cirrhosis and drunk driving are the most common causes of alcohol-related death or injury for Latino men. Many Latino women abstain. Many researchers agree that a major factor for alcohol problems in this ethnic group is the key role drinking plays in Latino culture.

Asian Americans have a very low rate of alcoholism. Social and cultural influences, such as strong kinship ties, are thought to discourage heavy drinking in Asian groups. Asians also have a genetic predisposition that might influence their low risk for alcohol abuse as well; for many, a defect in the gene that manufactures aldehyde dehydrogenase, a key enzyme in alcohol metabolism, leads to unpleasant side effects, making drinking a less pleasurable experience.[32]

Recovery

Despite growing recognition of our national alcohol problem, fewer than 10 percent of alcoholics in the United States receive any care. Factors contributing to this low figure include inability or unwillingness to admit to an alcohol problem; the social stigma attached to alcoholism; breakdowns in referral and delivery systems (failure of physicians or psychotherapists to follow up on referrals, failure of clients to follow through with recommended treatments, or failure of rehabilitation facilities to give quality care); and failure of the professional medical establishment to recognize and diagnose alcoholic symptoms among patients.

Most problem drinkers who seek help have experienced a turning point: a spouse walks out, taking children and possessions; the boss issues an ultimatum to dry out or ship out. Devoid of hope, physically depleted, and spiritually despairing, the alcoholic finally recognizes that alcohol controls his or her life. The first steps on the road to recovery are to regain that control and to assume responsibility for personal actions.

The Family's Role

Members of an alcoholic's family sometimes take action before the alcoholic does. They may go to an organization or a treatment facility to seek help for themselves and their relative. An effective method of helping an alcoholic to confront the disease is a process called **intervention.** Essentially, an intervention is a planned confrontation with the alcoholic that involves several family members and friends plus professional counselors. Family members express their love and concern, telling the alcoholic that they will no longer refrain from acknowledging the problem and affirming their support for appropriate treatment. A family intervention has been the turning point for a growing number of alcoholics.

Treatment Programs

The alcoholic who is ready for help has several avenues of treatment: psychologists and psychiatrists specializing in the treatment of alcoholism, private treatment centers, hospitals specifically designed to treat alcoholics, community mental health facilities, and support groups such as **Alcoholics Anonymous (AA).**

Private Treatment Facilities
Private treatment facilities have made concerted efforts to attract patients through radio and television advertising. Upon admission to the treatment facility, the patient receives a complete physical exam to determine whether underlying medical problems will interfere with treatment.

Alcoholics who decide to quit drinking will experience *detoxification,* the process by which addicts end their dependence on a drug. Withdrawal symptoms include hyperexcitability, confusion and agitation, sleep disorders, convulsions, tremors of the hands, depression, headache, and seizures. For a small percentage of people, alcohol withdrawal results in a severe syndrome known as **delirium tremens (DTs),** characterized by confusion, delusions, agitated behavior, and hallucinations.

Shortly after detoxification, alcoholics begin their treatment for psychological addiction. Most treatment facilities keep their patients from 3 to 6 weeks. Treatment at private treatment centers costs several thousand dollars, but some insurance programs or employers will assume most of this expense.

Family, Individual, and Group Therapy
In family therapy, the person and family members gradually examine the psychological reasons underlying the addiction. In individual and group therapy with fellow addicts, alcoholics learn positive coping skills for situations that have regularly caused them to turn to alcohol.

On some college campuses, the problems associated with alcohol abuse are so great that student health centers are opening their own treatment programs. The University of Texas offers a support service called Complete Recovery 101, and at other schools students in recovery live together in special housing. Because it can be difficult to recover from an alcohol abuse problem in college, support programs such as these hope to offer the support and comfortable environment recovering students need.

Relapse

Success in recovery varies with the individual. Roughly 60 percent of alcoholics relapse (resume drinking) within the first 3 months of treatment. Why is the relapse rate so high? Treating an addiction requires more than getting the addict to stop using a substance; it also requires getting the person to break a pattern of behavior that has dominated his or her life. Many alcoholics refer to themselves as "recovering" throughout their lifetime; they never use the word *cured.*

People who are seeking to regain a healthy lifestyle must not only confront their addiction, but also guard against the tendency to relapse. Drinkers with compulsive personalities need to learn to understand themselves and take control. To be effective, a recovery program must offer the alcoholic ways to increase self-esteem and resume personal growth.

---

intervention A planned confrontation with an alcoholic in which family members, friends, and professional counselors express their concern about the alcoholic's drinking.

Alcoholics Anonymous (AA) An organization whose goal is to help alcoholics stop drinking; includes auxiliary branches such as Al-Anon and Alateen.

delirium tremens (DTs) A severe state of confusion sometimes brought on by withdrawal from alcohol. Symptoms include hallucinations, anxiety, and trembling.

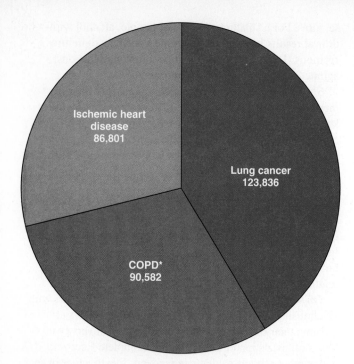

FIGURE 8.3 Annual Deaths Attributable to Smoking in the United States

*COPD = chronic obstructive pulmonary disease.

Source: Centers for Disease Control, "Annual Smoking-Attributable Mortality, Years of Potential Life Lost, and Economic Costs," *Morbidity and Mortality Weekly Report* 54, no. 25 (2005): 625–28.

Smoking in the United States

Tobacco use is the single most preventable cause of death in the United States.[33] While tobacco companies continue to publish full-page advertisements refuting the dangers of smoking, nearly 438,000 Americans die each year of tobacco-related diseases[34] **(Figure 8.3).** This is 50 times as many as will die from all illegal drugs combined. Moreover, another 10 million people will suffer from disorders caused by tobacco. To date, tobacco is known to cause about 25 diseases, and one in every five deaths in the United States is related to smoking. About half of all regular smokers die of smoking-related diseases. Therefore, any contention by the tobacco industry that tobacco use is not dangerous is irresponsible and ignores the scientific evidence.

In 1991, the Youth Risk Assessment Survey, which includes students in grades 9 through 12, indicated that 27.5 percent of teenagers smoked; by 2005, 23 percent were current smokers. This survey indicates a downward trend among adolescent smokers.[35] Every day, another 6,000 teens under the age of 18 smoke their first cigarette, and more than 3,000 others become daily smokers.[36] Cigarette use among teens is attributed to the ready availability of tobacco products through vending machines and the aggressive drive by tobacco companies to entice young people to smoke.

TABLE 8.4	Percentage of Population That Smokes (age 18 and older) among Select Groups in the United States

	Percentage
United States overall	20.9
Race	
Native American	32.0
Asian American/Pacific Islander	13.3
African American	21.5
Hispanic	16.2
White	21.9
Age	
18–24	24.4
25–44	24.1
45–64	21.9
65+	8.6
Sex	
Male	23.9
Female	18.1
Education	
Undergraduate	10.7
Some college	22.5
High school	24.6
9–11 years (no diploma)	32.6
Income Level	
Below poverty level	29.9
At or above poverty level	20.6

Source: Centers for Disease Control, "Tobacco Use Among Adults—United States, 2005," *Morbidity and Mortality Weekly Report* 55, no. 42 (2006): 1145–48.

Tobacco and Social Issues

The production and distribution of tobacco products in the United States and abroad involve many political and economic issues. Tobacco-growing states derive substantial income from tobacco production, and federal, state, and local governments benefit enormously from cigarette taxes. More recently, nationwide health awareness has led to a decrease in the use of tobacco products among U.S. adults. **Table 8.4** shows the percentages of Americans who smoke, by demographic group.

Advertising The tobacco industry spends an estimated $18 million per day on advertising and promotional materials. With the number of smokers declining by about 1 million each year, the industry must actively recruit new smokers. Campaigns are directed at all age, social, and ethnic groups, but because children and teenagers constitute 90 percent of all new smokers, much of the advertising has been directed toward them. Evidence of product recognition among underage smokers is clear: 86 percent of underage smokers prefer one of the three most heavily advertised brands—Marlboro, Newport, or Camel. One of the most blatant campaigns aimed at young adults was the popular Joe Camel ad campaign. After R. J. Reynolds introduced the cartoon figure, Camel's market share among underage smokers jumped from 3 to 13.3 percent in 3 years.

Advertisements in women's magazines imply that smoking is the key to financial success, independence, and social acceptance. Many brands also have thin spokeswomen pushing "slim" and "light" cigarettes to cash in on women's fear of gaining weight. These ads have apparently been working. From the mid-1970s through the early 2000s, cigarette sales to women increased dramatically. Not coincidentally, by 1987 cigarette-induced lung cancer had surpassed breast cancer as the leading cancer killer among women.

Women are not the only targets of gender-based cigarette advertisements. Men are depicted in locker rooms, charging over rugged terrain in off-road vehicles, or riding stallions into the sunset in blatant appeals to a need to feel and appear masculine. Minorities are often targeted, and so are college students.

Financial Costs to Society The use of tobacco products is costly to all of us in terms of lost productivity and lost lives. Estimates show that tobacco use causes over $167 billion in annual health-related economic losses.[37] The economic burden of tobacco use totals more than $75.5 billion in medical expenditures (costs include hospital, physician, and nursing home expenditures; prescription drugs; and home health care expenditures) and $92 billion in indirect costs (absenteeism, added cost of fire insurance, training costs to replace employees who die prematurely, disability payments, and so on). The economic costs of smoking are estimated to be about $3,391 per smoker per year.[38]

College Students and Smoking

Young people aged 18 to 24 are a popular target for tobacco advertisers. The tobacco industry has set up aggressive marketing promotions at bars, music festivals, and the like, specifically targeted to this age group. Peer influence and the desire to emulate peers can prompt a young person to start smoking. This potential impact is heightened by the fact that although over half of campuses claim to be smoke-free, they do permit smoking in residence hall rooms, student centers, and cafeterias, and many sell tobacco products in campus stores and student lounges.

College students may be especially vulnerable because they are in a new, often stressful social and academic environment. For many, the college years are their initial taste of freedom from parental supervision. Smoking may begin earlier, but most college students are a part of the age group in which people begin smoking and become hooked.

Cigarette smoking among U.S. college students has decreased slightly in recent years. In a 2005 study, about

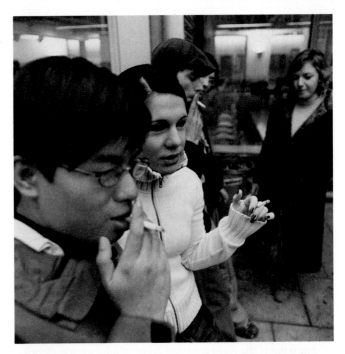

Despite all we know about the long-term health effects of smoking, young people continue to put their health at risk. Why?

18 percent of college students reported having smoked cigarettes in the past 30 days, down from about 30 percent in 1999. College men and women have nearly identical rates of cigarette smoking, but men use more cigars and smokeless tobacco.[39]

Social Smoking Many smokers describe themselves as "social smokers." One study defined *social smoking* as smoking when you are with people, rather than alone. Among people who smoked within the past 30 days, 51 percent were identified as social smokers. What differentiates a social smoker from a smoker? Social smokers smoke less often, and less intensely, and are less dependent on nicotine. Social smokers do not view themselves as being addicted to cigarettes, and they are less likely to quit the habit or have any intention to quit.[40]

However, even occasional smoking is not without risks. Social smoking in college can lead to a complete dependence on nicotine and, thus, all of the same health risks as smoking regularly. So why do college students become smokers? A survey identified four factors that contribute to smoking in college: a tendency toward risk taking, depression, social norms that tolerate or encourage smoking, and a lack of self-efficacy to resist peer pressure.[41]

Unlike social smokers, most students who smoke regularly and are nicotine dependent do want to stop smoking. One study reported that 70 percent of cigarette-smoking students had tried to quit smoking. Unfortunately, three out of four were still smokers.[42] It is important that colleges and universities engage in antismoking efforts, strictly control tobacco advertising, provide smoke-free residence halls, and offer greater access to smoking cessation programs.

what do you THINK?

Have you noticed a change in the number of your friends who are regular smokers or occasional smokers? ▪ How many of them smoked prior to coming to college, and how many picked up the habit at college? ▪ What are their reasons for smoking? ▪ What barriers keep your friends from quitting?

Tobacco and Its Effects

The chemical stimulant **nicotine** is the major psychoactive substance in all tobacco products. In its natural form, it is a colorless liquid that turns brown on exposure to air. When tobacco leaves are burned in a cigarette, pipe, or cigar, nicotine is released and inhaled into the lungs. Sucking or chewing tobacco releases nicotine into the saliva, and the nicotine is then absorbed through the mucous membranes in the mouth.

Smoking is the most common form of tobacco use. Smoking delivers a strong dose of nicotine to the user, along with an additional 4,700 chemical substances including arsenic, formaldehyde, and ammonia. Among these chemicals are various gases and vapors that carry particulate matter in concentrations that are 500,000 times greater than those of the most air-polluted cities in the world.[43]

Particulate matter condenses in the lungs to form a thick, brownish sludge called **tar.** Tar contains various carcinogenic (cancer-causing) agents, such as benzo[a]pyrene, and chemical irritants, such as phenol. Phenol has the potential to combine with other chemicals to contribute to the development of lung cancer.

In healthy lungs, millions of tiny hairlike projections (cilia) on the surfaces lining the upper respiratory passages sweep away foreign matter, which is expelled from the lungs by coughing. Nicotine impairs the cleansing function of the cilia by paralyzing them for up to 1 hour following the smoking of a single cigarette. This allows tars and other solids in tobacco smoke to accumulate and irritate sensitive lung tissue.

Tar and nicotine are not the only harmful chemicals in cigarettes. In fact, tars account for only 8 percent of tobacco smoke. The remaining 92 percent consists of various gases, the most dangerous of which is **carbon monoxide.** In tobacco smoke, the concentration of carbon monoxide is 800 times higher than the level considered safe by the U.S.

nicotine   The primary stimulant chemical in tobacco products.

tar   A thick, brownish substance condensed from particulate matter in smoked tobacco.

carbon monoxide   A gas found in tobacco smoke that binds at oxygen receptor sites in the blood.

Environmental Protection Agency (EPA). In the human body, carbon monoxide reduces the oxygen-carrying capacity of the red blood cells by binding with the receptor sites for oxygen, causing oxygen deprivation in many body tissues.

The heat from tobacco smoke is also harmful. Inhaling hot gases exposes sensitive mucous membranes to irritating chemicals that weaken the tissues and contribute to cancers of the mouth, larynx, and throat.

Tobacco Products

Tobacco comes in several forms. Cigarettes, cigars, pipes, and bidis are used for burning and inhaling tobacco. Smokeless tobacco is inhaled or placed in the mouth.

Cigarettes *Filtered cigarettes,* which are designed to reduce levels of gases such as hydrogen cyanide and carbon monoxide, may actually deliver more hazardous gases to the user than nonfiltered brands. Some smokers use low-tar and low-nicotine products as an excuse to smoke more cigarettes. This practice is self-defeating because they wind up exposing themselves to more harmful substances than they would with regular-strength cigarettes.

Clove cigarettes contain about 40 percent ground cloves (a spice) and about 60 percent tobacco. Many users mistakenly believe that these products are made entirely of ground cloves and that smoking them eliminates the risks associated with tobacco. In fact, clove cigarettes contain higher levels of tar, nicotine, and carbon monoxide than do regular cigarettes—and the numbing effect of eugenol, the active ingredient in cloves, allows smokers to inhale the smoke more deeply.

Cigars Those big stogies that we see celebrities and government figures puffing on these days are nothing more than tobacco fillers wrapped in more tobacco. Since 1991, cigar sales in the United States have increased dramatically. The fad, especially popular among young men and women, is fueled in part by the willingness of celebrities to be photographed puffing on one. Among some women, cigar smoking symbolizes an impulse to be slightly outrageous and liberated.

Many people believe that cigars are safer than cigarettes, when in fact nothing could be further from the truth.[44] Cigar smoke contains 23 poisons and 43 carcinogens. Smoking as little as one cigar per day can double the risk of several cancers, including cancer of the oral cavity (lip, tongue, mouth, and throat), esophagus, larynx, and lungs. Daily cigar smoking, especially for people who inhale, also increases the risk of heart disease (cigar smokers double their risk of heart attack and stroke) and a lung disease known as chronic obstructive pulmonary disease (COPD).

A common question is whether cigars are addictive. Most cigars contain as much nicotine as several cigarettes, and nicotine is highly addictive. When cigar smokers inhale, nicotine is absorbed as rapidly as it is with cigarettes. For those who don't inhale, nicotine is still absorbed through the mucous membranes in the mouth.

Bidis

Generally made in India or southeast Asia, **bidis** are small, hand-rolled, flavored cigarettes. They come in a variety of flavors, such as vanilla, chocolate, and cherry. Bidis resemble a marijuana joint or a clove cigarette and have become increasingly popular with college students, who view them as safer, cheaper, and easier to obtain than cigarettes. However, they are far more toxic than cigarettes. A study by the Massachusetts Department of Health found that bidis produced three times more carbon monoxide and nicotine and five times more tar than cigarettes. The leaf wrappers are nonporous, which means that smokers have to pull harder to inhale and inhale more to keep the bidi lit. During testing, it took an average of 28 puffs to smoke a bidi, compared to only 9 puffs for a regular cigarette. This results in much more exposure to the higher amounts of tar, nicotine, and carbon monoxide, and bidis lack any sort of filter to lower these levels. Bidi smokers face the same, if not higher, risk for coronary heart disease and cancer due to smoking.[45]

Spit (Smokeless) Tobacco

Approximately 5 million U.S. adults use smokeless tobacco. Most of them are teenaged (20 percent of male high school students) and young adult men, many of whom take up the habit to emulate a professional sports figure or family member. There are two types of smokeless tobacco: chewing tobacco and snuff.

Chewing tobacco is placed between the gums and teeth for sucking or chewing. It comes in three forms: loose leaf, plug, or twist. Chewing tobacco contains tobacco leaves treated with molasses and other flavorings. The user places a quid of tobacco in the mouth between the teeth and gums and then sucks or chews the quid to release the nicotine. Once the quid becomes ineffective, the user spits it out and inserts another. **Dipping** is another method of using chewing tobacco. The dipper places a small amount of tobacco between the lower lip and teeth to stimulate the flow of saliva and release the nicotine. Dipping rapidly releases nicotine into the bloodstream.

Snuff is a finely ground form of tobacco that can be inhaled, chewed, or placed against the gums. It comes in dry or moist powdered form or sachets (tea bag–like pouches). Usually snuff is placed inside the cheek.

Smokeless tobacco is just as addictive as cigarettes because of its nicotine content. There is nicotine in all tobacco products, but smokeless tobacco contains even more than cigarettes. Holding an average-sized dip or chew in the mouth for 30 minutes delivers as much nicotine as smoking four cigarettes. A two-can-a-week snuff user gets as much nicotine as a ten-pack-a-week smoker. Smokeless tobacco contains 10 times the amount of cancer-producing substances found in cigarettes and 100 times more than the U.S. Food and Drug Administration (FDA) allows in foods and other substances used by the public.

A major risk of chewing tobacco is **leukoplakia,** a condition characterized by leathery white patches inside the mouth produced by contact with irritants in tobacco juice. Three to 17 percent of diagnosed leukoplakia cases develop into oral cancer.

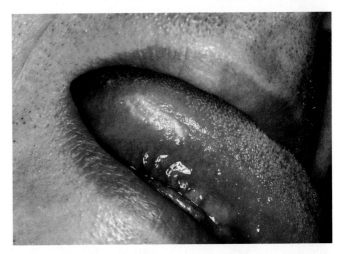

Leukoplakia can appear on the inside of the mouth or on the tongue, as shown here.

It is estimated that 75 percent of the estimated 34,360 oral cancer cases in the United States in 2007 resulted from either smokeless tobacco or cigarettes.[46] Users of smokeless tobacco are 50 times more likely to develop oral cancers than are nonusers. Warning signs include lumps in the jaw or neck; color changes or lumps inside the lips; white, smooth, or scaly patches in the mouth or on the neck, lips, or tongue; a red spot or sore on the lips or gums or inside the mouth that does not heal in 2 weeks; repeated bleeding in the mouth; and difficulty or abnormality in speaking or swallowing.

The lag time between first use and contracting cancer is shorter for smokeless tobacco users than for smokers because absorption through the gums is the most efficient route of nicotine administration. A growing body of evidence suggests that long-term use of smokeless tobacco also increases the risk of cancer of the larynx, esophagus, nasal cavity, pancreas, kidney, and bladder. Moreover, many smokeless tobacco users eventually "graduate" to cigarettes and further increase their risk for developing additional problems.

The stimulant effects of nicotine may create the same circulatory and respiratory problems for chewers as for smokers. Chronic smokeless tobacco use also delays wound healing and promotes peptic ulcers.

---

bidis   Hand-rolled flavored cigarettes.

chewing tobacco   A stringy type of tobacco that is placed in the mouth and then sucked or chewed.

dipping   Placing a small amount of chewing tobacco between the front lip and teeth for rapid nicotine absorption.

snuff   A powdered form of tobacco that is sniffed and absorbed through the mucous membranes in the nose or placed inside the cheek and sucked.

leukoplakia   A condition characterized by leathery white patches inside the mouth; produced by contact with irritants in tobacco juice.

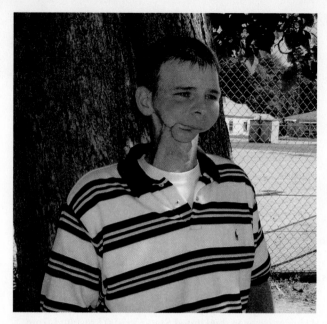

This 25-year-old cancer survivor has undergone surgery to remove neck muscles, lymph nodes, and his tongue. He began using smokeless tobacco at age 13; by age 17, he was diagnosed with squamous cell carcinoma. He now educates others about the dangers of chewing tobacco.

Like smoked tobacco, smokeless tobacco impairs the senses of taste and smell, causing the user to add salt and sugar to food, which may contribute to high blood pressure and obesity. Some smokeless tobacco products contain high levels of sodium (salt), which also promote high blood pressure. Dental problems are common among users of smokeless tobacco. Contact with tobacco juice causes receding gums, tooth decay, bad breath, and discolored teeth. Damage to both the teeth and jawbone can contribute to early loss of teeth. Users of any tobacco products may not be able to absorb the vitamins and other nutrients in food effectively.

Physiological Effects of Nicotine

Nicotine is a powerful CNS stimulant that produces a variety of physiological effects. Its stimulant action in the cerebral cortex produces an aroused, alert mental state. Nicotine also stimulates the adrenal glands, which increases the production of adrenaline. Nicotine stimulation increases heart and respiratory rate, constricts blood vessels, and, in turn, increases blood pressure because the heart must work harder to pump blood through the narrowed vessels.

Nicotine decreases blood sugar levels and the stomach contractions that signal hunger. These factors, along with

nicotine poisoning   Symptoms often experienced by beginning smokers, including dizziness, diarrhea, lightheadedness, rapid and erratic pulse, clammy skin, nausea, and vomiting.

decreased sensation in the taste buds, reduce appetite. For this reason, many smokers eat less than nonsmokers do and weigh, on average, 7 pounds less than nonsmokers.

Beginning smokers usually feel the effects of nicotine with their first puff. These symptoms, called **nicotine poisoning,** include dizziness, lightheadedness, rapid and erratic pulse, clammy skin, nausea, vomiting, and diarrhea. The effects of nicotine poisoning cease as tolerance to the chemical develops. Tolerance develops almost immediately in new users, perhaps after the second or third cigarette. In contrast, tolerance to most other drugs, such as alcohol, develops over a period of months or years. Regular smokers often do not experience the "buzz" of smoking. They continue to smoke simply because stopping is too difficult.

Health Hazards of Smoking

Cigarette smoking adversely affects the health of every person who smokes, as well as the health of everyone nearby. Each day, cigarettes contribute to more than 1,000 deaths from cancer, cardiovascular disease, and respiratory disorders.

Cancer

The American Cancer Society estimates that tobacco smoking causes 85 to 90 percent of all cases of lung cancer—fewer than 10 percent of cases occur among nonsmokers.[47] Lung cancer is the leading cause of cancer deaths in the United States. There were an estimated 213,380 *new* cases of lung cancer in the United States in 2007 alone, and an estimated 160,390 Americans died of the disease in 2007.[48] **Figure 8.4** illustrates how tobacco smoke damages the lungs.

Lung cancer can take 10 to 30 years to develop, and the outlook for its victims is poor. Most lung cancer is not diagnosed until it is fairly widespread in the body; at that point, the 5-year survival rate is only 13 percent. When a malignancy is diagnosed and recognized while still localized, the 5-year survival rate rises to 47 percent.

If you are a smoker, your risk of developing lung cancer depends on several factors. First, the number of cigarettes you smoke per day is important. Someone who smokes two packs a day is 15 to 25 times more likely to develop lung cancer than a nonsmoker. If you started smoking in your teens or if you inhale deeply when you smoke, you have a greater chance of developing lung cancer than people who started later. Occupational or domestic exposure to other irritants, such as asbestos and radon, will also increase your likelihood of developing lung cancer.

Tobacco is linked to other cancers as well. The rate of pancreatic cancer is more than twice as high for smokers as nonsmokers. Typically, people diagnosed with pancreatic cancer live about 3 months after their diagnosis. Cancers of the lip, tongue, salivary glands, and esophagus are five times more likely to occur among smokers than among nonsmokers.

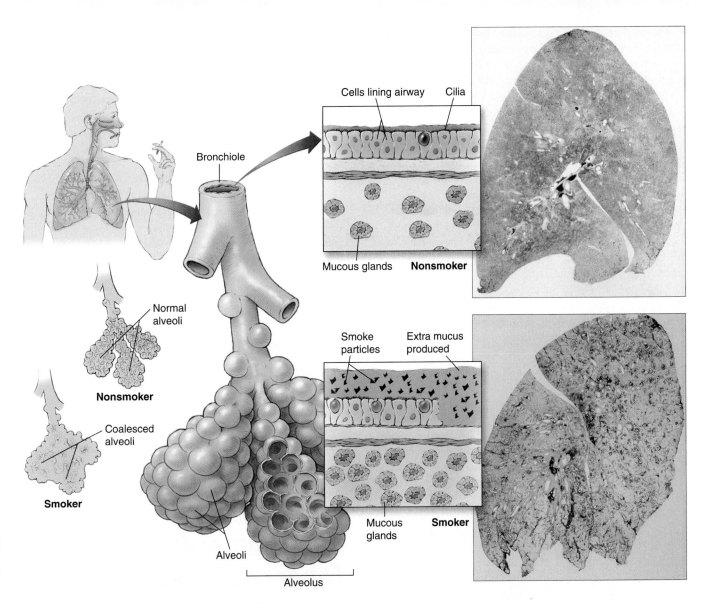

FIGURE 8.4 How Cigarette Smoking Damages the Lungs
Smoke particles irritate the lung pathways, causing excess mucus production. They also indirectly destroy the walls of the lungs' alveoli, which coalesce. Both factors reduce lung efficiency. Tar in tobacco smoke also has a direct cancer-causing action.

Smokers are also more likely to develop kidney, bladder, and larynx cancers.

Cardiovascular Disease

Over a third of all tobacco-related deaths occur from some form of cardiovascular disease.[49] Smokers have a 70 percent higher death rate from heart disease than nonsmokers do, and heavy smokers have a 200 percent higher death rate than moderate smokers do. In fact, smoking cigarettes poses as great a risk for developing heart disease as high blood pressure and high cholesterol levels do.

Smoking contributes to heart disease by adding the equivalent of 10 years of aging to the arteries.[50] One explanation is that smoking encourages the buildup of fatty deposits in the heart and major blood vessels (atherosclerosis). For unknown reasons, smoking decreases blood levels of HDLs, the "good cholesterol" that helps protect against heart attacks. Smoking also contributes to **platelet adhesiveness,** the sticking together of red blood cells that is associated with blood clots. The oxygen deprivation associated with smoking decreases the oxygen supplied to the heart and can weaken tissues. Smoking also contributes to irregular heart rhythms, which can trigger a heart attack. Both carbon monoxide and nicotine in cigarette smoke can precipitate angina attacks (pain spasms in the chest when the heart muscle does not get the blood supply it needs).

platelet adhesiveness   Stickiness of red blood cells associated with blood clots.

The number of years a person has smoked does not seem to bear much relation to cardiovascular risk. If a person quits smoking, the risk of dying from a heart attack falls by half after only 1 year without smoking and declines steadily thereafter. After about 15 years without smoking, the ex-smoker's risk of cardiovascular disease is similar to that of people who have never smoked.[51]

Stroke

Smokers are twice as likely to suffer strokes as nonsmokers are.[52] A stroke occurs when a small blood vessel in the brain bursts or is blocked by a blood clot, denying oxygen and nourishment to vital portions of the brain. Depending on the area of the brain affected, stroke can result in paralysis, loss of mental functioning, or death. Smoking contributes to strokes by raising blood pressure, which increases the stress on vessel walls. Platelet adhesiveness contributes to clotting. However, 5 to 15 years after they stop smoking, the risk of stroke for ex-smokers is the same as that for people who have never smoked.[53]

Respiratory Disorders

Smoking quickly impairs the respiratory system. Smokers can feel its impact in a relatively short period of time—they are more prone to breathlessness, chronic cough, and excess phlegm production than are nonsmokers their age. Smokers tend to miss work one-third more often than nonsmokers do, primarily because of respiratory problems, and they are up to 18 times more likely to die of lung disease.[54]

Chronic bronchitis is the presence of a productive cough that persists or recurs frequently. It may develop in smokers because their inflamed lungs produce more mucus and constantly try to rid themselves of this mucus and foreign particles. The effort to do so results in "smoker's hack," the persistent cough most smokers experience. Smokers are more prone than are nonsmokers to respiratory ailments such as influenza, pneumonia, and colds.

Emphysema is a chronic disease in which the alveoli (the tiny air sacs in the lungs) are destroyed, impairing the lungs' ability to obtain oxygen and remove carbon dioxide. As a result, breathing becomes difficult. Whereas healthy people expend only about 5 percent of their energy in breathing, people with advanced emphysema spend nearly 80 percent of

emphysema A chronic lung disease in which the tiny air sacs in the lungs are destroyed, making breathing difficult.

environmental tobacco smoke (ETS) Smoke from tobacco products, including secondhand and mainstream smoke.

mainstream smoke Smoke that is drawn through tobacco while inhaling.

secondhand smoke (sidestream smoke) The cigarette, pipe, or cigar smoke breathed by nonsmokers.

their energy. A simple movement such as rising from a seated position becomes painful and difficult for the emphysema patient. Because the heart has to work harder to do even the simplest tasks, it may become enlarged, and the person may die from heart damage. There is no known cure for emphysema, and once the damage is done, it is irreversible. Approximately 80 percent of all cases are related to cigarette smoking.

Sexual Dysfunction

Despite attempts by tobacco advertisers to make smoking appear sexy, research shows just the opposite: It can cause impotence in men. Several studies have found that male smokers are about two times more likely than are nonsmokers to suffer from some form of impotence. Toxins in cigarette smoke damage blood vessels, reducing blood flow to the penis and leading to an inadequate erection. It is thought that impotence may indicate oncoming cardiovascular disease.

Other Health Effects of Smoking

Gum disease is three times more common among smokers than among nonsmokers, and smokers lose significantly more teeth.[55] Smokers are also likely to use more medications. Nicotine and the other ingredients in cigarettes interfere with the metabolism of drugs. Nicotine speeds up the process by which the body uses and eliminates drugs, so that medications become less effective.

Environmental Tobacco Smoke

Although fewer than 30 percent of Americans smoke, air pollution from smoking in public places continues to be a problem. **Environmental tobacco smoke (ETS)** is divided into two categories: mainstream and sidestream smoke. **Mainstream smoke** refers to smoke drawn through tobacco while inhaling; **sidestream smoke** (commonly called secondhand smoke) refers to smoke from the burning end of a cigarette or smoke exhaled by a smoker. People who breathe smoke from someone else's smoking product are said to be *involuntary* or *passive* smokers. Nearly nine out of ten nonsmoking Americans are exposed to environmental tobacco smoke. In fact, measurable levels of nicotine were found in the blood of 88 percent of all nontobacco users.

Risks from Environmental Tobacco Smoke

Although involuntary smokers breathe less tobacco than active smokers do, they still face risks from exposure to tobacco smoke. Secondhand smoke actually contains more carcinogenic substances than the smoke that a smoker inhales. According to the American Lung Association, secondhand smoke has about 2 times more tar and nicotine, 5 times more carbon monoxide, and 50 times more ammonia than mainstream smoke. Every year, ETS is estimated to be responsible for approximately 3,000 lung cancer deaths, 46,000 coronary and heart disease deaths, and 430 deaths in newborns from sudden infant death sydrome.[56]

The Environmental Protection Agency has designated secondhand smoke as a known carcinogen (group A carcinogen). According to the Surgeon General's report titled *The Health Consequences of Involuntary Exposure to Tobacco Smoke,* there are more than 50 cancer-causing agents found in secondhand smoke.[57] The most likely mechanism whereby secondhand smoke causes lung cancer is continuous exposure to the carcinogens over time. There is also strong evidence that secondhand smoke interferes with normal functioning of the heart, blood, and vascular systems, significantly increasing the risk for heart disease and having immediate effects on the cardiovascular system.[58] Studies indicate that nonsmokers exposed to secondhand smoke were 20 to 30 percent more likely to have coronary heart disease than nonsmokers who are not exposed to smoke.[59]

Efforts to reduce the hazards associated with secondhand smoke have gained momentum in recent years. Groups such as GASP (Group Against Smokers' Pollution) and ASH (Action on Smoking and Health) have been working since the early 1970s to reduce smoking in public places. In response to their efforts, 35 states and the District of Columbia have enacted laws restricting smoking in public places such as restaurants, theaters, and airports. Of those 35 states, 17 have laws that make private workplaces smoke-free.[60] The Surgeon General has concluded that smoke-free workplace policies are the only effective way to eliminate secondhand smoke exposure in the workplace. Separating smokers from nonsmokers, cleaning the air, and ventilating buildings is not enough to eliminate exposure.[61] **Table 8.5** details measures you can take to protect yourself and others from secondhand smoke.

The hospitality industry has also taken steps to protect the health of nonsmokers. Hotels and motels now set aside rooms for nonsmokers, and many hotels are now becoming 100 percent smoke-free. Car rental agencies designate certain vehicles for nonsmokers. Smoking is banned on all U.S. airlines, and many other countries ban smoking on their airlines as well.

TABLE 8.5	Protecting Yourself and Others from Secondhand Smoke

Opening a window, sitting in a separate area, or using ventilation air conditioning, or a fan cannot eliminate secondhand smoke exposure.

You can protect yourself and others by

- Making your home and car smoke-free.
- Asking people not to smoke around you and your children.
- Making sure that your children's day care center or school is smoke free.
- Choosing smoke-free restaurants and other businesses. Thanking businesses for being smoke-free. Letting owners of businesses that are not smoke-free know that secondhand smoke is harmful to your health and the health of others.
- Teaching children to stay away from secondhand smoke.
- Avoiding secondhand smoke exposure if you or your children have respiratory conditions, you have heart disease, or you are pregnant.
- Talking to your doctor or health care provider more about the dangers of secondhand smoke.

If you are a smoker, the single best way to protect your family from secondhand smoke is to quit smoking. In the meantime, you can protect your family by making your home and vehicles smoke-free and smoking only outside. A smoke-free home rule can also help you quit smoking.

Source: Office on Smoking and Health, *The Health Consequences of Involuntary Exposure to Tobacco Smoke: A Report of the Surgeon General—Executive Summary.* (Washington DC: U.S. Department of Health and Human Services, 2006.)

Tobacco Use and Prevention Policies

It has been more than 40 years since the government began warning that tobacco use is hazardous to the health of the nation. Despite all the education on the health hazards of tobacco use, health care spending associated with smoking still exceeds $75.5 billion each year.[62] In response, 46 states have sued to recover health care costs related to treating smokers.

In 1998, the tobacco industry reached a Master's Settlement Agreement with 40 states. This agreement requires tobacco companies to pay approximately $206 billion over 25 years nationwide. The agreement also includes a variety of measures to support antismoking education and advertising and to fund research to determine effective smoking cessation strategies. The agreement also curbs tobacco industry billboard advertising and promotions and advertising that appeal to youth (including merchandise samples and use of cartoon characters in ads).

Unfortunately, most of the money designated for tobacco control and prevention at the state level has not been used for this purpose. Facing budget woes, many states have drastically cut spending on antismoking programs. In the few states that have spent the settlement money on smoking cessation programs, there has been some reported success in decreasing cigarette use.[63]

what do you THINK?

What rights, if any, should smokers have with regard to smoking in public places? ■ Does your campus allow smoking in residence halls? ■ Does your community have nonsmoking restaurants, or does it have only nonsmoking sections within restaurants? ■ Do you think your community would support nonsmoking restaurants and bars? Why or why not?

Quitting

Quitting smoking isn't easy. Smokers must break both the physical addiction to nicotine and the habit of lighting up at certain times of day. From what we know about successful quitters, quitting is often a lengthy process involving several unsuccessful attempts before success is finally achieved. Even successful quitters suffer occasional slips, which emphasizes the fact that stopping smoking is a dynamic process that occurs over time.

Approximately 70 percent of adult smokers in the United States want to quit smoking, and up to 40 percent make a serious attempt to quit each year. However, fewer than 5 percent succeed.[64]

The person who wishes to quit smoking has several options. Most people who are successful quit "cold turkey"— that is, they decide simply not to smoke again. Others resort to short-term programs, such as those offered by the American Cancer Society, which are based on behavior modification and a system of self-rewards. Still others turn to treatment centers that are part of large franchises, to a community outreach plan sponsored by a local medical clinic, or to a telephone quit line. Finally, some people work privately with their physicians to reach their goal.

Prospective quitters must decide which method or combination of methods will work best for them. Programs that combine several approaches have shown the most promise. Financial considerations, personality characteristics, and level of addiction are all factors to consider.

Breaking the Nicotine Addiction

Nicotine addiction may be one of the toughest addictions to overcome. Symptoms of **nicotine withdrawal** include irritability, restlessness, nausea, vomiting, and intense cravings for tobacco.

Nicotine Replacement Products
Nontobacco products that replace depleted levels of nicotine in the bloodstream have helped some people stop using tobacco. The two most common are nicotine chewing gum and the nicotine patch, both of which are available over-the-counter. The FDA has also approved a nicotine nasal spray and a nicotine inhaler.

Some patients use Nicorette, a prescription chewing gum containing nicotine, to reduce nicotine consumption over time. Under the guidance of a physician, the user chews 12 to 24 pieces of gum per day for up to 6 months. Nicorette delivers about as much nicotine as a cigarette does, but because it is absorbed through the mucous membrane of the mouth, it doesn't produce the same rush. Users experience no

---

withdrawal symptoms and fewer cravings for nicotine as the dosage is reduced until they are completely weaned.

Some controversy surrounds the use of nicotine replacement gum. Opponents believe that it substitutes one addiction for another. Successful users counter that it is a valid way to help break a deadly habit without suffering the unpleasant cravings that often lead to relapse.

The nicotine patch is generally used in conjunction with a comprehensive smoking-behavior cessation program. A small, thin, 24-hour patch placed on the smoker's upper body delivers a continuous flow of nicotine through the skin, helping to relieve cravings. The patch is worn for 8 to 12 weeks under the guidance of a clinician. During this time, the dose of nicotine is gradually reduced until the smoker is fully weaned from the drug. Occasional side effects include mild skin irritation, insomnia, dry mouth, and nervousness. The patch costs less than a pack of cigarettes—about $4—and some insurance plans will pay for it.

The nasal spray, which requires a prescription, is much more powerful and delivers nicotine to the bloodstream faster than gum or the patch. Patients are warned to be careful not to overdose; as little as 40 milligrams of nicotine taken at once could be lethal. The spray is somewhat unpleasant to use. The FDA has advised that it should be used for no more than 3 months and never for more than 6 months, so that smokers don't find themselves as dependent on nicotine in spray form as they were on cigarettes. The FDA also advises that no one who experiences nasal or sinus problems, allergies, or asthma should use it.

The nicotine inhaler, which also requires a prescription, consists of a mouthpiece and cartridge. By puffing on the mouthpiece, the smoker inhales air saturated with nicotine, which is absorbed through the lining of the mouth, not the lungs. This nicotine enters the body much more slowly than the nicotine in cigarettes does. Using the inhaler mimics the hand-to-mouth actions used in smoking and causes the back of the throat to feel as it would when inhaling tobacco smoke. Each cartridge lasts for 80 long puffs, and each cartridge is designed for 20 minutes of use.

Zyban, the smoking cessation pill, offers hope to many people who thought they could never quit. Zyban is thought to work on dopamine and norepinephrine receptors in the brain to decrease craving and withdrawal symptoms. Because of the way this prescription medication works, it is important to start the pills 1 to 2 weeks before the targeted quit date; it requires planning ahead.

A radical new way to help smokers quit is NicVAX, an antismoking vaccine due on the market very soon. The vaccination prevents nicotine from reaching the brain, making smoking less pleasurable and therefore easier to give up. A small amount may get to the brain, easing the discomfort of withdrawal. The vaccine differs from conventional cessation treatments by attacking the dependence in the brain, instead of just replacing the nicotine. One of the advantages of the vaccine over other forms of cessation methods is that it will reduce relapses by making the cigarette much less enjoyable when the quitter tries a cigarette again.[65]

---

nicotine withdrawal Symptoms, including nausea, headaches, irritability, and intense tobacco cravings, suffered by nicotine-addicted individuals who cease using tobacco.

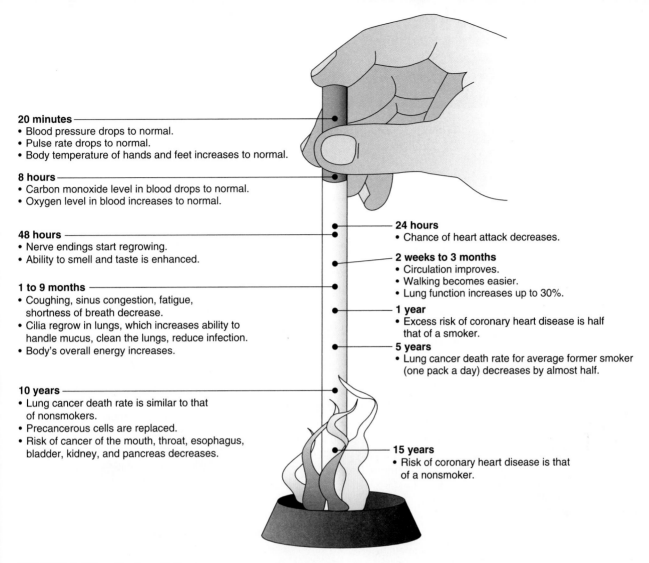

20 minutes
- Blood pressure drops to normal.
- Pulse rate drops to normal.
- Body temperature of hands and feet increases to normal.

8 hours
- Carbon monoxide level in blood drops to normal.
- Oxygen level in blood increases to normal.

48 hours
- Nerve endings start regrowing.
- Ability to smell and taste is enhanced.

1 to 9 months
- Coughing, sinus congestion, fatigue, shortness of breath decrease.
- Cilia regrow in lungs, which increases ability to handle mucus, clean the lungs, reduce infection.
- Body's overall energy increases.

10 years
- Lung cancer death rate is similar to that of nonsmokers.
- Precancerous cells are replaced.
- Risk of cancer of the mouth, throat, esophagus, bladder, kidney, and pancreas decreases.

24 hours
- Chance of heart attack decreases.

2 weeks to 3 months
- Circulation improves.
- Walking becomes easier.
- Lung function increases up to 30%.

1 year
- Excess risk of coronary heart disease is half that of a smoker.

5 years
- Lung cancer death rate for average former smoker (one pack a day) decreases by almost half.

15 years
- Risk of coronary heart disease is that of a nonsmoker.

FIGURE 8.5 When Smokers Quit
Within 20 minutes of smoking that last cigarette, the body begins a series of changes that continues for years. However, by smoking just one cigarette a day, the smoker loses all these benefits, according to the American Cancer Society.

Source: G. Hanson and P. Venturelli, *Drugs and Society,* 9th ed. Copyright © Jones and Bartlett Publishers, Sudbury, MA. www.jbpub.com. Reprinted with permission.

How effective are these therapies? The evidence is strong that consistent pharmacological treatments can help a smoker quit: an estimated 17 to 30 percent of people who have used these treatments continue to abstain from cigarettes.[66]

Breaking the Habit
For some smokers, the road to quitting includes antismoking therapy. Two common techniques are operant conditioning and self-control therapy. Pairing the act of smoking with an external stimulus is a typical example of an operant strategy. For example, one technique requires smokers to carry a timer that sounds a buzzer at different intervals. When the buzzer sounds, the patient is required to smoke a cigarette. Once the smoker is conditioned to associate the buzzer with smoking, the buzzer is eliminated, and, one hopes, so is the smoking. Self-control strategies view smoking as a learned habit associated with specific situations. Therapy is aimed at identifying these situations and teaching smokers the skills necessary to resist smoking.

The **Skills for Behavior Change** box on page 242 presents one of the American Cancer Society's approaches.

Benefits of Quitting
According to the American Cancer Society, many tissues damaged by smoking can repair themselves. As soon as smokers stop, the body begins the repair process **(Figure 8.5).** Within 8 hours, carbon monoxide and oxygen levels return to normal, and "smoker's breath" disappears. Often, within a month of quitting, the mucus that clogs airways is broken up and eliminated. Circulation and the senses of taste and smell improve within weeks. Many ex-smokers say they have more energy, sleep better, and feel more alert. By the end of 1 year, the risk for lung cancer and stroke decreases. Ex-smokers considerably reduce their risks of developing cancers of the mouth, throat, esophagus, larynx, pancreas, bladder, and cervix. They also cut their risk of peripheral artery disease, chronic obstructive lung disease, coronary heart disease, and ulcers. Women are less likely to

SKILLS FOR behavior change

DEVELOPING A PLAN TO KICK THE TOBACCO HABIT

There is no magic cure that can help you stop. Take the first step by answering this question: Why do I want to stop smoking? Write your reasons in the space below. Once you have prepared your list, carry a copy of it with you. Every time you are tempted to smoke, go over your reasons for stopping.

MY REASONS FOR STOPPING

1. _____
2. _____
3. _____
4. _____
5. _____

DEVELOP A PLAN; CHANGE SOME HABITS

Daily events such as finishing a meal, talking on the phone, drinking coffee, and chatting with friends can trigger the urge to smoke. Think about the times and places you usually smoke. What could you do instead of smoking at those times?

THINGS TO DO INSTEAD OF SMOKING

1. _____
2. _____
3. _____

THE BOTTOM LINE: COMMIT YOURSELF

There comes a time when you have to say good-bye to your cigarettes.

- Pick a day to stop smoking.
- Fill out the Behavior Change Contract.
- Have a family member or friend sign the contract.

Then

- Throw away all your cigarettes, lighters, and ashtrays at home and at work.
- Be prepared to feel the urge to smoke. The urge will pass whether you smoke or don't smoke. Use the "four Ds" to fight the urge:
  Delay
  Deep breathing
  Drink water
  Do something else

- Keep "mouth toys" handy: hard candies, gum, straws, and carrot sticks can help.
- If you've had trouble stopping before, ask your doctor about nicotine chewing gum, patches, nasal sprays, inhalers, or pills.
- Tell your family and friends that you've stopped smoking.
- Put "no smoking" signs in your car, work area, and house.
- Give yourself a treat for stopping. Go to a movie, go out to dinner, or buy yourself a gift.

FOCUS ON THE POSITIVES

Now that you have stopped smoking, your mind and your body will begin to feel better. Can you breathe more easily? Do you have more energy? Do you feel good about what you've done?

Make a list of the good things about not smoking. Carry a copy with you, and look at it when you have the urge to smoke.

---

bear babies with low birth weight. Within 2 years, the risk for heart attack drops to near normal. At the end of 10 smoke-free years, the ex-smoker can expect to live out his or her normal life span.

Caffeine

What is the most popular and widely consumed drug in the United States? Caffeine. Almost half of all Americans drink coffee every day, and many others consume caffeine in some other form, mainly for its well-known "wake-up" effect. Drink-ing coffee is legal, even socially encouraged. Many people believe caffeine is not a drug and not really addictive. Coffee, soft drinks, and other caffeine-containing products seem harmless. If you share these attitudes, think again; research in the past decade has linked caffeine to certain health problems.

Caffeine is a drug derived from the chemical family called **xanthines.** Two related chemicals, *theophylline* and *theobromine,* are found in tea and chocolate, respectively. The xanthines are mild CNS stimulants that enhance mental alertness and reduce feelings of fatigue. Other stimulant effects include increases in heart muscle contractions, oxygen consumption, metabolism, and urinary output. A person feels these effects within 15 to 45 minutes of ingesting a product that contains caffeine.

Side effects of the xanthines include wakefulness, insomnia, irregular heartbeat, dizziness, nausea, indigestion, and sometimes mild delirium. Some people also experience heartburn. As with some other drugs, the user's psychological outlook and expectations influence the effects.

caffeine   A stimulant found in coffee, tea, chocolate, and some soft drinks.

xanthines   The chemical family of stimulants to which caffeine belongs.

TABLE 8.6 Caffeine Content of Various Products

Product (Serving Size)	Caffeine Content (mg)
Coffees	
Starbucks Brewed Coffee (Grande) (16 oz.)	320
Coffee, generic brewed (8 oz.)	133 (range: 102–200)
Coffee, generic instant (8 oz.)	93 (range: 27–173)
Starbucks Espresso (1 oz.)	75
Espresso, generic (1 oz.)	40 (range: 30–90)
Coffee, generic decaffeinated (8 oz.)	5 (range: 3–12)
Starbucks Espresso decaffeinated (1 oz.)	4
Teas	
Starbucks Tazo Chai Tea Latte (Grande) (16 oz.)	100
Tea, brewed (8 oz.)	53 (range: 40–120)
Snapple: Lemon, Peach, Raspberry (and diet versions) (16 oz.)	42
Arizona Iced Tea, black (16 oz.)	32
Nestea (12 oz.)	26
Arizona Iced Tea, green (16 oz.)	15
Soft Drinks	
FDA official limit for cola and pepper soft drinks (12 oz.)	72
Jolt Cola (12 oz.)	72
Mountain Dew, regular or diet (12 oz.)	54 (20 oz. = 90)
Pepsi One (12 oz.)	54 (20 oz. = 90)
Diet Coke (12 oz.)	47 (20 oz. = 78)
Dr. Pepper, regular or diet (12 oz.)	41 (20 oz. = 68)
Pepsi (12 oz.)	38 (20 oz. = 63)
Diet Pepsi (12 oz.)	36 (20 oz. = 60)

Product (Serving Size)	Caffeine Content (mg)
Coca-Cola Classic (12 oz.)	35 (20 oz. = 58)
Barq's Root Beer, regular or diet (12 oz.)	23 (20 oz. = 38)
Energy Drinks	
Spike Shooter (8.4 oz.)	300
Full Throttle (16 oz.)	144
SoBe No Fear (8 oz.)	83
Red Bull (8.3 oz.)	80
Rockstar Energy Drink (8 oz.)	80
Glaceau Vitamin Water Energy Citrus (20 oz.)	50
Frozen Desserts	
Ben & Jerry's Coffee Heath Bar Crunch Ice Cream (8 fl. oz.)	84
Ben & Jerry's Coffee Flavored Ice Cream (8 fl. oz.)	68
Häagen-Dazs Coffee Ice Cream (8 fl. oz.)	58
Häagen-Dazs Coffee Frozen Yogurt (8 fl. oz.)	58
Starbucks Coffee Ice Cream (8 fl. oz.)	50–60
Chocolate	
Hershey's Special Dark Chocolate Bar (1.45 oz.)	31
Hershey's Chocolate Bar (1.55 oz.)	9
Hershey's Kisses (41 g; 9 pieces)	9
Hot cocoa (8 oz.)	9 (range: 3–13)
Over-the-Counter Drugs	
NoDoz (Maximum Strength) (1 tablet)	200
Vivarin (1 tablet)	200
Excedrin (Extra Strength) (2 tablet)	130

Serving sizes are based on commonly eaten portions, pharmaceutical instructions, or the amount of the leading-selling container size. For example, beverages sold in 16-ounce or 20-ounce bottles were counted as one serving.

Source: Center for Science in the Public Interest, "Caffeine Content of Food and Drugs," 2007, www.cspinet.org.

Different products contain different concentrations of caffeine. A 5-ounce cup of coffee contains 65 to 115 milligrams. Caffeine concentrations vary with the brand of the beverage and the strength of the brew. Small chocolate bars contain up to 15 milligrams of caffeine and theobromine. **Table 8.6** compares various caffeine-containing products.

Caffeine Addiction

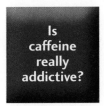

Is caffeine really addictive?

As the effects of caffeine wear off, users may feel let down—mentally or physically depressed, exhausted, and weak. To counteract this let-down, people commonly choose to drink another cup of coffee. Habitually engaging in this practice leads to tolerance and psychological dependence. Until the mid-1970s, caffeine was not medically recognized as addictive. Chronic caffeine use and its attendant behaviors were called "coffee nerves." This syndrome is now recognized as *caffeine intoxication,* or **caffeinism.**

Symptoms of caffeinism include chronic insomnia, jitters, irritability, nervousness, anxiety, and involuntary muscle twitches. Withdrawing the caffeine may compound the effects and produce severe headaches. (Some physicians ask their patients to take a simple test for caffeine addiction: don't consume anything containing caffeine, and if you get a severe headache within 4 hours, you are addicted.) Because caffeine meets the requirements for addiction—tolerance, psychological dependence, and withdrawal symptoms—it can be classified as addictive.

caffeinism Caffeine intoxication brought on by excessive caffeine use; symptoms include chronic insomnia, irritability, anxiety, muscle twitches, and headaches.

Although you would have to drink 67 to 100 cups of coffee in a day to produce a fatal overdose of caffeine, you may experience sensory disturbances after consuming only 10 cups of coffee within a 24-hour period. These symptoms include tinnitus (ringing in the ears), spots before the eyes, numbness in arms and legs, poor circulation, and visual hallucinations. Many people drink as many as 10 cups of coffee in one day, so such heavy caffeine intake may pose health threats.

Possible Health Concerns of Caffeine Use

Long-term caffeine use has been suspected of being linked to a number of serious health problems, ranging from heart disease and cancer to mental dysfunction and birth defects. However, no strong evidence exists to suggest that moderate caffeine use (less than 300 milligrams daily, approximately 3 cups of coffee) produces harmful effects in healthy, non-pregnant people.

It appears that caffeine does not cause long-term high blood pressure. It has not been linked to strokes, nor is there any evidence of a relationship between coffee and heart disease.[67] However, people who suffer from irregular heart-beat are cautioned against using caffeine because the resultant increase in heart rate might be life-threatening. Both decaffeinated and caffeinated coffee products contain ingredients that can irritate the stomach lining and be harmful to people with stomach ulcers.

For years, caffeine consumption was linked with fibrocystic breast disease, a condition characterized by painful, noncancerous lumps in the breast. Although these conclusions have been challenged, many clinicians advise patients with mammillary cysts to avoid caffeine. In addition, some reports indicate that very high doses of caffeine given to pregnant laboratory animals can cause stillbirths or offspring with low birth weights or limb deformations. Studies have found that moderate consumption of caffeine (less than 300 milligrams per day) did not significantly affect human fetal development.[68] However, women are usually advised to avoid or at least reduce caffeine use during pregnancy.

what do you THINK?

How much caffeine do you consume, and why? ▪ What is your pattern of caffeine consumption for the day? ▪ Have you ever experienced any ill effects after going without caffeine for a period of time?

TAKING charge

Summary

- Alcohol is a central nervous system (CNS) depressant used by 65 percent of all Americans and 90 percent of all college students; over 44 percent of college students are binge drinkers. Although consumption trends are slowly creeping downward, college students are under extreme pressure to consume alcohol.
- Alcohol's effect on the body is measured by the blood alcohol concentration (BAC), the ratio of alcohol to total blood volume. The higher the BAC, the greater the drowsiness and impairment of judgment and coordination.
- Negative consequences associated with alcohol use among college students include lower grade point averages, academic problems, traffic accidents, dropping out of school, unplanned sex, hangovers, and injury. Long-term alcohol overuse includes damage to the nervous system, cardiovascular damage, liver disease, and increased risk for cancer. Use during pregnancy can cause fetal alcohol effects (FAE) or fetal alcohol syndrome (FAS). Alcohol is also a causative factor in traffic accidents.
- Alcohol use becomes alcoholism when it interferes with school, work, or social and family relationships, or entails violations of the law. Causes of alcoholism include biological, family, social, and cultural factors. Alcoholism has far-reaching effects on families, especially on children. Treatment options for alcoholism include detoxification at

private medical facilities, therapy (family, individual, or group), and programs such as Alcoholics Anonymous.
- The use of tobacco involves many social and political issues, including advertising targeted at youth and women, the largest growing populations of smokers. Health care and lost productivity resulting from smoking cost the nation as much as $167 billion per year.
- Tobacco is available in smoking and smokeless forms, both of which contain addictive nicotine (a psychoactive substance). Smoking also delivers 4,000 other chemicals to the lungs of smokers.
- Health hazards of smoking include markedly higher rates of cancer, heart, and circulatory disorders, respiratory diseases, and gum diseases. Smoking during pregnancy presents risks for the fetus, including miscarriage and low birth weight. Smokeless tobacco dramatically increases risks for oral cancer and other oral problems. Environmental tobacco smoke (secondhand smoke) puts nonsmokers at risk for cancer and heart disease.
- Nicotine replacement products or the drug Zyban can help wean smokers off nicotine. Several therapy methods can help smokers break the habit.
- Caffeine is a widely used CNS stimulant. No long-term ill-health effects have been proven, although chronic users who try to quit may experience withdrawal.

Chapter Review

1. If a man and a woman drink the same amount of alcohol, the woman's BAC will be approximately
   a. the same as the man's BAC.
   b. 60% higher than the man's BAC.
   c. 30% higher than the man's BAC.
   d. 30% lower than the man's BAC.

2. The fastest-growing population of alcohol abusers are
   a. older adults.
   b. adolescents.
   c. women.
   d. immigrants.

3. Blood alcohol concentration (BAC) is the
   a. concentration of plant sugars in the blood stream.
   b. percentage of alcohol in a beverage.
   c. level of alcohol content in the blood.
   d. ratio of alcohol to the total blood volume.

4. Which of the following statements is *not* true?
   a. College students under 21 drink less often than older students but drink more heavily.
   b. College students tend to underestimate the amount that their peers drink.
   c. In the past 10 years, the number of college women who report being drunk 10 or more times has increased.
   d. Alcohol is involved in at least two-thirds of suicides on campus.

5. When Amanda goes out with her friends on the weekends, she usually has four to five beers in a row. This type of high-risk drinking is called
   a. tolerance.
   b. alcoholic addiction.
   c. alcohol overconsumption.
   d. binge drinking.

6. Jake was raised in an alcoholic family. To adapt to his father's alcoholic behavior, Jake played the obedient and good son to his parents. What role did Jake assume?
   a. family hero
   b. mascot
   c. scapegoat
   d. lost child

7. What age group is most targeted by tobacco advertisers?
   a. teenagers aged 14 to 17
   b. college students aged 18 to 24
   c. young adults aged 25 to 30
   d. married men aged 31 to 35

8. Which is the major psychoactive ingredient in tobacco products?
   a. carbon monoxide
   b. tar
   c. formaldehyde
   d. nicotine

9. What does nicotine do to the cilia hairs found in the lungs?
   a. instantly destroys the cilia hairs
   b. thickens the cilia hairs
   c. paralyzes the cilia hairs
   d. accumulates on the cilia hairs

10. Which type of tobacco product contains the ingredient eugenol, which allows smokers to inhale the smoke more deeply?
    a. bidis
    b. cigars
    c. snuff
    d. clove cigarettes

Answers to these questions can be found on page A-1.

Questions for Discussion and Reflection

1. When it comes to drinking alcohol, how much is too much? How can you avoid drinking amounts that will affect your judgment? When you see a friend having too many drinks at a party, what actions do you normally take? What actions could you take?
2. What are some of the most common negative consequences college students experience as a result of drinking? What are secondhand effects of binge drinking? Why do students tolerate negative behaviors of students who have been drinking?
3. Describe the difference between a problem drinker and an alcoholic. What factors can cause someone to slide from responsibly consuming alcohol to becoming an alcoholic? What effect does alcoholism have on an alcoholic's family?
4. Discuss short-term and long-term health hazards associated with tobacco. How will increased tobacco use among adolescents and college students impact the medical system in the future? Who should be responsible for the medical expenses of smokers? Insurance companies? Smokers themselves?
5. Restrictions on smoking are increasing in our society. Do you think these restrictions are fair? Do they infringe on people's rights? Are the restrictions too strict or not strict enough?
6. Describe the pros and cons of each method of tobacco cessation. Which would be most effective for you? Explain why.
7. Discuss problems related to caffeine use. How much caffeine do you consume? Why?

Accessing Your Health on the Internet

The following websites explore further topics and issues related to personal health. For links to the websites below, visit the Companion Website for *Health: The Basics,* Eighth Edition at www.aw-bc.com/donatelle.

1. *Alcoholics Anonymous.* Provides general information about AA and the 12-step program. www.alcoholics-anonymous.org
2. *American Lung Association.* This site offers a wealth of information regarding smoking trends, environmental smoke, and advice on smoking cessation. www.lungusa.org
3. *ASH (Action on Smoking and Health).* The nation's oldest and largest antismoking organization, ASH regularly takes hard-hitting legal actions and does other work to fight smoking and protect the rights of nonsmokers. www.ash.org
4. *College Drinking: Changing the Culture.* This online resource center is based on a series of reports published by the Task Force of the National Advisory Council on Alcohol Abuse and Alcoholism. It targets three audiences: the student population as a whole, the college and its surrounding environment, and the individual at-risk or alcohol-dependent drinker. www.collegedrinkingprevention.gov
5. *Had Enough.* This entertaining site is designed for college students who have suffered the secondhand effects (babysitting a roommate who has been drinking, having sleep interrupted, and so on) of other students' drinking.

It offers suggestions for taking action and being proactive about policy issues on your campus. http://gbgm-umc .org/mission_programs/cim/hadenough/home

6. *Higher Education Center for Alcohol and Other Drug Prevention.* This site is funded through the U.S. Department of Education and provides information relevant to colleges and universities. A specific site exists for students who are seeking information regarding alcohol. www.higheredcenter.org

7. *TIPS (Tobacco Information and Prevention Source).* This site provides access to a variety of information regarding tobacco use in the United States, with specific information for and about young people. www.cdc.gov/tobacco

Further Reading

Gately, I. *Tobacco: A Cultural History of How an Exotic Plant Seduced Civilization.* New York: Grove Press, 2003.

> *Tobacco has a sweeping history as the world's most prevalent addiction. The book begins with pre-Columbian America and continues through the tobacco litigation of the 1990s.*

Gilman, R. L. (Ed). *Smoke: A Global History of Smoking.* London: Reaktion Books, 2004.

> *An informative book that reviews human preoccupation with smoking over the past six centuries and explores issues relating to art, culture, and gender.*

Jersild, D. *Happy Hours: Alcohol in a Woman's Life.* New York: HarperCollins, 2001.

> *This book, a combination of cutting-edge research and personal stories of women who have struggled with alcohol problems, examines the role that alcohol plays in women's lives.*

Kuhn, C., S. Swartzwelder, W. Wilson, J. Foster, and L. Wilson. *Buzzed: The Straight Facts.* National Institute on Alcohol Abuse and Alcoholism (NIAAA) Research Monographs. Washington, DC: U.S. Department of Health and Human Services.

> *A series of publications containing the results of a number of studies conducted by research scientists under the auspices of NIAAA through 2002. These monographs address issues such as alcohol use among older adults, occupational alcoholism, social drinking, and the relationship between heredity and alcoholism.*

Sperber, M. *Beer and Circus: How Big Time College Sports Is Crippling Undergraduate Education.* New York: Henry Holt, 2000.

> *Sperber's book is an indictment of the attraction of undergraduates to schools based on the school's sports success and party reputations. He links student drinking behaviors to sports programs and argues that such an atmosphere shortchanges undergraduates of their education.*

Wechsler, H., and B. Wuethrich. *Dying to Drink: Confronting Binge Drinking on College Campuses.* Emmaus, PA: Rodale, 2002.

> *A report on the widespread alcohol culture that is prevalent on many campuses.*

Zailckas, K. *Smashed: A Story of a Drunken Girlhood.* New York: Viking, 2005.

> *A 24-year-old woman writes about her own experiences of drinking through high school and college.*

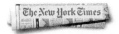

e-themes from *The New York Times*

For up-to-date articles about current health issues, visit www.aw-bc.com/donatelle, select *Health: The Basics,* Eighth Edition, Chapter 8, and click on "e-themes."

References

1. American College Health Association, "American College Health Association–National College Health Assessment (ACHA–NCHA) Spring 2006 Reference Group Data Report," *Journal of American College Health* 55, no. 4 (2007): 201.

2. R. Hingson et al., "Magnitude of Alcohol-Related Mortality and Morbidity among U.S. College Students Ages 18–24: Changes from 1998 to 2001," *Annual Review of Public Health* 26 (2005): 259–79.

3. H. Wechsler et al., "Trends in College Binge Drinking during a Period of Increased Prevention Efforts: Findings from Four Harvard School of Public Health College Study Surveys: 1993–2001," *Journal of American College Health* 50, no. 5 (2002): 207.

4. H. Wechsler et al., "College Binge Drinking in the 1990s: A Continuing Problem," *Journal of American College Health* 48, no. 10 (2000): 199–210.

5. M. Mohler-Kuo et al., "Correlates of Rape while Intoxicated in a National Sample of College Women," *Journal of Studies on Alcohol* 65, no. 1 (2004): 37.

6. Hingson et al., "Magnitude of Alcohol-Related Mortality and Morbidity."

7. N. E. Lakins et al., "Apparent Trends in per Capita Alcohol Consumption: National, State, and Regional Trends, 1977–2004," *Surveillance Report* no. 78 (2006), http://pubs.niaaa.nih.gov/publications/surveillance78/CONS04.htm.

8. J. Kinney et al., *Loosening the Grip,* 8th ed. (New York: McGraw-Hill, 2005).

9. S. MacDonald, "The Criteria for Causation of Alcohol in Violent Injuries in Six Countries," *Addictive Behaviors* 30, no. 1 (2005): 103–13.

10. J. Turner et al., "Serious Health Consequences Associated with Alcohol Use Among College Students: Demographic and Clinical Characteristics of Patients Seen in the Emergency Department," *Journal of Studies on Alcohol* 65, no. 2 (2004): 179.

11. K. Butler, "The Grim Neurology of Teenage Drinking," *New York Times,* July 4, 2006, www.nytimes.com/2006/7/04/04/health.

12. R. W. Hingson et al., "Age at Drinking Onset and Alcohol Dependence," *Archives of Pediatric and Adolescent Medicine* 160 (2006): 739–46.

13. National Institutes of Health, "Alcohol: A Women's Health Issue," 2005, http://pubs.niaaa.nih.gov/publications/brochurewomen/women.htm.

14. J. Theruvathu et al., "Polyamines Stimulate the Formation of Mutagenic 1, N2-Propanodeoxyguanosine Adducts from Acetaldehyde," *Nucleic Acids Research* 33, no. 11 (2005): 3513–20.

15. National Organization on Fetal Alcohol Syndrome, 2005, www.nofas.org.

16. National Highway Traffic Safety Administration, "Traffic Safety Facts, 2005: A Compilation of Motor Vehicle Crash Data from the Fatal Analysis Reporting System and General Estimates System," 2006, www.nhtsa.dot.gov.

17. National Highway Traffic Safety Administration, *Traffic Safety Facts, 1996—Alcohol* (Washington, DC: National Center for Statistics and Analysis, 1997).

18. R. Hingson et al. "Magnitude of Alcohol-related Mortality and Morbidity."

19. National Highway Traffic Safety Administration, "Traffic Safety Facts, 2005."

20. Insurance Institute for Highway Safety, "Fatality Facts: Alcohol 2005," 2007, www.iihs.org.

21. Ibid.

22. Ibid.

23. Substance Abuse and Mental Health Services Administration, "Results from the 2003 National Survey on Drug Use and Health: National Findings," Office of Applied Studies, NHSDA Series H-24, DHHS Publication No. SMA 04–3963 (Rockville, MD: U.S. Department of Health and Human Services, 2004).

24. J. Knight et al., "Alcohol Abuse and Dependence among U.S. College Students," *Journal of Studies on Alcohol* 63, no. 3 (2002): 263–70.

25. C. Wilson and J. Knight, "When Parents Have a Drinking Problem," *Contemporary Pediatrics* 18, no. 1, (January 2001): 67.

26. B. F. Grant, "Estimates of U.S. Children Exposed to Alcohol Abuse and Dependence in the Family," *American Journal of Public Health* 90, no. 1 (2000): 112–15.

27. National Institute on Alcohol Abuse and Alcoholism, *Alcohol Alert,* no. 51, January 2001.

28. T. R. Miller et al., "Societal Costs of Underage Drinking," *Journal of Studies on Alcohol* 67, no. 4 (2006): 519–28.

29. National Institutes of Health, "Alcohol: A Women's Health Issue," 2005, http://pubs.niaaa.nih.gov/publications/brochurewomen/women.htm.

30. F. Blow et al., "Use and Misuse of Alcohol Among Older Women," *Alcohol Research and Health* 26, no. 4 (2002): 308.

31. National Institute on Drug Abuse, "Info Facts: Treatment Methods for Women," August 30, 2004, www.nida.nih.gov/Infofax/treatwomen.html.

32. T. Wall et al., "ALDH2 Status and Conduct Disorder Mediate the Relationship Between Ethnicity and Alcohol Dependence in Chinese, Korean, and White American College Students," *Journal of Abnormal Psychology* 113, no. 2 (2004): 271–78.

33. Centers for Disease Control and Prevention, "Tobacco Information and Prevention Source: Fast Facts," March 2006, www.cdc.gov.

34. Ibid.

35. Centers for Disease Control and Prevention, "Cigarette Use Among High School Students—United States, 1991–2005," *Morbidity and Mortality Weekly Report* 55, no. 26 (2006): 724–26.

36. Office on Smoking and Health, *The Health Consequences of Smoking: What It Means to You* (Washington, DC: U.S Department of Health and Human Services, 2004).

37. American Cancer Society, *Cancer Facts and Figures, 2007* (Atlanta: American Cancer Society, 2007).

38. Centers for Disease Control and Prevention, "Annual Smoking-Attributable Mortality, Years of Potential Life Lost, and Productivity Losses—United States, 1997–2001," *Morbidity and Mortality Weekly Report* 54, no. 25 (2005): 625–28.

39. American College Health Association, "National College Health Assessment: Spring 2006 Reference Group Data," *Journal of American College Health* 55, no. 4 (2007): 195–206.

40. S. Moran et al., "Social Smoking Among U.S. College Students," *Pediatrics* 114 (2004): 1028–34.

41. M. E. Kear, "Psychosocial Determinants of Cigarette Smoking Among College Students," *Journal of Community Health Nursing,* 19, no. 4 (2002): 245.

42. S. A. Everett et al., "Smoking Initiation and Smoking Patterns among U.S. College Students," *Journal of American College Health* 48 (1999): 55.

43. American Cancer Society, "The Facts About Secondhand Smoke," 2004, www.cancer.org.

44. American Cancer Society, "Cigar Smoking," August 2006, www.cancer.org.

45. S. Hansen, "Bidis," University of Iowa's Student Health Service/Health Iowa, 2006, www.uiowa.edu/~shs.

46. American Cancer Society, *Cancer Facts and Figures, 2007.*

47. Ibid.

48. Ibid.

49. American Heart Association, "Heart Disease and Stroke Statistics: 2007 Update," 2007, www.americanheart.org.

50. Ibid.

51. American Lung Association, "Quit Smoking: Benefits," 2005, www.lungusa.org.

52. American Heart Association, "Stroke Risk Factors," 2007, www.americanheart.org.

53. Office on Smoking and Health, *The Health Consequences of Smoking: What It Means to You.*

54. American Cancer Society, *Cancer Facts and Figures, 2007.*

55. American Academy of Periodontology, "Tobacco Use and Periodontal Disease," 2004, www.perio.org.

56. Office on Smoking and Health, *The Health Consequences of Involuntary Exposure to Tobacco Smoke: A Report of the Surgeon General—Executive Summary* (Washington DC: U.S Department of Health and Human Services, 2006).

57. American Lung Association, "U.S. Surgeon General Releases Report on Health Consequences of Secondhand Smoke," 2006, www.lungusa.org.

58. Office on Smoking and Health, *The Health Consequences of Involuntary Exposure to Tobacco Smoke.*

59. Ibid.

60. American Nonsmokers' Rights Foundation, "Overview List: How Many Smokefree Laws?" 2007, www.no-smoke.org/pdf/mediaordlist.pdf.

61. Office on Smoking and Health, *The Health Consequences of Involuntary Exposure to Tobacco Smoke.*

62. Centers for Disease Control and Prevention, "Annual Smoking-Attributable Mortality."

63. M. Fogarty, "Public Health and Smoking Cessation," *The Scientist,* 17, no. 6 (2003), 23; Tobacco Control Research Center, Tobacco Litigation Documents, "Multistate Settlement with Tobacco Industry," 2004, www.library.ucsf.edu/tobacco/litigation; L. Robbins, "Balancing Smokers, Nonsmokers, and Health Concerns: Delaware and California Have Banned All Public Smoking," *State Legislatures,* 29, no. 1 (2003): 27.

64. U.S Department of Health and Human Services, "Effective Strategies for Tobacco Cessation Under Used," *National Institutes of Health News,* June 2006.

65. M. Marchione, "Doctors Test Stop Smoking Vaccine," *Corvallis Gazette Times,* Friday, July 28, 2006.

66. American Cancer Society, *Cancer Facts and Figures, 2007.*

67. Your Nutrition and Food Safety Resource, "Questions and Answers about Caffeine and Health," January 2003, http://ific.org.

68. Ibid.

9

Nutrition

EATING FOR OPTIMUM HEALTH

Do **carbohydrates** cause weight gain?

Are all **fats** bad for me?

Should I be taking **vitamin** supplements?

What does it mean if a food is **organic?**

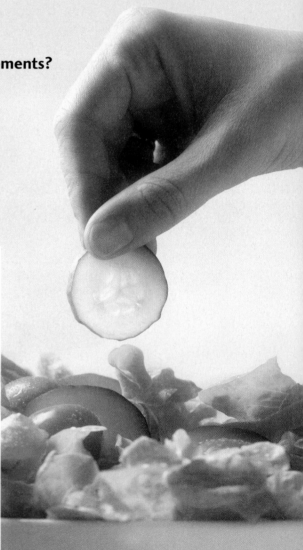

OBJECTIVES

- Understand the factors that influence dietary choices and the role essential nutrients play in maintaining our health.
- Discuss how to change old eating habits, improve dietary behaviors, and use the USDA MyPyramid Plan to make the best nutritional choices.
- Distinguish fact from fiction about trends in nutrition, potential risks versus benefits of food supplements, and the role of nutrition in fighting various diseases.
- Discuss issues surrounding gender, culture, and other factors that influence decision making about healthy nutrition.
- Discuss the unique challenges that college students face when trying to eat healthy foods and the actions they can take to eat healthfully.
- Explain food safety concerns facing Americans and people in other regions of the world.

When was the last time you ate something without thinking about how much fat or carbohydrates or how many calories it contained? Can you remember when you last went out to dinner with friends and didn't "think twice" before ordering the fried foods or high-calorie desserts? Do you eat "differently" around your health-conscious friends from when you eat alone? If so, you are not alone. Clearly, Americans are trying to heed expert advice and the multiple pressures to eat low-fat, high-fiber foods and to consume fewer calories overall. However, knowing what to eat, how much to eat, and how to choose from a media-driven array of foods and nutrition advice can be mind-boggling (see the **Health Headlines** box on page 252 for a discussion of some of the most recent nutritional claims).

The good news is that in survey after survey, 60 to 80 percent of food shoppers say they read food labels before selecting products; consume more vegetables, fruits, and lower-fat foods; and are cutting down on portion sizes and total calories. Diet book sales are at an all time high as millions of people make the leap toward healthy eating.[1] The not-so-good news is that overweight and obesity rates continue to rise, making the United States one of the "fattest" nations in the world. In fact, although we report that increasing numbers of us read labels and are trying to eat more healthfully, in the same surveys nearly 78% of all adults indicate that they were not eating the recommended servings of fruits and vegetables and that they are still eating too many refined carbohydrates and high-fat foods.[2]

Although the U.S. Food and Drug Administration (FDA), the U.S. Department of Agriculture (USDA), and several professional groups do a remarkable job in helping to protect our foods and supplements, recommending foods we should eat, and supporting research to provide sound dietary advice, they can't possibly regulate every dietary claim or food product on the market or monitor individual behaviors. That means that the responsibility for making wise dietary decisions is largely yours.

Just how important is sound nutrition? A landmark review of over 4,500 research studies concluded that widespread consumption of 5 to 6 servings of fruits and vegetables daily would lower cancer rates by over 20 percent in the global population.[3] Although no newer estimates of the global contribution of nutrition to cancer have been published, many documented studies and organizations indicate that undernutrition and overnutrition play major roles in global population health.[4] Indeed, undernutrition, overnutrition, and diet-related chronic diseases account for more than half of the world's diseases and hundreds of millions of dollars in public expenditure.[5]

Research has also emphasized the impact of diet and nutrition on cardiovascular disease, diabetes, and a host of other chronic and disabling conditions.[6] The evidence is compelling and clear. Your health depends largely on what you eat and how much you eat throughout your life.

The next three chapters focus on fundamental principles designed to help you eat more of the healthy foods, find strategies to improve your own nutritional status, exercise to reduce

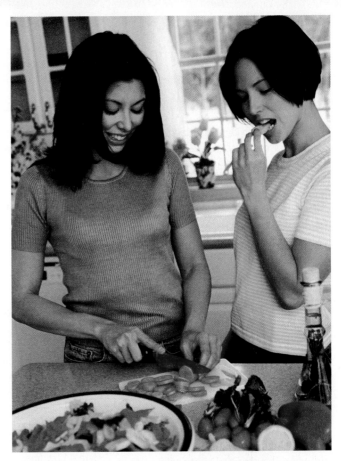

It takes information and planning to make healthy food choices, whether you are eating out, eating in the dining hall, or cooking your meals at home.

risks from excess calories, and improve your quality and quantity of life. In this chapter, we will discuss basic nutrition science and apply sound principles to lifestyle behaviors. You will also gain an appreciation for why you eat as you do, the role that your family of origin and basic biology play in determining your eating patterns and choices, and the resources that can help you change negative patterns while building on the healthy choices you are already making.

Assessing Eating Behaviors: Are You What You Eat?

True **hunger** occurs when there is a lack or shortage of basic foods needed to provide the energy and nutrients that support health.[7] When we are hungry, chemical messages in the brain,

hunger The physiological impulse to seek food, prompted by the lack or shortage of basic foods needed to provide the energy and nutrients that support health.

THE LATEST IN NUTRITIONAL SCIENCE: MAKING SENSE OF DIET HYPE

Frustrated by health food discoveries that seem to fizzle as fast as they burst on the scene? You're not alone. In the last decade, we've been bombarded with a wide variety of conflicting scientific evidence and claims about dietary choices we can make to reduce the risk of certain diseases and promote health.

The good news is that there are positive outcomes in all of this research, and positive health effects can be gained from proper nutrition. The bad news? With all of these studies also come conflicting reports that leave many of us scratching our heads. There are some promising new results coming out of the latest research. Let's take a closer look at a few.

THE SKINNY ON SOY

Soy and chemicals found in soy called isoflavones have gained considerable attention for their purported role in reducing the risk for various chronic diseases, most notably cardiovascular disease. A committee of the American Heart Association (AHA) completed a meta-analysis of years of studies on the benefits of soy and reached the following conclusions.

What soy doesn't do

- Soy foods do not lower cholesterol and triglycerides levels as much as previously believed and don't provide much benefit over milk or other protein. In fact, the AHA concludes that soy has no significant effects on HDL cholesterol, triglycerides, or blood pressure.

- Soy proteins don't prevent hot flashes and other symptoms in menopausal women.

What soy might do

- Soy may prevent postmenopausal bone loss in women.
- Recent research indicates that soy may lower total serum cholesterol and LDL cholesterol but has little effect on HDL cholesterol.

What soy probably does

- Soy foods are a good alternative for saturated animal fats. Soy is low in fat overall and contains an omega-3 fatty acid that has been independently shown to reduce risks for coronary diseases.
- Soy should be beneficial to some degree because of its high polyunsaturated fat, fiber, vitamin, and mineral content.

ARE THE BENEFITS OF FISH, FISHY?

Fish has been purported to reduce saturated fats and keep cholesterol levels down. In fact, it is recommended that most people eat fish at least twice per week in lieu of red meat and other high-fat foods.

For the most part, these claims have been upheld in a variety of studies, particularly those which point to the benefits of the high levels omega-3 fatty acids found in many types of fish. However, several studies have cautioned that eating farm-raised fish poses some risk because they

contain high levels of cancer-causing polychlorinated biphenyls (PCBs) and antibiotics. Other studies indicate that levels of PCBs and mercury are high in wild fish as well, because of environmental contamination.

According to Purdue University seafood expert Charles Santerre, the keys to minimizing risks for any food is variety. On his list of safe, low-mercury options: shrimp, salmon, pollock, farm-raised catfish, and tilapia. Finally, opt for the smaller-sized fish at the market: Smaller size means less exposure to ocean contaminants. For more information, check out the EPA website on fish advisories: www.epa.gov/waterscience/fish.

BONING UP ON CALCIUM

A large, randomized, double-blind, placebo-controlled trial of over 32,000 women who received calcium and vitamin D supplements as part of the Women's Health Initiative (WHI) Study yielded the following surprising findings:

- Women who received the calcium and vitamin D supplement over a 7-year period did not have any significantly reduced risk of colorectal cancer than those who received a placebo.
- In the same WHI study, women were assessed to see whether their risk of bone fracture was lower than the group who received no calcium or vitamin D supplements. Researchers were

---

especially in the hypothalamus, initiate a physiological response that prompts us to seek food.[8] Few Americans have experienced the type of hunger that continues for days and threatens survival. Most of us eat because of our **appetite,** a learned psychological desire to eat that may or may not have

anything to do with feeling hungry. Appetite can be triggered by smells, tastes, and other triggers such as certain times of day, special occasions, or proximity to a favorite food.

Hunger and appetite are not the only forces involved in our physiological drive to eat. Other factors that influence when, how, and what we eat include the following:

appetite The desire to eat; normally accompanies hunger but is more psychological than physiological.

- *Cultural and social meanings attached to food.* Cultural traditions and food choices give us many of our *food*

surprised that there was only a slight improvement in bone density of the hip, but no significant reductions in hip fracture, and a significantly increased risk of kidney stones in the group who received the treatment.

Most experts would tell you to continue to obtain calcium in your daily diet and to continue taking supplements. Although this was a large study, it studied only older women and examined only one form of calcium. As with all research, there is a potential for inaccuracy and factors that may skew results. More research is needed before we can change long-established recommendations, but these results pose interesting questions for future researchers.

THE LATEST ON MULTIVITAMIN SUPPLEMENTS

It's likely that most of the 52 percent of American adults who take multivitamins, at an annual cost of over $23 billion, assume that there is solid scientific evidence supporting these supplements' health benefits. However, according to a National Institute of Health panel, "The present evidence is insufficient to recommend either for or against the use of multivitamins and minerals by the American public to prevent chronic diseases." The committee concluded that much more research must be done to evaluate the huge amount of seemingly contradictory studies about using supplements individually or in combination.

MAKING SENSE OF CONFLICTING HEALTH INFORMATION

Even the big reports published in highly respected journals are only single blips on a radar screen full of other studies that have proven just the opposite. Here is what you really need to know about reports you hear and read about in the media:

1. Remember that any single study must be viewed with caution. Often, there are other studies that may prove opposite findings, and they are no less reputable.
2. Many of these studies are "meta-analyses." This means they summarize the results of many studies, often without regard to population, study design, age of the population studied, confounders (things that could influence effects), dosage, underlying bias of the population, and many other factors.
3. Information gained from the Women's Health Initiative about diet and exercise is based largely on self-reporting. Many people question the validity of some responses. Others point out that because this was such a long study, participants who actually followed through and participated over time might have very different health behaviors from the average person. Even randomized, controlled trials have limitations, and results should be viewed in light of potential limitations and the results of previous studies.
4. The best studies will conclude that more research must be done. Though

this may seem frustrating, and may not give the definitive answers we are looking for, this is the most current and accurate response that researchers can give.

The most sound advice? Make healthy changes that influence your entire lifestyle. Rather than popping ten different vitamin supplements each day, eat nutritious foods from each of the MyPyramid categories. Cut down on saturated animal fats, and use some soy and fish as part of a healthy diet.

Sources: F. Sacks et al., "Soy Proteins, Isoflavones, and Cardiovascular Health," Circulation 113 (2006): 1034–44; U.S. Food and Drug Administration, "Advisory on Mercury in Fish," March 2004, www.fda.gov; M. Callahan, "The Fish Conundrum," Cooking Light 19, no. 3 (2005): 52–56; J. Wactawshi-Wende et al., "Calcium plus Vitamin D Supplementation and the Risk of Colorectal Cancer," New England Journal of Medicine 354, no. 7 (2006): 684–96; R. Jackson et al., "Calcium plus Vitamin D Supplementation and the Risk of Fractures," New England Journal of Medicine 354, no. 7 (2006): 669–83; Tufts University Health and Nutrition Letter 24, no. 6 (August 2006): 1–2; National Institutes of Health "NIH State-of-the-Science Conference Statement on Multivitamin/Mineral Supplements and Chronic Disease Prevention," May 2006, http://consensus.nih.gov/2006/MVMFINAL080106.pdf. D. Mozaffarian, "Low-Fat Diet and Cardiovascular Disease," Journal of the American Medical Association 296 (2006): 279–80; Linus Pauling Diet and Optimum Health Conference, Portland, Oregon, May 2007; K. Taku et al., "Soy Isoflavones Lower Serum Total and LDL Cholesterol in Humans: A Meta-Analysis of 11 Randomized Controlled Trials," American Journal of Clinical Nutrition 85 (2007): 1148–56.

preferences. We learn to like the tastes of certain foods, especially the foods we grew up eating. A yearning for sweet, salty, or high-fat foods can evolve from our earliest days.
- Convenience and advertising. That juicy burger on TV looked really good. You've got to have it.
- Habit or custom. Often we select foods because they are familiar and fit religious, political, or spiritual views.

- Emotional comfort. Eating it makes you feel better—a form of reward and security. We derive pleasure or sensory delight from eating the foods and reward ourselves with foods.
- Nutritional value. You think the food is good or bad for you, or it may help you maintain your weight.
- Social interaction. Eating out or having company over for a meal is an enjoyable social event.
- Regional/seasonal trends. Some foods may be favored in your area by season or overall climate.

With all of the factors that influence our dietary choices and the wide array of foods available, the challenge of eating for health increases daily. Fortunately, we have a wealth of solid information that serves as a foundation for our decisions. **Nutrition** is the science that investigates the relationship between physiological function and the essential elements of the foods we eat. With our country's overabundance of food and vast array of choices, media that "prime" us to want the tasty morsels shown in advertisements, and easy access to almost every type of **nutrient** (proteins, carbohydrates, fats, vitamins, minerals, and water), Americans should have few nutritional problems. However, these "diets of affluence" contribute to many major diseases, including obesity-related problems with heart disease; cancer; diabetes; high blood pressure; cirrhosis of the liver; varicose veins; gout; gallbladder disease; respiratory problems; abdominal hernias; flat feet; injuries to the knees, hips, and other weight-bearing joints; complications in pregnancy and surgery; and even higher accident rates, to name but a few.

Eating for Health

Generally, a healthful diet provides the proper combination of energy and nutrients. It is sufficient to keep us functioning well in our daily activities. A healthful diet should be[9]

- *Adequate.* It provides enough of the energy, nutrients, and fiber to maintain health and essential body functions. A **calorie** is the unit of measurement used to quantify the amount of energy we obtain from a particular food. Everyone's energy needs differ (**Table 9.1**). For example, a small woman who has a sedentary lifestyle may need only 1,700 calories of energy to support her body's functions, whereas a professional biker may need several thousand calories of energy to be up for his competition.
- *Moderate.* The quantity of food you consume can cause you to gain weight. Moderate caloric consumption, portion control, and awareness of the total amount of nutrients in the foods you eat are key aspects of dietary health.
- *Balanced.* Your diet should contain the proper combination of foods from different groups. Following the

nutrition The science that investigates the relationship between physiological function and the essential elements of foods eaten.

nutrients The constituents of food that sustain humans physiologically: proteins, carbohydrates, fats, vitamins, minerals, and water.

calorie A unit of measure that indicates the amount of energy obtained from a particular food.

TABLE 9.1	Estimated Daily Calorie Needs		
	Calorie Range		
	Sedentary[a]	→	**Active**[b]
Children			
2–3 years	1,000	→	1,400
Females			
4–8 years	1,200	→	1,800
9–13	1,600	→	2,200
14–18	1,800	→	2,400
19–30	2,000	→	2,400
31–50	1,800	→	2,200
51+	1,600	→	2,200
Males			
4–8 years	1,400	→	2,000
9–13	1,800	→	2,600
14–18	2,200	→	3,200
19–30	2,400	→	3,000
31–50	2,200	→	3,000
51+	2,000	→	2,800

[a] A lifestyle that includes only the light physical activity associated with typical day-to-day life.
[b] A lifestyle that includes physical activity equivalent to walking more than 3 miles per day at 3 to 4 miles per hour, in addition to the light physical activity associated with typical day-to-day life.

Source: Department of Agriculture Center for Nutrition Policy & Promotion, April 2005, www.MyPyramid.gov.

recommendations for the MyPyramid plan, discussed later in the chapter, should help you achieve balance.
- *Varied.* Eat a lot of different foods each day. Variety helps you avoid boredom and can make it easier to keep your diet interesting and in control.
- *Nutrient dense.* Nutrient density refers to the proportion of vitamins, minerals, and other nutrients compared to the number of calories. In short, the foods you eat should have the biggest nutritional bang for the calories consumed. Making each bite count and not wasting calories on foods that give you little nutritional value are also keys to healthful eating.

In a 30-year study of changes in consumption, women's overall caloric intake increased by 22 percent and men's by 7 percent.[10] Are we eating more food, or is it what we are eating? Trends indicate that it isn't actual amounts of food, but the number of calories in the foods we choose to eat (**Figure 9.1**). When these trends are combined with our increasingly sedentary lifestyle, it is not surprising that we have seen a dramatic rise in obesity.

Americans typically get approximately 38 percent of their calories from fat, 15 percent from proteins, 22 percent from complex carbohydrates, and 24 percent

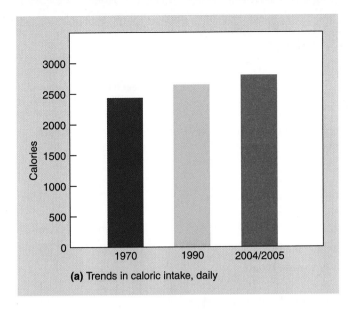

(a) Trends in caloric intake, daily

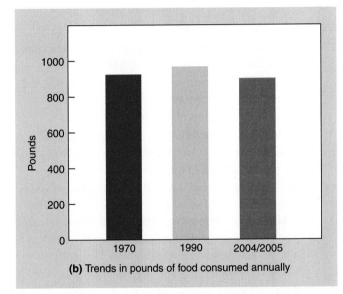

(b) Trends in pounds of food consumed annually

FIGURE 9.1 Trends in Caloric Intake and Food Consumption

Source: United States Department of Agriculture, "Food Consumption Patterns: How We've Changed, 1970–2005," December 2005, www.usda.gov.

from simple sugars.[11] Nearly one-third of the calories we consume come from junk foods with no real nutritional value. Sweets and desserts, soft drinks, sugary fruit juice beverages, and alcoholic beverages make up 25 percent of those calories, and another 5 percent come from salty snacks and fruit-flavored drinks. In sharp contrast, healthy foods such as vegetables and fruit make up only 10 percent of our total calories.[12]

How much do you know about nutrition and healthy eating? Find out by completing the quiz in the **Assess Yourself** box on page 256.

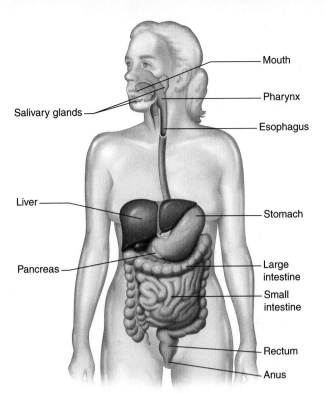

FIGURE 9.2 The Digestive Process
Your mouth prepares for food by increasing production of saliva, which contains enzymes that begin the digestive process. From the mouth, food passes down the esophagus to the stomach. Here, food is mixed by muscular contractions and is broken down by enzymes and stomach acids. Further digestive activity and absorption of nutrients take place in the small intestine, aided by enzymes from the liver and the pancreas. Next, water and salts are absorbed by the large intestine, and then solid waste moves into the rectum and is passed out through the anus. The entire digestive process takes approximately 24 hours.

Source: Adapted from M. Johnson, *Human Biology: Concepts and Current Issues,* 3rd ed. (San Francisco: Benjamin Cummings, 2006), 314.

Obtaining Essential Nutrients

The Digestive Process

Food provides the chemicals we need for activity and body maintenance. Because our bodies cannot synthesize or produce certain essential nutrients, we must obtain them from the foods we eat. Before the body can use foods properly, the digestive system must break down the larger food particles into smaller, more usable forms. The sequence of functions by which the body breaks down foods and either absorbs or excretes them is known as the **digestive process (Figure 9.2).**

digestive process The process by which the body breaks down foods and either absorbs or excretes them.

(Text continues on page 259.)

ASSESS yourself

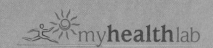

WHAT'S YOUR EQ (EATING QUOTIENT)?

Fill out this assessment online at www.aw-bc.com/myhealthlab or www.aw-bc.com/donatelle.

Keeping up with the latest on what to eat—or not eat—isn't easy. If you think a few facts might have slipped past you, this quiz should help. There's only one correct answer for each question.

	True	False
1. Fresh fruits and vegetables contain more nutrients than canned or frozen varieties.	☐	☐
2. While you are shopping, it makes a difference what area of the store you start in, in terms of keeping your foods safe.	☐	☐
3. Fruit drinks count as a serving from the fruit group in the MyPyramid Plan.	☐	☐
4. Baked potatoes have a higher glycemic index (carbohydrate's ability to raise blood sugar levels quickly) than sweet potatoes or apples.	☐	☐
5. A late dinner is more likely to cause weight gain than eating the same meal earlier in the day.	☐	☐
6. Nuts are okay to eat if you are trying to stick to a low-fat diet.	☐	☐
7. Certain foods, such as grapefruit, celery, or cabbage soup, can burn fat and make you lose weight.	☐	☐

8. Which of the following has the most fiber?
   a. chuck roast
   b. dark-meat chicken with skin
   c. skinless chicken wing
   d. they are all about the same

9. Which of the following is the strongest predictor of obesity in America today?
   a. region of the country you live in
   b. ethnicity/culture
   c. lack of exercise
   d. socioeconomic status

10. When you eat a meal, how long does it take for your brain to get the message that you are full?
    a. 10 minutes
    b. 20 minutes
    c. at least an hour
    d. 2 hours or more

11. Which of the following are at the *top* of the list in bacterial levels among domestically grown vegetables?
    a. green onions, cantaloupe, and cilantro
    b. beets, potatoes, and summer squash
    c. celery, leaf lettuce, and parsley
    d. strawberries, apples, and tomatoes

12. Which of the following foods contains the most grams of fiber per serving?
    a. ½ cup of strawberries
    b. ½ cup of kidney beans
    c. 1 cup popcorn
    d. 1 medium banana

13. To ensure that you are getting your antioxidants each day, which tip below would be most helpful?
    a. Eat several dark green vegetables and orange, red, and yellow fruits and vegetables.
    b. Eat at least 2 servings of lean red meat per day.
    c. Eat whole-grain foods with at least 2 grams of fiber per serving.
    d. Eat several servings of tuna and salmon per week.

14. Olive oil, one of the heart-healthy monounsaturated fats, is a great source for antioxidants. To reap the most benefits from olive oil, which recommendation should you follow?
    a. Buy it only in amounts that you will use relatively quickly. Nutrients are lost quickly after 12 months sitting on the shelf.
    b. If you buy larger bottles, separate it into smaller bottles and keep the lid on tightly to reduce oxidation from air contact. Refrigerate if possible. Refrigeration causes cloudiness but doesn't affect quality.
    c. Store it in opaque airtight glass bottles or metal tins away from heat and light.
    d. All of the above.

15. Which strategy will help you identify high-fiber breads to maximize your quality carbohydrate intake?
    a. Choose a whole-grain bread that lists a whole grain as the first ingredient.
    b. Try to purchase breads with 1 to 2 grams of fiber per slice.
    c. Look for bread that is dark colored. The darker it is, the greater the chance that it has lots of good-quality fiber in its recipe.
    d. All of the above.

Answers

1. *False:* There is usually little difference, depending on how produce is handled and how quickly it reaches your supermarket. Canned and frozen produce is typically picked at its peak and may contain more nutrients than fresh produce that was picked overripe or too early, sat in a warehouse, spent days in transit, or sat at improper temperatures for prolonged periods. However, canned or frozen fruits and vegetables may have added salt or sugar, so check labels carefully. Whenever possible, buy local produce fresh from the fields or neighboring areas.

2. *True:* As a general rule, milk, meat, and other perishables that have been left at room temperature for more than 2 hours have a significant risk of conveying a foodborne illness. Be sure to factor in the time that you spend driving home from the store or running other errands. Start your shopping in the canned and nonrefrigerated sections of the store, and save your meat and dairy products and frozen foods until last. Run your other errands before you shop for food, and if you know it will take time to get home, bring a cooler with ice.

3. *False:* Even if fruit juice is an actual ingredient (often it is not), most fruit drinks consist primarily of water and high fructose corn syrup or other sweeteners, colorings, and fruit flavoring. It is always better to eat the whole fruit, because you will get added fiber, more nutrients, and other benefits. Next best are 100 percent fruit juices, preferably with added vitamin C. Lowest on the nutrient quality list are the sweetened, flavored fruit drinks.

4. *True:* Unfortunately, we'd probably be better off with a sweet potato or apple instead of substituting baked potatoes for fries if we are trying to keep our blood sugar levels down or control diabetes. For more information, check the glycemic index reference books available at most bookstores, or use the handy guide found at www .diabetesnet.com/diabetes_food_diet/glycemic_index.php.

5. *False:* It's not when you eat but what you eat that makes a difference in weight gain. If you ate a 500-calorie salad at 10 PM and it was your only meal, you wouldn't gain weight. However, a 5,000 calorie pizza for breakfast, followed by a big lunch and dinner would provide enough total calories to put more than muscle on the hips, buttocks, and waist.

6. *True:* Although they are high in fat, nuts contain mostly unsaturated (good) fat and are good sources of protein, magnesium, and the antioxidants vitamin E and selenium. Moderation is the key.

7. *False:* No foods can burn fat. Some foods with caffeine may speed up your metabolism for a short time but do not cause weight loss. One of the best ways to boost your metabolism is to increase your muscle mass through weight training and exercise—not by eating specific foods.

8. *d:* There is no fiber in animal foods. Fiber is found only in plants and plant-based foods such as fruits, beans, whole grains, and vegetables.

9. *d:* Although the other responses are all contributors to obesity, the greatest single predictor of obesity is low socioeconomic status. Although related factors such as education play a role, the poor nutritional quality of foods commonly eaten when people are forced to stretch their food budget—high-fat meats, hot dogs, inexpensive white breads and pastries, and other high-calorie, low-fiber foods—often increases the risk of obesity.

10. *b:* It takes about 20 minutes for your brain to get the message that you are full. To make sure you don't gorge yourself, eat slowly, talk with others, put your fork down after taking a bite, take a drink of water, or do other things to delay your meal. Let your brain catch up to your fork, and slow it down!

11. *a:* The bad news is that in a recent government study of bacterial levels found in domestic produce, green onions, cantaloupe, and cilantro scored the highest in positive tests for two common bacteria: *Salmonella* and *Shigella*. The good news is that out of nearly 1,100 samples, only 2 to 3 percent were contaminated, but washing your produce (even the bagged and washed variety) is still a must; run a heavy stream of water over the produce while rubbing the outside under the water.

12. *b:* One-half cup of kidney beans provides 4.5 grams of fiber; the medium banana has 2 grams of fiber; strawberries and popcorn each have 1 gram of fiber per serving.

13. *a:* Antioxidants, particularly vitamins C and E, the mineral selenium, and plant pigments known as carotenoids (which include beta-carotene) are found in green leafy vegetables and orange, yellow, and red vegetables and fruit. Eating several servings of these per day may help avoid risks from selected health problems.

14. *d:* Olive oil does lose nutrients over time, with one year being the general guesstimate of "use by" time. Keeping it in the refrigerator helps prolong shelf life. If the oil smells

(continued)

rancid or if you note mold or other discoloration, discard the bottle.

15. *a:* A true whole-grain bread clearly says so on the label (e.g., "100 percent whole wheat" or "100 percent stone-ground whole wheat"). If all the ingredients aren't whole grain, then it's not a true whole-grain bread. The more fiber in each slice, the better; look for a minimum of 3 grams per slice. Color is not a good indicator of nutrient value. Dyes and coloring may make even the whitest white bread brown.

Scoring

If you answered all of the above correctly, congratulations! You clearly have a good sense of some of the current issues and facts surrounding dietary choices. If you missed one or more questions, read the corresponding section of this chapter to find out more. Don't despair. Nutrition information changes rapidly, and there is a wealth of information available. Check with your instructor for courses you can take to increase your nutritional knowledge. Review the resources that are recommended, and work hard to stay current.

MAKE *it* happen!

ASSESSMENT: The Assess Yourself activity gave you the chance to test your knowledge of some of the health effects of various foods. Now that you have considered these results, you can decide whether you need to do more to keep up on what to eat and what to avoid for long-term health.

MAKING A CHANGE: To change your behavior, you need to develop a plan. Follow these steps below and complete your Behavior Change Contract to take action.

1. Evaluate your behavior, and identify patterns and specific things you are doing. What can you change now? What can you change in the near future?

2. Select one pattern of behavior that you want to change.

3. Fill out the Behavior Change Contract found at the front of your book. It should include your long-term goals for change, your short-term goals, the rewards you'll give yourself for reaching these goals, potential obstacles along the way, and strategies for overcoming these obstacles. For each goal, list the small steps and specific actions that you will take.

4. Chart your progress in a journal. At the end of a week, consider how successful you were in following your plan. What helped you be successful? What made change more difficult? What will you do differently next week?

5. Revise your plan as needed. Are the short-term goals attainable? Are the rewards satisfying?

EXAMPLE: Tara discovered that she had very little idea about what foods to eat and which ones to avoid for long-term health. She decided to keep track of her normal diet for a week and then evaluate it in light of some of the guidelines in this chapter. She considered her diet fairly balanced and was surprised to find that she was eating fewer than 2 servings of vegetables a day, instead of the recommended 3 to 5. Tara looked at her eating patterns and identified several times when she snacked on foods that could be replaced with healthier snacks. She decided to cut carrots up into sticks that she could toss into her backpack. They stayed fresh all day and made a good snack between classes instead of a candy bar from the vending machine. She also found that her favorite Mexican restaurant offered a vegetarian burrito full of black beans (not refried), squash, tomatoes, and other vegetables that was even tastier than her usual pork burrito. At the end of the first week, Tara and her friends decided to order pizza after a late night of studying. Instead of getting pepperoni or sausage, Tara suggested a pizza with green peppers, spinach, and onions as toppings. Tara did have a setback when she went to a baseball game and ate peanuts and hot dogs all day, but the next day she had a salad for lunch and saw that her vegetable consumption was almost at her goal.

Tara's goal for the next week is to continue to substitute healthy snacks and to look for healthy alternatives when she is eating out. When she is consistently eating the recommended servings of vegetables each week, she will start focusing on other parts of her diet that could use improvement. She is already thinking about how to replace some of the white bread and sugary breakfast cereals she eats now with more whole wheat and whole grains.

Water: A Crucial Nutrient

You may be surprised to learn that you could survive much longer without food than you could without water. Even in severe conditions, the average person can go for weeks without certain vitamins and minerals before experiencing serious deficiency symptoms. However, **dehydration** (abnormal depletion of body fluids) can cause serious problems within a matter of hours, and death after a few days without water.

The human body consists of 50 to 60 percent water by weight. The water in our bodies bathes cells, aids in fluid and electrolyte balance, maintains pH balance, and transports molecules and cells throughout the body. Water is the major component of our blood, which carries oxygen and nutrients to the tissues and is responsible for maintaining cells in working order.

Individual needs for water vary drastically according to dietary factors, age, size, overall health, environmental temperature and humidity levels, and exercise. Certain diseases, such as diabetes and cystic fibrosis, cause people to lose fluids at a rate necessitating a higher volume of fluid intake.

Proteins

Next to water, **proteins** are the most abundant substances in the human body. Proteins are major components of nearly every cell and have been called the "body builders" because of their role in developing and repairing bone, muscle, skin, and blood cells. They are the key elements of the antibodies that protect us from disease, of enzymes that control chemical activities in the body, and of hormones that regulate body functions. Proteins help transport iron, oxygen, and nutrients to all body cells and supply another source of energy to cells when fats and carbohydrates are not readily available. In short, adequate amounts of protein in the diet are vital to many body functions and ultimately to survival.

Whenever you consume proteins, your body breaks them down into smaller molecules known as **amino acids**, the building blocks of protein. Nine of the 20 different amino acids are termed **essential amino acids**, which means the body must obtain them from the diet; the other 11 can be produced by the body.

Dietary protein that supplies all of the essential amino acids is called **complete (high-quality) protein.** Typically, protein from animal products is complete. When we consume foods that are deficient in some of the essential amino acids, the total amount of protein that can be synthesized from the other amino acids is decreased. For proteins to be complete, they also must be present in digestible form and in amounts proportional to body requirements.

What about plant sources of protein? Proteins from plant sources are often **incomplete proteins** in that they may lack one or two of the essential amino acids. Nevertheless, it is relatively easy for the non–meat eater to combine plant foods effectively and eat complementary sources of plant protein **(Figure 9.3)**. An excellent example of this mutual supplementation process is eating peanut butter on whole-grain bread. Although each of these foods lacks certain essential amino acids, eating them together provides complete protein.

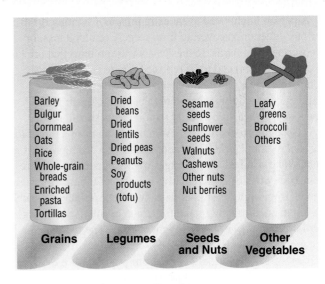

FIGURE 9.3 Complementary Proteins

Source: Adapted from J. Thompson and M. Manore, *Nutrition: An Applied Approach.* Copyright © 2005. Reprinted by permission of Pearson Education, Inc.

Plant sources of protein fall into three general categories: *legumes* (beans, peas, peanuts, and soy products), *grains* (such as wheat, corn, rice and oats), and *nuts and seeds.* Certain vegetables, such as leafy green vegetables and broccoli, also contribute valuable plant proteins. Mixing two or more foods from each of these categories during the same meal will provide all of the essential amino acids necessary to ensure adequate protein absorption. People who are not interested in obtaining all of their protein from plants can combine incomplete plant proteins with complete low-fat animal proteins, such as chicken, fish, turkey, and lean red meat. Low-fat or nonfat cottage cheese, skim milk, egg whites, and nonfat dry milk all provide complete proteins and have few calories and little dietary fat.

---

dehydration Abnormal depletion of body fluids; a result of lack of water.

proteins The essential constituents of nearly all body cells; necessary for the development and repair of bone, muscle, skin, and blood; the key elements of antibodies, enzymes, and hormones.

amino acids The building blocks of protein.

essential amino acids Nine of the basic nitrogen-containing building blocks of protein, which must be obtained from foods to ensure health.

complete (high-quality) proteins Proteins that contain all nine of the essential amino acids.

incomplete proteins Proteins that lack one or more of the essential amino acids.

A person might need to eat extra protein if fighting off a serious infection, recovering from surgery or blood loss, or recovering from burns. In these instances, proteins that are lost to cellular repair need to be replaced. There is considerable controversy over whether someone in high-level physical training needs additional protein to build and repair muscle fibers or whether normal daily requirements should suffice.

Although protein deficiency continues to pose a threat to the global population, few Americans suffer from protein deficiencies. In fact, the average American consumes more than 100 grams of protein daily, and about 70 percent of this comes from high-fat animal flesh and dairy products.[13] The recommended protein intake for adults is only 0.8 gram (g) per kilogram (kg) of body weight per day. The typical recommendation is that in a 2,000-calorie diet, 10 to 35 percent of calories should come from protein, for a total average of 50 to 175 grams per day (a 6-ounce steak contains 53 grams of protein—more than the daily needs of an average-sized woman!). See **Figure 9.4** to determine your daily protein requirement.

Carbohydrates

Although we should not underestimate the importance of proteins in the body, it is **carbohydrates** that supply us with the energy needed to sustain normal daily activity. Carbohydrates can actually be metabolized more quickly and efficiently than proteins and are a quick source of energy for the body, being easily converted to glucose, the fuel for the body's cells. These foods also play an important role in the functioning of internal organs, the nervous system, and the muscles. They are the best fuel for endurance athletics because they provide both an immediate and a time-released energy source; they are digested easily and then consistently metabolized in the bloodstream.

Not all carbohydrates are the same. There are two major types of carbohydrates: **simple sugars,** which are found primarily in fruits, and **complex carbohydrates,** which are found in grains, cereals, dark green leafy vegetables, yellow fruits and vegetables (carrots, yams), *cruciferous* vegetables (such as broccoli, cabbage, and cauliflower), and certain tuberous vegetables, such as potatoes. Most of us do not get enough complex carbohydrates in our daily diets.

carbohydrates Basic nutrients that supply the body with glucose, the energy form most commonly used to sustain normal activity.

simple sugars A major type of carbohydrate, which provide short-term energy.

complex carbohydrates A major type of carbohydrate, which provide sustained energy.

monosaccharides Simple sugars that contain only one molecule of sugar.

disaccharides Combinations of two monosaccharides.

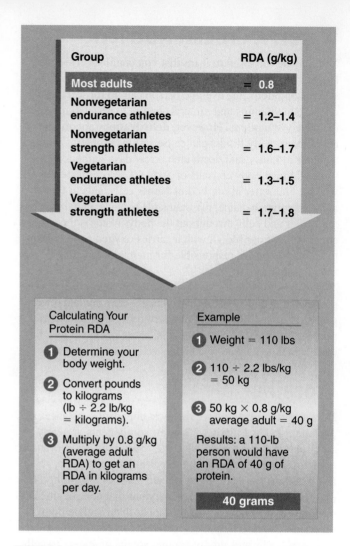

Group	RDA (g/kg)
Most adults	= 0.8
Nonvegetarian endurance athletes	= 1.2–1.4
Nonvegetarian strength athletes	= 1.6–1.7
Vegetarian endurance athletes	= 1.3–1.5
Vegetarian strength athletes	= 1.7–1.8

Calculating Your Protein RDA

1 Determine your body weight.
2 Convert pounds to kilograms (lb ÷ 2.2 lb/kg = kilograms).
3 Multiply by 0.8 g/kg (average adult RDA) to get an RDA in kilograms per day.

Example

1 Weight = 110 lbs
2 110 ÷ 2.2 lbs/kg = 50 kg
3 50 kg × 0.8 g/kg average adult = 40 g

Results: a 110-lb person would have an RDA of 40 g of protein.

40 grams

FIGURE 9.4 Calculating Your Protein RDA (Recommended Dietary Allowance)

Source: Adapted from J. Thompson and M. Manore, *Nutrition: An Applied Approach.* Copyright © 2005. Reprinted by permission of Pearson Education, Inc.

A typical American diet contains large amounts of simple sugars. The most common form is *glucose.* Eventually, the human body converts all types of simple sugars to glucose to provide energy to cells. In its natural form, glucose is sweet and is obtained from substances such as corn syrup, honey, molasses, vegetables, and fruits. *Fructose* is another simple sugar found in fruits and berries. Glucose and fructose are **monosaccharides**—they contain only one molecule of sugar.

Disaccharides are combinations of two monosaccharides. Perhaps the best-known example is granulated table sugar (*sucrose*). *Lactose* (milk sugar), found in milk and milk products, and *maltose* (malt sugar) are other examples of common disaccharides. Disaccharides must be broken down into monosaccharides before they can be used by the body.

Controlling the amount of sugar in your diet can be difficult because it is often present in food products that you might not expect to contain it. Such diverse items as ketchup, barbecue sauce, and flavored coffee creamers derive 30 to 65 percent of their calories from sugar. Read food labels carefully before purchasing.

Complex carbohydrates, or **polysaccharides,** are formed by long chains of sugar molecules. Like disaccharides, they must be broken down into simple sugars before the body can use them. There are two major forms of complex carbohydrates: *starches* and *fiber,* or **cellulose.**

Starches make up the majority of the complex carbohydrate group. Starches in our diet come from flours, breads, pasta, potatoes, and related foods. The body breaks these complex carbohydrates down into glucose, which can be easily absorbed by cells to use as energy. Polysaccharides can also be stored in body muscles and the liver as **glycogen.** When the body requires a sudden burst of energy, it breaks down glycogen into glucose.

Carbohydrates and Athletic Performance
In the past decade, carbohydrates have become the "health food" of many athletes. Some fitness enthusiasts consume concentrated sugary foods or drinks before or during athletic activity, thinking that the sugars provide extra energy. This may actually be counterproductive.

One possible problem involves the gastrointestinal tract. If your intestines react to activity (or the nervousness before competition) by moving material through the small intestine more rapidly than usual, undigested disaccharides and/or unabsorbed monosaccharides will reach the colon, which can result in an inopportune bout of diarrhea.

Consuming large amounts of sugar during exercise also can have a negative effect on hydration. Concentrations exceeding 24 grams of sugar per 8 ounces of fluid can delay stomach emptying and hence absorption of water. Some fruit juices, fruit drinks, and other sugar-sweetened beverages have more than this amount of sugar. If you use these products, dilute them with ice cubes or water.

Marathon runners and other people who require reserves of energy for demanding tasks often attempt to increase stores of glycogen in the body by *carbohydrate loading.* This process involves modifying the nature of both workouts and diet, usually during the week or so before competition. The athletes train very hard early in the week while eating small amounts of carbohydrates. Right before competition, they dramatically increase their intake of carbohydrates to force the body to store more glycogen to be used during endurance activities (such as the last miles of a marathon).

Carbohydrates and Weight Loss
The low-carb craze captured the attention of millions of would-be dieters

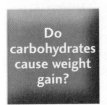
Do carbohydrates cause weight gain?

who started dumping their carbohydrates for programs such as the Atkins Diet, Protein Power, The Zone, South Beach, and other diet plans. As Americans bought into the low-carb diet trend, sales of items such as white bread and pasta took a dive, while an entire low-carb/no-carb industry emerged. Though the interest in extreme carb-reduction plans has waned, one positive legacy of these diet plans is that they

educated consumers and the food industry on the importance of whole grains, high fiber, and low-sugar food choices. (For more on these and other fad diets, see Chapter 10.)

Fiber

Fiber, often referred to as "bulk" or "roughage," is the indigestible portion of plant foods that helps move foods through the digestive system, delays absorption of cholesterol and other nutrients, and softens stools by absorbing water. Fiber also appears to reduce risk from heart disease[14] and helps to control weight by creating a feeling of fullness without adding extra calories. *Insoluble fiber,* which is found in bran, whole-grain breads and cereals, and most fruits and vegetables, is associated with these gastrointestinal benefits and has been found to reduce the risk for several forms of cancer. *Soluble fiber* appears to be a factor in lowering blood cholesterol levels and reducing risk for cardiovascular disease. Major sources of soluble fiber in the diet include oat bran, dried beans (such as kidney, garbanzo, pinto, and navy beans), and some fruits and vegetables.

A few years ago, fiber was thought to be the remedy for just about everything. Much of this hope was probably unrealistic, although research does support many benefits of fiber:[15]

■ *Protection against colon and rectal cancer.* One of the leading causes of cancer deaths in the United States, colorectal cancer is much rarer in countries having diets high in fiber and low in animal fat. Several studies have contributed to the theory that fiber-rich diets, particularly those including insoluble fiber, prevent the development of precancerous growths. Whether this is because more fiber helps to move foods through the colon faster (thereby reducing the colon's contact time with cancer-causing substances) or because insoluble fiber reduces bile acids and certain bacterial enzymes that may promote cancer remains in question.

■ *Protection against breast cancer.* Research into the effects of fiber on breast cancer risk is inconclusive. However, some studies indicate that wheat bran (rich in insoluble fiber) reduces blood estrogen levels, which may affect the risk for breast cancer. Another theory is that people who eat more fiber have proportionally less fat in their diets and that this is what reduces overall risk.

---

polysaccharides Complex carbohydrates formed by the combination of long chains of sugar molecules.

cellulose Fiber; a major form of complex carbohydrates.

glycogen The polysaccharide form in which glucose is stored in the liver and, to a lesser extent, in muscles.

fiber The indigestible portion of plant foods that helps move food through the digestive system and softens stools by absorbing water.

- *Protection against constipation.* Insoluble fiber, consumed with adequate fluids, is the safest, most effective way to prevent or treat constipation. The fiber acts like a sponge, absorbing moisture and producing softer, bulkier stools that are easily passed. Fiber also helps produce gas, which in turn may initiate a bowel movement.
- *Protection against diverticulosis.* About one in ten Americans over the age of 40 and at least one in three over age 50 suffers from *diverticulosis,* a condition in which tiny bulges or pouches form on the large intestinal wall. These bulges can become irritated and cause chronic pain if under strain from constipation. Insoluble fiber helps to reduce constipation and discomfort.
- *Protection against heart disease.* Many studies have indicated that soluble fiber (as in oat bran, barley, and fruit pectin) helps reduce blood cholesterol, primarily by lowering low-density lipoprotein (LDL, or "bad") cholesterol. Whether this reduction is a direct effect or occurs through the displacement of fat calories by fiber calories or through intake of other nutrients (such as iron) remains in question.
- *Protection against diabetes.* Some studies suggest that soluble fiber improves control of blood sugar and can reduce the need for insulin or medication in people with diabetes. Soluble fiber seems to delay the emptying of the stomach and slow the absorption of glucose by the intestine.
- *Protection against obesity.* Because most high-fiber foods are high in carbohydrates and low in fat, they help control *caloric* intake. Many take longer to chew, which slows you down at the table, and fiber stays in the digestive tract longer than other nutrients, making you feel full sooner.

In spite of a growing amount of evidence supporting the benefits of whole grains and high-fiber diets, intake among the general public remains low. The most recent National Health and Nutrition survey indicated that only 8 percent of Americans consumed three or more servings of whole grains each day.[16] Most experts believe that Americans should double their current consumption of dietary fiber—to 20 to 35 grams per day for most people and perhaps to 40 to 50 grams for others. (A large bowl of high-fiber cereal with a banana provides close to 20 grams.) What's the best way to increase your intake of dietary fiber? Eat more complex carbohydrates, such as whole grains, fruits, vegetables, dried peas and beans, nuts, and seeds. As with most nutritional advice, however, too much of a good thing can pose problems. Sudden increases in dietary fiber may cause flatulence (intestinal gas), cramping, or a bloated feeling. Consume plenty of water or other liquids to reduce such side effects.

Fats

Fats, or *lipids,* another group of basic nutrients, are perhaps the most misunderstood of the body's required energy sources. Fats play a vital role in maintaining healthy skin and hair, insulating body organs against shock, maintaining body temperature, and promoting healthy cell function. Fats make foods taste better and carry the fat-soluble vitamins A, D, E, and K to the cells. They also provide a concentrated form of energy in the absence of sufficient amounts of carbohydrates and make you feel full after eating.

If fats perform all these functions, why are we constantly urged to cut back on them? Although moderate consumption of fats is essential to health, overconsumption can be dangerous. **Triglycerides,** which make up about 95 percent of total body fat, are the most common form of fat circulating in the blood. When we consume too many calories, the liver converts the excess into triglycerides, which are stored throughout our bodies.

The remaining 5 percent of body fat is composed of substances such as **cholesterol,** which can accumulate on the inner walls of arteries and narrow the channels through which blood flows. This buildup, called **plaque,** is a major cause of *atherosclerosis* (the depositing of fatty substances that leads to blockage of vessels), a component of cardiovascular disease.

The ratio of total cholesterol to a group of compounds called **high-density lipoproteins (HDLs)** is important to determining risk for heart disease. Lipoproteins facilitate the transport of cholesterol in the blood. High-density lipoproteins are capable of transporting more cholesterol than are **low-density lipoproteins (LDLs).** Whereas LDLs transport cholesterol to the body's cells, HDLs apparently transport circulating cholesterol to the liver for metabolism and elimination from the body. People with a high percentage of HDLs therefore appear to be at lower risk for developing cholesterol-clogged arteries. Regular vigorous exercise plays a part in reducing cholesterol by increasing high-density lipoproteins.

fats Basic nutrients composed of carbon and hydrogen atoms; needed for the proper functioning of cells, insulation of body organs against shock, maintenance of body temperature, and healthy skin and hair.

triglycerides The most common form of fat in the body; excess calories consumed are converted into triglycerides and stored as body fat.

cholesterol A form of fat circulating in the blood that can accumulate on the inner walls of arteries, causing a narrowing of the channel through which blood flows.

plaque Cholesterol buildup on the inner walls of arteries; a major cause of atherosclerosis.

high-density lipoproteins (HDLs) Compounds that facilitate the transport of cholesterol in the blood to the liver for metabolism and elimination from the body.

low-density lipoproteins (LDLs) Compounds that facilitate the transport of cholesterol in the blood to the body's cells.

Types of Fats Fat cells consist of chains of carbon and hydrogen atoms. Those that are unable to hold any more hydrogen in their chemical structure are labeled **saturated fats.** They generally come from animal sources, such as meat, poultry, and dairy products, and are solid at room temperature. **Unsaturated fats,** which come from plants and include most vegetable oils, are generally liquid at room temperature and have room for additional hydrogen atoms in their chemical structure.

MUFAs and PUFAs: Unsaturated "Good Guys" The terms *monounsaturated fat* (MUFA) and *polyunsaturated fat* (PUFA) refer to the relative number of hydrogen atoms that are missing in an unsaturated fat. Peanut and olive oils are high in monounsaturated fats, whereas corn, sunflower, and safflower oils are high in polyunsaturated fats.

There is currently a great deal of controversy about which type of unsaturated fat is most beneficial. Many nutritional researchers believe that PUFAs may decrease beneficial HDL levels as well as the harmful LDL. PUFAs come in two forms: omega-3 fatty acids and omega-6 fatty acids. MUFAs, such as olive oil, seem to lower LDL levels and increase HDL levels and thus are currently the preferred, or least harmful, fats. MUFAs are also resistant to oxidation, a process that leads to cell and tissue damage. For a breakdown of the types of fats in common vegetable oils, see **Figure 9.5.**

> **Are all fats bad for me?**

Avoiding *Trans* Fatty Acids For decades, Americans have shunned saturated fats found in butter, certain cuts of red meat, and a host of other foods. What they didn't know is that foods low in saturated fat, such as margarine, can be just as bad for us. As early as the 1990s Dutch researchers reported that a form of fat known as *trans* fats increased LDL cholesterol levels while decreasing HDL cholesterol. In a more recent study, researchers concluded that just a 2 percent caloric intake of *trans* fats was associated with an increased risk for heart disease of 23 percent and a 47 percent increased chance of sudden cardiac death. Most significantly, they estimated that nearly 228,000 deaths related to coronary and heart disease in the United States could be averted each year by reducing Americans' consumption of *trans* fats.[17]

What are ***trans* fats (*trans* fatty acids)**? *Trans* fats are fatty acids that are produced by adding hydrogen molecules to liquid oil to make the oil into a solid. Unlike regular fats and oils, these "partially hydrogenated" fats stay solid or semisolid at room temperature. They change into irregular shapes at the molecular level, priming them to clog up arteries. *Trans* fats are used in margarines, many commercial baked goods, and restaurant deep-fried foods.

In 2006, the Food and Drug Administration began to require labeling that tells consumers how much *trans* fat is in that cookie they are putting in their mouths. The evidence against *trans* fats was too overwhelming to ignore any longer. However, keep in mind that the new labels don't

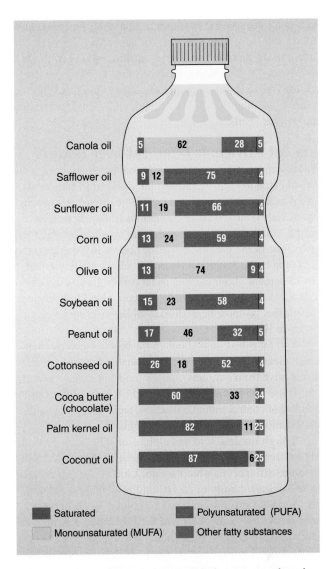

FIGURE 9.5 Percentages of Saturated, Polyunsaturated, and Monounsaturated Fats in Common Vegetable Oils

require listing *trans* fats for foods containing less than 500 milligrams per serving. If a product claims no *trans* fats, it could just contain less than 500 mg. In spite of labeling, *trans* fat hasn't gone away. Foods such as canned frosting, apple turnovers, and stick margarines are still loaded with *trans* fats, and many restaurants still fry their

saturated fats Fats that are unable to hold any more hydrogen in their chemical structure; derived mostly from animal sources; solid at room temperature.

unsaturated fats Fats that do have room for more hydrogen in their chemical structure; derived mostly from plants; liquid at room temperature.

***trans* fats (*trans* fatty acids)** Fatty acids that are produced when polyunsaturated oils are hydrogenated to make them more solid.

foods and make pastries using it. Remember, however, that a food label indicating that the product has no *trans* fat doesn't mean that the product is "healthy." Many of these products are high in sugar, saturated fats, and sodium. In fact, low-fat foods often compensate for bland taste and texture by adding these flavor enhancers at levels way above their former levels.

New Fat Advice: Is More Fat Ever Better?

Although most of this section has promoted the long-term recommendation to reduce saturated fat, avoid *trans* fatty acids, and eat more monounsaturated fats, some researchers worry that we have gone too far in our anti-fat frenzy. In fact, according to some experts, our zeal to eat no-fat or low-fat foods may be one of the greatest causes of obesity in America today. According to the American Heart Association, eating fewer than 15 percent of our calories as fat (fewer than 34 g a day on a 2,000-calorie diet) can actually increase blood triglycerides to levels that promote heart disease while lowering levels of protective HDLs.

Not all fat is bad. In addition to the benefits already mentioned, dietary fat supplies the two essential fatty acids that we must receive from our diets, *linoleic acid* and *alpha-linolenic acid*. These two fats are needed to make hormonelike compounds that control immune function, pain perception, and inflammation, to name a few key benefits.[18]

Although linoleic acid and alpha-linolenic acid are both polyunsaturated fats and have similar names, they are actually quite different in what they do. Linoleic acid, a member of the omega-6 family of fats (found in soybeans, peanuts, corn, and sunflower seeds), reduces blood levels of total cholesterol and "bad" cholesterol (LDL) when consumed in reasonable amounts. Alpha-linolenic acid is part of the omega-3 family of fats and is found in flax, canola oil, sardines, spinach, kale, green leafy vegetables, walnuts, and wheat germ. Alpha-linolenic acid is converted to two other beneficial omega-3 fats in the body, but you get a much bigger dose of those nutrients by eating cold-water fish, such as salmon and tuna, that have abundant supplies of omega-3. Today, Americans eat much more omega-6 than omega-3 fats, and most experts agree that we need a more balanced approach.

How can you add appropriate amounts of essential fatty acids to your diet?

- Eat fatty fish (bluefish, herring, mackerel, salmon, sardines, or tuna) at least twice weekly.
- Substitute soy and canola oils for corn, safflower, and sunflower. Keep using olive oil, too.
- Add healthy doses of green leafy vegetables, walnuts, walnut oil, and ground flaxseed to your diet to increase intake of alpha-linolenic acid.

---

vitamins Essential organic compounds that promote growth and help maintain life and health.

There is still much research to be done on the benefits versus the risks of consuming large amounts of omega-3 fatty acids. Stay informed on this issue to be a wise consumer and to make wise dietary choices.

Reducing Total Fat in Your Diet What's the bottom line on fat? Moderation in all fat intake is the best rule of thumb. Remember that no more than 7 to 10 percent of your total calories should come from saturated fat and that no more than 30 percent should come from all forms of fat. Want to cut the fat from your diet? These guidelines offer a good place to start.

- *Know what you are putting in your mouth.* Read food labels. Be wary of fried foods cooked in restaurants, and avoid prepared cakes, cookies, potato chips, and anything else that lists "partially hydrogenated oils" as an ingredient.
- *Use olive oil for baking and sautéing.* Animal studies have shown that olive oil doesn't raise cholesterol or promote the growth of tumors.
- *Avoid margarine products with* trans *fatty acids.* Whenever possible, opt for other condiments on your bread, such as fresh vegetable spreads, sugar-free jams, fat-free cheese, and other toppings.
- *Choose lean meats, fish, or poultry.* Remove skin. Broil or bake whenever possible. Drain off fat after cooking.
- *Choose fewer cold cuts, bacon, sausages, hot dogs, and organ meats.* Be careful of products claiming to be "95 percent fat-free"—they may still have high levels of fat.
- *Select nonfat dairy products whenever possible.* Part-skim-milk cheeses, such as mozzarella, farmer's, Lappi, and ricotta are good choices.
- *When cooking, use substitutes for butter, margarine, oils, sour cream, mayonnaise, and salad dressings.* Chicken broths, wine, vinegar, and low-calorie dressings provide flavor with less fat.
- *Think of your food intake as an average over a day or a couple of days.* If you have a high-fat breakfast or lunch, balance it with a low-fat dinner.

Vitamins

Vitamins are potent and essential organic compounds that promote growth and help maintain life and health. Every minute of every day, vitamins help maintain nerves and skin, produce blood cells, build bones and teeth, heal wounds, and convert food energy to body energy—and they do all this without adding any calories to your diet.

Vitamins can be classified as either *fat soluble,* which means they are absorbed through the intestinal tract with the help of fats, or *water soluble,* which means they are dissolved easily in water. Vitamins A, D, E, and K are fat soluble; B-complex vitamins and vitamin C are water soluble. Fat-soluble vitamins tend to be stored in the body, and toxic accumulations in the liver may cause cirrhosis-like symptoms. Water-soluble vitamins generally are excreted and cause few toxicity problems. See **Table 9.2** (page 266) and the section on functional foods (page 274) for more information on the benefits and dangers of specific vitamins.

Despite media suggestions to the contrary, few Americans suffer from true vitamin deficiencies if they eat a diet containing all of the food groups at least part of the time. Nevertheless, Americans continue to purchase large quantities of vitamin supplements. For the most part, vitamin supplements are unnecessary and even, in certain instances, harmful. Overusing them can lead to a toxic condition known as **hypervitaminosis.** See the section on supplements (page 276) for a further discussion of this issue.

Minerals

Minerals are the inorganic, indestructible elements that aid physiological processes within the body. Without minerals, vitamins could not be absorbed. Minerals are readily excreted and are usually not toxic. **Macrominerals** are those minerals that the body needs in fairly large amounts: sodium, calcium, phosphorus, magnesium, potassium, sulfur, and chloride. **Trace minerals** include iron, zinc, manganese, copper, and iodine. Only very small amounts of trace minerals are needed, and serious problems may result if excesses or deficiencies occur (**Table 9.3,** page 268).

Sodium Sodium is necessary for the regulation of blood and body fluids, transmission of nerve impulses, heart activity, and certain metabolic functions. It enhances flavors, balances the bitterness of certain foods, acts as a preservative, and tenderizes meats, so it's often present in high quantities in many of the foods we eat. As a result, most of us consume far too much sodium. Today, the Institute of Medicine, the American Heart Association, the FDA, and the USDA are among the many professional organizations that recommend that healthy people consume fewer than 2,300 milligrams of sodium each day. What does that really mean? For most of us, that means consuming less than 1 teaspoon of table salt per day! Recent studies indicate that, on average, we eat nearly twice that amount each day.[19]

A common misconception is that salt and sodium are the same thing. However, table salt accounts for only 15 percent of sodium intake. The majority of sodium in our diet comes from highly processed foods that are infused with sodium to enhance flavor and preservation. Pickles, salty snack foods, processed cheeses, canned soups and frozen dinners, many breads and bakery products, and smoked meats and sausages often contain several hundred milligrams of sodium per serving.

Why is high sodium intake a concern? Many experts believe that there is a link between excessive sodium intake and hypertension (high blood pressure). Although this theory is controversial, it is recommended that hypertensive Americans cut back on sodium to reduce their risk for cardiovascular disorders including stroke, debilitating bone fractures, and other health problems.[20]

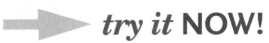
try it NOW!

Shake your salt habit! Extra salt can be found in almost everything from cereal to bread to snack foods. Take simple steps today to reduce your overall sodium intake: read food labels and choose products labeled as low-sodium (containing fewer than 500 mg per serving) or sodium/salt-free. Order your popcorn without salt, and, when dining out, ask the restaurant to cook with low-sodium products and hold the monosodium glutamate (MSG). Switch to kosher salt— it has 25 percent less sodium than regular table salt. Instead of adding salt to food you prepare, try using fresh or prepackaged herb blends to season foods. Try to train yourself to taste the natural flavors of the foods. Once you cut your sodium intake, you'll taste the difference the next time you eat a sodium-heavy product.

Calcium The issue of calcium consumption has gained national attention with the rising incidence of osteoporosis among older adults. Although calcium plays a vital role in building strong bones and teeth, muscle contraction, blood clotting, nerve impulse transmission, regulating heartbeat, and fluid balance within cells, most Americans do not consume the recommended 1,200 mg of calcium per day.[21]

It is critical to consume the minimum required amount each day. Milk is one of the richest sources of dietary calcium. Calcium-fortified orange juice and soy milk are good alternatives if you do not drink dairy milk. Many green leafy vegetables are good sources of calcium, but some contain oxalic acid, which makes their calcium harder to absorb. Spinach, chard, and beet greens are not particularly good sources of calcium, whereas broccoli, cauliflower, and many peas and beans offer good supplies (pinto beans and soybeans are among the best). Many nuts, particularly almonds, Brazil nuts, and hazelnuts, and seeds such as sunflower and sesame contain good amounts of calcium. Molasses is fairly high in calcium, and some fruits—citrus, figs, raisins, and dried apricots—have moderate amounts. Bone meal is not a recommended calcium source because of possible contamination.

It is generally best to take calcium throughout the day, consuming it with foods containing protein, vitamin D, and vitamin C for optimum absorption. Many dairy products are fortified with vitamin D, which is known to improve

hypervitaminosis A toxic condition caused by overuse of vitamin supplements.

minerals Inorganic, indestructible elements that aid physiological processes.

macrominerals Minerals that the body needs in fairly large amounts.

trace minerals Minerals that the body needs in only very small amounts.

TABLE 9.2　A Guide to Vitamins

Vitamin	Best Sources	Chief Functions in the Body
Water-Soluble Vitamins		
Vitamin B$_1$ (thiamin) 1.5 mg (RDA + RDI)	Meat, pork, liver, fish, poultry, whole-grain and enriched breads, cereals, pasta, nuts, legumes, wheat germ, oats	Helps carbohydrate convert to energy; supports normal appetite and nervous system function
Vitamin B$_2$ (riboflavin) 1.7 mg (RDA + RDI)	Milk, dark green vegetables, yogurt, cottage cheese, liver, meat, whole-grain or enriched breads and cereals	Helps carbohydrates, fat, and protein convert to energy; promotes healthy skin and normal vision
Niacin 20 mg NE (RDA + RDI)	Meat, eggs, poultry, fish, milk, whole-grain and enriched breads and cereals, nuts, legumes, peanuts, nutritional yeast, all protein foods	Helps convert nutrients to energy; promotes health of skin, nerves, and digestive system
Vitamin B$_6$ (pyridoxine) 2.0 mg (RDA + RDI)	Meat, poultry, fish, shellfish, legumes, whole-grain products, green leafy vegetables, bananas	Protein and fat metabolism; formation of antibodies and red blood cells; helps convert tryptophan to niacin
Folate 400 μg (DFE + RDA)	Green leafy vegetables, liver, legumes, seeds	Red blood cell formation; protein metabolism; new cell division; prevents neural tube birth defects
Vitamin B$_{12}$ (cobalamin) 2.4 mg (RDA)	Meat, fish, poultry, shellfish, milk, cheese, eggs, nutritional yeast	Maintenance of nerve cells; red blood cell formation; synthesis of genetic material
Pantothenic acid 5–7 mg (AI)	Widespread in foods	Coenzyme in energy metabolism
Biotin 30 μg (AI)	Widespread in foods	Coenzyme in energy metabolsim; fat synthesis; glycogen formation
Vitamin C (ascorbic acid) 60 mg (RDI + RDA)	Citrus fruits, cabbage-type vegetables, tomatoes, potatoes, dark green vegetables, peppers, lettuce, cantaloupe, strawberries	Heals wounds, maintains bones and teeth, strengthens blood vessels; antioxidant; strengthens resistance to infection; aids iron absorption
Fat-Soluble Vitamins		
Vitamin A 5,000 IU	Fortified milk and margarine, cream, cheese, butter, eggs, liver, spinach, and other dark leafy greens, broccoli, deep orange fruits and vegetables (carrots, sweet potatoes, peaches)	Vision; growth and repair of body tissues; reproduction; bone and tooth formation; immunity; cancer protection; hormone synthesis
Vitamin D 400–600 IU (RDA + RDI)	Self-synthesis with sunlight; fortified milk, fortified margarine, eggs, liver, fish	Calcium and phosphorus metabolism (bone and tooth formation); aids body's absorption of calcium
Vitamin E 30 IU (RDA + RDI)	Vegetable oils, green leafy vegetables, wheat germ, whole-grain products, butter, liver, egg yolk, milk fat, nuts, seeds	Protects red blood cells; antioxidant; stabilization of cell membranes
Vitamin K 70–140 μg	Liver, green leafy, and cabbage-type vegetables; milk	Bacterial synthesis in digestive tract; synthesis of blood-clotting proteins and a blood protein that regulates blood calcium

calcium absorption. We also know that sunlight increases the manufacture of vitamin D in the body and is therefore like an extra calcium source. Expert opinions vary on which type of supplemental calcium is most readily and efficiently absorbed, although aspartate and citrate salts of calcium are often recommended. As with all nutrients, the best way to obtain calcium is to consume it as part of a balanced diet.

Do you consume carbonated soft drinks? Be aware that the added phosphoric acid (phosphate) in these drinks can cause you to excrete extra calcium, which may result in calcium loss from your bones. A recent study of 2,500 men and women found that in women who consumed at least three cans of cola per week, even diet cola, bone density of the hip was 4 to 5 percent lower than in women who drank fewer than one cola per month. Colas did not seem to have the same effect on men.[22] In addition to the above, calcium-phosphorus imbalance may lead to kidney stones and other calcification problems and to increased atherosclerotic plaque.

Iron Worldwide, iron deficiency is the most common nutrient deficiency, affecting more than 2 billion people, nearly 30 percent of the world's population. In the United States iron deficiency is less prevalent, but it is still the most common micronutrient deficiency.[23] How much iron do we need? Women aged 19 to 50 need about 18 mg per day, and men aged 19 to 50 need about 10 mg.

Iron deficiency frequently leads to *iron-deficiency anemia*. **Anemia** is a problem resulting from the body's inability to produce hemoglobin (the bright red oxygen-carrying component of the blood). When iron-deficiency anemia occurs, body cells receive less oxygen, and carbon dioxide wastes are removed less efficiently. As a result, the iron-deficient person feels tired and run down. Iron deficiency in

anemia　Iron-deficiency disease that results from the body's inability to produce hemoglobin.

Deficiency Symptoms	Toxicity Symptoms
Beriberi, edema, heart irregularity, mental confusion, muscle weakness, low morale, impaired growth	Rapid pulse, weakness, headaches, insomnia, irritability
Eye problems, skin disorders around nose and mouth	None reported, but an excess of any of the B vitamins can cause a deficiency of the others
Pellagra: skin rash on parts exposed to sun, loss of appetite, dizziness, weakness, irritability, fatigue, mental confusion, indigestion	Flushing, nausea, headaches, cramps, ulcer irritation, heartburn, abnormal liver function, low blood pressure
Nervous disorders, skin rash, muscle weakness, anemia, convulsions, kidney stones	Depression, fatigue, irritability, headaches, numbness, damage to nerves, difficulty walking
Anemia, heartburn, diarrhea, smooth tongue, depression, poor growth	Diarrhea, insomnia, irritability, may mask a vitamin B_{12} deficiency
Anemia, smooth tongue, fatigue, nerve degeneration progressing to paralysis	None reported
Rare; sleep disturbances, nausea, fatigue	Occasional diarrhea
Loss of appetite, nausea, depression, muscle pain, weakness, fatigue, rash	None reported
Scurvy, anemia, depression, frequent infections, bleeding gums, loosened teeth, muscle degeneration, rough skin, bone fragility, poor wound healing	Nausea, abdominal cramps, diarrhea, breakdown of red blood cells in persons with certain genetic disorders; deficiency symptoms may appear at first on withdrawal of high doses
Night blindness, rough skin, susceptibility to infection, impaired bone growth, vision problems	Nosebleeds, abdominal cramps, nausea, diarrhea, weight loss, blurred vision, irritability, bone pain, rashes, cessation of menstruation, growth retardation
Rickets in children; osteomalacia in adults; abnormal growth, joint pain, soft bones	Raised blood calcium, constipation, weight loss, irritability, weakness, nausea, kidney stones, mental and physical retardation
Muscle wasting, weakness, red blood cell breakage, anemia, hemorrhaging, fibrocystic breast disease	Interference with anticlotting medication, general discomfort
Hemorrhaging	Interference with anticlotting medication; may cause jaundice

Note: Values increase among women who are pregnant or lactating.

Source: From J. Thompson and M. Manore, *Nutrition: An Applied Approach.* Copyright © 2005. Reprinted by permission of Pearson Education, Inc.

the diet is a common cause, but not the only cause, of anemia; anemia can also result from blood loss, cancer, ulcers, and other conditions. Generally, women are more likely to develop iron deficiency problems because they typically eat less than men and their diets contain less iron. Women having heavy menstrual flow may be at greater risk.

Iron overload or iron toxicity due to ingesting too many iron-containing supplements remains the leading cause of accidental poisoning in small children in the United States. Symptoms of toxicity include nausea, vomiting, diarrhea, rapid heartbeat, weak pulse, dizziness, shock, and confusion. Children have died from taking as few as five iron tablets containing as little as 200 mg of iron. Excess iron intake has also been associated with other problems: a recent study of over 45,000 men indicated that those who consumed excess heme iron—the kind found in meat, seafood, and poultry—

had a 20 percent higher risk of gallstones than those who consumed low-iron foods or got their iron from supplements.[24]

Determining Your Nutritional Needs

Historically, dietary guidelines were developed to reduce the public's risk of diseases from nutrient deficiency. Known as the **Recommended Dietary Allowances (RDAs)**, these

Recommended Dietary Allowances (RDAs) The average daily intakes of energy and nutrients considered adequate to meet the needs of most healthy people in the United States under usual conditions.

TABLE 9.3   A Guide to Minerals

Mineral	Significant Sources	Chief Functions in the Body
Calcium AI: 1,000 mg/day (men and women aged 19 to 50); 1,200 mg/day (men and women over 50)	Milk and milk products, small fish (with bones), tofu, greens, legumes	Principal mineral of bones and teeth; involved in muscle contraction and relaxation, nerve function, blood clotting, blood pressure
Phosphorus RDA = 700 mg/day	All animal tissues	Part of every cell; involved in acid-base balance
Magnesium RDA = 400 mg/day (men); 310 mg/day (women)	Nuts, legumes, whole grains, dark green vegetables, seafood, chocolate, cocoa	Involved in bone mineralization, protein synthesis, enzyme action, normal muscular contraction, nerve transmission
Sodium AI: 1.5 g/day	Salt, soy sauce; processed foods; cured, canned, and pickled foods	Helps maintain normal fluid and acid-base balance
Chloride AI: 2.3 g/day	Salt, soy sauce; processed foods	Part of stomach acid, necessary for proper digestion, fluid balance
Potassium AI: 4.7 g/day	All whole foods: meats, milk, fruits, vegetables, grains, legumes	Facilitates many reactions including protein synthesis, fluid balance, nerve transmission, and contraction of muscles
Iodine RDA = 150 μg	Iodized salt, seafood	Part of thyroxine, which regulates metabolism
Iron RDA = 8 mg/day (men; women over 51); 18 mg/day (women aged 19 to 50)	Beef, fish, poultry, shellfish, eggs, legumes, dried fruits	Hemoglobin formation; part of myoglobin; energy use
Zinc RDA = 11 mg/day (men); 8 mg/day (women)	Protein-containing foods: meats, fish, poultry, grains, vegetables	Part of many enzymes; present in insulin; involved in making genetic material and proteins, immunity, vitamin A transport, taste, wound healing, sperm creation, normal fetal development
Fluoride AI: 3 to 4 mg/day	Drinking water (if naturally fluoride-containing or fluoridated), tea, seafood	Formation of bones and teeth; helps make teeth resistant to decay and bones resistant to mineral loss
Selenium RDA = 55 μg	Seafood, meats, grains	Helps protect body compounds from oxidation

guidelines have provided Americans and Canadians with recommended intake levels necessary to meet the nutritional needs for about 97 percent of healthy individuals. More recently, the U.S. Food and Nutrition Board replaced and expanded upon the RDAs by creating new **Dietary Reference Intakes (DRIs),** a list of 26 nutrients essential to maintaining health. The DRIs identify recommended and maximum safe intake levels for healthy people and establish the amount of a nutrient needed to prevent deficiencies or to reduce the risk of chronic disease. DRIs are considered the umbrella guidelines under which the following categories fall:

- **U.S. Recommended Daily Allowances (USRDAs)**—The reference standard for intake levels necessary to meet the nutritional needs of 97 to 98 percent of healthy individuals.
- **Adequate Intake (AI)**—The recommended average daily nutrient intake level of a nutrient by healthy people when there is not enough research to determine the full RDA.
- **Tolerable Upper Intake Level (UL)**—The highest amount of a nutrient an individual can consume daily without the risk of adverse health effects.

Dietary Reference Intakes (DRIs) A set of nutritional values; a new combined listing, including more than 26 essential vitamins and minerals, that applies to healthy people.

U.S. Recommended Daily Allowances (USRDAs) Dietary guidelines developed by the Food and Drug Administration (FDA) and the U.S. Department of Agriculture (USDA).

Adequate Intake (AI) Best estimates of nutritional needs.

Tolerable Upper Intake Level (UL) The highest amount of a nutrient that an individual can safely consume daily without risking adverse health effects.

Reference Daily Intakes (RDIs) Recommended amounts of 19 vitamins and minerals, also known as micronutrients.

Reading Labels for Health To help consumers determine the nutritional values of foods, the FDA and the USDA developed the **Reference Daily Intakes (RDIs)** and

Deficiency Symptoms	Toxicity Symptoms
Stunted growth in children; bone loss (osteoporosis) in adults	Excess calcium is excreted except in hormonal imbalance states
Unknown	Can create relative deficiency of calcium
Weakness, confusion, depressed pancreatic hormone secretion, growth failure, behavioral disturbances, muscle spasms	Pharmacological overuse can cause nausea, cramps, dehydration
Muscle cramps, mental apathy, loss of appetite	Hypertension (in salt-sensitive persons)
Growth failure in children, muscle cramps, mental apathy, loss of appetite	Normally harmless (different from poisonous chlorine gas); disturbed acid-base balance; vomiting
Muscle weakness, paralysis, confusion; can cause death, accompanies dehydration	Causes muscular weakness; triggers vomiting; if given into a vein, can stop the heart
Goiter, cretinism	Very high intakes depress thyroid activity
Anemia: weakness, pallor, headaches, reduced resistance to infection, inability to concentrate	Nausea, vomiting, dizziness, damage to organs, death
Growth failure in children, delayed development of sexual organs, loss of taste, poor wound healing	Fever, nausea, vomiting, diarrhea
Susceptibility to tooth decay and bone loss	Fluorosis (discoloration of teeth)
Impaired immune function, depression, muscle pain	Vomiting, nausea, rash, brittle hair and nails

Note: RDA = Recommended Daily Allowance; AI = Adequate Intakes. Values are for all adults aged 19 and older, except as noted.

Source: From J. Thompson and M. Manore, *Nutrition: An Applied Approach.* Copyright © 2005. Reprinted by permission of Pearson Education, Inc.

Daily Reference Values (DRVs). RDIs are the recommended daily amounts of 19 vitamins and minerals, also known as micronutrients, and DRVs are the recommended amounts for macronutrients, such as total fat, saturated fat, cholesterol, total carbohydrates, dietary fiber, sodium, potassium, and protein.

Confused by all of these values? Don't despair—many people are confused by all the numbers, percentages, and serving sizes that make up today's labels. Just remember this: together, RDIs and DRVs make up the **Daily Values (DVs).** These are the percentages that you will find listed as "% DV" on food and supplement labels **(Figure 9.6).** In addition to the percentage of nutrients found in a serving of food, labels also include information on the serving size, calories, calories from fat per serving, and percentage of *trans* fats in a food.

The New MyPyramid Food Guide

In 2005, the Food Guide Pyramid underwent a landmark overhaul to account more completely for the variety of nutritional needs throughout the United States population **(Figure 9.7).** This new pyramid, called the MyPyramid Plan, replaced the

Daily Reference Values (DRVs)   Recommended amounts for macronutrients such as total fat, saturated fat, and cholesterol.

Daily Values (DVs)   Percentages listed as "% DV" on food and supplement labels; made up of the RDIs and DRVs together.

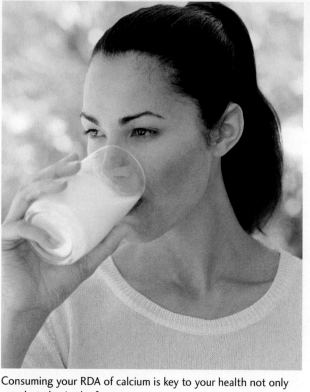

Consuming your RDA of calcium is key to your health not only now, but also in the future.

former Food Guide Pyramid promoted since 1993 by the USDA and incorporated the *2005 Dietary Guidelines for Americans.*[25] Although the former pyramid emphasized variety in daily intake, it did not reflect what we now know about restricting fats, eating more fruits and vegetables, and consuming whole grains. The MyPyramid Plan also takes into consideration the various dietary and caloric needs for a variety of individuals (such as people over 65, children, and active adults) as well as activity levels.

Goals of the MyPyramid Plan

The MyPyramid Plan is meant to encourage consumers to make healthier food choices and to be active every day. It promotes personalizing dietary and exercise recommendations based on individual needs.[26]

MyPyramid strives to illustrate the following:

- *Personalization* is demonstrated by the MyPyramid website, www.MyPyramid.gov. The website offers personalized recommendation of the kinds and amounts of food to eat each day, tips and ideas for achieving a healthy diet, and interactive assessments based on an individual's gender, age, and activity level.
- *Gradual improvement* encourages individuals to take small steps to improve their diet and lifestyle each day.
- *Physical activity,* represented by the person climbing steps, reminds us about the importance of daily physical activity in maintaining a healthy weight, improving overall health, and preventing disease.

Sample label for macaroni and cheese

Nutrition Facts

Serving size 1 cup (228g)
Servings Per Container 2

Amount Per Serving

Calories 250 — Calories from Fat 110

% Daily Value*

Total Fat 12g	**18%**
Saturated Fat 3g	**15%**
Trans Fat 1.5g	
Cholesterol 30mg	**10%**
Sodium 470mg	**20%**
Total Carbohydrate 31g	**10%**
Dietary Fiber 0g	**0%**
Sugars 5g	
Protein 5g	

Vitamin A	4%
Vitamin C	2%
Calcium	20%
Iron	4%

* Percent Daily Values are based on a 2,000 calorie diet. Your Daily Values may be higher or lower depending on your calorie needs:

	Calories:	2,000	2,500
Total Fat	Less than	65g	80g
Sat Fat	Less than	20g	25g
Cholesterol	Less than	300mg	300mg
Sodium	Less than	2,400mg	2,400mg
Total Carbohydrate		300g	375g
Dietary Fiber		25g	30g

Labels pointing to the nutrition facts:
- **Start here**
- **Limit these nutrients**
- **Get enough of these nutrients**
- **Quick guide to % DV:**
  - 5% or less is low
  - 20% or more is high

FIGURE 9.6 Reading a Food Label

Source: Center for Food Safety and Applied Nutrition, "Questions and Answers about *Trans* Fat Nutrition Labeling," 2006, www.cfsan.fda.gov/~dms/qatrans2.html.

- *Variety* is represented by the six color bands. It is important to eat foods from each group every day so that you obtain the proper nutrients for overall health.
- *Moderation* in food intake is represented by the narrowing of each color band from bottom to top. You should select foods with little or no fat or sugar more often to get the most from the foods you eat.
- *Proportionality* is symbolized by the varying width of each color band. A wider band generally suggests you should choose more foods from that group, whereas a narrow band suggests you limit your intake of foods from the corresponding group.

Using the New MyPyramid Plan

Understanding serving sizes, daily physical activity, and eating a nutritionally balanced diet are key components to using the MyPyramid Plan recommendations successfully. Though these elements are not new to the 2005 pyramid, they have been updated to reflect the latest in nutritional science.

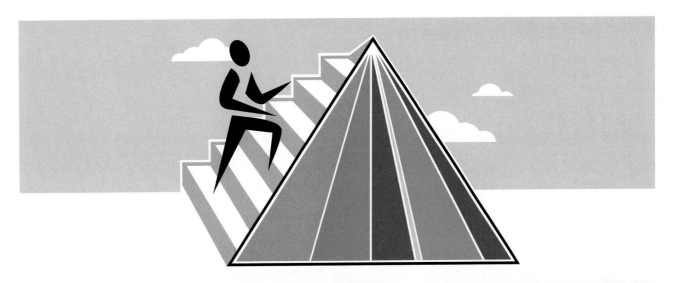

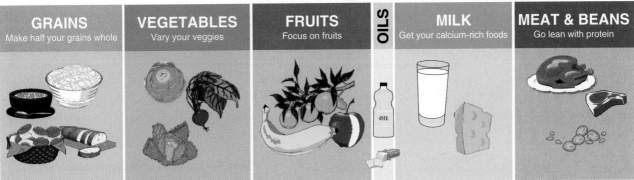

FIGURE 9.7 MyPyramid Plan
The USDA MyPyramid Plan takes a new approach to dietary and exercise recommendations. Each colored section of the pyramid represents a food group, with the specific needs of individuals in mind. Figure 9.9 on page 273 can help you determine the right number of servings from each food group for you.

Source: United States Department of Agriculture, 2005, www.MyPyramid.gov.

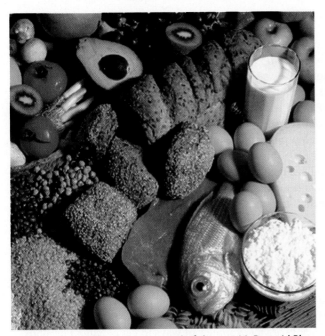

Eating a variety of foods is a key goal of the new MyPyramid Plan.

Understanding Serving Sizes How much is one serving? Is it different from a portion? Although these two terms are often used interchangeably, they actually mean very different things. It is important to understand the difference to use the MyPyramid Plan and other nutrition guidelines effectively. A *serving* is the recommended amount you should consume, whereas a *portion* is the amount you choose to eat at any one time and may be more or less than a serving. Most of us select portions that are much bigger than servings. According to a survey conducted by the American Institute for Cancer Research (AICR), respondents were asked to estimate the standard servings defined by the old USDA Food Guide Pyramid for eight different foods. Only 1 percent of those surveyed correctly answered all serving size questions, and nearly 65 percent answered five or more of them incorrectly.[27] See **Figure 9.8** for a handy pocket guide with tips on recognizing serving sizes.

Unfortunately, we don't always get a clear picture from food producers and advertisers about what a serving really is. Consider a bottle of soda: the food label may list one serving

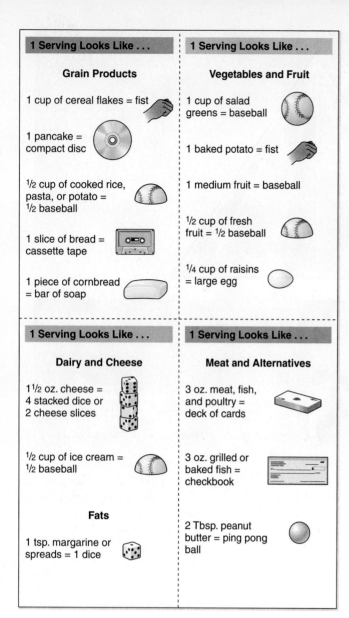

1 Serving Looks Like . . .	1 Serving Looks Like . . .
Grain Products	**Vegetables and Fruit**
1 cup of cereal flakes = fist	1 cup of salad greens = baseball
1 pancake = compact disc	1 baked potato = fist
½ cup of cooked rice, pasta, or potato = ½ baseball	1 medium fruit = baseball
1 slice of bread = cassette tape	½ cup of fresh fruit = ½ baseball
1 piece of cornbread = bar of soap	¼ cup of raisins = large egg

1 Serving Looks Like . . .	1 Serving Looks Like . . .
Dairy and Cheese	**Meat and Alternatives**
1½ oz. cheese = 4 stacked dice or 2 cheese slices	3 oz. meat, fish, and poultry = deck of cards
½ cup of ice cream = ½ baseball	3 oz. grilled or baked fish = checkbook
Fats	
1 tsp. margarine or spreads = 1 dice	2 Tbsp. peanut butter = ping pong ball

FIGURE 9.8 Serving Size Card
One of the challenges of following a healthy diet is judging how big a portion size should be and how many servings you are really eating. The comparisons on this card can help you recall what a standard food serving looks like. For easy reference, photocopy or cut out this card, fold on the dotted lines, and keep it in your wallet. You can even laminate it for long-term use.

Source: National Heart, Lung, and Blood Institute, "Portion Distortion," 2007, http://hp2010.nhlbihin.net/portion.

size as 8 fluid ounces and 100 calories. However, note the size of the entire bottle; the bottle may hold 20 ounces, and drinking the entire bottle serves up a whopping 250 calories.

Be sure to eat at least the lowest number of servings from the major food groups; you need them for the nutrients they provide. If you eat a large portion, count it as more than one serving. **Figure 9.9** lists the suggested daily amount of food from each group for a variety of calorie intake levels. Examples of one serving from each food group in MyPyramid follow.

Grains

- 1 slice of bread or ½ English muffin
- ½ cup cooked rice, pasta, or hot cereal
- 1 cup ready-to-eat cereal

Fruits

- 1 small apple or 1 large banana
- 1 cup of raw, cooked, or canned fruit
- 1 cup of fruit juice
- ½ cup dried fruit

Vegetables

- 1 cup raw greens or 2 cups cooked greens
- 1 cup beans, peas, or carrots (raw or cooked)
- 1 medium baked potato

Meat and Beans

- 1 ounce lean meat, poultry, or fish
- 1 tablespoon peanut butter
- ¼ cup tofu or cooked beans
- 1 egg

Milk

- 1 cup milk or yogurt
- 1½ ounces natural cheese or ⅓ cup shredded cheese
- 2 ounces processed cheese

Oil

- 1 tablespoon margarine or mayonnaise equals 2½ teaspoons of oil
- ½ avocado equals 3 teaspoons of oil
- 2 tablespoons Italian dressing equals 2 teaspoons oil

Discretionary Calories Every day you must consume a certain number of nutrient-rich foods to maintain health. *Discretionary calories* are those obtained from foods that do not provide a significant amount of nutritional value. Most of us have a very small discretionary caloric allowance at the end of the day. For example, suppose you are on a 2000-calorie diet and have eaten wisely all day, choosing whole-grain, low-fat, and low-sugar food items, so your calorie balance for the day is 1,800. This means you can spend the remaining 200 calories on what might be considered luxury indulgences. This might include a soda, a small serving of ice cream, or a higher fat cheese or meat than you would normally consume.

Physical Activity Strive to be physically active for at least 30 minutes daily, preferably with moderate to vigorous activity levels on most days. Physical activity does not mean you have to go to the gym, jog 3 miles a day, or hire a personal trainer. Any activity that gets your heart pumping (such as gardening, playing basketball, heavy yard work, and dancing) are all examples of ways to get moving. For more on physical fitness, see Chapter 11.

	1,200	1,400	1,600	1,800	2,000	2,200	2,400	2,600	2,800	3,000
Fruits	1 cup	1.5 cups	1.5 cups	1.5 cups	2 cups	2 cups	2 cups	2 cups	2.5 cups	2.5 cups
Vegetables	1.5 cups	1.5 cups	2 cups	2.5 cups	2.5 cups	3 cups	3 cups	3.5 cups	3.5 cups	4 cups
Grains	4 oz.-eq.	5 oz.-eq.	5 oz.-eq.	6 oz.-eq.	6 oz.-eq.	7 oz.-eq.	8 oz.-eq.	9 oz.-eq.	10 oz.-eq.	10 oz.-eq.
Meat and Beans	3 oz.-eq.	4 oz.-eq.	5 oz.-eq.	5 oz.-eq.	5.5 oz.-eq.	6 oz.-eq.	6.5 oz.-eq.	6.5 oz.-eq.	7 oz.-eq.	7 oz.-eq.
Milk	2 cups	2 cups	3 cups	3 cups	3 cups	3 cups	3 cups	3 cups	3 cup	3 cups
Oils	4 tsp.	4 tsp.	5 tsp.	5 tsp.	6 tsp.	6 tsp.	7 tsp.	8 tsp.	8 tsp.	10 tsp.
Discretionary calorie allowance	171	171	132	195	267	290	362	410	426	512

FIGURE 9.9 Nutritional Needs for Different Groups
Once you've determined your daily caloric requirements (Table 9.1), use this chart to determine how many servings of each food group you need per day to maintain good health.

Eating Nutrient-Dense Foods Although eating the proper number of servings from MyPyramid is important, it is also important to recognize that there are large caloric, fat, and energy differences among foods within a given food group. For example, fish and hot dogs provide vastly different fat and energy levels per ounce, with fish providing better energy and caloric value per serving. Nutrient density is even more important for someone who is ill and unable to keep food down. It is important to eat foods that have a high nutritional value for their caloric content. Avoid "empty calories," that is, high-calorie foods that have little nutritional value.

Vegetarianism: Eating for Health

For ethical, economic, personal, health, cultural, or religious reasons, some people choose specialized diets. Today, 5 to 15 percent of Americans identify themselves as vegetarians, and the number continues to rise. Normally, vegetarianism provides a superb alternative to our high-fat, high-calorie, meat-based cuisine. But without proper information and food choices, vegetarians can develop serious dietary problems in much the same way as their meat-eating counterparts.

The term **vegetarian** means different things to different people. Strict vegetarians, or *vegans,* avoid all foods of animal origin, including dairy products and eggs. Vegans must be careful to obtain all of the necessary nutrients. Far more common are *lacto-vegetarians,* who eat dairy products but avoid flesh foods. Their diet can be low in fat and cholesterol, but only if they consume skim milk and other low-fat or nonfat products. *Ovo-vegetarians* add eggs to their diet, and *lacto-ovo-vegetarians* eat both dairy products and eggs. *Pesco-vegetarians* eat fish, dairy products, and eggs, and *semivegetarians* eat chicken, fish, dairy products, and eggs. Some people in the semivegetarian category prefer to call themselves "non–red meat eaters."

Generally, people who follow a balanced vegetarian diet weigh less and have better cholesterol levels, fewer problems with irregular bowel movements (constipation and diarrhea), and a lower risk of heart disease than do nonvegetarians. The benefits of vegetarianism also include a reduced risk of some cancers, particularly colon cancer, and a reduced risk of kidney disease.[28]

Although in the past vegetarians often suffered from vitamin deficiencies, most vegetarians today are adept at combining the right types of foods and eating a variety of different foods to ensure proper nutrient intake. In fact, whereas vegans typically get 50 to 60 grams of protein per day, lacto-ovo-vegetarians normally consume between 70 and 90 grams per day, well beyond the RDA. Vegan diets may be deficient in vitamins B_2 (riboflavin), B_{12}, and D. Riboflavin is found mainly in meat, eggs, and dairy products; but broccoli, asparagus, almonds, and fortified cereals are also good sources. Vitamins B_{12} and D are found primarily in dairy products and fortified products such as soy milk. Vegans are also at risk for deficiencies of calcium, iron, zinc, and other minerals but can obtain these nutrients from supplements. Strict vegans have to pay much more attention to what they eat than the average person does, but by eating complementary combinations of plant products, they can receive adequate amounts of essential amino acids. Eating a full variety of grains, legumes, fruits, vegetables, and seeds each day will keep even the strictest vegetarian in excellent

vegetarian A term with a variety of meanings. *Vegans* avoid all foods of animal origin; *lacto-vegetarians* do not eat meat or eggs but do eat dairy products; *ovo-vegetarians* avoid flesh foods and dairy products but do eat eggs; *lacto-ovo-vegetarians* avoid flesh foods but eat both dairy products and eggs; *pesco-vegetarians* avoid red meat but eat fish, dairy products, and eggs; *semivegetarians* eat chicken, fish, dairy products, and eggs.

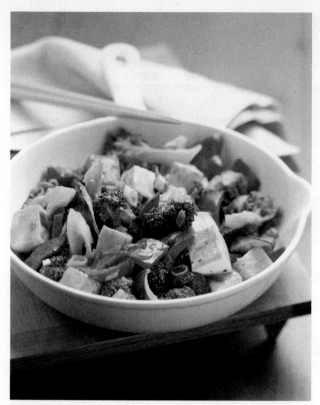

Meals like this tofu and vegetable stir-fry provide the vegetarian with essential vitamins and protein. Adding a whole grain, such as brown rice, would further enhance this meal by making use of complementary plant proteins.

health. For more information on plant source of protein, see the proteins section on page 259. Pregnant women, older adults, sick people, and children who are vegans need to take special care to ensure that their diets are adequate. In all cases, seek advice from a health care professional if you have questions.

Adapting MyPyramid for Vegetarians

As mentioned above, vegetarian diets can easily meet all of the recommendations for nutrient needs. As we learn more about the health benefits of high-fiber, low-fat diets—and as we better understand the importance of eating foods that take fewer resources to produce—researchers and professional groups are increasingly promoting vegetarian options. Options for soy-based products have increased in direct response to

functional foods Foods believed to have specific health benefits and/or to prevent disease.

antioxidants Substances believed to protect active people from oxidative stress and resultant tissue damage at the cellular level.

consumer demand. By focusing on nonmeat sources of protein, iron, calcium, zinc, and vitamin B_{12} while paying attention to personalized serving size and physical activity guidelines, vegetarians can be just as healthy as omnivores.

 what do you THINK?

Why are so many people today becoming vegetarians? ■ How easy is it to be a vegetarian on your campus? ■ What concerns about vegetarianism would you be likely to have, if any?

Functional Foods: Can Food Have Medicinal Value?

The old adage "you are what you eat" is indeed a motto to live by. Beneficial foods are termed **functional foods** based on the ancient belief that eating the right foods not only may prevent disease, but also actually cure it. This perspective is gaining credibility among the scientific community. The American Heart Association recommends dietary changes to reduce cholesterol and control diabetes **(Table 9.4)**. This is just the beginning of the functional food trend.

Antioxidants and Your Health

Many people today believe that **antioxidants** are wonder nutrients that will prevent just about anything. Although these substances do appear to protect people from the ravages of oxidative stress and resultant tissue damage at the cellular level, you may want to take a step back and consider all of the evidence. First, it is important to understand what *oxidative stress* really is. This damage occurs in a complex process in which *free radicals* (molecules with unpaired electrons that are produced in excess when the body is overly stressed) either damage or kill healthy cells, cell proteins, or genetic material in the cells. Antioxidants produce enzymes that scavenge free radicals, slow their formation, and/or actually repair oxidative stress damage. Thus, the theory goes that if you consume lots of antioxidants, you will nullify or greatly reduce the negative effects of oxidative stress. Among the more commonly cited nutrients touted as providing a protective effect are vitamin C, vitamin E, beta-carotene and other carotenoids, and the mineral selenium.

How valid is the theory? To date, many claims about the benefits of antioxidants in reducing the risk of heart disease, improving vision, and slowing the aging process have not been fully investigated, and conclusive statements about their true benefits are difficult to find. Large, longitudinal epidemiological studies support the hypothesis that antioxidants in foods, mostly fruits and vegetables, help protect against

TABLE 9.4	American Heart Association's Recommended Dietary Patterns to Improve Health		

Eating Pattern	DASH[a]	TLC[b]	Serving Sizes
Grains[c]	6 to 8 servings per day	7 servings[d] per day	1 slice bread; 1 oz dry cereal;[e] $\frac{1}{2}$ cup cooked rice, pasta, or cereal
Vegetables	4 to 5 servings per day	5 servings[d] per day	1 cup raw leafy vegetable, $\frac{1}{2}$ cup cut up raw or cooked vegetable, $\frac{1}{2}$ cup vegetable juice
Fruits	4 to 5 servings per day	4 servings[d] per day	1 medium fruit; $\frac{1}{4}$ cup dried fruit; $\frac{1}{2}$ cup fresh, frozen, or canned fruit $\frac{1}{2}$ cup fruit juice
Fat-free or low-fat milk and milk products	2 to 3 servings per day	2 to 3 servings per day	1 cup milk, 1 cup yogurt, 1 $\frac{1}{2}$ oz cheese
Lean[f] meats, poultry, and fish	<6 oz per day	≤5 oz per day	
Nuts, seeds, and legumes	4 to 5 servings per week	Counted in vegetable servings	$\frac{1}{3}$ cup (1 $\frac{1}{2}$ oz), 2 Tbsp peanut butter, 2 Tbsp or $\frac{1}{2}$ oz seeds, $\frac{1}{2}$ cup dry beans or peas
Fats and oils	2 to 3 servings[g] per day	Amount depends on daily calorie level	1 tsp soft margarine, 1 Tbsp mayonnaise, 2 Tbsp salad dressing, 1 tsp vegetable oil
Sweets and added sugars	5 or fewer servings per week	No recommendation	1 Tbsp sugar, 1 Tbsp jelly or jam, $\frac{1}{2}$ cup sorbet and ices, 1 cup lemonade.

[a] Dietary Approaches to Stop Hypertension. For more information, please visit www.nhlbi.nih.gov/resources/deca/descriptions/dashs.htm.

[b] Therapeutic Lifestyle Changes. For more information, please visit www.nhlbi.nih.gov/cgi-bin/chd/step2intro.cgi. TLC includes two therapeutic diet options: plant stanol/sterol (add 2 g per day) and soluble fiber (add 5 to 10 g per day).

[c] Whole-grain foods are recommended for most grain servings to meet fiber recommendations.

[d] This number can be lower or higher depending on other food choices to meet 2,000 calories.

[e] Equals $\frac{1}{2}$ to 1 $\frac{1}{4}$ cups, depending on cereal type. Check the product's Nutrition Facts label.

[f] Lean cuts include sirloin tip, round steak, and rump roast; extra lean hamburger; and cold cuts made with lean meat or soy protein. Lean cuts of pork are center-cut ham, loin chops, and pork tenderloin.

[g] Fat content changes serving counts for fats and oils: For example, 1 Tbsp of regular salad dressing equals 1 serving; 1 Tbsp of low-fat dressing equals $\frac{1}{2}$ serving; 1 Tbsp of fat-free dressing equals 0 servings.

cognitive decline and risk of Parkinson's disease. However, because of problems with design and difficulties in isolating dietary effects from supplement effects, it is difficult to assess overall neurological benefits of antioxidants.[29] Other studies indicate that these vitamins, particularly when taken as supplements, have no effect on atherosclerosis.[30]

Some studies indicate that when people's diets include foods rich in vitamin C, they seem to develop fewer cancers, but other studies detect no effect from dietary vitamin C.[31] Recent studies indicate that high-dose vitamin C given intravenously, rather than orally, may be effective in treating cancer[32] and providing protection from diseases affecting the central nervous system.[33]

Possibilities of vitamin E benefits are even more controversial. It has long been theorized that because many cancers result from DNA damage, and because vitamin E appears to protect against DNA damage, vitamin E would also reduce cancer risk. Surprisingly, the great majority of studies has demonstrated no effect or, in some cases, a negative effect, prompting the American Heart Association to advise people to get their antioxidants from a balanced diet, rather than from supplements in pill form.[34]

Carotenoids are part of the red, orange, and yellow pigments found in fruits and vegetables. They are fat soluble, transported in the blood by lipoproteins, and stored in

the fatty tissues of the body. Beta-carotene, the most researched carotenoid, is a precursor of vitamin A. This means that vitamin A can be produced in the body from beta-carotene; like vitamin A, beta-carotene has antioxidant properties. Although there are over 600 carotenoids in nature, two that have received a great deal of attention are *lycopene* (found in tomatoes, papaya, pink grapefruit, and guava) and *lutein* (found in green, leafy vegetables such as spinach, broccoli, kale, and brussels sprouts). Both are believed to be more beneficial than beta-carotene in preventing disease.

The National Cancer Institute and the American Cancer Society have endorsed lycopene as a possible factor in reducing the risk of cancer. A landmark study assessing the effects of tomato-based foods reported that men who ate 10 or more servings of lycopene-rich foods per week had a 45 percent lower risk of prostate cancer.[35] Subsequent research has questioned the benefits of lycopene, and some professional groups are modifying their endorsements of

carotenoids Fat-soluble compounds with antioxidant properties.

tomato-based products. Lutein is most often touted as a means of protecting the eyes, particularly from age-related macular degeneration (ARMD), a leading cause of blindness for people aged 65 and over. Although there is considerable controversy over many of the benefits of these nutrients in protecting against selected illnesses, experts generally agree that the best way to obtain these nutrients is through foods rather than pills. Eating a wide range of fruits and vegetables, trying to eat vegetables of different colors and fruits in their whole form rather than from high-sugar juices, is the best rule of thumb. It is recommended that adults take 500 milligrams of vitamin C and 400 to 800 IU of vitamin E, plus 10 milligrams of beta-carotene, daily. Researchers agree that intake should vary based on physical activity levels and overall health and that moderation is probably the best strategy.

Folate

In 1998, the FDA began requiring *folate* fortification of all bread, cereal, rice, and pasta products sold in the United States. This practice, which boosts folate intake by an average of 100 micrograms daily, is expected to decrease the number of infants born with spina bifida and other neural tube birth defects.

Folate is a form of vitamin B that was widely studied in the late 1990s and was believed to decrease blood levels of *homocysteine,* an amino acid that has been linked to vascular diseases, and to protect against cardiovascular disease. More recent research has raised questions about the benefits of the B vitamins in reducing risks of CVD or stroke, leading researchers to question these earlier results.[36] See Chapter 12 for more on homocysteine.

Although the amount of folate needed to protect the heart has not been determined, many people have jumped on the folate bandwagon and take daily folate supplements of up to 800 micrograms. Recently, a new *dietary folate equivalent (DFE)* was established to distinguish folate in food from its synthetic counterpart, *folic acid.* As a food additive or a supplement, folic acid is absorbed about twice as efficiently as folate. The DFE for folate in women aged 19 or older is approximately 400 micrograms, with higher levels for pregnant or lactating women. (See Table 9.2 for

folate A type of vitamin B believed to decrease levels of homocysteine, an amino acid that has been linked to vascular diseases.

probiotics Live microorganisms found in or added to fermented foods; they optimize the bacterial environment in our intestines.

dietary supplements Vitamins and minerals taken by mouth that are intended to supplement existing diets.

daily recommended amounts of other B vitamins.) Potential dangers of taking too much folate include masking of vitamin B_{12} deficiencies and resulting problems, ranging from nerve damage, immunodeficiency problems, anemia, fatigue, and headache, to constipation, diarrhea, weight loss, gastrointestinal disturbances, and a host of neurological symptoms.[37]

Probiotics

Probiotics are currently receiving much attention as natural healers. Probiotics are live microorganisms found in or added to fermented foods that optimize the bacterial environment in our intestines. Commonly, they are found in fermented milk products such as yogurt, and you will see them labeled as *Lactobacillus* or *Bifidobacterium* in a product's list of ingredients. Although thousands of studies of various supplements and functional foods have been done, no single supplement has been proven effective, particularly in long-term studies in which daily intake is monitored over time. Probiotics do not typically pose harm to healthy humans. However, it is possible that someone with a compromised immune system could have complications over time.

Supplements: Research on the Daily Dose

Dietary supplements are products—usually vitamins and minerals—taken by mouth and intended to supplement existing diets. Ingredients range from vitamins, minerals, and herbs to enzymes, amino acids, fatty acids, and organ tissues. They come in tablet, capsule, liquid, powder, and other forms. Because of their potential for influencing health, sales of dietary supplements have skyrocketed in the last decade. An important thing to remember about all dietary supplements is that they are not regulated like other food and drug products. The FDA does not evaluate the safety and efficacy of supplements prior to their marketing; it can take action to remove a supplement from the market only after it has been proven harmful. Currently, the United States has no formal guidelines for their sale and safety, and supplement manufacturers are responsible for self-monitoring their activities.

Should I be taking vitamin supplements?

For years, health experts had touted the benefits of eating a balanced diet over popping a vitamin-mineral supplement, so it came as a surprise when a 2001 article in the *Journal of the American Medical Association (JAMA)* recommended that "a vitamin/mineral supplement a day just might be important in keeping the doctor away, particularly for some groups of people."[38] The article indicated that older adults, vegans, alcohol-dependent individuals, and patients with malabsorption problems may be at particular risk of deficiency of several vitamins. Although the article acknowledged a possible risk of overdosing on fat-soluble vitamins, it noted that preliminary research has linked inadequate amounts of vitamins B_6, B_{12}, D, and E and lycopene to chronic diseases, including coronary heart disease, cancer, and osteoporosis. As a result of this study, *JAMA* advised that all adults take a basic multivitamin.

If you are in doubt about which supplements might be best for you, make sure you eat from the major food groups. If you are facing extreme stressors on the body from physical endurance events, illness, or other nutrient-depleting events, supplements might be beneficial; in general, a multivitamin added to a balanced diet is likely to do more good than harm. In all cases, beware of megadoses and overdosing on vitamin supplements.

Gender and Nutrition

Men and women differ in body size, body composition, and overall metabolic rates. They therefore have differing needs for most nutrients throughout the life cycle (see Tables 9.2 and 9.3 on vitamin and mineral requirements) and face unique difficulties in keeping on track with their dietary goals. Some of these differences have already been discussed, but some factors need further consideration. Have you ever wondered why men can eat more than women without gaining weight? Although there are many possible reasons, one factor is that women have a lower ratio of lean body mass to adipose (fatty) tissue at all ages and stages of life. Also, after sexual maturation, the rate of metabolism is higher in men, meaning that they will burn more calories doing the same activities.

Different Cycles, Different Needs

In addition to the above mentioned differences, women have many "milestone" times in life when their nutritional requirements vary significantly from requirements at other times. From menarche to menopause, women undergo cyclical physiological changes that can exert dramatic effects on metabolism and nutritional needs. For example, during pregnancy and lactation, women's nutritional requirements increase substantially. Those who are unable to follow the strict dietary recommendations of their doctors may find themselves gaining much more weight during pregnancy and retaining it afterward. During the menstrual cycle, many women report significant food cravings. Later in life, with the advent of menopause, nutritional needs again change rather dramatically. With depletion of the hormone estrogen, the body's need for calcium to ward off bone deterioration becomes pronounced. Women must pay closer attention to exercising and getting enough calcium through diet or dietary supplements, or they run the risk of osteoporosis.

Changing the "Meat-and-Potatoes" American

Since our earliest agrarian years, many Americans, especially men, have relied on a "meat-and-potatoes" diet. What's wrong with all those hamburgers and french fries? Heart disease, stroke, and cancer are probably the greatest threats. Add increased risks for colon and prostate cancer, and the rationale for dietary change becomes even more compelling. Consider the following points.

- Heavy red meat eaters are more than twice as likely to get prostate cancer and nearly five times more likely to develop colon cancer.
- For every three servings of fruits or vegetables they consume per day, men can expect a 22 percent lower risk of stroke.
- Diets high in fruit and vegetables may lower the risk of lung cancer in smokers from 20 times the risk of nonsmokers to "only" 10 times the risk. Such diets may also protect against oral, throat, pancreatic, and bladder cancers, all of which are more common among smokers.
- The fastest-rising malignancy in the United States is cancer of the lower esophagus, particularly among white men. Though obesity seems to be a factor, fruits and vegetables are the protectors. (The average American man eats fewer than three servings per day, although five to nine servings are recommended. Women average three to seven servings per day.)

Does something in meat make it inherently bad? The saturated fat content of meat and fried potatoes and the potential carcinogenic substances produced through cooking have been implicated. Probably something more basic is also involved. By eating so much protein, a person fills up sooner and never gets around to the fruits and vegetables. Thus, the potential protective value of consuming these foods is lost.

Improved Eating for the College Student

College students often face a challenge when trying to eat healthy foods. Some students live in dorms and do not have their own cooking or refrigeration facilities. Others live in crowded apartments where everyone forages in the refrigerator for everyone else's food. Still others eat at university food services where food choices may be overwhelming. Nearly all have financial and time constraints that make buying, preparing, and eating healthy food a difficult task. What's a student to do?

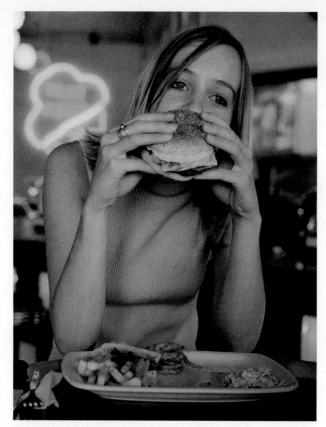

Meals like this one might be convenient, but they are high in fat and calories. Even when you are short on time and money, it is possible—and worthwhile—to make healthier choices.

When Time Is Short: Eating On the Run

Many college students may find it hard to fit a well-balanced meal into the day, but eating breakfast and lunch are important to keep energy levels up and get the most out of your classes. If your campus is like many others, you've probably noticed a distinct move toward fast-food restaurants in your student unions to meet students' needs for a fast bite of food at a reasonable price between classes. Eating a complete breakfast that includes complex carbohydrates and protein and bringing a small healthy snack (such as carrots, an apple, or even a small sandwich on whole-grain bread) to class are ways to ensure you fit meals into your day. If you must eat fast food, follow the tips below (and see the **Skills for Behavior Change** box on page 280 for more ideas about how to eat healthily while eating out).

- Ask for nutritional analyses of items. Most fast-food chains now have them.
- Order salads, but be careful about what you add to them. Taco salads and Cobb salads are often high in fat, calories, and sodium. Ask for dressing on the side, and use sparingly. Try the vinaigrette or low-fat alternative dressings. Stay away from eggs and other high-fat add-ons, such as bacon bits, croutons, and crispy noodles.

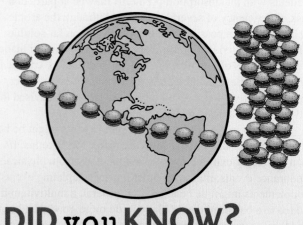

DID you KNOW?

U.S. college students consume an estimated 2 billion hamburgers each year. That's enough burgers to circle the earth nearly 5 times.

Source: Based on an estimated 14 million college students in the United States, consuming an average of three hamburgers per week. *Cornell Hotel and Restaurant Administration Quarterly,* June 2000.

- If you must have fries, check to see what type of oil is used to cook them. Avoid lard-based or other saturated-fat products and *trans* fats. Some fast-food restaurants offer "baked" fries, which may be lower in fat.
- Avoid giant sizes, and refrain from ordering extra sauce, bacon, cheese, dressings, and other extras that add additional calories, sodium, carboydrates, and fat.
- Limit beverages and foods high in added sugars. Common forms of added sugars include sucrose, glucose, fructose, maltose, dextrose, corn syrups, concentrated fruit juices, and honey.
- At least once per week, substitute a vegetable-based meat substitute into your fast-food choices. Most places now offer Gardenburgers, Boca burgers, and similar products, which provide excellent sources of protein and often have considerably less fat and fewer calories.

When Funds Are Short

Maintaining a nutritious diet within the confines of student life can be challenging. However, if you take the time to plan healthy meals, you will find that you are eating better, enjoying your food more, and actually saving money. Follow these steps to ensure a healthy but affordable diet at home, and see **Table 9.5** for ideas on how to eat healthily in the dining hall.

- Buy fruits and vegetables in season whenever possible for their lower cost, higher nutrient quality, and greater variety. Wash all produce, even bagged items, before eating. Don't bother buying veggie washes and other products. A fast-flowing water faucet, brisk rubbing with your

TABLE 9.5 | Eating Well in the Dining Hall

- Choose lean meats, grilled chicken, fish, or vegetable dishes. Avoid fried chicken, fatty cuts of red meat, or meat dishes smothered in creamy or oily sauce.
- Hit the salad bar and load up on leafy greens, beans, tuna, or tofu. Choose items such as avocado or nuts for a little "good" fat, and go easy on the dressing.
- Get creative: Choose items such as a baked potato with salsa, or add a grilled chicken breast to your salad. Toast some bread, and top it with vegetables, hummus, or grilled chicken or tuna.
- When choosing foods from a made-to-order food station ask the preparer to hold the butter or oil, mayonnaise, sour cream, or cheese or cream-based sauce. Do ask for extra servings of vegetables and lean meat or white-meat chicken.
- Avoid going back for seconds and consuming large portions. Many colleges limit the number of visits you make each day to the dining hall, but don't view this as a reason to overeat.
- If there is something you'd like but don't see in your dining hall, or if you are vegetarian and feel that your food choices are limited, speak to your food services manager and provide suggestions.
- Pass on high-calorie, low-nutrient foods such as sugary cereals, soft-serve ice cream, waffles, and other sweet treats. Choose fruit or low-fat yogurt to satisfy your sweet tooth.

hands, soaking in salt water, or other cleaning techniques are more effective and cost less.

- Buy locally, whenever possible. Fresh produce is often higher in nutrients and, if organic, has fewer pesticides and other chemicals. Shop early in the day, and bring produce home for refrigeration as soon as possible.
- Use coupons and specials to get price reductions. Plan your menu for the week, make a list, and stick to it so you can avoid impulse shopping. No food is cheap if you don't eat it.
- Shop at discount warehouse food chains; capitalize on volume discounts and no-frills products. However, don't buy more than you can reasonably use before "shelf life" expirations.
- Purchase meats and other products in volume; freeze portions in vacuum-packed bags or freezer bags, put dates on them, and save for future needs. Or, purchase small amounts of meats and other expensive proteins and combine them with beans and plant proteins for lower cost, calories, and fat.
- Drain off extra fat after cooking. Save juices to use in soups and other dishes.
- If you find that you have no money for food, talk to staff at your county or city health department. They may know of ways for you to get assistance.
- Plan your shopping list so that it includes ample quantities of foods from the various food pyramid groupings. If you don't have it on hand, you can't eat it.
- Invest in storage containers that hold up well to microwaving and dishwashing. Cook larger quantities at a time, and freeze leftovers.

Food Safety: A Growing Concern

Foodborne Illnesses

Are you concerned that the chicken you are buying doesn't look pleasingly pink or that your "fresh" fish smells a little *too* fishy? Are you sure that your apple juice is free of animal waste? You may have good reason to be worried. In increasing numbers, Americans are becoming sick from what they eat, and many of these illnesses are life-threatening. Scientists estimate, based on several studies conducted over the past 10 years, that foodborne pathogens sicken over 76 million people and cause some 400,000 hospitalizations and 5,000 deaths in the United States annually.[39] Because most of us don't go to the doctor every time we feel ill, we may not make a connection between what we eat and later symptoms.

Signs of foodborne illnesses vary tremendously and usually include one or several symptoms: diarrhea, nausea, cramping, and vomiting. Depending on the amount and virulence of the pathogen, symptoms may appear as early as 30 minutes after eating contaminated food or as long as several days or weeks later. Most of the time, symptoms occur 5 to 8 hours after eating and last only a day or two. For certain populations, however, including the very young, older adults, and people with severe illnesses such as cancer, diabetes, kidney disease, or AIDS, foodborne diseases can be fatal.

Several factors may be contributing to the increase in foodborne illnesses. The movement away from a traditional meat-and-potato American diet to "heart-healthy" eating—increased consumption of fruits, vegetables, and grains—has spurred demand for fresh foods that are not in season most of the year. This means that we must import fresh fruits and vegetables, thus putting ourselves at risk for ingesting exotic pathogens or even pesticides that have been banned in the United States for safety reasons. Depending on the season, up to 70 percent of the fruits and vegetables consumed in the United States come from Mexico alone. Although we are told when we travel to developing countries, "boil it, peel it, or don't eat it," we bring these foods into our kitchens at home and eat them, often without even washing them. Food can become contaminated by being watered with contaminated water, being fertilized with animal manure, being picked by people who have not washed their hands properly after using the toilet, or by not being subjected to the same rigorous pesticide regulations as American-raised produce. To give you an idea of the implications, studies have shown that *Escherichia coli* (a lethal bacterial pathogen) can survive in cow manure for up to 70 days and can multiply in foods grown with manure unless heat or additives such as salt or preservatives are used to kill the microbes.[40] There are no regulations that prohibit farmers from using animal manure to fertilize crops. Additionally, *E. coli* actually increases in summer months

SKILLS FOR behavior change

WHAT'S GOOD ON THE MENU?

Although some restaurants offer hints for health-conscious diners, you're on your own most of the time. To help you order wisely, here are lighter options and high-fat pitfalls. "Best" choices contain fewer than 30 grams of fat, a generous meal's worth for an active, medium-sized woman. "Worst" choices have up to 100 grams of fat.

FAST FOOD

Best Grilled chicken sandwich; lean roast beef sandwich; single hamburger with lettuce and tomato (hold the cheese and mayo!); salad with light vinaigrette

Worst Bacon burger; double cheeseburger; french fries; onion rings

Tips Order sandwiches without mayo or special sauce. Avoid deep-fried items such as fish fillets, chicken nuggets, and french fries.

ITALIAN

Best Pasta with red or white clam sauce; spaghetti with marinara or tomato-and-meat sauce. Order sauce on the side and use less than the portion provided. Even tomato sauce calories add up.

Worst Eggplant parmigiana; fettuccine alfredo; fried calamari; lasagna

Tips Stick with plain bread instead of garlic bread made with butter or oil. If you need something on your bread, opt for olive oil or canola oil and use it sparingly. Ask for the waiter's help in avoiding cream- or egg-based sauces. Try vegetarian pizza, and don't ask for extra cheese. Feta or other strong cheeses can perk up flavor and allow you to use less cheese overall.

MEXICAN

Best Black or pinto bean burrito (not refried) without cheese; chicken fajitas

Worst Beef chimichanga; chile relleno; quesadilla; refried beans

Tips Choose soft tortillas (not fried) with fresh salsa, not guacamole. Special-order grilled shrimp, fish, or chicken. Ask for beans made without lard or fat, and ask for cheeses and sour cream on the side or left out altogether.

CHINESE

Best Hot-and-sour soup; stir-fried vegetables; shrimp with garlic sauce; Szechuan shrimp; wonton soup

Worst Crispy chicken; kung pao chicken; moo shu pork; sweet-and-sour pork

Tips Share a stir-fry; ask for brown rice rather than steamed rice. Ask for vegetables steamed or stir-fried with less oil. Order moo shu vegetables instead of pork. Avoid fried rice, breaded dishes, egg rolls, spring rolls, crispy noodles, and nuts. Avoid high-sodium sauces.

JAPANESE

Best Steamed rice and vegetables; low-fat tofu as a substitute for meat; broiled or steamed chicken and fish

Worst Fried rice dishes; miso (very high in sodium); tempura

Tips Avoid soy sauces. Use caution in eating sashimi and sushi (raw fish) dishes to avoid possible bacteria or parasites.

THAI

Best Clear-broth soups; stir-fried chicken and vegetables; grilled meats

Worst Coconut milk; peanut sauces; deep-fried dishes

Tips Avoid coconut-based curries. Ask for steamed, not fried, rice.

BREAKFAST

Best Hot or cold cereal with skim or 1 percent milk; pancakes or French toast (use syrup sparingly); scrambled eggs with hash browns and plain toast (ask for a combination of egg substitute mixed with eggs to cut cholesterol levels)

Worst Belgian waffle with sausage; sausage and eggs with biscuits and gravy; ham-and-cheese omelette with hash browns and toast

Tips Ask for whole-grain cereal, oatmeal, or shredded wheat with skim or 1 percent milk or whole-wheat toast without butter or margarine. Order omelettes without cheese, and fried eggs without bacon or sausage.

SANDWICHES

Best Ham and Swiss cheese; roast beef; turkey

Worst Tuna salad; Reuben sandwich; submarine

Tips Ask for mustard; hold the mayo and cheese. If you must use mayo, go for the light versions, or opt for fat-free. See whether turkey ham is available.

SEAFOOD

Best Broiled bass, halibut, or snapper; grilled scallops; steamed crab or lobster

Worst Fried seafood platter; blackened catfish

Tips Order fish broiled, baked, grilled, or steamed—not pan-fried or sautéed. Ask for fresh lemon instead of tartar sauce. Avoid creamy and buttery sauces.

Sources: American Dietetic Association, 2007, www.eatright.org.; R. L. Duyff, *American Dietetic Association Complete Food and Nutrition Guide* (Hoboken, NJ: John Wiley & Sons, 2006).

as cows await slaughter in crowded, overheated pens. This increases the chance of meat going to market already contaminated.[41]

Other key factors associated with the increasing spread of foodborne diseases include inadvertent introduction of pathogens into new geographic regions and insufficient education about food safety.[42]

Responsible Use: Avoiding Risks in the Home

Part of the responsibility for preventing foodborne illness lies with consumers—more than 30 percent of such illnesses result from unsafe handling of food at home.

- When shopping for fish, buy from markets that get their supplies from state-approved sources. Check for cleanliness at the salad bar and at the meat and fish counters.
- Keep most cuts of meat, fish, and poultry in the refrigerator no more than 1 or 2 days. Check the shelf life of all products before buying.
- Eat leftovers within 3 days.
- Keep hot foods hot and cold foods cold.
- Use a meat thermometer to ensure that meats are completely cooked. Beef and lamb steaks and roasts should be cooked to at least 145°F; ground meat, pork chops, ribs, and egg dishes to 160°F; ground poultry and hot dogs to 165°F; chicken and turkey breasts to 170°F; and chicken and turkey legs, thighs, and whole birds to 180°F.
- Fish is done when the thickest part becomes opaque and the fish flakes easily when poked with a fork.
- Never leave cooked food standing on the stove or table for more than 2 hours.
- Never thaw frozen foods at room temperature. Put them in the refrigerator for a day to thaw, or thaw in cold water, changing the water every 30 minutes.
- Wash your hands and countertop with soap and water when preparing food, particularly after handling meat, fish, or poultry.
- When freezing chicken and other raw foods, make sure juices can't spill over into ice cubes or into other areas of the refrigerator.

Food Irradiation: How Safe Is It?

Food irradiation is a process that involves treating foods with invisible waves of energy that damage microorganisms. These energy waves are actually low doses of radiation, or ionizing energy, which breaks chemical bonds in the DNA of harmful bacteria, destroying the pathogens and keeping them from replicating. The rays essentially pass through the food without leaving any radioactive residue.

Irradiation lengthens food products' shelf life and prevents the spread of deadly microorganisms, particularly in high-risk foods such as ground beef and pork. Thus, the minimal costs

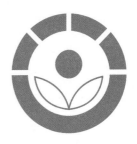

FIGURE 9.10 Label for Irradiated Foods

Source: Center for Food Safety and Applied Nutrition, "Food Safety A to Z Reference Guide," 2004, www.cfsan.fda.gov/~dms/a2z-i.html.

of irradiation should result in lower overall costs to consumers and reduce the need for toxic chemicals now used to preserve foods and prevent contamination from external pathogens. Some environmentalists and consumer groups have raised concerns; however, food irradiation is now common in over 40 countries. Foods that have been irradiated are marked with the "radura" logo (**Figure 9.10**).

Food Additives

Additives are substances added to food to reduce the risk of foodborne illness, prevent spoilage, and enhance the look and taste of foods. Additives can also enhance nutrient value, especially to benefit the general public. Good examples include the fortification of milk with vitamin D and of grain products with folate. Although the FDA regulates additives according to effectiveness, safety, and ability to detect them in foods, questions have been raised about those additives put into foods intentionally and those that get in unintentionally before or after processing. Whenever these substances are added, consumers should take the time to determine what they are and whether there are alternatives. As a general rule, the fewer chemicals, colorants, and preservatives, the better. Also, it should be noted that certain foods and additives can interact with medications. To be a smart consumer, be aware of the potential dietary interactions. Examples of common additives include the following:

- *Antimicrobial agents.* Substances such as salt, sugar, nitrates, and others that tend to make foods less hospitable for microbes.
- *Antioxidants.* Substances that preserve color and flavor by reducing loss due to exposure to oxygen. Vitamins C and E are among the antioxidants believed to reduce the risk of cancer and cardiovascular disease. The additives BHA and BHT are also antioxidants.
- *Artificial colors, nutrient additives, and flavor enhancers such as MSG (monosodium glutamate).*

food irradiation Treating foods with gamma radiation from radioactive cobalt, cesium, or other sources of X rays to kill microorganisms.

- *Sulfites.* Used to preserve vegetable color; some people have severe allergic reactions to them.
- *Dioxins.* Found in coffee filters, milk containers, and frozen foods.
- *Methylene chloride.* Found in decaffeinated coffee.
- *Hormones.* Bovine growth hormone (BGH) found in animal meat and milk.

Food Allergy or Food Intolerance?

At some point, nearly everyone will believe that they are experiencing a *food allergy* or *food intolerance reaction.* You eat something, develop gas, or have an unpleasant visit to the bathroom, and you assume that it is a food allergy. One out of every three people today either say they have a food allergy or avoid something in their diet because they think they are allergic to it; however, in fact, only 2 percent of adults and 5 percent of all children experience genuine allergic reactions to what they eat.[43] Surprised? Most people are when they hear this.

A **food allergy,** or hypersensitivity, is an abnormal response to a food that is triggered by the immune system. Reactions range from minor rashes to severe swelling in the mouth, tongue, and throat, to violent vomiting and diarrhea and occasionally death.

In 2004, congress passed the Food Allergies Labeling and Consumer Protection Act (FALCPA), which requires food manufacturers to clearly label foods containing ingredients that are common allergens and foods that could have been contaminated by a major allergen. The most common allergens are milk, eggs, fish and shellfish, nuts, wheat and soybeans.[44]

In contrast to allergies, **food intolerance** can cause you to have symptoms of gastric upset, but it is not the result of an immune system response. Probably the best example of a food intolerance is *lactose intolerance,* a problem that affects about one in every ten adults. Lactase is an enzyme in the lining of the gut that degrades lactose, which is in dairy products. If you don't have enough lactase, you cannot digest lactose, and it remains in the gut to be used by bacteria. Gas is formed, and you experience bloating, abdominal pain, and sometimes diarrhea. Food intolerance also occurs in response to some food additives, such as the flavor enhancer MSG, certain dyes, sulfites, gluten, and

food allergies Overreaction by the body to normally harmless proteins, which are perceived as allergens. In response, the body produces antibodies, triggering allergic symptoms.

food intolerance Adverse effects resulting when people who lack the digestive chemicals needed to break down certain substances eat those substances.

organic Grown without use of pesticides, chemicals, or hormones.

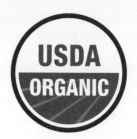

FIGURE 9.11 Label for Certified Organic Foods
This seal indicates that a product is at least 95 percent organic according to USDA guidelines.
Source: USDA Agriculture Marketing Program, The National Organic Program, "Organic Food Standards and Labels: The Facts," updated 2007, www.ams.usda.gov/nop.

other substances. In some cases, the food intolerance may have psychological triggers.

If you suspect that you have an actual allergic reaction to food, see an allergist to be tested to determine the source of the problem. Because there are several diseases that share symptoms with food allergies (ulcers and cancers of the gastrointestinal tract can cause vomiting, bloating, diarrhea, nausea, and pain), you should have persistent symptoms checked out as soon as possible. If particular foods seem to bother you consistently, look for alternatives or modify your diet. In true allergic instances, you may not be able to consume even the smallest amount safely.

Is Organic for You?

Mounting concerns about food safety and the health impacts of chemicals used in the growth and production of food have led many people to refuse to buy processed foods and mass-produced agricultural products. Instead, they purchase foods that are **organic**—foods and beverages developed, grown, or raised without the use of synthetic pesticides, chemicals, or hormones.

Less than a decade ago, buying organic foods meant going to a specialty store and paying premium prices for products that came with no guarantee that they were really grown in organic environments. People who bought these foods did so out of a desire to eat healthier produce and avoid the chemicals that they were increasingly being told caused cancer, immune system problems, and a host of other ailments. Enter the organics of the twenty-first century—larger, fresher looking, more affordable, and produced according to more reliable guidelines.

What does it mean if a food is organic?

As of 2002, any food sold as organic has to meet criteria set by the USDA under the National Organic Rule and can carry a USDA seal verifying products as "certified organic" **(Figure 9.11).** Under this rule, a product that is certified may carry one of the following terms: "100 percent Organic" (100 percent compliance with organic criteria), "Organic" (must contain at least 95 percent organic materials), "Made with Organic Ingredients" (must contain at least 70 percent organic ingredients), or "Some Organic Ingredients" (contains less than 70 percent organic ingredients—usually listed individually). To be labeled with any of the above terms, the foods must be produced without hormones, antibiotics, herbicides, insecticides, chemical fertilizers, genetic modification, or germ-killing radiation. However, reliable monitoring systems to ensure credibility are still under development.

Is buying organic really better for you? Perhaps if we could put a group of people in a pristine environment and ensure that they never ate, drank, or were exposed to chemicals, we could test this hypothesis. In real life, however, it is almost impossible to assess the health impact of organic versus nonorganic foods. Nevertheless, the market for organics has been increasing by over 20 percent per year—five times faster than food sales in general. Nearly 40 percent of U.S. consumers now reach occasionally for something labeled organic; by 2010, organic food sales are expected to reach $23.8 billion.[45]

In 2007, several reports by consumer groups questioned the nutrient value of organic foods. Some sources actually indicated that smaller, organic farmers may have more trouble getting their produce to market in the proper climate-controlled vehicles. As such, their foods might lose valuable nutrients while sitting in warm trucks or at a roadside stand as compared to the refrigerated section of a local supermarket. In general, the closer to the field you can purchase produce and the faster you can get it home and in the refrigerator, the more nutritious the foods will be.

TAKING charge

Summary

- Recognizing that we eat for more reasons than just survival is the first step toward changing our health.
- The major nutrients that are essential for life and health include water, proteins, carbohydrates, fiber, fats, vitamins, and minerals. MyPyramid provides guidelines for healthy eating.
- Vegetarianism can provide a healthy alternative for people wishing to reduce animal consumption from their diets. The MyPyramid Plan may be adapted to help vegetarians obtain needed nutrients.
- Men and women have differing needs for most nutrients throughout the life cycle because of different body size and composition.
- Experts are interested in the role of food as medicine and the benefits of "functional foods." These foods may play an important role in improving certain conditions, such as hypertension.
- College students face unique challenges in eating healthfully. Learning to make better choices at fast-food restaurants, to eat healthfully when funds are short, and to eat nutritionally in the dorm are all possible when you use the information in this chapter.
- Foodborne illnesses, food irradiation, food allergies, and other food safety and health concerns are becoming increasingly important to health-wise consumers. Recognizing potential risks and taking steps to prevent problems are part of a sound nutritional plan.

Chapter Review

1. What type of carbohydrates is found primarily in fruits?
   a. glucose
   b. dextrose
   c. simple carbohydrates
   d. complex carbohydrates

2. Which of the following foods would be considered a healthy, *nutrient-dense* food?
   a. nonfat milk
   b. cheddar cheese
   c. soft drink
   d. potato chips

3. What is the most crucial nutrient?
   a. water
   b. fiber
   c. minerals
   d. starch

4. Which of the following nutrients moves food through the digestive tract?
   a. fat
   b. fiber
   c. minerals
   d. starch

5. Which of the following nutrients is required for the repair and growth of body tissue?
   a. carbohydrates
   b. protein
   c. vitamins
   d. fats

6. What substance plays a vital role in maintaining healthy skin and hair, insulating body organs against shock, maintaining body temperature, and promoting healthy cell function?
   a. fats
   b. fibers
   c. proteins
   d. carbohydrates

7. What substance supplies us with the energy needed to sustain normal daily activity?
   a. fats
   b. fibers
   c. proteins
   d. carbohydrates

8. What is the most common nutrient deficiency worldwide?
   a. fat deficiency
   b. iron deficiency
   c. fiber deficiency
   d. calcium deficiency

9. Carrie eats fish, dairy products, and eggs, but she does not eat red meat. Carrie is considered a(n)
   a. vegan.
   b. lacto-vegetarian.
   c. ovo-vegetarian.
   d. pesco-vegetarian.

10. Which of the following fats is a healthier fat to include in the diet?
    a. *trans* fats
    b. saturated fats
    c. unsaturated fats
    d. hydrogenated fats

Answers to these questions can be found on page A-1.

Questions for Discussion and Reflection

1. Which factors influence the dietary patterns and behaviors of the typical college student? What factors have been the greatest influences on your eating behaviors?
2. What are the six major food groups in MyPyramid? From which groups do you eat too few servings? What can you do to increase or decrease your intake of selected food groups? How can you remember the six groups?
3. What are the major types of nutrients that you need to obtain from the foods you eat? What happens if you fail to get enough of some of them? Are there significant differences between men and women in particular areas of nutrition?
4. Distinguish between the different types of vegetarianism. Which types are most likely to lead to nutrient deficiencies? What can be done to ensure that even the most strict vegetarian receives enough of the major nutrients?
5. What are the major problems that many college students face when trying to eat the right foods? List five actions that you and your classmates could take immediately to improve your eating.
6. What are the major risks for foodborne illnesses, and what can you do to protect yourself? How do food illnesses differ from food allergies?

Accessing Your Health on the Internet

The following websites explore further topics and issues related to personal health. For links to the websites below, visit the Companion Website for *Health: The Basics,* Eighth Edition at www.aw-bc.com/donatelle.

1. *American Dietetic Association (ADA).* Provides information on a full range of dietary topics, including sports nutrition, healthful cooking, and nutritional eating. Links to scientific publications and information on scholarships and public meetings. www.eatright.org
2. *American Heart Association (AHA).* Includes information about a heart-healthy eating plan and an easy-to-follow guide to healthy eating. www.americanheart.org
3. *U.S. Food and Drug Administration (FDA).* Provides information for consumers and professionals in the areas of food safety, supplements, and medical devices. Links to other sources of information about nutrition and food. www.fda.gov
4. *Food and Nutrition Information Center.* Offers a wide variety of information related to food and nutrition. http://fnic.nal.usda.gov
5. *National Institutes of Health: Office of Dietary Supplements.* Site of the International Bibliographic Information on Dietary Supplements (IBIDS), updated quarterly. http://dietary-supplements.info.nih.gov
6. *U.S. Department of Agriculture (USDA).* Offers a full discussion of the USDA Dietary Guidelines for Americans. www.usda.gov
7. *National Center for Complementary and Alternative Medicine (NCCAM).* Includes information on new research results for supplements and functional foods. http://nccam.nih.gov

Further Reading

Center for Science in the Public Interest. *Nutrition Action Healthletter.* Washington, DC: Center for Science in the Public Interest.

This newsletter, published ten times a year, contains up-to-date information on diet and nutritional claims and current research issues. The newsletter can be obtained by writing to the Center for Science in the Public Interest, 1501 16th St. NW, Washington, DC 20036.

Duyff, R. L. *American Dietetic Association Complete Food and Nutrition Guide,* 3rd ed. Hoboken, NJ: John Wiley & Sons, 2006.

The most up-to-date dietary guidelines from the American Dietetic Association. Offers quick access to timely advice on a multitude of food and nutrition topics. Includes chapters on food for fitness, healthy weight, vegetarian eating, and nutrition for every stage of life.

Schlosser, E. *Chew on This.* Boston: Houghton Mifflin, 2006.

Overview of fast foods and their effect on health and well-being in America, with a special focus on children.

Selkowitz, A. *The College Student's Guide to Eating Well on Campus,* 2nd ed. Bethesda, MD: Tulip Hill Press, 2005.

Revised and expanded edition has the need-to-know information to take you through college in top form: how to beat the Freshman Fifteen and make the most of dorm or restaurant offerings. Tips on how to be a healthy vegetarian and how to help a friend with an eating disorder.

Tufts University Health and Nutrition Letter.

An excellent source for quick "fixes" on current nutritional topics. Reputable sources and information. Subscribe at http://healthletter.tufts.edu or phone (800) 274–7581.

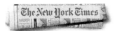

e-themes from *The New York Times*

For up-to-date articles about current health issues, visit www.aw-bc.com/donatelle, select *Health: The Basics,* Eighth Edition, Chapter 9, and click on "e-themes."

References

1. Centers for Disease Control and Prevention, "Behavioral Risk Factor Surveillance System (BRFSS)," 2007, www.cdc.gov/brfss.
2. Ibid.
3. American Institute of Cancer Research, *Food, Nutrition, and the Prevention of Cancer: A Global Perspective* (Washington, DC: American Institute of Cancer Research, 1997).
4. World Health Organization, *Nutrition for Health and Development: Challenges,* January 2007, www.who.int/nutrition/.
5. Ibid.
6. K. Flegal et al., "Excess Death Associated with Underweight, Overweight, and Obesity," *Journal of the American Medical Association* 293 (2005): 1861–67.
7. J. Thompson, M. Manore, and L. Vaughn, *The Science of Nutrition* (San Francisco: Benjamin Cummings, 2008).
8. Ibid.
9. Ibid.
10. U.S. Department of Agriculture, "Food Consumption Patterns: How We've Changed, 1970–2005," December 2005, www.usda.gov.
11. Thompson et al., *The Science of Nutrition.*
12. National Center for Health Statistics, *National Health and Nutrition Examination Survey, 2005–2006,* 2007, www.cdc.gov/nchs/nhanes .htm; G. Block, "Foods Contributing to Energy Intake in the U.S.: Data from NHANES III and NHANES 1999–2000," *Journal of Food Composition and Analysis* 17, nos. 3–4 (2004): 439–47.
13. Food and Agriculture Organization of the United Nations, "Food Security Statistics," 2006, www.fao.org/faostat/foodsecurity/.
14. P. B. Mellen, T. Walsh, and D. Herrington, "Whole Grain Intake and Cardiovascular Disease: A Meta-Analysis," *Nutrition, Metabolism & Cardiovascular Diseases,* doi: 10.1016/j.numecd.2006.12.008 (April 19, 2007), published online ahead of print.
15. M. Pereira et al., "Dietary Fiber and Risk of Coronary Heart Disease: A Pooled Analysis of Cohort Studies," *Archives of Internal Medicine* 164, no. 4 (2004): 370–76.
16. National Center for Health Statistics, *National Health and Nutrition Examination Survey, 2005–2006.*
17. D. Mozaffarian et. al., "*Trans* Fatty Acids and Cardiovascular Disease," *New England Journal of Medicine* 354 (2006): 1601–13.
18. B. McKevith, "Review: Nutritional Aspects of Oilseeds," *Nutrition Bulletin* 30 no. 1 (2005): 13–14.
19. H. Cohen et al., "Sodium Intake and Mortality in the NHANES II Follow-Up Study," *American Journal of Medicine* 119, no. 275 (2006): e7–14.
20. H. Cohen et al., "Sodium Intake and Mortality," e7–14; J. Feng et al., "Salt Intake and Cardiovascular Mortality," *American Journal of Medicine* 120, no. 1 (2007): e5–7; H. Harpannen and E. Mervaala, "Sodium Intake and Hypertension," *Progress in Cardiovascular Diseases* 49, no. 2 (2006): 59–75.
21. J. Ma, R. Johns, and R. Stafford, "Americans Are Not Meeting Current Calcium Recommendations," *American Journal of Clinical Nutrition* 85 (2007): 1361–66.
22. K. Tucker et al., "Colas, But Not other Carbonated Beverages, Are Associated with Low Bone Mineral Density in Older Women: The Framingham Osteoporosis Study," *American Journal of Clinical Nutrition* 84 (2006): 936–42.

23. World Health Organization, "Miconutrient Deficiencies," 2007, www.who.int/nutrition/topics/ida/en/index.html.

24. C. Tsai et al., "Heme and non-Heme Iron Consumption and Risk of Gallstone Disease in Men," *American Journal of Clinical Nutrition* 85 (2007): 518–22.

25. U.S. Department of Health and Human Services and U.S. Department of Agriculture, *Dietary Guidelines for Americans, 2005* (Washington, D.C.: Government Printing Office, 2005).

26. United States Department of Agriculture, "Johanns Reveals USDA's Steps to a Healthier You," Press Release, April 19, 2005.

27. B. Black, "Healthgate: Just How Much Food IS on that Plate? Understanding Portion Control," 2004. EBSCO Publishing.

28. J. Thompson and M. Manore, *Nutrition: An Applied Approach* (San Francisco: Benjamin Cummings, 2005).

29. A. Asherio, "Dietary Antioxidant Intakes and Neurological Disease Risks," Paper presented at the Linus Pauling Diet and Optimum Health Annual Conference, Portland, OR, May 2007.

30. J. Bleys et al., "Vitamin-Mineral Supplementation and the Progression of Atherosclerosis: A Meta-Analysis of Randomized Controlled Trials," *American Journal of Clinical Nutrition* 84 (2006): 880–87.

31. Thompson and Manore, *Nutrition: An Applied Approach.*

32. M. Levine, "Pharmacologic Ascorbate Concentrations Selectively Kill Cancer Cells: Ascorbic Acid as a Pro-Drug for Ascorbate Radical and/or H_2O_2 Delivery to Tissues," Paper presented at the Linus Pauling Diet and Optimum Health Annual Conference, Portland, OR, May 2007.

33. J. May, "Ascorbic Acid Transporters in Health and Disease," Paper presented at the Linus Pauling Diet and Optimum Health Annual Conference, Portland, OR, May 2007.

34. G. Bjelakovic and C. Gluud, "Surviving Antioxidant Supplements," *Journal of the National Cancer Institute* 99, no. 10 (2007): 742–43; E. Miller et al., "Meta-Analysis: High-Dosage Vitamin E Supplementation May Increase All-Cause Mortality," *Annals of Internal Medicine* 142 (2005): 37–46.

35. J. Chan and E. Giovannucci, "Vegetables, Fruits, Associated Micronutrients and Risk of Prostate Cancer," *Epidemiology Review* 23, no.1 (2001): 82–86.

36. J. Manson et al., "A Randomized Trial of Folic Acid and B-Vitamins in the Secondary Prevention of Cardiovascular Events in Women: Results From the Women's Antioxidant and Folic Acid Cardiovascular Study (WAFACS)," *Circulation* 114, no. 22 (2006): 2424; J. Manson et al., "A Randomized Factorial Trial of Vitamins C, E, and Beta-Carotene in the Secondary Prevention of Cardiovascular Events in Women: Results from the Women's Antioxidant Cardiovascular Study (WACS)," *Circulation* 114, no. 22 (2006): 2424.

37. R. Malinow, "Homocysteine, Folic Acid, and CVD," Linus Pauling Institute International Conference on Diet and Optimum Health, Portland, OR, May 2001.

38. K. M. Fairfield and R. H. Fletcher, "Vitamins for Chronic Disease Prevention in Adults: Scientific Review," *Journal of the American Medical Association* 287, no. 23 (2001): 3116–26.

39. Centers for Disease Control and Prevention, Division of Bacterial and Mycotic Diseases, "Food Borne Illnesses," 2005, www.cdc.gov/ncidod/dbmd/diseaseinfo/foodborneinfections_g.htm.

40. Centers for Disease Control and Prevention, Foodborne and Diarrheal Disease Branch, "*E. coli*," 2007, www.cdc.gov/ecoli.

41. Ibid.

42. P. Morris, Y. Motarjemi, and F. Kaferstein, "Emerging Foodborne Diseases," *World Health* 50 (1997): 16–22; Centers for Disease Control and Prevention, Division of Bacterial and Mycotic Diseases, "Food Borne Illnesses," 2005, www.cdc.gov/ncidod/dbmd/diseaseinfo/foodborneinfections_g.htm.

43. U.S. Food and Drug Administration, Center for Food Safety and Applied Nutrition, "Information for Consumers: Food Allergy Labeling," 2006, www.cfsan.fda.gov/.

44. Ibid.

45. United States Department of Agriculture, Economic Research Services, "Food Consumption," 2007, www.ers.usda.gov/briefing/consumption.

Managing Your Weight

FINDING A HEALTHY BALANCE

What are the **health** risks of being overweight?

How can I tell if I have too much **body fat?**

Is there a best **diet plan** for losing weight?

How can I help a friend who has an **eating disorder?**

OBJECTIVES

- Define *obesity*, describe the current epidemic of obesity in the United States, and understand risk factors associated with obesity.

- Explain why so many people are obsessed with thinness.

- Discuss reliable options for determining body fat content and the right weight for you.

- Describe factors that place people at risk for problems with obesity. Distinguish factors that can and cannot be controlled.

- Discuss the roles of exercise, dieting, nutrition, lifestyle modification, fad diets, and other strategies of weight control, and evaluate which methods are most effective.

- Describe major eating disorders, explain their health risks, and indicate the factors that make people susceptible to them.

O ver the past 20 years, the United States has become known as one of the fattest nations on earth. From young children to seniors, virtually no segment of the populace is immune to the epidemic of overweight and obesity **(Figure 10.1).** Just how serious is the problem?

According to a national survey of health behaviors and nutrition, 66 percent of American adults are considered overweight or obese, with obesity rates alone in excess of 32 percent.[1] Even more alarming is the rapid rise in overweight and obesity among U.S. children; it is estimated that over 17 percent of all youth are overweight, and there is a clear trend of young people becoming obese with increasing age.[2] Obesity rates have been rising dramatically in nearly every state. In a recent report, Mississippi ranked as the heaviest state, and Colorado ranked as the least heavy state. Experts predict that at the current pace, 50 percent of Americans will be obese by the year 2025.[3]

What does all of this excess weight mean to the health of our population? Recent studies indicate that obesity is one

What are the health risks of being overweight?

of the top underlying preventable causes of death in the United States. Obesity and inactivity increase the risks from three of our leading killers: heart disease, cancer, and cerebrovascular ailments, including strokes.[4] Other associated health risks of obesity include diabetes, gallstones, sleep apnea, osteoarthritis, and several cancers **(Table 10.1).** Some experts predict that the number of Americans diagnosed with diabetes, a major obesity-associated problem, will increase by a whopping 165 percent, from 15 million in 2005 to well over 30 million in 2030.[5] It is noteworthy that other nations, such as Canada, have already seen a rise of 69 percent in diabetes rates in just the last decade, indicating that global rates may well exceed even the most dire predictions for the next 20 to 30 years.[6]

Short- and long-term health consequences of obesity are not our only concern: the estimated annual cost of obesity in the United States exceeds $152 billion in medical expenses and lost productivity.[7] Of course, it is impossible to place a dollar value on a life lost prematurely due to diabetes, stroke, or heart attack or to assess the cost of social isolation and discrimination against overweight individuals. Of growing importance is the recognition that obese individuals suffer significant disability during their lives, in terms of both mobility and activities of daily living.

This chapter will help you understand why we have such a weight problem in America today and provide simple strategies to help you manage your own weight. (See the **Assess Yourself** box on page 294 to obtain a better understanding of your own dietary habits.) It will also help you understand what *underweight, normal weight, overweight,* and *obesity* really mean and why managing your weight is essential to overall health and well-being.

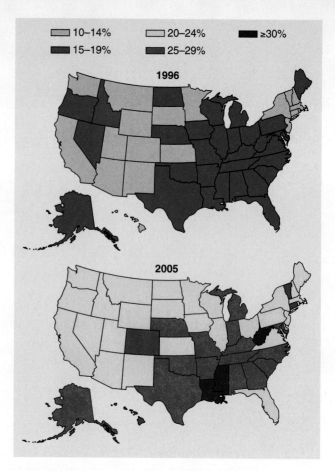

FIGURE 10.1 Obesity Trends Among U.S. Adults, 1996 and 2005
This map indicates the percentage of population in each state that is considered obese, based on a BMI of 30 or higher, or about 30 pounds overweight for a person 5 feet, 4 inches tall.
Source: Centers for Disease Control and Prevention, "U.S. Obesity Trends: 1985–2005," 2007, www.cdc.gov/nccdphp/dnpa/obesity/trend.

Determining the Right Weight for You

What weight is right for you? This depends on a wide range of variables, including your body structure, height, weight distribution, and the ratio of fat to lean tissue. In fact, weight can be a deceptive indicator. Many extremely muscular athletes would be considered overweight based on traditional height–weight charts. Many young women think that they are the right weight based on charts but are shocked to discover that 35 to 40 percent of their weight is body fat!

In general, weights at the lower end of the range on these charts are recommended for individuals with a low ratio of muscle and bone to fat; those at the upper end are advised for people with more muscular builds **(Table 10.2).** However, because actual body composition is hard to determine, most charts give a general range.

TABLE 10.1 Selected Health Consequences of Overweight and Obesity

Premature Death

- Obese individuals have a 50–100% increased risk of death from all causes compared with people of normal weight. Among 25- to 35-year-olds, severe obesity increases the risk of death by a factor of 12.
- At least 300,000 deaths per year may be attributable to obesity.
- The risk of death rises with increasing weight.
- Even moderate excess weight (10–20 pounds for a person of average height) increases risk of death.

Cardiovascular Disease

- High blood pressure is twice as common in obese adults as it is in those who are at healthy weights.
- Incidence of all forms of heart disease is increased among overweight and obese people.
- Obesity is associated with elevated triglycerides and decreased HDLs ("good" cholesterol).

Diabetes

- A weight gain of 11–18 pounds increases a person's risk of developing type 2 diabetes to twice that of individuals who have not gained weight.
- More than 80% of people with diabetes are overweight or obese.

Cancer

- Overweight and obesity are associated with increased risk of endometrial, colon, gallbladder, prostate, kidney, uterine, and postmenopausal breast cancer.
- Women gaining more than 20 pounds between age 18 and midlife double their risk of postmenopausal breast cancer compared with women whose weight remains stable.

Additional Health Consequences

- Sleep apnea and asthma are both associated with obesity.
- For every 2-pound increase in weight, the risk of developing arthritis increases by 9–13%.
- Obesity related complications during pregnancy include increased risk of fetal and maternal death, labor and delivery complications, and increased risk of birth defects.
- Increased risk of osteoarthritis, especially in weight-bearing joints such as knees and hips.

Sources: Mayo Clinic, "Obesity Consequences," 2006, www.mayoclinic.com; National Institutes of Health, "Summary of Obesity," 2005; S. J. Olshansky et al., "A Potential Decline in Life Expectancy in the U.S. in the 21st Century," *New England Journal of Medicine* 352 (2005): 1103–10.

Overweight or Obese?

Most of us cringe at the thought of being labeled as one of the "O" words. What is the distinction between the two? **Overweight** refers to increased body weight in relation to height when compared to a standard such as the height–weight charts in Table 10.2. The excess weight may come from muscle, bone, fat, and/or water. Historically, health experts have defined *overweight* as being 1 to 19 percent above one's ideal weight and *obese* as over 19 percent.

Another measurement of overweight and obesity is a mathematical formula known as **body mass index (BMI),** which represents weight levels associated with the lowest overall risk to health (see page 291 to calculate your BMI). Desirable BMI levels may vary with age.[8] About 34 percent of all Americans are classified as being overweight using BMI calculations.

A person may be classified as overweight using these standards even if the weight gain is due to an increase in lean muscle mass. For example, an athlete may be very lean and muscular, with very little body fat, yet she may weigh a lot more than others of the same height who have little muscle tissue. Conversely, a person may proudly proclaim that he weighs the same that he did in high school but have a much greater proportion of body fat, particularly in the hips, buttocks, or thighs, than he did at a younger age. Therefore, BMI is a useful guideline, but by itself it is not diagnostic of a person's overall fitness and health status.[9]

Obesity is defined as an excessively high amount of body fat (adipose tissue) in relation to lean body mass or a BMI of 30 or more. In determining obesity, it is important to consider both the distribution of fat throughout the body and the size of the adipose tissue deposits. Body fat distribution can be estimated in a variety of ways, as will be discussed shortly. By traditional standards, people 20 to 40 percent above their ideal weight are labeled as *mildly obese* (90 percent of the obese fall into this category). Those 41 to 99 percent above their ideal weight are described as *moderately obese* (about 7 to 8 percent of the obese fit into this category), and increasing numbers of people are in the *severely, morbidly,* or *grossly obese* category, meaning that they are 100 percent or more above their ideal weight (with a BMI greater than 40). Nearly 3 percent of obese men and almost 7 percent of obese women are in this category.[10] In the last decade, more and more

overweight Increased body weight in relation to height.

body mass index (BMI) A technique of weight assessment based on the relationship of weight to height.

obesity A weight disorder characterized by an accumulation of fat beyond that considered normal for a person based on age, sex, and body type. Obesity is generally defined as a body mass index of 30 or more.

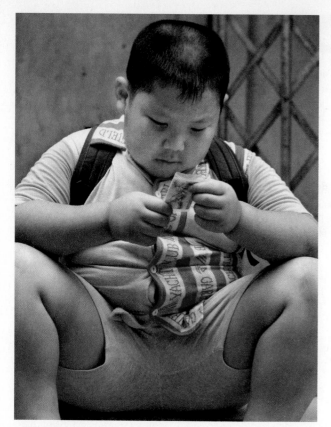

Obesity is increasing especially dramatically among children. Being overweight or obese from an early age can have devastating physical and emotional consequences.

TABLE 10.2 Healthy Weight Ranges*

Height without Shoes	Weight† without Clothes
4'10"	91–119
4'11"	94–124
5'0"	97–128
5'1"	101–132
5'2"	104–137
5'3"	107–141
5'4"	111–146
5'5"	114–150
5'6"	118–155
5'7"	121–160
5'8"	125–164
5'9"	129–169
5'10"	132–174
5'11"	136–179
6'0"	140–184
6'1"	144–189
6'2"	148–195
6'3"	152–200
6'4"	156–205
6'5"	160–211
6'6"	164–216

*Each data entry applies to both men and women.

†In pounds

Source: Center for Nutrition Policy and Promotion, "Dietary Guidelines for Americans, 2005," www.cnpp.usda.gov/DietaryGuidelines.htm.

people have reached the moderate and severe levels of obesity, meaning increased risks at all ages and stages of their lives.[11]

The difficulty with defining obesity lies in determining what is normal. To date, there are no universally accepted standards for the most "desirable" or "ideal" body weight or *body composition* (the ratio of lean body mass to fat body mass). Although sources vary slightly, most agree that men's bodies should contain between 11 and 15 percent total body fat and that women should be within the range of 18 to 22 percent body fat. At various ages and stages of life, these ranges also vary, but generally, men who exceed 20 percent body fat and women who exceed 30 percent body fat have slipped into obesity.

Lean body mass consists of the structural and functional elements in cells, body water, muscle, bones, and other body organs such as the heart, liver, and kidneys. Body fat is composed of two types: essential and storage fat. Essential fat is necessary for normal physiological functioning, such as nerve conduction. Essential fat makes up approximately 3 to 7 percent of total body weight in men and approximately 15 percent of total body weight in women. Storage fat, the part that many of us try to shed, makes up the remainder of our fat reserves. It accounts for only a small percentage of total body weight for very lean people, and 5 to 25 percent of body weight of most American adults. Female bodybuilders, who are among the leanest of female athletes, may have body fat percentages of 8 to 13 percent, nearly all of which is essential fat.

Too Little Fat?

A certain amount of body fat is necessary for insulating the body, cushioning parts of the body and vital organs, and maintaining body functions. In men, this lower limit is approximately 3 to 4 percent. Women generally should not go below 8 percent. Excessively low body fat in females may lead to amenorrhea, a disruption of the normal menstrual cycle. The critical level of body fat necessary to maintain normal menstrual flow is believed to be 8 to 13 percent, but many additional factors can affect the menstrual cycle. Under extreme circumstances, such as starvation diets and certain diseases, the body uses all available fat reserves and begins to break down muscle tissue as a last-ditch effort to obtain nourishment.

The fact is that too much fat and too little fat are both potentially harmful. The key is to find a healthy level at which you are comfortable with your appearance and your ability to be as active as possible. Many options are available for determining your body fat and weight.

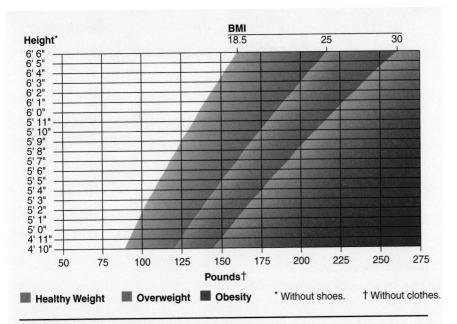

Height*

| | | BMI |
| 6' 6" | | 18.5 ... 25 ... 30 |

Pounds†

50 75 100 125 150 175 200 225 250 275

■ **Healthy Weight**   ■ **Overweight**   ■ **Obesity**   * Without shoes.   † Without clothes.

FIGURE 10.2 **Body Mass Index: Are You at a Healthy Weight?**

Source: National Heart, Lung, and Blood Institute, 2007.

Directions: Find your weight on the bottom of the graph. Go straight up from that point until you come to the line that matches your height. Then look to find your weight group.

➢ BMI of 25 defines the upper boundary of healthy weight
➢ BMI of higher than 25 to 30 defines overweight
➢ BMI of higher than 30 defines obesity

Assessing Fat Levels

Today, most weight-control authorities believe that looking at where you fall on some arbitrary chart may not be helpful.

> **How can I tell if I have too much body fat?**

Height–weight charts may lead some people to think they are overweight when they are not and others to think that they are okay when, in fact, they may be at risk. Other measures exist for calculating body content, and some provide a very precise calculation of body fat. They include body mass index, waist circumference, waist-to-hip ratio, and various measures of body fat.

Body Mass Index

A useful index of the relationship of height and weight, BMI is a standard measurement used by obesity researchers and health professionals. It is not gender specific. Although it does not directly measure percentage of body fat, it does provide a more accurate measure of overweight and obesity than weight alone.[12]

We find BMI by dividing a person's weight in kilograms by height in meters squared. The mathematical formula is

$$\text{BMI} = \text{weight (kg)} \div \text{height squared (m}^2)$$

To determine BMI using pounds and inches, see **(Figure 10.2).** The BMI calculator also is available at the National Heart, Lung,

and Blood Institute (NHLBI) website at www.nhlbisupport.com/bmi.

Healthy weights are defined as those associated with BMIs of 18.5 to 25, the range of lowest statistical health risk.[13] The desirable range for women falls between 21 and 23; for men, between 22 and 24.[14] A BMI greater than 25 indicates overweight and potentially significant health risks. A body mass index of 30 or more is considered obese.[15] **Table 10.3** summarizes the various weight classifications, their health risks, and the BMI and waist measurements associated with them.

Calculating BMI is simple, quick, and inexpensive—but it does have limitations. One problem is that very muscular people may fall into the overweight category when they are actually healthy and fit. In addition, certain population groups, such as Asians, tend to have higher-than-healthy body fat at normal BMI levels, whereas other groups, such as Polynesians, have somewhat lower body fat than other populations at the same BMI.[16]

These standards may seem almost impossible for people who consistently exceed the target weights and who have difficulty keeping off any lost weight. Constant failure may lead them to stop trying. The secret lies in establishing a healthful weight at a young age and maintaining it—a task easier said than done. The *U.S. Dietary Guidelines for Americans* encourage a weight gain of no more than ten pounds after reaching adult height and endorse small weight losses of one-half to one pound per week, if needed,

TABLE 10.3 Classification of Overweight and Obesity by BMI and Waist Circumference, and Associated Disease Risks

	BMI (kg/m^2)	Obesity Class	Disease Risk* Relative to Normal Weight and Waist Circumference	
			Men: 102 cm (40 in.) or less Women: 88 cm (35 in.) or less	Men: > 102 cm (40 in.) Women: > 88 cm (35 in.)
Underweight	< 18.5		-	-
Normal	18.5–24.9		-	-
Overweight	25.0–29.9		Increased	High
Obesity	30.0–34.9	I	High	Very high
	35.0–39.9	II	Very high	Very high
Extreme Obesity	40.0†	III	Extremely high	Extremely high

*Disease risk for type 2 diabetes, hypertension, and cardiovascular disease (CVD).

†Increased waist circumference can also be a marker for increased risk even in persons of normal weight.

Source: National Heart, Lung, and Blood Institute, 2007.

as well as smaller weight losses of 5 to 10 percent to make a difference toward health.[17]

Waist Circumference and Ratio Measurements

Waist circumference measurement is a useful tool for assessing abdominal fat. Research indicates that a waistline greater than 40 inches (102 cm) in men and 35 inches (88 cm) in women may indicate greater health risk. If a person is under 5 feet tall or has a BMI of 35 or above, waist circumference standards used for the general population might not apply.[18] Measure waist circumference by wrapping a tape measure comfortably around the smallest area below the rib cage and above the belly button.

waist circumference measurement Assessment of healthy body fat by measurement of the circumference of the waist.

waist-to-hip ratio Ratio that indicates increased risks due to unhealthy fat distribution.

hydrostatic weighing techniques Method of determining body fat by measuring the amount of water displaced when a person is completely submerged.

skinfold caliper technique A method of determining body fat whereby folds of skin and fat at various points on the body are grasped between thumb and forefinger and measured with calipers.

dual energy X-ray absorptiometry (DEXA) Technique using low-dose X rays that read bone and soft tissue mass at the same time.

The **waist-to-hip ratio** measures regional fat distribution. A waist-to-hip ratio greater than 1.0 in men and 0.8 in women indicates increased health risks.[19] Therefore, knowing where your fat is carried may be more important than knowing your total fat content. Men and postmenopausal women tend to store fat in the upper regions of their body, particularly in the abdominal area. Premenopausal women usually store their fat in lower regions of their bodies, particularly the hips, buttocks, and thighs.

Measures of Body Fat

Hydrostatic Weighing Techniques From a clinical perspective, **hydrostatic weighing techniques** offer the most accurate method of measuring body fat. This method measures the amount of water a person displaces when completely submerged. Because fat tissue is less dense than muscle or bone tissue, a relatively accurate indication of actual body fat can be computed by comparing underwater and out-of-water weights.

Pinch and Skinfold Measures The most accurate method of measuring body fat using the skinfold measurement technique is the **skinfold caliper technique.** A specially calibrated instrument called a *skinfold caliper* is used to measure the fat layer. In making this assessment, a technician pinches a fold of skin on a predetermined body location, such as the triceps area or waist, with the calipers. Special formulas are employed to arrive at a combined prediction of total body fat.

Dual Energy X-Ray Absorptiometry One of the newer technologies available for assessing body fat, **dual energy X-ray absorptiometry (DEXA)** is also among the most accurate and precise. Essentially, DEXA is a whole-body scanning technique involving two low-dose

X rays that read bone and soft tissue mass at the same time. DEXA is more precise than other methods and is relatively easy for anyone to have done. The downside is that it isn't as accurate for extremely obese individuals, and it is expensive because of the high cost of the machines. Many universities have DEXA machines in their exercise physiology or biomechanics labs.

Near-Infrared Interactance

Another newer technique is **near-infrared interactance (NIR),** in which a fiberoptic probe is connected to a digital analyzer that indirectly measures tissue composition (both fat and water). Usually, the biceps are used to assess fatness; once measures are taken, an equation that includes your height, weight, frame size, and level of activity is used to calculate body fat. It is relatively inexpensive and fast, but it is not nearly as accurate as the other methods described above. Very fat and very lean, muscular people are likely to have inaccurate measures.

Magnetic Resonance Imaging

Magnetic resonance imaging (MRI) uses magnetic fields to assess how much fat a person has and where it is deposited. Generally MRIs are not performed solely for the purpose of measuring body fat; however, if you were having a full body MRI for diagnosis of other illnesses, it is possible that you could ask the technician to determine your body fat.

The Bod Pod and Pea Pod

The **Bod Pod** (for adults) and **Pea Pod** (for children) are relative newcomers on the body fat assessment scene. Both are egg-shaped chambers. The person sits inside, and then the pod is closed with a tight seal, so that the machine can measure the amount of air the body displaces. Bod Pods use this air displacement measure, along with body weight, to assess overall body fat.

Bioelectrical Impedance Analysis

Essentially, **bioelectrical impedance analysis (BIA)** measures how lean you are, rather than how fat you are, yet the net results are just as informative. This is the only method based on measuring electrical signals as they pass through fat, lean mass, and water in the body, rather than estimating fat from other measures. BIA reliability is related to the sophistication of the machine doing the testing and the knowledge of the technician.

Total Body Electrical Conductivity

Much like an MRI, **total body electrical conductivity (TOBEC)** uses an electromagnetic force field to assess relative body fat. Also like MRI, it requires elaborate, expensive equipment and therefore is not practical for most people.

Although all of these methods can be useful, they also can be inaccurate and even harmful unless the testers are skillful and well trained. Before undergoing any procedure, make sure you understand the expense, potential for accuracy, risks, and training of the tester.

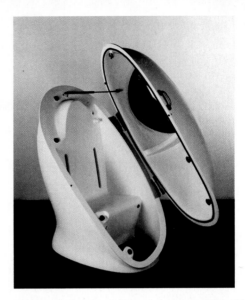

The Bod Pod is a new fat assessment machine with a chamber in which a person sits, and the air displaced by the body is measured to determine body fat.

Risk Factors for Obesity

In spite of efforts to keep Americans fit and in good health, obesity is the most common nutritional disorder in the United States, with rates that have increased dramatically among children and adults in recent decades.[20] The prevalence of obesity and overweight is generally higher among minorities, especially minority women.[21]

In a major report, the U.S. Surgeon General stated it quite plainly: overweight and obesity result from an energy imbalance. This means eating too many calories and not getting enough exercise.[22] However, many have criticized such a simplistic view. If it were that simple, Americans would merely reevaluate their diets, reduce the amount they eat, and exercise more.

What are some of these factors that influence our collective trend toward overweight and obesity? We know that body

(Text continues on page 298.)

near-infrared interactance (NIR) Fiberoptic measurement of tissue composition.

magnetic resonance imaging (MRI) Diagnostic technique using magnetic fields, which can be used to measure body fat.

Bod Pod/Pea Pod A body fat assessment tool that measures the air your body displaces in a sealed chamber.

bioelectrical impedance analysis (BIA) A technique of body fat assessment in which electrical currents are passed through fat and lean tissue.

total body electrical conductivity (TOBEC) Technique using an electromagnetic force field to assess relative body fat.

ASSESS yourself

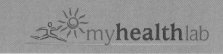

READINESS FOR WEIGHT LOSS

Fill out this assessment online at
www.aw-bc.com/myhealthlab
or www.aw-bc.com/donatelle.

How well do your attitudes equip you for a weight-loss program? For each question, circle the answer that best describes your attitude. As you complete each section, tally your score, and analyze it according to the scoring guide.

I. GOALS, ATTITUDES, AND READINESS

1. Compared to previous attempts, how motivated are you to lose weight this time?

1	2	3	4	5
Not at all motivated	Slightly motivated	Somewhat motivated	Quite motivated	Extremely motivated

2. How certain are you that you will stay committed to a weight-loss program for the time it will take to reach your goal?

1	2	3	4	5
Not at all certain	Slightly certain	Somewhat certain	Quite certain	Extremely certain

3. Considering all outside factors at this time in your life—stress at work, family obligations, and so on—to what extent can you tolerate the effort required to stick to a diet?

1	2	3	4	5
Cannot tolerate	Can tolerate somewhat	Uncertain	Can tolerate well	Can tolerate easily

4. Think honestly about how much weight you hope to lose and how quickly you hope to lose it. Figuring a weight loss of 1 to 2 pounds per week, how realistic is your expectation?

1	2	3	4	5
Very unrealistic	Somewhat unrealistic	Moderately unrealistic	Somewhat realistic	Very realistic

5. While dieting, do you fantasize about eating a lot of your favorite foods?

1	2	3	4	5
Always	Frequently	Occasionally	Rarely	Never

6. While dieting, do you feel deprived, angry, and/or upset?

1	2	3	4	5
Always	Frequently	Occasionally	Rarely	Never

Analyzing This Section

6 to 16: This may not be a good time for you to start a diet. Inadequate motivation and commitment and unrealistic goals could block your progress. Think about what contributes to your unreadiness, and consider changing these factors before undertaking a diet.

17 to 23: You may be close to being ready to begin a program but should think about ways to boost your readiness.

24 to 30: The path is clear: you can decide how to lose weight in a safe, effective way.

II. HUNGER AND EATING CUES

7. When food comes up in conversation or in something you read, do you want to eat, even if you are not hungry?

1	2	3	4	5
Never	Rarely	Occasionally	Frequently	Always

8. How often do you eat for a reason other than physical hunger?

1	2	3	4	5
Never	Rarely	Occasionally	Frequently	Always

9. Do you have trouble controlling your eating when your favorite foods are around the house?

1	2	3	4	5
Never	Rarely	Occasionally	Frequently	Always

Analyzing This Section

3 to 6: You might occasionally eat more than you should, but apparently not because you are highly responsive to environmental cues. Controlling the attitudes that make you eat may be especially helpful.

7 to 9: You may have a moderate tendency to eat just because food is available. Losing weight may be easier for you if you try to resist external cues and eat only when you are physically hungry.

10 to 15: Some or much of your eating may be in response to thinking about food or exposing yourself to temptations to eat. Think of ways to minimize your exposure to temptations so you eat only in response to physical hunger.

III. CONTROLLING OVEREATING

If the following situations occurred while you were on a diet, would you be likely to eat more or less immediately afterward and for the rest of the day?

10. Although you planned to skip lunch, a friend talks you into going out for a midday meal.

1	2	3	4	5
Would eat much less	Would eat somewhat less	Would make no difference	Would eat somewhat more	Would eat much more

11. You "break" your plan by eating a fattening, "forbidden" food.

1	2	3	4	5
Would eat much less	Would eat somewhat less	Would make no difference	Would eat somewhat more	Would eat much more

12. You have been following your diet faithfully and decide to test yourself by eating something you consider a treat.

1	2	3	4	5
Would eat much less	Would eat somewhat less	Would make no difference	Would eat somewhat more	Would eat much more

Analyzing This Section

3 to 7: You recover rapidly from mistakes. However, if you frequently alternate between eating that is out of control and dieting very strictly, you may have a serious eating problem and should get professional help.

8 to 11: You do not seem to let unplanned eating disrupt your program. This is a flexible, balanced approach.

12 to 15: You may be prone to overeat after an event breaks your control or throws you off the track. Your reaction to these problem-causing events can be improved.

IV. BINGE EATING AND PURGING

13. Aside from holiday feasts, have you ever eaten a large amount of food rapidly and felt afterward that this eating incident was excessive and out of control?

2	0
Yes	No

14. If you answered yes to question 13, how often have you engaged in this behavior during the past year?

1	2	3	4	5	6
Less than once a month	About once a month	A few times a month	About once a week	About 3 times a week	Daily

15. Have you purged (used laxatives or diuretics, or induced vomiting) to control your weight?

5	0
Yes	No

16. If you answered yes to question 15, how often have you engaged in this behavior during the past year?

1	2	3	4	5	6
Less than once a month	About once a month	A few times a month	About once a week	About 3 times a week	Daily

(continued)

Analyzing This Section

0: It appears that binge eating and purging are not problems for you.

2 to 11: Pay attention to these eating patterns. Should they arise more frequently, get professional help.

12 to 19: You show signs of having a potentially serious eating problem. See a counselor experienced in evaluating eating disorders right away.

V. EMOTIONAL EATING

17. Do you eat more than you would like to when you have negative feelings such as anxiety, depression, anger, or loneliness?

1	2	3	4	5
Never	Rarely	Occasionally	Frequently	Always

18. Do you have trouble controlling your eating when you have positive feelings—do you celebrate feeling good by eating?

1	2	3	4	5
Never	Rarely	Occasionally	Frequently	Always

19. When you have unpleasant interactions with others in your life or after a difficult day at work, do you eat more than you'd like?

1	2	3	4	5
Never	Rarely	Occasionally	Frequently	Always

Analyzing This Section

3 to 8: You do not appear to let your emotions affect your eating.

9 to 11: You sometimes eat in response to emotional highs and lows. Monitor this behavior to learn when and why it occurs, and be prepared to find alternate activities.

12 to 15: Emotional ups and downs can stimulate your eating. Try to deal with the feelings that trigger the eating and find other ways to express them.

VI. EXERCISE PATTERNS AND ATTITUDES

20. How often do you exercise?

1	2	3	4	5
Never	Rarely	Occasionally	Somewhat frequently	Frequently

21. How confident are you that you can exercise regularly?

1	2	3	4	5
Not at all confident	Slightly confident	Somewhat confident	Highly confident	Completely confident

22. When you think about exercise, do you develop a positive or negative picture in your mind?

1	2	3	4	5
Completely negative	Somewhat negative	Neutral	Somewhat positive	Completely positive

23. How certain are you that you can work regular exercise into your daily schedule?

1	2	3	4	5
Not at all certain	Slightly certain	Somewhat certain	Quite certain	Extremely certain

Analyzing This Section

4 to 10: You're probably not exercising as regularly as you should. Determine whether attitude about exercise or your lifestyle is blocking your way, then change what you must and put on those walking shoes!

11 to 16: You need to feel more positive about exercise so you can do it more often. Think of ways to be more active that are fun and fit your lifestyle.

17 to 20: It looks as if the path is clear for you to be active. Now think of ways to get motivated.

After scoring yourself in each section of this questionnaire, you should be able to better judge your dieting strengths and weaknesses. Remember that the first step in changing eating behavior is to understand the conditions that influence your eating habits.

Source: From "The Diet Readiness Test," in Kelly D. Brownell, "When and How to Diet," *Psychology Today,* June 1989, 41–46. Copyright © 1989 Sussex Publishers, Inc. Reprinted with permission from *Psychology Today* Magazine.

MAKE it happen!

ASSESSMENT: The Assess Yourself activity identified six areas of importance in determining your readiness for weight loss. If you want to lose weight to improve your health, understanding your attitudes about food and exercise will help you succeed in your plan.

MAKING A CHANGE: To change your behavior, you need to develop a plan. Follow these steps below and complete your Behavior Change Contract to take action.

1. Evaluate your behavior, and identify patterns and specific things you are doing. What can you change now? What can you change in the near future?

2. Select one pattern of behavior that you want to change.

3. Fill out the Behavior Change Contract found at the front of your book. It should include your long-term goals for change, your short-term goals, the rewards you'll give yourself for reaching these goals, potential obstacles along the way, and strategies for overcoming these obstacles. For each goal, list the small steps and specific actions that you will take.

4. Chart your progress in a journal. At the end of a week, consider how successful you were in following your plan. What helped you be successful? What made change more difficult? What will you do differently next week?

5. Revise your plan as needed. Are the short-term goals attainable? Are the rewards satisfying?

EXAMPLE: Shannon had gained the "freshman 15" and wanted to put together a weight-management plan. She assessed her readiness for weight loss and saw that her scores highlighted areas that she needed to improve. Shannon saw that she was not always aware of the eating cues and emotions that caused her to overeat (sections II, III, and V). Although she hadn't realized it, she tended to do most of her snacking while she was studying at night. No matter what else she had eaten during the day, she would end up eating candy and chips from the vending machines. When she was anxious about an upcoming test or bored by her reading, she would eat even though she was already full. Shannon also noted her strengths: she had never binged and purged (section IV), she had strong motivation (section I), and she already had an enjoyable, regular exercise program (section VI).

Shannon made a plan that would help her manage her weight by controlling snacking. She set up a series of small steps to help her become aware of what she was eating and how it was contributing to her weight gain. First, she went through her cupboards and got rid of any unhealthy snacks. The she bought some study snacks that were healthier choices than chips and candy, such as grapes and low-fat granola. She then created a schedule that included meal times and snack times. Shannon planned to note whether she was eating out of hunger or mindlessly on this schedule. If she was snacking because she was bored or anxious, she would try to restrict her snack to a predetermined amount or to wait until she really was hungry.

Shannon tried this plan for 2 weeks. At the end of 2 weeks, she saw that she had lost 3 pounds. She decided she wanted to address another of her eating habits, which was ordering pizza with her roommates when they watched their favorite TV shows during the week. Even after she had eaten a full dinner, Shannon found herself eating two or three slices of pizza in front of the TV. Shannon suggested to her roommates that if they already had eaten dinner, they pop some popcorn to eat instead of the pizza. This not only was healthier, but also cost less than having a pizza delivered.

weight is a result of genes, metabolism, behavior, environment, culture, and socioeconomic status. Of these, behavior and environment are the easiest to change.

Heredity and Genetic Factors

Are some people born to be fat? Several factors appear to influence why one person becomes obese and another remains thin; genes seem to interact with many of these factors. Over 250 gene markers have shown positive association to obesity in over 400 separate studies.[23]

Body Type and Genes In some animal species, the shape and size of the individual's body are determined largely by its parents' shape and size. Many scientists have explored the role of heredity in determining human body shape. Children whose parents are obese also tend to be overweight. In fact, a family history of obesity has long been thought to increase one's chances of becoming obese. Researchers have found that adopted individuals tend to be similar in weight to their biological parents and that identical twins are twice as likely to weigh the same as are fraternal twins, even if they are raised separately.[24]

Genes play a significant role in how the body balances calories and energy. Although the exact mechanism remains unknown, it is believed that genes set metabolic rates, influencing how the body handles calories. Some genes, such as the CD36 gene, may influence our cravings for fatty foods.[25] Also, by influencing the amount of body fat and fat distribution, genes can make a person more susceptible to gaining weight.[26]

Specific Obesity Genes? In the past decade, more and more research has pointed to the existence of a "fat gene." Rather than inheriting a particular body type that predisposes us to overweight, it may be that our genes predispose us toward certain satiety and feeding behaviors. This "I need to eat" gene may account for up to one-third of our risk for obesity.[27] The most promising candidate is the GAD2 gene. For some individuals, a variation in this gene increases the production of a chemical that boosts appetite and signals a person to eat.[28]

Another gene getting a lot of attention is an Ob gene (for obesity), which is believed to disrupt the body's "I've had enough to eat" signaling system and may prompt individuals to keep eating past the point of being comfortably full. Research on Pima Indians, who have an estimated 75 percent obesity rate (nine out of ten are overweight),

points to an Ob gene that is a "thrifty gene." It is theorized that because their ancestors struggled through centuries of famine, during which the Ob gene prompted them to eat as much as possible whenever food was available, their basal metabolic rates slowed, allowing them to store precious fat for survival. Survivors may have passed these genes on to their children, which would explain the lower metabolic rates found in Pimas today and their tendency toward obesity.[29]

Endocrine Influence: The Hungry Hormones

Over the years, many people have attributed obesity to problems with their thyroid gland and resultant hormone imbalances. They believed that an underactive thyroid impeded their ability to burn calories. Today most authorities agree that less than 2 percent of the obese population have a thyroid problem and can trace their weight problems to a metabolic or hormone imbalance.[30] However, researchers are investigating the impact various hormones have on a person's ability to lose weight, control appetite, and sense fullness.

One such hormone researchers suspect may play a role in our ability to keep weight off is *ghrelin,* which is produced in the stomach. Researchers at the University of Washington studied a small group of obese people who had lost weight over a 6-month period.[31] They noted that ghrelin levels rose before every meal and fell drastically shortly afterward, suggesting that the hormone plays a role in appetite stimulation. Subsequent studies will test the impact of ghrelin-blocking drugs in controlling appetite as a form of intervention.

Another hormone that has been the focus of some study is *leptin,* which scientists believe serves as a form of satiety signal, telling the brain when you are full and need to stop eating.[32] Other scientists have isolated a hormone called *GLP-1,* which is known to slow down the passage of food through the intestines to allow the absorption of nutrients. Research suggests that the GLP-1 hormone may stimulate insulin production and may eventually be a key factor in preventing and controlling diabetes and obesity.[33] It is speculated that leptin and GLP-1 might play complementary roles in weight control. Leptin and its receptors may regulate body weight over the long term, calling on fast-acting appetite suppressants such as GLP-1 when necessary.

Hunger, Appetite, and Satiety

Scientists distinguish **hunger,** an inborn physiological response to nutritional needs, from **appetite,** a learned response to food that is tied to an emotional or psychological craving and is often unrelated to nutritional needs. Obese people may be more likely than are thin people to satisfy their appetite and eat for reasons other than nutrition.

In some instances, the problem with overconsumption may be more related to **satiety** than to appetite or hunger. People generally feel satiated, or full, when they have satisfied their nutritional needs and their stomach signals "no more." For

hunger An inborn physiological response to nutritional needs.

appetite A learned response that is tied to an emotional or psychological craving for food; often unrelated to nutritional needs.

satiety The feeling of fullness or satisfaction at the end of a meal.

undetermined reasons, obese people may not feel full until much later than thin people do. The leptin and GLP-1 studies seem to support this theory.

Theories abound concerning the mechanisms that regulate food intake. Some sources indicate that the hypothalamus (the part of the brain that regulates appetite) closely monitors levels of certain nutrients in the blood. When these levels fall, the brain signals us to eat. According to one theory, in the obese person this monitoring system does not work properly, and the cues to eat are more frequent and intense than they are in people of normal weight.

Metabolic Rates and Weight

Even at rest, the body consumes a certain amount of energy. The amount of energy your body uses at complete rest is your **basal metabolic rate (BMR).** About 60 to 70 percent of all the calories you consume on a given day go to support your basal metabolism: heartbeat, breathing, maintaining body temperature, and so on. So if you consume 2,000 calories per day, between 1,200 and 1,400 of those calories are burned without your doing any significant physical activity. But unless you exert yourself enough to burn the remaining 600 to 800 calories, you will gain weight.

Your BMR can fluctuate considerably, with several factors influencing whether it slows down or speeds up. In general, the younger you are, the higher your BMR, partly because in young people cells undergo rapid subdivision, which consumes a good deal of energy. BMR is highest during infancy, puberty, and pregnancy, when bodily changes are most rapid.

Body composition also influences BMR. Muscle tissue is highly active—even at rest—compared to fat tissue. In essence, the more lean tissue you have, the greater your BMR; and the more fat tissue you have, the lower your BMR. Men have a higher BMR than women do, at least partly because of their greater proportion of lean tissue. (This is another reason why developing muscular strength and endurance is so important to weight loss and obesity reduction plans.[34])

Age is another factor. After age 30, BMR slows down by about 1 to 2 percent a year. Therefore, people over 30 commonly find that they must work harder to burn off an extra helping of ice cream than they did when in their teens. "Middle-aged spread," a reference to the tendency to put on weight later in life, is partly related to this change. A slower BMR, coupled with less activity, shifting priorities (family and career become more important than fitness), and loss in muscle mass, puts the weight of many middle-aged people in jeopardy.

In addition, the body has self-protective mechanisms that signal BMR to speed up or slow down. For example, when you have a fever, the energy needs of your cells increase, which generates heat and speeds up your BMR. In starvation situations, the body protects itself by slowing down BMR to conserve precious energy. Thus, when people repeatedly resort to extreme diets, it is believed that their bodies "reset" their BMRs at lower rates. **Yo-yo diets,** in which people repeatedly gain weight and then starve themselves to lose it, are doomed to fail. When dieters resume eating after their

weight loss, their BMR is set lower, making it almost certain that they will regain the pounds they just lost. After repeated cycles of dieting and regaining weight, these people find it increasingly hard to lose weight and increasingly easy to regain it, so they become heavier and heavier.

Environmental Factors

With all our twenty-first-century conveniences, environmental factors have come to play a large role in weight maintenance. Automobiles, remote controls, office jobs where we sit all day, and spending time on the Internet all impact how much we move, and this lack of physical activity causes a decrease in energy expenditure.[35] Time our grandparents spent going for a walk after dinner we now spend watching our favorite television shows. Our culture has urged us not only to move less, but also to eat more. There is a long list of environmental factors that encourage us to increase our consumption:

- Bombardment with advertising designed to increase energy intake—ads for high-calorie foods at a low price, marketing super-sized portions (see the **Spotlight on Your Health** box on page 300). They hit us at an early age and market to our vulnerabilities when it comes to foods we love. Prepackaged meals, fast food, and soft drinks are all increasingly widespread. High-calorie drinks such as coffee lattes and energy drinks add to daily caloric intake.[36]
- Changes in the number of working women, leading to greater consumption of restaurant meals, fast foods, and convenience foods. As society eats out more, higher-calorie, high-fat foods become the norm, and increased weight is the result.
- Bottle-feeding of infants, which may increase energy intake relative to breast-feeding.[37]
- Misleading food labels that confuse consumers about portion and serving sizes.
- Increased opportunities for eating. Fast-food restaurants, cafes, vending machines, and food stores are everywhere, offering easy access to high-calorie foods and beverages. Meals, mini-meals, and snacks have become common diversions for many of us.

 what do you THINK?

In addition to those listed, can you think of other environmental factors that contribute to obesity?
- What actions could you take to reduce your risk for each of these factors?

basal metabolic rate (BMR) The energy expenditure of the body under resting conditions at normal room temperature.

yo-yo diets Cycles in which people repeatedly gain weight and then starve themselves to lose weight. This lowers their BMR, which makes regaining weight even more likely.

ARE SUPER-SIZED MEALS SUPER-SIZING AMERICANS?

Today, super-sized meals are the norm at many restaurants. Consider the 25-ounce prime rib dinner served at a local steak chain. At nearly 3,000 calories and 150 grams of fat for the meat alone, this meal both slams shut arteries and adds on pounds. Add a baked potato with sour cream and/or butter, a salad loaded with creamy salad dressing, and fresh bread with real butter, and the meal may surpass the 5,000-calorie mark and ring in at close to 300 grams of fat. In other words, it exceeds what most adults should eat in 2 days!

And this is just the beginning. Soft drinks, once commonly served in 12-ounce sizes, now come in 1-liter bottles. Cinnamon buns now come in giant 700-calorie portions. What is the result? Super-sized portions consumed by super-sized Americans. "People are eating a ton of extra calories," says Donna Skoda, a dietitian and chair of the Ohio State University Extension Service. "Ironically, although the U.S. fat intake has dropped in the past 20 years from an average of 40 to 33 percent of calories, the daily calorie intake has risen from 1,852 calories per day to over 2,000 per day. In theory, this translates into a weight gain of 15 pounds a year."

Skoda and others say that the main reason that Americans are gaining weight is that people no longer know what a normal serving size is. The National Heart, Lung, and Blood Institute has developed a pair of "Portion Distortion" quizzes that show how today's portions compare to those of 20 years ago. Test yourself online at

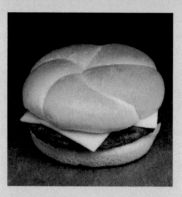

20 years ago

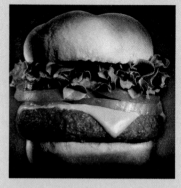

Today

http://hp2010.nhlbihin.net/portion/ to see whether you can guess the differences between today's supersized meals and those once considered normal. Just one example is the difference between an average cheeseburger 20 years ago (left photo) and the typical cheeseburger of today (right). According to the "Portion Distortion" quiz, today's cheeseburger has 590 calories—257 more calories than the cheeseburger of 20 years ago!

Carrie Wiatt, a Los Angeles dietitian and author of *Portion Savvy,* explains that a telling marker of the big-food trend is that restaurant plates have grown from an average of 9 to 13 inches in the past decade. Studies show that people eat 40 to 50 percent more than they normally would now that large portions are available.

How can you reduce your own risk of super-sizing? Follow these strategies:

- Avoid super-sizing anything. Order the smallest size available when dining out.
- Chew your food, and avoid the urge to wash it down with high-calorie drinks.
- Serve food on a small or medium plate.

- Always order dressings, gravies, and sauces on the side. Sprinkle these added calories on carefully. Remember that a tablespoon of gravy could mean an hour on the treadmill to burn off its 200+ calories!
- Avoid appetizers in restaurants. They are expensive, not only in terms of money, but also in calories and fat content.
- Share your dinner with a friend, and order a side salad for each of you. Alternatively, eat only half of your dinner and save the rest to take home and eat another day.
- Avoid buffets and all-you-can-eat establishments. Most of us can eat two to three times what we need—or more.

Source: E. J. Fried, "The Potential for Policy Initiatives to Address the Obesity Epidemic in the United States," in *Obesity Prevention and Public Health,* ed. D. Crawford and R. W. Jeffrey (New York: Oxford University Press, 2005); K. D. Brownell et al., "Does a Toxic Environment Make Obesity Inevitable?" *Obesity Management* 1(2005): 52–55; National Heart, Lung, and Blood Institute, "Portion Distortion," 2007, http://hp2010.nhlbihin.net/portion/.

Psychological Factors

The relationship of weight problems to deeply rooted emotional insecurities, needs, and wants remains uncertain. Food often is used as a reward for good behavior in childhood. As adults face unemployment, broken relationships, financial uncertainty, fears about health, and other problems, the bright spot in the day is often "what's on the table for dinner" or "we're going to that restaurant tonight." Again, the research underlying this theory is controversial. What is certain is that eating tends to be a focal point of people's lives; eating is essentially a social ritual associated with companionship, celebration, and enjoyment. For many people, the psycho-social aspect of the eating experience is a major obstacle to successful weight control.

Early Sabotage: Obesity in Youth

Another major factor is the pressure placed on us by the food industry's sophisticated marketing campaigns. There may be salad bars at the local fast-food joints, but customers have to run the gauntlet of starchy, beefy delights and high-fat fries to find them. The food and restaurant industries spend billions each year on ads to entice hungry people to forgo fresh fruit and sliced vegetables for Ring Dings and Happy Meals. Children are among the most vulnerable to these ads.

Children's impulses to eat junk food haven't changed much in recent decades. However, as noted earlier, they are eating larger portions. Social forces—the decline of home cooking, increased production of calorie- and fat-laden fast foods, and video technology that encourages kids to surf the Internet rather than ride their bicycles—have converged to increase the number of overweight young Americans. As a direct consequence, over 17 percent of U.S. children and adolescents are now overweight or obese enough to endanger their health. Millions of others are on the threshold, and the problem is growing more extreme daily. Obese children suffer both physically and emotionally throughout childhood, and those who stay heavy in adolescence tend to stay fat as adults.[38]

Lifestyle

Of all the factors affecting obesity, perhaps the most critical is the relationship between activity levels and calorie intake. Obesity rates are rising. But how can this be happening? Aren't more people exercising than ever before?

Though the many advertisements for sports equipment and the popularity of athletes may give the impression that Americans love a good workout, the facts are not so positive. Data from the National Health Interview Survey show that four in ten adults in the United States *never* engage in any exercise, sports, or physically active hobbies in their leisure time.[39] Women (43.2 percent) were somewhat more likely than men (36.5 percent) to be sedentary, a finding that was consistent across all age groups. Among both men and women, black and Hispanic adults were more sedentary than white adults.[40] Leisure-time physical activity was also strongly associated with level of education. About 72 percent of adults who never attended high school were sedentary, declining steadily to 45 percent among high school graduates and about 24 percent among adults with graduate-level college degrees.[41]

Do you know people who seemingly can eat whatever they want without gaining weight? With few exceptions, if you were to follow them around for a typical day and monitor the level and intensity of their activity, you would discover the reason. Even if their schedule does not include jogging or

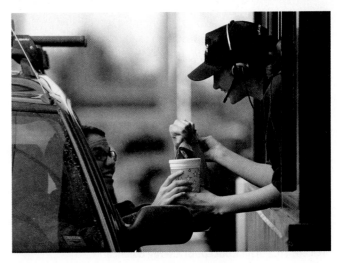

Modern conveniences support a sedentary lifestyle and unhealthy eating choices. Small changes to your daily habits can help to increase your activity level, improve your diet, and impact your health positively.

intense exercise, it probably includes a high level of activity. Walking up a flight of stairs rather than taking the elevator, speeding up the pace while mowing the lawn, getting up to change the TV channel rather than using the remote, and doing housework all burn extra calories.

Actually, it may even go beyond that. In studies of calorie burning by individuals placed in a controlled respiratory chamber environment where calories consumed, motion, and overall activity were measured, it was found that some people are better fat burners than others. It is possible that low fat burners may not produce as many of the enzymes needed to convert fat to energy. They may not have as many blood vessels supplying fatty tissue, making it tougher for them to deliver fat-burning oxygen; or, perhaps in subtle ways, these people burn more calories through extra motions. Clearly, any form of activity that burns additional calories helps maintain weight.

Smoking Women who smoke tend to weigh 6 to 10 pounds less than nonsmokers do. After they quit, their weight generally increases to the level found among nonsmokers. Weight gain after smoking cessation may be partly due to nicotine's ability to raise a body's metabolic rate. When smokers stop, they burn fewer calories. Another reason former smokers often gain weight is that they generally eat more to satisfy free-floating cravings.[42]

Gender and Obesity

Throughout our lives, issues of appearance and attractiveness are constantly in the foreground. In spite of the prevalence of overweight in our society, a severe social stigma is attached to it, particularly for women. Yet, women are also disadvantaged biologically when it comes to losing weight. Compared to men, they have a lower ratio of lean body mass to fatty mass, in part because of differences in bone size and mass, muscle size, and other variables. Because men have more muscle, and

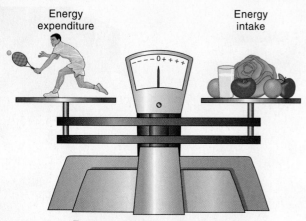

Energy expenditure = Energy intake

FIGURE 10.3 The Concept of Energy Balance
How many calories do you need each day? If you consume more calories than you burn, you will gain weight. If you burn more than you consume, you will lose weight. If both are equal, your weight will not change, according to this concept.

Source: From S. Powers and S. Dodd, *Total Fitness and Wellness,* 5th ed. Copyright © 2009 Benjamin Cummings. Reprinted by permission of Pearson Education, Inc.

muscle uses more energy than fat does, they burn 10 to 20 percent more calories than women do during rest.[43] (See Chapter 11 for an overview of the role that increased muscle mass plays on weight reduction.) After sexual maturity, men have higher metabolic rates, making it easier for them to burn off excess calories. Women also face greater potential for weight fluctuation because of hormonal changes, pregnancy, and other conditions that increase the likelihood of weight gain. Also, men are more socialized into physical activity from birth. Strenuous work and play are encouraged for men, whereas women's roles have typically been more sedentary and required a lower level of caloric expenditure.

Not only are women more vulnerable to weight gain, but also pressures to maintain and/or lose weight make them more likely to take dramatic measures to lose weight. For example, eating disorders are more prevalent among women, and more women than men take diet pills.

However, men experience these pressures, too. The male image is becoming more associated with the bodybuilder shape and size, and men are becoming more preoccupied with their own physical form. Thus eating disorders, exercise addictions, and other maladaptive responses are on the increase among men as well.

Of increasing concern is an emerging problem seen in both young men and women, known as **social physique anxiety (SPA),** in which the desire to "look good" has a destructive and sometimes disabling effect on one's ability to function effectively in relationships and interactions with others. Peo-

social physique anxiety (SPA) A desire to look good that has a destructive effect on a person's ability to function effectively in social interactions and relationships.

ple suffering from SPA may spend a disproportionate amount of time fixating on their bodies, working out, and performing tasks that are ego-centered and self-directed, rather than focusing on interpersonal relationships and general tasks.[44] Incessant worry about their bodies and their appearance permeates their lives. Overweight and obesity are clear risks for these people, and experts speculate that this anxiety may contribute to eating-disorder behaviors.

what do you THINK?

Can you think of other reasons why men and women may differ in how much weight they gain and how easily they are able to lose it? ■ What historical patterns may have contributed to this trend?

Managing Your Weight

At some point in our lives, almost all of us will decide to go on a diet, and many will meet with mixed success. The problem is probably related to the fact that we think about losing weight in terms of dieting rather than in terms of adjusting lifestyle and eating behaviors. It is well documented that low-calorie diets produce only temporary losses and may actually lead to disordered binge eating or related problems. Repeated bouts of restrictive dieting may be physiologically harmful; moreover, the sense of failure that we get each time we try and don't lose the weight can also exact far-reaching psychological costs. Drugs and intensive counseling can contribute to positive weight loss, but even then, many people regain weight after treatment.

Keeping Weight Control in Perspective

Weight loss is difficult for many people and may require supportive friends, relatives, and community resources, plus extraordinary efforts to prime the body for burning extra calories. Although experts say that losing weight simply requires burning more calories than are consumed, putting this principle into practice is far from simple (**Figure 10.3**). Sure, calories in minus calories out equals weight, but people of the same age, sex, height, and weight can have differences of as much as 1,000 calories a day in resting metabolic rate—this may explain why one person's gluttony is another's starvation, even if it results in the same readout on the scale. And whereas people of normal weight average 25 to 35 billion fat cells, obese people can inherit a billowing 135 billion. Other factors such as depression, stress, culture, and available foods can also affect a person's ability to lose weight. It is important to remember that being overweight does not mean that a person is weak-willed or lazy.

To reach and maintain the weight at which you will be healthy and feel best, you need to develop a program of exercise and healthy eating behaviors that will work for you now and in the long term. See the **Skills for Behavior Change** box on page 304 for strategies to make your weight management program succeed. To become a wise food consumer, you also need to become familiar with important concepts in weight control.

Understanding Calories

A **calorie** is a unit of measure that indicates the amount of energy gained from food or expended through activity. One pound of body fat contains approximately 3,500 calories. Each time you consume 3,500 calories more than your body needs to maintain weight, you gain a pound. Conversely, each time your body expends an extra 3,500 calories, you lose a pound. So if you drink an extra can of a soft drink (140 calories) every day and make no other changes in diet or activity, you would gain a pound in 25 days (3,500 calories ÷ 140 calories/day = 25 days; see Did You Know?). Conversely, if you walk for an extra half an hour each day at a pace of 15 minutes per mile (172 calories burned), you would lose one pound in approximately 20 days (3,500 calories ÷ 172 calories/day = 20.3 days). The two ways to lose weight, then, are to lower calorie intake (through better eating habits) and to increase exercise (thereby expending more calories).

 try it NOW!

Set SMART goals for weight loss. Give your goals a reality check: are they Specific, Measurable, Achievable, Relevant, and Time specific? For example, rather than aiming to lose 15 pounds this month (which probably wouldn't be healthy or achievable), set a comfortable goal to lose 5 pounds in a month. Realistic goals will encourage weight-loss success by boosting your confidence in your ability to make life-long healthy changes.

Adding Exercise

Approximately 90 percent of the daily calorie expenditures of most people is due to the **resting metabolic rate (RMR).** Slightly higher than the BMR, the RMR includes the BMR plus any additional energy expended through daily sedentary activities such as food digestion, sitting, studying, or standing. Because lean muscle tissue appears to influence metabolic rates, increasing muscle mass may be a factor in burning calories throughout the day (see Chapter 11). The **exercise metabolic rate (EMR)** accounts for the remaining 10 percent of all daily calorie expenditures; it refers to the energy expenditure that occurs during physical exercise. For most of us, these calories come from light daily activities,

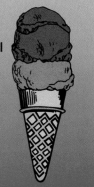

DID you KNOW?

Want to avoid the "freshman 15"? Skip dessert. There are 130 calories in a typical half-cup serving of ice cream. You could gain 14 pounds if you indulge in this treat every day for a year.

such as walking, climbing stairs, and mowing the lawn. If we increase the level of physical activity to moderate or heavy, however, our EMR may be 10 to 20 times greater and can contribute substantially to weight loss.

Increasing BMR, RMR, or EMR levels will help burn calories. Any increase in the intensity, frequency, and duration of daily exercise levels can have a significant impact on total calorie expenditure.

Physical activity makes a greater contribution to metabolic rate when large muscle groups are used. The energy spent on physical activity is the energy used to move the body's muscles—the muscles of the arms, back, abdomen, legs, and so on—and the extra energy used to speed up heartbeat and respiration rate. The number of calories spent depends on three factors:

1. The amount of muscle mass moved
2. The amount of weight moved
3. The amount of time the activity takes

An activity involving both the arms and legs burns more calories than one involving only the legs. An activity performed by a heavy person burns more calories than the same activity performed by a lighter person. And an activity performed for 40 minutes requires twice as much energy as the same activity performed for only 20 minutes. Thus, an obese person walking for 1 mile burns more calories than does a slim person walking the same distance. It also may take overweight people longer to walk the mile, which means that they are burning energy for a longer time and therefore expending more overall calories than the thin walkers.

calorie   Unit of measurement indicating the amount of energy in a particular food that can be supplied to the body.

resting metabolic rate (RMR)   The energy expenditure of the body under BMR conditions plus other daily sedentary activities.

exercise metabolic rate (EMR)   The energy expenditure that occurs during exercise.

TIPS FOR SENSIBLE AND SAFE WEIGHT MANAGEMENT

Rather than thinking about the best diet, the key to successful weight management is finding a sustainable way to control food: one that will work for you. Combine the following strategies with a Behavior Change Contract to develop a weight-management plan that is right for you. Remember, you are not going on a diet that you will quit someday. You are making lifelong changes that will result in weight loss.

BEFORE YOU BEGIN YOUR PLAN

- *Talk with your health care provider.* Tell your health care provider that you would like to lose weight. Be sure to discuss any medical condition you have or medicines you take.
- *Ask yourself some key questions.* Why do you want to make this change? Is your weight affecting your health and quality of life? What are your weight loss goals? Are you ready to change your eating habits and incorporate physical activity into your lifestyle?
- *Assess where you are.* Monitor your eating habits for 2 to 3 days, taking careful note of the good things you are doing and the things that need improvement.

MAKE A PLAN

- *Think of it as a way of life.* This is a way of improving your body and your health rather than a punishment or a diet.
- *Set realistic goals.* No matter what you do, you may not have a perfect body. Establish short-term goals on the way to the final goal. Make changes that are comfortable for you (parking farther from a destination and walking, eating

cereal and juice for breakfast, walking 3 days per week, and so on).
- *Establish a plan.* What are three dietary changes you can make today? What exercise will you do tomorrow, the next day, and sustain for 1 week? Once you do 1 week, plot a course for 2 weeks. Jot down how you feel after each week's activity.
- *Look for balance in what you do.* Remember that it's more about balance than about giving things up. If you must have that piece of chocolate cake, enjoy it, but then be responsible for doing the extra exercise it takes to burn off the calories or for limiting caloric intake the next day. Remember that it's calories taken in and burned over time that makes the difference.
- *Stay positive.* Focus on the positive steps you are taking and the healthy things you do each week rather than the less healthy things.
- *Be patient and persistent.* You didn't develop a weight problem overnight. Don't expect instant results.
- *Reward success.* Set short-term goals and reward yourself when you've reached them—new shoes, a new CD, or whatever else it takes to keep you motivated.

CHANGE YOUR DIET

- *Be adventurous.* Expand your usual meals and snacks to enjoy a wide variety of different options.
- *Do not constantly deprive yourself of favorite foods or set unrealistic guidelines.* If you slip and eat something you know you shouldn't, just be more careful the next day.
- *Eat only when you are hungry.* Do not skip meals or let yourself get too hungry.

- *Eat breakfast.* This will prevent you from being too hungry and overeating at lunch.
- *Plan ahead and be prepared for when you might get hungry.* Always have good food available when and where you get hungry.

MODIFY YOUR LEVEL OF ACTIVITY

- *Be active, and slowly increase activity.* If you stick to something, it will gradually take less and less effort to walk that mile, for example. Gradually increase your speed and/or distance (see Chapter 11). Purchasing an inexpensive pedometer and recording your daily steps is an excellent way to monitor and improve your level of activity.
- *Be creative with your physical activity.* Find activities that you really love, and stick to them. If you hate to walk in the rain but love to shop, walk in a covered mall and then shop! Try things you haven't tried before.
- *Pick an activity that is inexpensive and does not require fancy equipment.* This means you will maintain your fitness program even when you are away from home.
- *Find an exercise partner to help you stay motivated.* Don't pick your fittest friend. Choose someone who also wants to become more active and commit to helping each other.

Sources: Adapted in part from M. Manore and J. Thompson, "Table 15.3: Techniques to Help an Active Individual Identify and Maintain a Healthy Body Weight Throughout the Life Cycle" in *Sport Nutrition for Health and Performance* (Champaign, IL: Human Kinetics Publishing, 2000), 417; Weight Control Information Network, "Choosing a Safe and Successful Weight-Loss Program," NIH Publication no. 03-3700, February 2006.

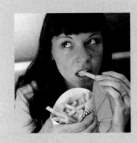

What triggers your "Eat" response?

• Nervousness/
  anxiety/stress
• Hormonal fluctuations
	• Time of day
	• Mood
	• Boredom
	• Peer/family pressure
	• Inattentiveness
	• Habit
	• Hunger/appetite
	• Low self-esteem
	• Environment
	• Sight and smell
	  of favorite foods

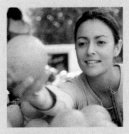

What stops your "Eat" response?

• Acting responsibly in
  assessing foods
• Practicing stress
  management
• Breaking the habit
• Remaining active
• Analyzing emotional
  problems
• Making a conscious effort
• Recognizing true hunger
• Avoiding environment that
  causes "eat" response
	• Selecting alternatives
	• Recognizing triggers
	• Planning

FIGURE 10.4 The "Eat" Response
Learn to understand what triggers and stops your "eat" response by keeping a daily log.

Improving Your Eating Habits

At any given time, many Americans are trying to lose weight. Given the hundreds of different diets and endless expert advice available, why do we find it so difficult?

Determining What Triggers an Eating Behavior Before you can change a behavior, you must first determine what causes it. Many people have found it helpful to keep a chart of their eating patterns: when they feel like eating, where they are when they decide to eat, the amount of time they spend eating, other activities they engage in during the meal (watching television or reading), whether they eat alone or with others, what and how much they consume, and how they felt before they took their first bite. If you keep a detailed daily log of eating triggers for at least a week, you will discover useful clues about what in your environment or your emotional makeup causes you to want food **(Figure 10.4)**. Typically, these dietary triggers center on problems in everyday living rather than on real hunger pangs. Many people find that they eat compulsively when stressed. For other people, the same circumstances diminish their appetite, which causes them to lose weight.

Changing Your Triggers
Once you recognize the factors that cause you to overeat, removing the triggers or substituting other activities for them will help you develop more sensible eating patterns. Here are some examples of substitute behaviors:

- When eating dinner, turn off all distractions, including phones, computers, television, and radio.
- Replace snack breaks or coffee breaks with exercise breaks. Seek healthy snacks if you must eat something. Fruits, vegetables, and low-fat proteins are good starting places.
- Instead of gulping your food, chew each bite slowly, and savor it. Put your fork down between bites.

- Vary mealtimes. Instead of eating by the clock, do not eat until you are truly hungry. Allow yourself only a designated amount of time for eating—but do not rush. Try to become more aware of true feelings of hunger.
- If you find that you generally eat all that you can cram on a plate, use smaller plates. Put your dinner plates away, and use the salad plates instead.
- Stop buying high-calorie foods that tempt you to snack, or store them in an inconvenient place. (Having to run upstairs for the potato chips will force you to think twice before munching them.) Buy the new 100-calorie snack foods that force you to limit how much you eat . . . eat only one, and put the rest away.

See **Table 10.4** for ideas on sensible snacking, and refer to the Skills for Behavior Change box for more weight management tips.

 ***try it* NOW!**

Make healthy substitutions at meal time—that's the key to successful weight maintenance! The next time you make dinner, take a look at the proportions on your plate. Veggies and whole grains should take up the most space; if not, substitute 1 cup of the meat, pasta, or cheese on your plate for 1 cup of legumes, salad greens, or a favorite vegetable. You'll reduce the number of calories in your meal while eating the same amount of food.

Selecting a Nutritional Plan

Seek assistance from reputable sources in selecting a dietary plan that is nutritious and easy to follow, such as the MyPyramid Plan discussed in Chapter 9. Registered dietitians, some physicians (not all doctors have a strong background in nutrition), health educators and exercise

TABLE 10.4 Tips for Sensible Snacking

According to the American Heart Association and other professional groups focused on nutrition, these healthy snacks can help curb your hunger pangs, keep your blood glucose from spiking, and will stay with you for longer periods of time.

- **Keep healthy munchies around.** Buy whole-wheat breads and if you need something to spice that up, buy low-fat or soy cheese, low-fat cream cheese or other healthy favorites and use them.

- **Keep crunchies on hand.** Apples, pears, green pepper sticks, popcorn, carrots, and celery all are good choices. Wash them and cut them up to carry with you or eat when you feel a snack attack coming on.

- **Quench your thirst with hot drinks.** Hot tea, heated milk, decaffeinated coffee, hot chocolate made with nonfat milk or water, or soup broths will help keep you satisfied.

- **Choose natural beverages.** Drink plain water, natural 100% juice drinks, tomato juice, or other low-sugar choices to satisfy your thirst.

- **Eat nuts instead of candy.** If you have to have a piece of chocolate, keep that piece small, preferably dark chocolate.

- **Avoid high-calorie energy bars** unless you are really exercising hard and don't have an opportunity to eat normal food. If you buy energy bars, look for a good mixture of fiber, protein, low-fat, and low-calorie options.

physiologists with nutritional training, and other health professionals can provide reliable information. Beware of people who call themselves nutritionists. There is no such official designation, which leaves the door open for just about anyone to call himself or herself a nutritional expert. Avoid weight-loss programs that promise quick, "miracle" results.

Before engaging in any weight-loss program, ask about the credentials of the adviser; assess the nutrient value of the prescribed diet; verify that dietary guidelines are consistent with reliable nutrition research; and analyze the suitability of the diet to your tastes, budget, and lifestyle. Any diet that requires radical behavior changes is likely to be doomed to failure. The most successful plans allow you to make food choices and do not ask you to sacrifice everything you enjoy. See the **Consumer Health** box for ratings of some of the more popular diets being marketed today.

Reward yourself when you lose pounds. If you binge and go off your nutrition plan, get right back on it the next day.

very-low-calorie diets (VLCDs) Diets with a daily caloric value of 400 to 700 calories.

ketosis A condition in which the body adapts to prolonged fasting or carbohydrate deprivation by converting body fat to ketones, which can be used as fuel for some brain activity.

Remember that you did not gain 40 pounds in 8 weeks, so it is unrealistic to punish your body by trying to lose that amount of weight in a short time.

Considering Drastic Weight-Loss Measures

When nothing seems to work, people often become willing to take significant risks to lose weight. Dramatic weight loss may be recommended in cases of extreme health risk. However, even in such situations, drastic dietary, pharmacological, or surgical measures should be considered carefully and discussed with several knowledgeable health professionals.

Fad Diets Fasting, starvation diets, and other forms of **very-low-calorie diets (VLCDs)** have been shown to cause significant health risks. Typically, depriving the body of food for prolonged periods forces it to make adjustments to prevent the shutdown of organs. The body depletes its energy reserves to obtain necessary fuels. To maintain its supply of glucose, one of the first reserves the body turns to is lean, protein tissue. As this occurs, the body loses weight rapidly because protein contains only half as many calories per pound as fat. At the same time, the body loses significant water stores. Over time, the body begins to run out of liver tissue, heart muscle, blood, and so on, because the body burns these readily available substances to supply energy. Only after depleting the readily available proteins from these sources does the body begin to burn fat reserves. In this process, known as **ketosis**, the body adapts to prolonged fasting or carbohydrate deprivation by converting body fat to ketones, which can be used as fuel for some brain cells. Within about 10 days after the typical adult begins a complete fast, the body will have used many of its energy stores, and death may occur.

In very-low-calorie diets, powdered formulas are usually given to patients under medical supervision. These formulas have daily values of 400 to 700 calories plus vitamin and mineral supplements. Although these diets may be beneficial for people who have failed at all conventional weight-loss methods and who face severe health risks due to obesity, they never should be undertaken without strict medical supervision. Problems associated with fasting, VLCDs, and other forms of severe calorie deprivation include blood sugar imbalance, cold intolerance, constipation, decreased BMR, dehydration, diarrhea, emotional problems, fatigue, headaches, heart irregularity, ketosis, kidney infections and failure, loss of lean body tissue, weakness, and eventual weight gain due to the yo-yo effect and other variables. Also consider the nutritional quality of packaged "low-fat" foods commonly used as part of a low-calorie diet. Many of these foods have a high sugar and sodium content to make the food taste better. They might be low in fat, but generally they are full of salt and empty calories from sugar.

Drug Treatment When used as part of a long-term, comprehensive weight-loss program, drugs can help people who are severely obese lose up to 10 percent of their weight and maintain the loss. The challenge is to develop an effective drug that can be used over time without adverse effects or abuse, and no such drug currently exists.

A classic example of supposedly safe drugs that later were found to have dangerous side effects were Pondimen and Redux, known as *fen-phen* (from their chemical names, fenfluramine and phentermine), two of the most widely prescribed diet drugs in U.S. history. When they were found to damage heart valves and contribute to pulmonary hypertension, a massive recall and lawsuit occurred.

Other diet drugs that you should view with caution include sibutramine, orlistat, herbal weight-loss aids, and over-the-counter (OTC) drugs. Sibutramine (Meridia) is an appetite suppressant that works by increasing serotonin levels in the brain. Orlistat (Xenical) is a drug that blocks fat absorption. It has recently been approved by the FDA for over-the-counter sale (brand name Alli) in a smaller dose than the prescription dose. Though these drugs have been found to minimize weight regain in people following low-calorie diets, they can have negative side effects, and their long-term safety and effectiveness are still unknown.

Surgery When all else fails, particularly for people who are severely overweight and have weight-related diseases such as diabetes or hypertension, a person may be a candidate for weight-loss surgery. Generally, these surgeries fall into one of two major categories: *restrictive surgeries,* such as *gastric banding,* or *malabsorption surgeries,* such as *gastric bypass.*

In gastric banding and other restrictive surgeries, the surgeon uses an inflatable band to partition off part of the stomach. The band is wrapped around that part of the stomach and is pulled tight, like a belt, leaving only a small opening between the two parts of the stomach. The upper part of the stomach is smaller, so the person feels full more quickly, and food digestion slows so that the person also feels full longer. Although the bands are designed to stay in place, they can be removed surgically. Weight loss is slower than with gastric bypass surgery, but risks are fewer, particularly because it is a less invasive surgical procedure.

In contrast, gastric bypass is designed to restrict drastically the amount of food a person can eat and absorb. It is done with general anesthesia, hospitalization is required, and it is irreversible. Results are fast and dramatic, but there are many risks, including blood clots in the legs, a leak in a

(Text continues on page 312.)

CONSUMER health

ANALYZING POPULAR DIETS

Many college students, like countless Americans, are in an ongoing quest to lose weight. However, many college-aged men and women not only choose unhealthy options, such as skipping breakfast or smoking cigarettes to control hunger, but also must negotiate a myriad of seemingly reputable diets. Are any of these diet plans really the miracles they often claim to be?

Virtually anyone can write a book making diet claims. These arguments may be based on unproven science or faulty scientific reasoning. Although health claims should be published only after solid research has proven the results repeatedly with different populations, this happens all too infrequently. The most recent ratings from *Consumer Reports* of some of the most popular diets and diet books follows.

DIET PLANS: WHAT THE STUDIES SAY

All of the diets in **Table 1** on page 308 have been tested in clinical trials published in scientific journals. *Consumer Reports* rated them through an evaluation of published study results and an analysis of nutritional quality based on the 2005 *U.S. Dietary Guidelines for Americans.* Overall score is based on adherence to nutritional guidelines and the results of published randomized clinical studies (exception noted in footnote) that reported 3- to 6-month short-term results and 1-year long-term results, and that together studied at least 40 subjects per diet.

Plans are listed in rank order of overall score. Even the highest-rated diets generally produced less than a 10 percent

weight loss after a year and had dropout rates of more than one in five participants. Weight Watchers, Jenny Craig, and Slim-Fast scores were very close together.

DIET BOOKS: WHAT THE EXPERTS SAY

The diet books rated in **Table 2** on page 310 have never been tested in a large clinical trial. *Consumer Reports* rated them through an expert-panel questionnaire and an analysis of nutritional quality based on the 2005 *U.S. Dietary Guidelines for Americans.* Books are listed in rank order of overall score, though scores of *Eat, Drink, and Weigh Less; You on a Diet;* and *The Abs Diet* were very close to one another.

(continued)

ANALYZING POPULAR DIETS (continued)

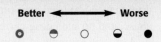

Better ◀——————▶ Worse

Table 1 *Consumer Reports* Ratings of Clinically Tested Diets

VOLUMETRICS

What It Is Based on research at Penn State, diet aims to maximize the amount of food available per calorie, mainly by use of reduced-fat products, liberal addition of vegetables, and low-fat cooking techniques. Encourages first course of broth-based soup or low-calorie salad to take the edge off appetite.

Pros and Cons Recent clinical trials show best overall weight loss of any diet evaluated. We judged the recipes appetizing but somewhat time-consuming to prepare.

WEIGHT WATCHERS

What It Is Venerable program uses weekly meetings and weigh-ins for motivation and behavioral support for diet and exercise changes, or you can sign up for similar support online. Dieters either earn or spend "points" with food and exercise or consume specified foods with "Core" plan. Vegetarian menu available.

Pros and Cons Behavioral support is proven to increase adherence to any diet. Scored average on weight loss in this group but first in long-term adherence. We judged recipes to be appetizing and fairly easy to prepare.

JENNY CRAIG

What It Is Dieters sign up for individual counseling and meal plans at company outlets, by phone, or online. Centerpiece of diet is eating Jenny Craig-prepared foods of single-serving entrées and snacks, supplemented by dairy products, salads, and other vegetables you prepare yourself. Vegetarian menu available.

Pros and Cons Diet requires minimal food preparation and meets dietary guidelines. Published study of actual client histories revealed high dropout rate, though those who stuck with plan lost considerable weight. Clinical trial had better adherence.

SLIM-FAST

What It Is Brand line of controlled-calorie shakes and bars, widely available in drugstores and supermarkets. Company website provides weekly menus. On standard meal plan, a bar or shake for breakfast and lunch, with additional food. For dinner, a low-calorie meal you fix yourself.

Pros and Cons Menu we analyzed meets dietary guidelines. Convenient for people with little time or inclination to cook. Clinical studies show above-average long-term weight loss but high long-term dropout rate.

	VOLUMETRICS	WEIGHT WATCHERS	JENNY CRAIG	SLIM-FAST
Rating				
Overall score	◒	◒	◒	◒
Study results				
Short-term				
Weight loss	◒	○	◒	◒
Drop-out rate	◒	○	○	◒
1 year				
Weight loss	◒	○	◒	◒
Drop-out rate	○	○	○	●
Nutrition analysis	◉	◉	◉	◉
Percentage of calories				
Fat	23	24	18	22
Saturated fat	7	7	7	6
Carbohydrates	55	56	62	57
Protein	22	20	20	21
Fiber g/1,000 cal,	20	20	16	21
Fruits & veg., daily serv.	14	11	6	12
Average daily calories	1,500	1,450	1,520	1,540

Guide to the Ratings

Overall score is based on adherence to nutritional guidelines and the results of published randomized clinical studies (exception noted in footnote) that reported three- to six-month short-term and one-year long-term results and together studied at least 40 subjects per diet. **Study results,** including short- and long-term weight-loss and dropout rates, were derived from published studies of each diet. **Nutrition analysis,** done in 2005, was based on a week of menus from each book or program, using The Food Processor software from ESHA Research. For diets that had a short introductory phase and a longer weight-loss phase, we evaluated the latter. Higher scores went to menus that conformed most closely to the recommendations of the 2005 U.S. Dietary Guidelines for Americans: 20 to 35 percent of calories from fat, with less than 10 percent from saturated fat; 45 to 65 percent from carbohydrates; 10 to 35 percent from protein; more than 14 grams of fiber per 1,000 calories. **Average daily calories** and servings of fruits and vegetables are listed for information only and are not part of the overall nutrition score. Guidelines call for the 6 to 9 servings in a 1,400- to 1,900-calorie diet.

Better ◄———► Worse   ◉ ◓ ○ ◒ ●

eDIETS

What It Is Well-established online subscription diet site offers 24 meal plans customized for various eating preferences and desired weight loss. Membership includes access to support groups, experts, menu plans, recipes. The standard eDiets.com weekly menu we analyzed met dietary guidelines and delivered the number of calories promised.

Pros and Cons Customizable plans are appealing, especially for those with wheat or lactose intolerances, but clinical studies find average adherence and below-average weight loss.

THE ZONE DIET(men's menu)†

What It Is The "Zone," as conceived by Barry Sears, is the ideal balance of foods to keep your blood sugar and hormones ready to fight obesity and diseases. To stay in the Zone, every meal must consist of 30% fat calories, 30% protein, and 40% carbs. Diet allows many fruits and practically no grains except oatmeal.

Pros and Cons We judged the recipes simple to prepare and the meal plan to have a good nutritional profile, but figuring out the diet without a meal plan involves a lot of math. Weight loss below average.

ORNISH DIET

What It Is Ultra–low-fat vegetarian regimen bans all meat, fish, oils, alcohol, sugar, and white flour. Ornish's clinical studies have shown that strictly following the diet can prevent or reverse disease. He believes it's easier to make drastic changes in diet than small ones.

Pros and Cons Provides the most food per calorie of any diet evaluated. Lower in fat than guidelines recommend. Studies show average long-term weight loss and below-average long-term adherence.

ATKINS DIET

What It Is This granddaddy of low-carb diets starts with a 2-week induction period that bans practically all carbs. The longer "ongoing weight loss" phase is only slightly less restrictive, gradually adding more vegetables, fruit, and wine.

Pros and Cons There's growing evidence that dieters aren't as hungry on Atkins as on some other diets. But many find it too restrictive, so long-term adherence is below average; long-term weight loss is average. Its nutritional profile is far outside dietary guidelines.

	eDIETS	THE ZONE DIET	ORNISH DIET	ATKINS DIET
Rating				
Overall score	◓	◓	○	◒
Study results				
Short-term				
Weight loss	◒	○	○	◓
Drop-out rate	○	○	○	○
1 year				
Weight loss	◒	◒	○	○
Drop-out rate	○	○	◒	◒
Nutrition analysis	◉	◉	○	●
Percentage of calories				
Fat	23	27	6	60
Saturated fat	5	7	1	20
Carbohydrates	53	42	77	11
Protein	24	30	16	29
Fiber, g/1,000 cal,	19	21	31	12
Fruits & veg.,daily serv.	12	17	17	6
Average daily calories	1,450	1,660	1,520	1,520

*One study used was a longitudinal study of all enrollees in Jenny Craig's premium plan for a 1-year period, published in the February 2007 *International Journal of Obesity.*

†Women's menu in The Zone was similar, but about 1,300 calories.

Source: "Diet Plans: What the Studies Say" © 2007 by Consumers Union of U.S., Inc. Yonkers, NY 10703-1057, a nonprofit organization. Reprinted with permission from the June 2007 issue of *Consumer Reports*® for educational purposes only. No commercial use or reproduction permitted. www.ConsumerReports.org.

Better ◄——► Worse

◉ ◓ ○ ◑ ●

Table 2 *Consumer Reports* Ratings of Untested Diet Books

THE BEST LIFE DIET
by Bob Greene

What It Is The diet's first phase involves exercise and a recommended eating schedule. Calorie reduction starts in phase two. You eat enough healthful foods to satisfy hunger, but no more. Includes tools to customize diet and exercise plans.

Pros and Cons Reviewers liked personalized advice and section on exercise. Extensive discussion of "emotional eating" might help some. Dieters might be discouraged when they don't lose weight in phase one. Straightforward recipes use common ingredients.

EAT, DRINK, & WEIGH LESS
by Mollie Katzen and Walter Willett, MD

What It Is Harvard nutrition researcher Walter Willett teamed up with cookbook author Mollie Katzen for this book based on the Mediterranean diet. Premise is that by "mindfully" following this diet, you can lose weight while enjoying eating. Little full-fat dairy or red meat. Up to one egg and one glass of wine a day.

Pros and Cons Sample diet had 1,910 calories per day—too many to allow most people to lose weight. Reviewers liked book's scientific accuracy but thought the exercise chapter too brief.

YOU ON A DIET
by Michael F. Roizen, MD, and Mehmet C. Oz, MD

What It Is The physician-authors devote more than half the book to background on appetite, metabolism, and behavior. Diet starts with a 2-week "rebooting program." Monotonous breakfasts and lunches cut down cravings. Sugar, saturated fat, and refined flour products are banned.

Pros and Cons Most reviewers thought the diet lacked detail and was too restrictive, and some were skeptical that habits can change for good in 2 weeks. Most recipes were very simple.

THE ABS DIET
by David Zinczenko with Ted Spiker

What It Is Written by the editor of *Men's Health* magazine, the diet promises "a six-pack in 6 weeks" by eating 6 meals a day featuring "power 12" foods. Includes about 100 pages of illustrated exercises.

Pros and Cons Reviewers were skeptical of the promise of rapid weight loss and disliked emphasis on whey supplements. Fitness program deemed easy to follow but possibly too strenuous for beginners and more appealing to men.

	THE BEST LIFE DIET	EAT, DRINK, & WEIGH LESS	YOU ON A DIET	THE ABS DIET
Rating				
Overall score	◑	◑	◑	◑
Expert evaluation	◑	◑	○	○
Science	◑	◑	◑	○
Nutrition	◑	◑	◑	○
Exercise	◑	○	◑	◑
Ease of use	◑	◑	○	○
Meal plans	◑	◑	○	○
Nutrition analysis	◉	◉	◉	◉
Percent of calories				
Fat	30	39	33	27
Saturated fat	6	8	6	7
Carbohydrates	47	45	48	49
Protein	23	17	19	24
Fiber, g/1,000 cal	22	19	18	20
Fruits & veg., daily serv.	8	16	13	7
Average daily calories	1,520	1,910	1,520	1,890

Guide to the Ratings

Overall score is based on adherence to nutritional guidelines and the results of expert evaluations of each diet book. **Expert evaluation** ratings are derived from results of panel survey on the books' nutritional and scientific information, exercise recommendations, ease of use, menus, and meal plans. **Nutrition analysis** was based on a week of menus from each book, using The Food Processor software from ESHA Research. For diets that had a short introductory phase and a longer weight-loss phase, we evaluted the latter. Higher scores went to menus that conformed most closely to the recommendations of the 2005 U.S. Dietary Guidelines for Americans: 20 to 35 percent of calories from fat, with less than 10 percent from saturated fat; 45 to 65 percent from carbohydrates; 10 to 35 percent from protein; more than 14 grams of fiber per 1,000 calories. **Average daily calories** and servings of fruits and vegetables are listed in the Ratings for information only and are not part of the overall nutrition score. Guidelines call for 6 to 9 servings in a 1,400 to 1,900 calorie diet.

THE SOUTH BEACH DIET
by Arthur Agatston, MD

What It Is Slightly more permissive version of the Atkins diet is based on the premise that eating low-glycemic foods decreases cravings for sugar and refined carbs. In the first phase, fruits, sugar, and grains are banned. Phase two allows some fruit, high-fiber grains, and dark chocolate.

Pros and Cons Reviewers thought the simplicity of diet would appeal to some but criticized overuse of the glycemic index and the too-short exercise section. Recipes seemed easy to prepare, but some called for unusual ingredients.

Rating

Overall score	◓
Expert evaluation	○
Science	○
Nutrition	○
Exercise	◒
Ease of use	◓
Meal plans	◓
Nutrition analysis	◓

Percent of calories

Fat	39
Saturated fat	9
Carbohydrates	38
Protein	22
Fiber, g/1,000 cal	19
Fruits & veg., daily serv.	13
Average daily calories	1,340

THE SONOMA DIET
by Connie Gutterson, RD, PhD

What It Is An updated lower-carb diet with a Mediterranean theme, its 10-day "wave 1" bans most sweet or refined foods. The longer wave 2, where most weight loss takes place, permits fruits and wine. You calculate portions by filling sectors of small plates with specified food categories.

Pros and Cons Reviewers found the overall diet healthful but complex and needlessly restrictive. They felt the book stinted on exercise. Recipes were rather elaborate to prepare.

Rating

Overall score	◓
Expert evaluation	○
Science	○
Nutrition	◓
Exercise	◒
Ease of use	○
Meal plans	○
Nutrition analysis	◓

Percent of calories

Fat	36
Saturated fat	8
Carbohydrates	39
Protein	24
Fiber, g/1,000 cal	20
Fruits & veg., daily serv.	10
Average daily calories	1,390

ULTRA-METABOLISM
by Mark Hyman, MD

What It Is The author designed the diet around his theory that people get fat because their systems become toxic, inflamed, stressed, and imbalanced. Initial "detox" phase and longer "rebalancing" phase. Eliminates white rice, refined grains, grain-fed or processed red meats, caffeinated beverages.

Pros and Cons Reviewers felt book's theory goes beyond scientific evidence and was overly restrictive and complicated. Exercise section judged somewhat brief but practical.

Rating

Overall score	○
Expert evaluation	◒
Science	◒
Nutrition	○
Exercise	◒
Ease of use	◒
Meal plans	◒
Nutrition analysis	◓

Percent of calories

Fat	41
Saturated fat	8
Carbohydrates	41
Protein	18
Fiber, g/1,000 cal	22
Fruits & veg., daily serv.	12
Average daily calories	1,660

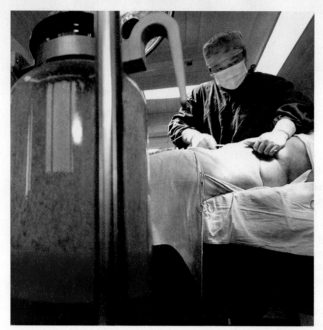

Liposuction is a surgical procedure that removes fat cells from specific areas of the body. It is not a solution for long-term weight loss.

| TABLE 10.5 | Putting on the Pounds: Tips for Gaining Weight |

- Eat at regularly scheduled times, whether hungry or not.
- Eat more frequently, spend more time eating, eat the high-calorie foods first if you fill up fast, and always start with the main course. Take time to shop, to cook, and to eat slowly. Put extra spreads such as peanut butter, cream cheese, or cheese on your foods. Make your sandwiches with extra-thick slices of bread, and add more fillings. Take seconds whenever possible, and eat high-calorie snacks during the day.
- Supplement your diet. Add high-calorie drinks that have a healthy balance of nutrients.
- Try to eat with people you are comfortable with. Avoid people who you feel are analyzing what you eat or make you feel like you should eat less.
- If you are sedentary, be aware that exercise can increase appetite. If you are exercising or exercising to extremes, moderate your activities until you've gained some weight.
- Avoid diuretics, laxatives, and other medications that cause you to lose body fluids and nutrients.
- Relax. Many people who are underweight operate at high gear most of the time. Slow down, get more rest, and control stress.

staple line in the stomach, pneumonia, infection, and death. Because the stomach pouch that remains after surgery is so small (about the size of a lime), the person can drink only a few tablespoons of liquid and consume only a very small amount of food at a time. For this reason, possible side effects include nausea and vomiting (if the person consumes too much), vitamin and mineral deficiencies, and dehydration (if the patient cannot eat or drink enough).

Keep in mind that it is always best to lose weight through a healthy diet and regular physical activity. Ironically, even after going through surgery, people must learn to eat healthy foods and exercise. Otherwise, they can continue to gain weight, even returning to their original weight. There are no quick fixes for weight control problems.

Liposuction is a surgical procedure in which fat cells are removed from specific areas of the body. Generally, liposuction is considered cosmetic surgery rather than weight-loss surgery and is used for spot-reducing and body contouring. Although this technique has garnered much attention, it too is not without risk: infections, severe scarring, and even death have resulted. In many cases, people who have liposuction regain fat in those areas or require multiple surgeries to repair lumpy, irregular surfaces from which the fat was removed.

Trying to Gain Weight

For some people, trying to gain weight is a challenge for a variety of metabolic, hereditary, psychological, and other reasons. If you are one of these individuals, the first priority is to determine why you cannot gain weight. For example,

among older adults, the senses of taste and smell may decline, which makes food taste differently and be less pleasurable. Visual problems and other disabilities may make meals more difficult to prepare, and dental problems may make eating more difficult. People who engage in sports that require extreme nutritional supplementation may be at risk for nutritional deficiencies, which can lead to immune system problems and organ dysfunction, weakness that leads to falls and fractures, slower recovery from diseases, and a host of other problems. **Table 10.5** details some weight-gaining strategies.

Thinking Thin: Body Image Disorders

Waif-like celebrities such as Kate Moss and Nicole Richie dominate fashion and the media. These images set the standard for what we find attractive, leading some people to go to impossible extremes to be the perfect size 0 or have the biggest biceps. Most of us think of this obsession with weight control as a recent phenomenon. However, an obsession with being thin has long been part of our culture. During the Victorian era, women wore corsets to achieve unrealistically tiny waists. By the 1920s, it was common knowledge that obesity was linked to poor health. In the 1960s, rail-thin supermodel Twiggy emerged on the scene.

Today more than ever before, underweight models and celebrities exemplify desirability and success, delivering the subtle message that thin is best. Some of these distorted

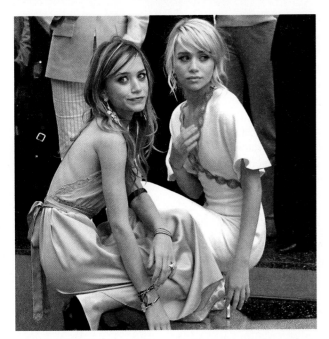

Pressures from society, especially on women, can have a detrimental effect on body image. Mary-Kate Olsen is one celebrity struggling with an eating disorder.

views of self-image arise from misinterpreting height–weight charts, making some people strive for the lower readings stipulated for a light-boned person when determining their own normal weight. Increasing numbers of people are so preoccupied with trying to be "model-thin" that they make themselves ill.

Social Bias against the Overweight

Although much has been written about the potentially devastating physical consequences of being overweight or obese, an area that is often brushed under the table relates to the social consequences of excess weight. Difficulty in finding a job, workplace discrimination, and problems in just about every avenue of one's social life have been noted for people who are obese.

Research increasingly points to a nation of weight **bias,** generally referring to negative attitudes that affect our interpersonal interactions and activities in a detrimental way. Stigma against heavy people may come in several forms, including verbal types of bias (such as ridicule, teasing, insults, stereotypes, derogatory names, or pejorative language), physical stigma (such as touching, grabbing, or other aggressive behaviors), or other barriers and obstacles for obese people, such as seats in movie theaters, stadiums, or airplanes that are too small for many overweight people. In an extreme form, stigma can result in subtle and overt forms of discrimination, such as denial of a promotion or a raise.[45]

Bias and stigmatization can lead to social isolation and a host of other problems for obese individuals. People who experience it have higher rates of depression, poorer psychological adjustment, and higher rates of suicide. They may feel that they are "unlovable" and have difficulties in relationships. They also may have higher rates of disordered eating, issues with self-esteem, more difficulties in their medical encounters, and a host of other problems.[46]

 what do you THINK?

Are you biased against overweight and obese people? ▪ When you see someone who is extremely obese, do you make any judgments about that person? ▪ If you see someone with very obese children, what do you think about them? ▪ How many of your really close friends are obese? ▪ Would you date someone who is overweight? ▪ Are there some jobs that you think overweight or obese people should not hold? Why?

Eating Disorders

For an increasing number of people, particularly young women, an obsessive relationship with food develops into **anorexia nervosa,** a persistent, chronic eating disorder characterized by deliberate food restriction and severe, life-threatening weight loss. **Bulimia nervosa** involves frequent bouts of binge eating followed by purging (self-induced vomiting), laxative abuse, or excessive exercise. **Binge eating disorder (BED)** also involves episodes of binge eating, but unlike bulimics, binge eaters do not purge after a binge episode.

In the United States, as many as 24 million people meet the established criteria for one of these disorders, and their numbers appear to be increasing; it has been estimated that up to 4.5 percent of all individuals have experienced an eating disorder at some time in their lives.[47] It is estimated that 19 to 30 percent of all female college students suffer from

bias Negative or unfair attitudes or actions stemming from prejudice.

anorexia nervosa Eating disorder characterized by excessive preoccupation with food, self-starvation, and/or extreme exercising to achieve weight loss.

bulimia nervosa Eating disorder characterized by binge eating followed by inappropriate measures, such as purging, to prevent weight gain.

binge eating disorder (BED) Eating disorder characterized by recurrent binge eating, without excessive measures to prevent weight gain.

some type of eating disorder, with athletes among those at highest risk. Some suffer from lesser forms of these conditions—not enough for a true diagnosis but dangerously close to the precipice that will ultimately lead to life-threatening results. Some of the physical complications associated with eating disorders include osteoporosis, heart attack, seizures, anemia, electrolyte imbalances, and tooth erosion. The severity of these conditions varies with the degree and duration of the eating disorder.

Anorexia Nervosa

Anorexia nervosa involves self-starvation motivated by an intense fear of gaining weight, along with an extremely distorted body image. Nearly 1 percent of girls in late adolescence meet the full criteria for anorexia; many others suffer from significant symptoms.

Initially, most people with anorexia lose weight by reducing total food intake, particularly of high-calorie foods, eventually leading to restricted intake of almost all foods. What they do eat, they often purge through vomiting or using laxatives. Although they lose weight, people with anorexia never seem to feel thin enough and constantly identify body parts that are "too fat." Anorexia has the highest death rate (20 percent) of any psychological illness.

Bulimia Nervosa

People with bulimia nervosa often binge and then take inappropriate measures, such as secret purging (vomiting), taking laxatives, or excessive exercise, to lose the calories they have just acquired. Up to 3 percent of adolescents and young women are bulimic; rates among men are about 10 percent of the rate among women. People with bulimia are also obsessed with their bodies, weight gain, and their appearance. Unlike people with anorexia, people with bulimia are often "hidden" from the public eye because their weight may vary only slightly or fall within a normal range. Also, treatment appears to be more effective for bulimia than for anorexia.

One of the more common symptoms of bulimia is tooth erosion, which results from the excessive vomiting associated with this disorder. Chronic regurgitation causes hydrochloric acid (stomach acid) to break down the enamel of the teeth.[48]

Binge Eating Disorder

Individuals with binge eating disorder binge like their bulimic counterparts but do not take excessive measures to lose the weight that they gain. Often they are clinically obese, and they tend to binge much more often than the typical obese person. Binge eating episodes are often characterized by eating rapidly, eating large amounts of food even when not feeling hungry, and feeling guilty or depressed after overeating. Though it is not currently recognized as

an official mental disorder by the American Psychiatric Association, evidence suggests that binge eating disorder is becoming increasingly common. In fact, a national survey on eating disorders conducted by Harvard-affiliated McLean Hospital reported that binge eating disorder is more prevalent than either anorexia or bulimia. The survey showed that 3.5 percent of women and 2 percent of men experience binge eating disorder at some point in their lives, as contrasted with lifetime rates of 0.9 percent of women and 0.3 percent of men for anorexia, and 1.5 percent of women and 0.5 percent of men for bulimia.[49]

Who's at Risk?

There's no simple explanation for why intelligent, often highly accomplished people spiral downward into the destructive behaviors associated with eating disorders. One factor is a desperate need to win social approval or gain control of their lives through food. Many people with disordered eating patterns also suffer from other problems: many are clinically depressed, suffer from obsessive-compulsive disorder, and have other health problems. One recent study of college-aged women who purge regularly indicated that this group is also at high risk for alcohol abuse and other negative consequences from alcohol.[50] In addition, studies have shown that individuals with low self-esteem, negative body image, and a high tendency for perfectionism are also at risk.[51] **Figure 10.5** details the characteristic body image issues and eating patterns of people at risk for an eating disorder. Where do you fall on this continuum?

Disordered eating, defined as bulimia, exercise bulimia, anorexia, and abuse of diet pills, affects roughly 62 percent of college athletes in sports such as gymnastics, wrestling, swimming, and figure skating. Of those 62 percent, 86 percent reported onset of disordered eating before the age of 20.[52] Athletes participating in sports that have weight class guidelines are particularly likely to develop eating disorders. Women aged 12 to 25 make up more than 90 percent of people with an eating disorder,[53] but women aren't the only ones at risk: eating disorders are on the rise among young men. Men represent up to 25 percent of anorexia and bulimia patients and almost 40 percent of binge eaters.[54] Many men suffering from eating disorders fail to seek treatment because eating disorders are traditionally thought of as a female problem and treatment centers are often geared to female patients.

Treatment for Eating Disorders

How can I help a friend who has an eating disorder?

Because eating disorders result from many factors spanning many years of development, there are no quick or simple solutions. **Table 10.6** details what you can do to help a friend or family member who has an

• I am not concerned about what others think regarding what and how much I eat. • I feel no guilt or shame no matter how much I eat or what I eat. • Food is an important part of my life but only occupies a small part of my time. • I trust my body to tell me what and how much to eat.	• I pay attention to what I eat in order to maintain a healthy body. • I may weigh more than what I like, but I enjoy eating and balance my pleasure in eating with my concern for a healthy body. • I am moderate and flexible in goals for eating well. • I try to follow the *Dietary Guidelines* for healthy eating.	• I think about food a lot. • I feel I don't eat well most of the time. • It's hard for me to enjoy eating with others. • I feel ashamed when I eat more than others or more than what I feel I should be eating. • I am afraid of getting fat. • I wish I could change how much I want to eat and what I am hungry for.	• I have tried diet pills, laxatives, vomiting, or extra time exercising in order to lose or maintain my weight. • I have fasted or avoided eating for long periods of time in order to lose or maintain my weight. • I feel strong when I can restrict how much I eat. • Eating more than I wanted to makes me feel out of control.	• I regularly stuff myself and then exercise, vomit, use diet pills or laxatives to get rid of the food or calories. • My friends/family tell me I am too thin. • I am terrified of eating fat. • When I let myself eat, I have a hard time controlling the amount of food I eat. • I am afraid to eat in front of others.
FOOD IS NOT AN ISSUE	**CONCERNED WELL**	**FOOD PREOCCUPIED/ OBSESSED**	**DISRUPTIVE EATING PATTERNS**	**EATING DISORDERED**
BODY OWNERSHIP	**BODY ACCEPTANCE**	**BODY PREOCCUPIED/ OBSESSED**	**DISTORTED BODY IMAGE**	**BODY HATE/ DISASSOCIATION**
• Body image is not an issue for me. • My body is beautiful to me. • My feelings about my body are not influenced by society's concept of an ideal body shape. • I know that the significant others in my life will always find me attractive. • I trust my body to find the weight it needs to be so I can move and feel confident of my physical body.	• I base my body image equally on social norms and my own self-concept. • I pay attention to my body because it is important to me, but it only occupies a small part of my day. • I nourish my body so it has the strength and energy to achieve my physical goals. • I am able to assert myself and maintain a healthy body without losing my self-esteem.	• I spend a significant time viewing my body in the mirror. • I spend a significant time comparing my body to others. • I have days when I feel fat. • I am preoccupied with my body. • I accept society's ideal body shape and size as the best body shape and size. • I'd be more attractive if I were thinner, more muscular, etc...	• I spend a significant amount of time exercising and dieting to change my body. • My body shape and size keeps me from dating or finding someone who will treat me the way I want to be treated. • I have considered changing or have changed my body shape and size through surgical means so I can accept myself. • I wish I could change the way I look in the mirror.	• I often feel separated and distant from my body—as if it belongs to someone else. • I hate my body and I often isolate myself from others. • I don't see anything positive or even neutral about my body shape and size. • I don't believe others when they tell me I look OK. • I hate the way I look in the mirror.

FIGURE 10.5 The Eating Issues and Body Image Continuum
Individuals whose responses fall to the far left side of the continuum have normal eating patterns and are not at risk for an eating disorder. Individuals whose answers fall to the far right of this continuum likely suffer from an eating disorder. Where are your responses on the continuum?

Source: Smiley, King, Avery: Campus Health Service. Original Continuum, C. Schislak: *Preventive Medicine and Public Health.* Copyright © 1997. Arizona Board of Regents. Used with permission.

eating disorder. Treatment often focuses first on reducing the threat to life; once the patient is stabilized, long-term therapy involves family, friends, and other significant people in the individual's life. Therapy focuses on the psychological, social, environmental, and physiological factors that have led to the problem. Finding a therapist who really understands the multidimensional aspects of the problem is a must. Therapy allows the patient to focus on building new eating behaviors, recognizing threats, building self-confidence, and finding other ways to deal with life's problems. Support groups often help the family and the individual gain understanding and emotional support and learn self-development techniques designed to foster positive reactions and actions. Treatment of underlying depression may also be a focus.

what do you THINK?

Which groups or individuals on your campus appear to be at greatest risk for eating disorders? ■ What social factors might encourage this? ■ Why do you think society tends to overlook eating disorders in men?

TABLE 10.6 **Does Someone Close to You Have an Eating Disorder?**

Although every situation is different, there are several things that you can do if you suspect someone is struggling with an eating disorder.

- Learn as much as you can about eating disorders ahead of time.

- Check out resources on your campus and in your local community. Talk to professionals about what approaches and treatments have been most successful. Have a list of referrals ready to give to the person. Be armed with information.

- Set up a time to meet and share your concerns openly, honestly, and in a caring and supportive way. Be a good listener, and don't give advice unless asked.

- Provide examples of why you think there might be a disordered eating problem. Talk about health, relationship, and changes in behaviors.

- Avoid conflicts or a battle of the wills with this person. If he or she denies that there is a problem or minimizes it, repeat your concerns in a nonjudgmental way. You want the person to feel comfortable talking to you—not to drive him or her away.

- Never nag, plead, beg, bribe, threaten, or manipulate. Be straightforward, acknowledge it will be hard but that you know he or she can work through this.

- Don't get involved in endless conversation about diet, fatness, or exercise.

- Don't talk about how thin they are or focus on weight, diets, or exercise. Remember that the person wants to hear he or she is thin, and if you say it's good he or she is gaining weight, he or she will try to lose it.

- If the person is nervous about seeing a counselor, offer to go along as a support.

- Avoid placing shame, guilt, or accusations. Use "I" statements (such as, "I am worried that you won't be able to do such and such if you don't eat,") rather than "you" statements (e.g., "you need to eat or you are going to make yourself really sick").

- Stay calm and realize your own limitations. Be patient and supportive and be there in an emergency if the person asks for your help.

Sources: Adapted from National Eating Disorders Association, "How to Help a Friend with Eating and Body Image Issues," 2006; and National Eating Disorders Association, "What Should I Say? Tips for Talking to a Friend Who May Be Struggling with an Eating Disorder," 2006, www.nationaleatingdisorders.org.

TAKING charge

Summary

- Overweight, obesity, and weight-related problems appear to be on the rise in the United States. Obesity is now defined in terms of fat content rather than in terms of weight alone.

- There are many different methods of assessing body fat. Body mass index (BMI) is one of the most commonly accepted measures of weight based on height. Body fat percentages more accurately indicate how fat or lean a person is.

- Many factors contribute to one's risk for obesity, including genetics, developmental factors, endocrine influences, psychosocial factors, eating cues, lack of awareness, metabolic changes, lifestyle, and gender. Women often have considerably more difficulty losing weight.

- Exercise, dieting, diet pills, surgery, and other strategies are used to maintain or lose weight. However, sensible eating behavior and adequate exercise offer the best options.

- Eating disorders consist of severe disturbances in eating behaviors, unhealthy efforts to control body weight, and abnormal attitudes about body and shape. Anorexia nervosa, bulimia nervosa, and binge eating disorder are the three main eating disorders. Eating disorders are prevalent among young women, athletes, and increasing numbers of young men.

Chapter Review

1. Essential fat makes up approximately _____ percent of total body weight in men and approximately _____ percent of total body weight in women.
   a. 3 to 5; 18
   b. 3 to 7; 15
   c. 5 to 25; 13
   d. 3 to 5; 7

2. The method of determining body fat by measuring the amount of water displaced when a person is completely submerged is called the
   a. skinfold caliper test.
   b. body mass index.
   c. hydrostatic weighing technique.
   d. bioelectrical impedance analysis.

3. What technique of weight assessment is based on the relationship of weight to height?
   a. body composition index
   b. body mass index
   c. hydrostatic weight
   d. waist-to-hip ratio

4. At what body mass index (BMI) is a person considered to be overweight but not obese?
   a. BMI of 18 to 24
   b. BMI of 25 to 29
   c. BMI of 30 to 39
   d. BMI greater than 40

5. What percent of all the calories you consume on a given day go to support your basal metabolism?
   a. 10 to 20 percent
   b. 30 to 40 percent
   c. 60 to 70 percent
   d. 80 to 90 percent

6. Jenny binge eats and then secretly vomits. What eating disorder does she suffer from?
   a. compulsive overeating
   b. anorexia nervosa
   c. bulimia nervosa
   d. binge eating disorder

7. Which of the following is not a characteristic of women suffering from anorexia?
   a. increased sensitivity to cold
   b. absence of menstruation
   c. gaining more weight
   d. abnormal sense of taste

8. Tim's desire to look good interferes with his relationship with others. Rather than spending his leisure time with family and friends, he spends a disproportionate amount of time exercising excessively at the gym and worrying about how his body looks. Tim suffers from
   a. social physique anxiety.
   b. appearance anxiety.
   c. obesity anxiety.
   d. anorexia nervosa.

9. What is the death rate for anorexia nervosa?
   a. 1 percent
   b. 5 percent
   c. 10 percent
   d. 20 percent

10. One pound of body fat contains
    a. 1,500 calories.
    b. 3,500 calories.
    c. 5,000 calories.
    d. 7,000 calories.

Answers to these questions can be found on page A-1.

Questions for Discussion and Reflection

1. Discuss the pressures, if any, you feel to change the shape of your body. Do these pressures come from media, family, friends, and other external sources, or from concern for your personal health?
2. What type of measurement would you choose to assess your fat levels? Why?
3. List the risk factors for obesity. Evaluate which seem to be most important in determining whether you will be obese in middle age.
4. Create a plan to help someone lose the "freshman 15" over the summer vacation. Assume that the person is male, weighs 180 pounds, and has 15 weeks to lose the excess weight.
5. Differentiate among the three major eating disorders. Why are women more prone to anorexia and bulimia than men are?

Accessing Your Health on the Internet

The following websites explore further topics and issues related to personal health. For links to the websites below, visit the Companion Website for *Health: The Basics,* Eighth Edition at www.aw-bc.com/donatelle.

1. *American Dietetic Association.* Includes recommended dietary guidelines and other current information about weight control. www.eatright.org
2. *Duke University Diet and Fitness Center.* Includes information about one of the best programs in the country; focuses on helping people live healthier, fuller lives through weight control and lifestyle change. www.cfl.duke.edu/dfc
3. *Weight-Control Information Network.* Excellent resource for diet and weight control information. Offers practical strategies and current information on research. http://win.niddk.nih.gov

4. *Yale Center for Eating and Weight Disorders.* Operated by the Yale University psychology department, this center offers services to people who experience problems with weight and food. A good source of information on eating disorders. www.yale.edu/ycewd

5. *The Rudd Center for Food Policy and Obesity.* Website for the research center at Yale University. Provides excellent information on the latest in obesity research, public policy, and ways we can put a stop to the obesity epidemic at the community level. www.yaleruddcenter.org

Further Reading

Brownell, K. and K. Horgen. *Food Fight: The Inside Story of the Food Industry, America's Obesity Crisis, and What We Can Do about It.* New York: McGraw-Hill, 2004.

> *Director of the Yale Center for Eating and Weight Disorders, Brownell critiques the way that food is marketed and sold to children and places much of the blame for childhood obesity on advertising and unhealthy foods being offered in schools.*

Brownell, K. D. et al. (eds.), *Weight Bias: Nature, Consequences and Remedies* (New York: Guilford Press, 2005).

> *Expert review of issues surrounding weight stigma, bias, and discrimination, as well as possible solutions to these problems.*

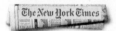

e-themes from *The New York Times*

For up-to-date articles about current health issues, visit www.aw-bc.com/donatelle, select *Health: The Basics,* Eighth Edition, Chapter 10, and click on "e-themes."

References

1. National Center for Health Statistics, *National Health and Nutrition Examination Survey (NHANES) 2003–2004* (Hyattsville, MD: U.S. Department of Health and Human Services, 2005); C. L. Ogden et al., "Prevalence of Overweight and Obesity in the U.S. 1999–2004," *Journal of the American Medical Association* 295, no. 13 (April 2006):1549–55; J. Wang and R. Beydoun, "The Obesity Epidemic in the United States—Gender, Age, Socioeconomic, Racial/Ethnic and Geographic Characteristics: A Systematic Review and Meta-Regression Analysis," *Epidemiological Review,* doi:10.1093/epirev/mxm007 (May 2007) published online ahead of print.
2. L. Fontana, "Excessive Adiposity, Calorie Restriction, and Aging," *Journal of the American Medical Association* 295 (2006):1577–78.
3. Trust for America's Health, 2005, www.healthyamericans.org. Specific information about how your state ranks is available at www.healthyamericans.org.; Department of Health and Children, National Task Force on Obesity, *Obesity: The Policy Challenges* (Dublin, Ireland: Department of Health and Children, 2005), www.dohc.ie/publications.
4. K. Flegal et al., "Excess Deaths Associated with Underweight, Overweight and Obesity," *Journal of the American Medical Association* 293 (2005): 1861–67.
5. N. Pandey and V. Gupta, "Trends in Diabetes," *Lancet* 369, no. 14 (2007): 1256–57.
6. L. Lipscombe and J. Hux, "Trends in Diabetes Prevalence, Incidence, and Mortality in Ontario, Canada, 1995–2005: A Population-Based Study," *Lancet* 369, no. 14 (2007): 750–56.
7. E. Finkelstein et al., "Economic Causes and Consequences of Obesity," *Annual Reviews of Public Health* 26 (2005): 239–57; Division of Nutrition and Physical Activity, National Center for Chronic Disease Prevention and Health Promotion, "Economic Consequences," 2007, www.cdc.gov/nccdphp/dnpa/obesity/economic_consequences.htm.
8. U.S. Department of Health and Human Services and U.S. Department of Agriculture, *Dietary Guidelines for Americans 2007,* www.healthierus.gov/dietaryguidelines.
9. Weight-Control Information Network, "Statistics Related to Overweight and Obesity," 2006, http://win.niddk.nih.gov/statistics.
10. Ogden et al, "Prevalence of Overweight and Obesity in the United States, 1999–2004."
11. Weight-Control Information Network, "Statistics Related to Overweight and Obesity"; Ogden et al., "Prevalence of Overweight and Obesity in the United States, 1999–2004."
12. Weight-Control Information Network, "Statistics Related to Overweight and Obesity."
13. American Obesity Association, "AOA Fact Sheets: What Is Obesity?" May 2005, www.obesity.org.
14. National Center for Health Statistics, *Prevalence of Overweight and Obesity Among Adults: United States, 1999–2002* (Hyattsville, MD: National Center for Health Statistics, 2004).
15. American Obesity Association, "AOA Fact Sheets: What Is Obesity?"
16. D. Eberwine, "Globesity: The Crisis of Growing Proportions," *Perspectives in Health* 7, no. 3 (2003): 9.
17. U.S Department of Health and Human Services, U.S Department of Agriculture, *Dietary Guidelines for Americans 2007.*
18. Ibid.

19. Rush University, "Waist to Hip Ratio Calculator," 2005, www.rush.edu/itools/hip/hipcalc.html.

20. Wang and Beydoun, "The Obesity Epidemic in the United States"; S. Kautiainen et al., "Use of Information and Communication Technology and Prevalence of Overweight and Obesity Among Adolescents," *International Journal of Obesity* 29 (2005): 925–33.

21. Wang and Beydoun, "The Obesity Epidemic in the United States."

22. U.S. Department of Health and Human Services, *Surgeon General's Call to Action to Prevent and Decrease Overweight and Obesity* (Washington, DC: U.S. Department of Health and Human Services, 2001).

23. T. Rankinen et al., "The Human Obesity Gene Map: 2005 Update," *Obesity* 14 (2006): 529–644.

24. D. Cummings and M. Schwartz, "Genetics and Pathophysiology of Human Obesity," *Annual Review of Medicine* 54 (2003): 453–71.

25. N. Abumad, "*CD36* May Determine Our Desire for Dietary Fats," *Journal of Clinical Nutrition* 115 (2005): 2965–67.

26. C. Bell et al., "The Genetics of Obesity," *Nature Reviews Genetics* 6 (2005): 221–34.

27. Rankinen et al., "The Human Obesity Gene Map."

28. Ibid.

29. J. Loos and C. Bouchard, "Obesity—Is It a Genetic Disorder?" *Journal of Internal Medicine* 254 (2003): 401–25.

30. Mayo Clinic, "Special Report: Weight Control," 2005, www.mayoclinic.com.

31. D. E. Cummings et al., "Plasma Ghrelin Levels after Diet-Induced Weight Loss or Gastric Bypass Surgery," *New England Journal of Medicine* 346, no. 21 (2002): 1623–30.

32. V. Paracchini, P. Pedotti, and E. Taioli, "Genetics of Leptin and Obesity: A HuGE Review," *American Journal of Epidemiology* 162, no. 2 (2005): 101–14.

33. D. Williams, D. Baskin, and M. Schwartz, "Leptin Regulation of Anorexic Responses to Glucogan-like Peptide-1 Receptor Stimulation," *Diabetes* 55, no. 12 (2006): 3387–93.

34. Centers for Disease Control and Prevention, "Growing Stronger: Strength Training for Older Adults—Why Strength Training?" April 2005, www.cdc.gov/nccdphp/dnpa/physical/growing_stronger/why.htm.

35. American Obesity Association, "Obesity: A Global Epidemic," May 2005, www.obesity.org.

36. J. Powell et al., "Exposure to Food Advertising on Television Among U.S. Children," *Archives of Pediatrics & Adolescent Medicine* 161 (2007): 553–60.

37. T. Harder et al., "Duration of Breast Feeding and Risk of Overweight," *American Journal of Epidemiology* 162, no. 5 (2005): 397–403.

38. Ogden et al., "Prevalence of Overweight and Obesity in the U.S., 1999–2004."

39. National Center for Health Statistics, "Prevalence of Sedentary Leisure Time Behavior Among Adults in the United States," February 2005, www.cdc.gov/nchs.

40. Ibid.

41. Ibid.

42. National Institute of Diabetes and Digestive and Kidney Diseases, Weight Control Information Network, "You Can Control Your Weight as You Quit Smoking," 2006, http://win.niddk.nih.gov/publications/smoking.htm

43. Mayo Clinic, "Special Report: Weight Control."

44. G. Flett and P. Hewitt, "The Perils of Perfectionism in Sports and Exercise," *Current Directions in Psychological Science* 14, no. 1 (2005): 14–22; P. Crocker et al., "Examining Current Ideal Discrepancy Scores and Exercise Motivations as Predictors of Social Physique Anxiety in Exercising Females," *Journal of Sport Behavior* 28 (2005): 63–72.

45. North American Association for the Study of Obesity (NAASO), The Obesity Society, "Obesity, Bias, and Stigmatization," 2007, www.naaso.org/information/weight_bias.asp.

46. N. Amy et al., "Barriers to Routing Gynecological Cancer Screening for White and African-American Obese Women, *Journal of Obesity Research*, 30 (2006): 147–55; NAASO, The Obesity Society, "Obesity, Bias, and Stigmatization."

47. "Disordered Eating Statistics (U.S.)," 2007, www.disordered-eating.co.uk/eating-disorders-statistics/eating-disorders-statistics-us.html; National Eating Disorder Association, "Statistics: Eating Disorders and their Precursors," 2002, www.nationaleatingdisorders.org.

48. M. P. Faine, "Recognition and Management of Eating Disorders in the Dental Office," *The Dental Clinics of North America* 47, no. 2 (2003): 395–410.

49. J. Hudson et al., "The Prevalence and Correlates of Eating Disorders in the National Comorbidity Survey Replication," *Biological Psychiatry* 61, no. 3 (2007): 348–58.

50. T. Adams and T. Araas, "Purging and Alcohol Related Effects in College Women," *International Journal of Eating Disorders* 39, no. 3 (2006): 240–44.

51. S. Forsberg and J. Lock, "The Relationship between Perfectionism, Eating Disorders and Athletes: A Review," *Minerva Pediatrica* 58, no. 6 (2006): 525–34.

52. K. Beals and A. Hill, "The Prevalence of Disordered Eating, Menstrual Dysfunction, and Low Bone Mineral Density among U.S. Collegiate Athletes," *International Journal of Sport Nutrition and Exercise Metabolism* 16, no. 3 (2006): 1–23; American College of Sports Medicine (ACSM), "Female Athlete Health Challenges Prevalent but Misunderstood: Study Shows Too Few Coaches Aware of Conditions, Implications," June 2006, www.acsm.org; L. Ronco, "The Female Athlete Triad: When Women Push Their Limits in High-Performance Sports," *American Fitness* 25, no. 2 (2007): 22–24.

53. "Disordered Eating Statistics (U.S.)."

54. E. Bernstein, "Men, Boys Lack Options to Treat Eating Disorders," *Wall Street Journal*, April 17, 2007, D1–D2.

11

Personal Fitness

IMPROVING HEALTH THROUGH EXERCISE

Can I lose **weight** with exercise alone?

What types of exercises can I do to **improve** my muscular strength?

How can I go about developing a **fitness** plan?

What can I do to charge up my **exercise** routine and prevent boredom?

OBJECTIVES

- Distinguish among physical activity for health, for fitness, and for performance.
- Describe the benefits of regular physical activity, including improvements in physical health, mental health, stress management, and life span.
- Explain the components of an aerobic exercise program, a strength-training program, and a stretching program.
- Summarize ways to prevent and treat common fitness injuries.
- Summarize the key components of a personal fitness program, and design a program that works for you.

A century ago in the United States, just to survive meant you had to perform physical labor on a daily basis. However, science and technology have transformed our lives. Today most adults in our country lead sedentary lifestyles and perform little physical labor or exercise. Students are no different; a recent survey indicated that 29 percent of college women and 21 percent of college men participate in no moderate or vigorous physical activities.[1] The growing percentage of Americans who live sedentary lives has been linked to dramatic increases in the incidence of obesity, diabetes, and other chronic diseases.[2] More than 108 million Americans are overweight or obese, 65 million have high blood pressure, 7.2 million suffer a heart attack in any given year, 21 million have diabetes, and approximately 41 million have "prediabetes."[3]

Decades of research show that physical activity has tremendous health-promoting and disease-preventing benefits.[4] Now is an excellent time to develop exercise habits that will improve the quality and duration of your own life.

Physical Activity for Health, Fitness, and Performance

Generally speaking, **physical activity** is defined as any bodily movement that is produced by the contraction of skeletal muscles and that substantially increases energy expenditure.[5] Walking, swimming, heavy lifting, and housework are all examples of physical activity. Physical activities also may vary by intensity. For example, walking to class may require little effort, but walking to class up a hill while carrying a heavy backpack makes the activity more intense. There are three general categories of physical activity defined by the purpose for which they are done: physical activity for health, physical activity for fitness, and physical activity for performance.

Physical Activity for Health

Research shows that just about everyone can improve general health by increasing overall physical activity, even if it doesn't involve going to the gym. Just adding more physical movement to your day can benefit your health. A physically active lifestyle might include choices such as parking further away from your destination, taking walking breaks while studying, or choosing to take the stairs instead of the elevator. In addition to these incidental ways to increase activity, there are lots of ways you can enjoy being physically active in recreation. Going dancing, playing Frisbee, or walking your dog are all good examples of recreational physical activity. The good

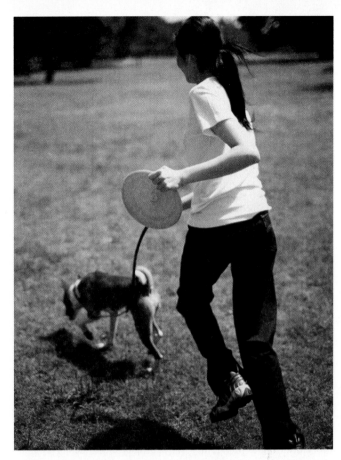

Exercise does not have to involve going to the gym; activities such as playing with your dog do count toward your daily physical activity.

thing about lifestyle physical activity is that you don't necessarily have to sustain your activity for an extended period of time to get a health benefit. Research shows that accumulating overall activity throughout the day can contribute to overall health and well-being.

Physical Activity for Fitness

The term **exercise** is a bit more specific than the term *physical activity*. Although all exercise is physical activity, not all physical activity may be exercise. For example, walking from your car to class is physical activity, but going for a brisk 30-minute walk is considered exercise. *Exercise* is defined as planned, structured, and repetitive bodily movement done to improve or maintain one or more components

physical activity Any bodily movement that is produced by the contraction of skeletal muscles and that substantially increases energy expenditure.

exercise Planned, structured, and repetitive bodily movement done to improve or maintain one or more components of physical fitness.

TABLE 11.1 | Components of Physical Fitness

Cardiorespiratory fitness	Ability to sustain moderate-intensity whole-body activity for extended time periods
Flexibility	Ability to move a joint or series of joints fluidly through the complete range of motion
Muscular strength and endurance	Maximum force applied with single muscle contraction; ability to perform repeated high-intensity muscle contractions
Body composition	A composite of total body mass, fat mass, fat-free mass, and fat distribution

Source: "ACSM Position Stand on the Recommended Quantity and Quality of Exercise for Developing and Maintaining Cardiorespiratory and Muscular Fitness and Flexibility in Adults," *Medicine and Science in Sports and Exercise* 30 (1998): 975–91. Copyright © 1998 American College of Sports Medicine.

of physical fitness, such as endurance, flexibility, and strength.[6] **Physical fitness** is the ability to perform moderate to vigorous physical activity on a regular basis without excessive fatigue. **Table 11.1** identifies the major health-related components of physical fitness.

If you want to become physically fit, you'll need to do more than make physically active lifestyle choices. You'll need to increase the frequency, intensity, and duration of your exercise. The Centers for Disease Control and Prevention (CDC) and American College of Sports Medicine (ACSM) recommend that adults engage in moderate-intensity physical activities for at least 30 minutes on most days of the week.[7] This amount of physical activity will not prepare you for running a marathon, but it can improve your overall health and can result in some cardiovascular improvements. The ACSM and CDC recommend that if you want to improve your cardiorespiratory fitness even more, you need to perform vigorous physical activities (for example, jogging or running, walking hills, circuit weight training, singles tennis) at least 3 days per week for at least 20 minutes at a time; if losing weight is your goal, you need to add to your daily routine moderate to vigorous exercise for 60 to 90 minutes.

Some people have physical limitations that make achieving these recommendations difficult, but they can still be physically active and reap the benefits of a regular exercise program. For example, a woman with arthritis in

physical fitness The ability to perform regular moderate to vigorous levels of physical activity without excessive fatigue.

cardiorespiratory fitness The ability of the heart, lungs, and blood vessels to supply oxygen to skeletal muscles during sustained physical activity.

the knee and hip joints might not be able to jog without extreme pain, but she can engage in water exercise in a swimming pool. The water will help relieve much of the stress on her joints, and she can improve her range of motion. Similarly, a man who uses a wheelchair may be unable to walk or run, but he can stay physically fit by playing wheelchair basketball.

Physical Activity for Performance

People who want to take their fitness level one step further can add exercise to improve performance. Specific programs can be designed to increase speed, strength, or overall performance. One example of a common activity used in performance training programs is plyometrics. *Plyometrics* are exercises that contract muscles in a certain order to increase power. An example of a plyometric activity is doing push-ups with a clap between each push-up. Plyometrics can help improve body control and the speed at which you physically change directions. Additionally, recreational exercisers and athletes alike utilize interval training to improve speed and cardiovascular fitness.

Performance training is meant for people who already have a high level of physical fitness and are training to enhance some aspect of their ability. Those who engage in this level of activity will achieve a high level of fitness but are also more prone to risk of injury and overtraining.

what do you THINK?

Which of the key aspects of physical fitness do you currently possess? ■ Which ones would you like to improve or develop? ■ What types of activities could you do to improve your fitness level?

Benefits of Regular Physical Activity

Regular physical activity has been shown to improve more than 50 different physiological, metabolic, and psychological aspects of human life.[8] **Figure 11.1** summarizes some of the major health-related benefits of regular physical activity and exercise.

Improved Cardiorespiratory Fitness

Cardiorespiratory fitness is the ability to perform exercise using large-muscle groups at moderate to high intensity for prolonged periods.[9] Because it requires the circulatory and respiratory systems to supply oxygen to the

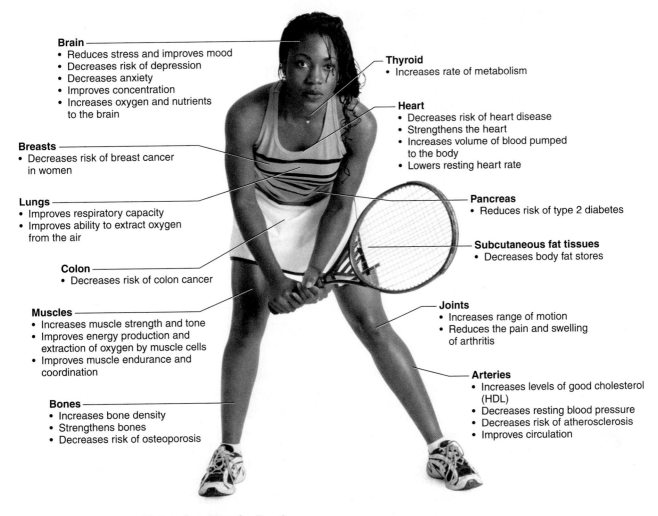

FIGURE 11.1 Some Health Benefits of Regular Exercise

Brain
- Reduces stress and improves mood
- Decreases risk of depression
- Decreases anxiety
- Improves concentration
- Increases oxygen and nutrients to the brain

Breasts
- Decreases risk of breast cancer in women

Lungs
- Improves respiratory capacity
- Improves ability to extract oxygen from the air

Colon
- Decreases risk of colon cancer

Muscles
- Increases muscle strength and tone
- Improves energy production and extraction of oxygen by muscle cells
- Improves muscle endurance and coordination

Bones
- Increases bone density
- Strengthens bones
- Decreases risk of osteoporosis

Thyroid
- Increases rate of metabolism

Heart
- Decreases risk of heart disease
- Strengthens the heart
- Increases volume of blood pumped to the body
- Lowers resting heart rate

Pancreas
- Reduces risk of type 2 diabetes

Subcutaneous fat tissues
- Decreases body fat stores

Joints
- Increases range of motion
- Reduces the pain and swelling of arthritis

Arteries
- Increases levels of good cholesterol (HDL)
- Decreases resting blood pressure
- Decreases risk of atherosclerosis
- Improves circulation

body during sustained physical activity, it is a good indicator of overall health. Low levels or cardiorespiratory fitness are associated with increased risk of premature death and disease.[10]

Regular exercise makes the circulatory and respiratory systems more efficient by enlarging the heart muscle, enabling more blood to be pumped with each stroke and increasing the number of *capillaries* (small blood vessels that allow gas exchange between blood and surrounding tissues) in trained skeletal muscles, which supply more blood to working muscles. Exercise also improves the respiratory system by increasing the amount of oxygen that is inhaled and distributed to body tissues.[11]

Reduced Risk of Heart Disease Your heart is a muscular organ made up of highly specialized tissue. Because muscles become stronger and more efficient with use, regular exercise strengthens the heart, which enables it to pump more blood with each beat. This increased efficiency means that the heart requires fewer beats per minute to circulate blood throughout the body. A stronger, more efficient heart is better able to meet the ordinary demands of life.

Prevention of Hypertension *Blood pressure* refers to the force exerted by blood against blood vessel walls, generated by the pumping action of the heart. *Hypertension,* the medical term for abnormally high blood pressure, is a significant risk factor for cardiovascular disease and stroke. Hypertension is particularly prevalent in adult African Americans. People with consistently elevated blood pressure are more susceptible to heart disease and die at a younger age than people with normal blood pressure.[12] Studies report that moderate exercise can reduce both diastolic and systolic blood pressure by 7 mm Hg.[13]

Improved Blood Lipid and Lipoprotein Profile Lipids are fats that circulate in the bloodstream and are stored in various places in the body. Regular exercise is known to increase the number of high-density lipoproteins (HDLs, or "good cholesterol") in the blood.[14] Higher HDL levels are associated with lower risk for artery disease because they remove some of the "bad" cholesterol from artery walls and hence prevent clogging. The bottom line: regular exercise lowers the risk of cardiovascular disease. (For more on cholesterol and blood pressure, see Chapter 12.)

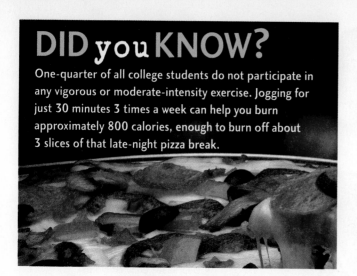

Source: American College Health Association, *American College Health Association–National College Health Assessment: Reference Group Data Report, Fall 2006* (Baltimore: American College Health Association, 2007).

Reduced Cancer Risk

Regular physical activity appears to lower the risk for some types of cancer. There is strong evidence that physical activity reduces the risk of breast cancer. Research on exercise and breast cancer risk has found that the earlier in life a woman starts to exercise, the lower the breast cancer risk.[15]

Regular exercise is also associated with lower risk for colon cancer. One theory is that exercise reduces colon cancer risk by increasing intestinal transit time. Experts say that because physical activity makes food move more quickly through your digestive system, there is less time for the body to absorb potential carcinogens and for potential carcinogens to be in contact with the digestive tract. Physical activity also decreases the levels of prostaglandins, substances found in cells of the large intestine that are implicated in cancer.[16]

Improved Bone Mass

A common affliction among older adults is **osteoporosis,** a disease characterized by low bone mass and deterioration of bone tissue, which increase fracture risk. Bone, like other human tissues, responds to the demands placed upon it. Women (and men) have much to gain by remaining physically active as they age—bone mass levels are significantly higher among active than among sedentary women.[17] New research indicates that by "surprising" bone (by jumping and other sudden activities), young children may improve their bone density.[18] Regular weight-bearing exercise, when

osteoporosis A disease characterized by low bone mass and deterioration of bone tissue, which increase risk of fracture.

combined with a balanced diet containing adequate calcium, helps keep bones healthy.[19]

Improved Weight Control

Many people start exercising because they want to lose weight. Level of physical activity has a direct effect on metabolic rate and can raise it for several hours following a vigorous workout. An effective method for losing weight combines regular endurance-type exercises with a moderate decrease in food intake (see Did You Know?). In addition to helping you lose weight, increased physical activity also improves your chances at keeping the weight off once you have lost it.[20]

The ACSM recommends 30 minutes of moderate physical activity daily with an intake between 1,500 to 2,000 calories per day.[21] Cutting daily caloric intake beyond this range ("severe dieting") actually decreases metabolic rate by up to 20 percent and makes weight loss more difficult. Although combining exercise and dietary changes works best for weight loss, research shows that exercise alone can reduce obesity. For example, in a study of obese men, those who exercised at a moderate intensity for 60 minutes 5 times a week with no dietary changes significantly decreased their body fat and increased muscle mass.[22] However, remember that if you want to lose weight only through physical activity, you will have to spend more time exercising than if you reduce your calories at the same time.

Can I lose weight with exercise alone?

Improved Health and Increased Life Span

Prevention of Diabetes Noninsulin-dependent diabetes (type 2 diabetes) is a complex disorder that affects millions of Americans, many of whom have no idea that they have the disease (see Chapter 12). Risk factors for this type of diabetes include obesity, high blood pressure, and high cholesterol, as well as a family history of the disease.[23] Physicians suggest exercise combined with weight loss and healthy diet to prevent diabetes. In a major national clinical trial, researchers found that exercising 150 minutes per week while eating fewer calories and less fat could prevent or delay the onset of type 2 diabetes.[24] Some researchers say that increasing physical activity is one of the most effective strategies both for preventing type 2 diabetes and for managing it once it is present.[25]

Longer Life Span Several large studies that followed groups of people over time found that those who exercised or were more fit lived longer.[26] In a study of over 5,000 middle-aged and older Americans, researchers found that those who had moderate to high levels of activity lived 1.3 to 3.7 years longer than those who got little exercise. Study subjects who exercised at a more intense level outlived sedentary subjects by 3.5 to 3.7 years.[27]

Improved Immunity to Disease Regular, consistent exercise promotes a healthy immune system. Research shows that moderate exercise gives the immune system a temporary boost in the production of the cells that attack bacteria.[28] But whereas moderate amounts of exercise can be beneficial, extreme exercise may actually be detrimental. For example, athletes engaging in marathon-type events or very intense physical training have an increased risk of colds and flu.[29]

Just how exercise alters immunity is not well understood. We do know that brisk exercise temporarily increases the number of white blood cells (WBCs), the blood cells responsible for fighting infection.[30] The largest changes in immunity are seen in people who are sedentary and begin a moderately energetic program. Because their fitness level is low when they embark on an exercise program, they gain a high number of WBCs. Interestingly, those who participate in regular, long-term heavy exercise, such as marathon runners, experience a decrease in their immune function. If you are feeling worn-down, your body could be trying to tell you to take a break and prevent overtraining.[31]

Improved Mental Health and Stress Management

People who engage in regular physical activity also notice psychological benefits. Regular vigorous exercise has been shown to "burn off" the chemical by-products of the stress response and increase endorphins, giving your mood a natural boost. Regular exercise improves a person's physical appearance by toning and developing muscles and reducing body fat. Feeling good about personal appearance boosts self-esteem. At the same time, as exercisers come to appreciate the improved strength, skills, and flexibility that accompany fitness, they often become less obsessed with physical appearance.[32]

what do you THINK?

Among the many benefits to be derived from physical activity, which two are most important to you? Why? ■ After exercising regularly for several weeks, what benefits do you notice?

Improving Cardiorespiratory Fitness

There are many options for improving cardiorespiratory fitness. Swimming, cycling, jogging, and in-line skating are just a few options for **aerobic exercise.** The term *aerobic* means "with oxygen" and describes any type of exercise, typically

performed at moderate levels of intensity for extended periods of time, that increases your heart rate. A person said to be in good shape has an above-average **aerobic capacity**—a term used to describe the functional status of the cardiorespiratory system (heart, lungs, and blood vessels). Aerobic capacity (commonly written as $\dot{V}O_2$max) is defined as the maximum volume of oxygen consumed by the muscles during exercise.

To measure your maximal aerobic capacity, an exercise physiologist or physician will typically perform a **graded exercise test** (sometimes called a *stress test*). This is a diagnostic exam used to evaluate your level of fitness, heart rate, and blood pressure response to activity and the adequacy of blood supply to your heart. The test is performed on a treadmill or stationary bicycle. Participants start out slowly and gradually increase the speed, resistance, or elevation. Generally, the higher your cardiorespiratory endurance level, the more oxygen you can transport to exercising muscles and the longer you can exercise without becoming exhausted. In other words, the higher the $\dot{V}O_2$max value, the higher your level of aerobic fitness.

You can test your own cardiorespiratory fitness by using either the 1.5-mile walk or run endurance test described in the **Assess Yourself** box on page 326. However, do not take this test if you are just starting to exercise. Progress slowly through a walking/jogging program at low intensities before measuring your fitness with one of these tests. If you have any medical conditions, such as asthma, diabetes, heart disease, or obesity, consult your physician before beginning any exercise program.

Aerobic Fitness Programs

The most beneficial aerobic exercises are total body activities involving all the large muscle groups of your body, for example, swimming, cross-country skiing, and rowing. If you have been sedentary for quite a while, simply initiating a physical activity program may be the hardest task you'll face. The key is to begin at a very low intensity, progress slowly, and stay with it!

There are three main dimensions to an aerobic exercise program: frequency, intensity, and duration. The characteristics of these dimensions vary by individual exercise goal and beginning fitness level. These same dimensions also apply to

(Text continues on page 328.)

---

aerobic exercise Any type of exercise that increases heart rate.

aerobic capacity The current functional status of a person's cardiovascular system; measured as $\dot{V}O_2$max.

graded exercise test A test of aerobic capacity administered by a physician, exercise physiologist, or other trained person; two common forms are the treadmill running test and the stationary bike test.

ASSESS yourself

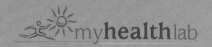

HOW PHYSICALLY FIT ARE YOU?

Fill out this assessment online at
www.aw-bc.com/myhealthlab or
www.aw-bc.com/donatelle.

EVALUATING YOUR MUSCULAR ENDURANCE (THE 1-MINUTE SIT-UP TEST)

Abdominal muscle strength and endurance are important for core stability and back support. This sit-up test measures the strength and endurance of your abdominals and hip flexor muscles.

Description/Procedure

Lie on a carpeted or cushioned floor with your knees bent at approximately right angles and your feet flat on the ground. Rest your hands on your thighs. Squeeze your stomach, push your back flat, and raise yourself high enough for your hands to slide along your thighs to touch the tops of your knees. Don't pull with your neck or head, and keep your lower back on the floor. Then return to the starting position. Have a partner time you and count how many sit-ups you can do in 1 minute.

Fitness Category	Age 18–25	Age 26–35	Age 36–45	Age 46–55	Age 56–65	Age 65+
Men						
Excellent	>49	>45	>41	>35	>31	>28
Good	44–49	40–45	35–41	29–35	25–31	22–28
Above average	39–43	35–39	30–34	25–28	21–24	19–21
Average	35–38	31–34	27–29	22–24	17–20	15–18
Below average	31–34	29–30	23–26	18–21	13–16	11–14
Poor	25–30	22–28	17–22	13–17	9–12	7–10
Very poor	<25	<22	<17	<9	<9	<7
Women						
Excellent	>43	>39	>33	>27	>24	>23
Good	37–43	33–39	27–33	22–27	18–24	17–23
Above average	33–36	29–32	23–26	18–21	13–17	14–16
Average	29–32	25–28	19–22	14–17	10–12	11–13
Below average	25–28	21–24	15–18	10–13	7–9	5–10
Poor	18–24	13–20	7–14	5–9	3–6	2–4
Very poor	<18	<20	<7	<5	<3	<2

Source: Golding et al., *The Y's Way to Physical Fitness, 1991.*

EVALUATING YOUR FLEXIBILITY (THE SIT-AND-REACH TEST)

This test measures the flexibility of the lower back and hamstring muscles.

Description/Procedure

Sit on the floor with your legs straight out in front of you, toes pointed up. Place a yardstick between your feet on the floor so that the 23 cm mark is at your heels. Hold your knees flat against the floor. With hands on top of each other and palms facing down, reach forward along the measure of the yardstick, as far as possible. Take three practice stretches. On the fourth stretch, hold for 2 seconds, and record the distance you reach. Make sure that you make no jerky movements and that your fingertips remain level and your legs flat. Record the score to the nearest centimeter as the distance before (negative) or beyond (positive) the toes. (Because your toes are at the 23 cm mark, you need to subtract 23 from your measurement to calculate your score.) The table below gives you a guide for expected scores (in cm.).

Flexibility Level	Men	Women
Super	> +27	> +30
Excellent	+17 to +27	+21 to +30
Good	+6 to +16	+11 to +20
Average	0 to +5	+1 to +10
Fair	−8 to −1	−7 to 0
Poor	−19 to −9	−14 to −8
Very poor	< −20	< −15

EVALUATING YOUR CARDIORESPIRATORY ENDURANCE

This test assesses your cardiorespiratory endurance level.

Description/Procedure

Find a local track, typically one-quarter mile per lap, to perform your test. You may either *run or walk* for 1.5 miles; use a stopwatch to measure how long it takes to reach that distance. If you become extremely fatigued during the test, slow your pace or walk—do not overstress yourself! If you feel faint or nauseated or experience any unusual pains in your upper body, stop and notify your instructor. Use the following chart to estimate your cardiorespiratory fitness level based on your age and sex. Note that women have lower standards for each fitness category because they have higher levels of essential fat than men do.

Fitness Category	Age 18–29	Age 30–39	Age 40–49	Age 50+
Men				
Good	<11:27	<12:06	<12:32	<13:50
Adequate	11:28–12:58	12:07–13:37	12:33–14:03	13:25–15:21
Borderline	12:59–13:25	13:38–14:04	14:04–14:30	14:56–15:48
Poor	>13:25	>14:04	>14:30	>15:22
Women				
Good	<13.24	<14.03	<14:29	<15:21
Adequate	13:25–14:55	14:04–15:21	14:30–15:47	15:22–16:39
Borderline	14:56–15:22	15.22–15:48	15:48–16:14	16:40–17:06
Poor	>15:22	>15:48	>16:14	>17:06

Source: From E. T. Howley and B. D. Franks, *Health Fitness Instructor's Handbook*, 4th ed., p. 75, table 5.2. Copyright © 2003 by Edward T. Howley and B. Don Franks. Reprinted with permission from Human Kinetics (Champaign, IL).

MAKE it happen!

ASSESSMENT: Complete the Assess Yourself activity to determine your current fitness levels. Your results may indicate that you should take steps to improve one or more components of your physical fitness.

MAKING A CHANGE: To change your behavior, you need to develop a plan. Follow these steps below and complete your Behavior Change Contract to take action.

1. Evaluate your behavior, and identify patterns and specific things you are doing. What can you change now? What can you change in the near future?

2. Select one pattern of behavior that you want to change.

3. Fill out the Behavior Change Contract found at the front of your book. It should include your long-term goals for change, your short-term goals, the rewards you'll give yourself for reaching these goals, potential obstacles along the way, and strategies for overcoming these obstacles. For each goal, list the small steps and specific actions that you will take.

4. Chart your progress in a journal. At the end of a week, consider how successful you were in following your plan. What helped you be successful? What made change more difficult? What will you do differently next week?

5. Revise your plan as needed. Are the short-term goals attainable? Are the rewards satisfying?

EXAMPLE: Chris was dissatisfied with his scores on the various fitness assessments—he'd scored average on muscular endurance, but only fair on flexibility and borderline on cardiorespiratory endurance. Chris had played sports throughout high school and had considered himself to be in good physical shape. However, he realized he had stopped exercising regularly in his freshman year of college when he didn't make the baseball team.

Chris decided to start by incorporating more activity into his daily routine. He tended to drive even to places that he could walk or bicycle to as easily. His friends had invited him to join in the pick-up basketball games they played on Saturday afternoons, but he had turned them down to play video games with his roommate. Chris filled out a Behavior Change Contract with a goal to ride his bicycle the 3 miles to and from campus three times a week and to play basketball every Saturday. He also set a goal to stretch before each of these activities. If he did this consistently every week, he would reward himself with a new CD. After a month of this increased activity, Chris was already feeling more fit and was ready to add another aerobic activity. With winter weather coming, he thought he should add an indoor activity, so he started swimming laps at the school pool. He found swimming boring, so when he realized he was making excuses not to go, Chris switched to using a stair-climbing machine, which he could do while reading *Sports Illustrated* or watching ESPN. He was able to stick to doing this 3 times a week and made a commitment to go a fourth time whenever he missed his Saturday basketball game.

	Cardiorespiratory endurance	Strength	Flexibility
Frequency	3–5 days a week	2–3 nonconsecutive days a week	Minimum of 2–3 days a week
Intensity	55/65–90% of maximum heart rate	70–85% of maximal resistance. Sufficient resistance to enhance strength and endurance	Sufficient to develop and maintain full range of motion
Time	20–60 minutes continuous aerobic activity	1 or more sets (8–12 repetitions) of 8–10 exercises conditioning all the major muscle groups	2–4 repetitions of each stretch held for 15–30 seconds
Type	Continuous aerobic activity that uses large-muscle groups	Resistance exercises in a full range of motion for all major muscle groups	Stretching for all major joints and muscle groups

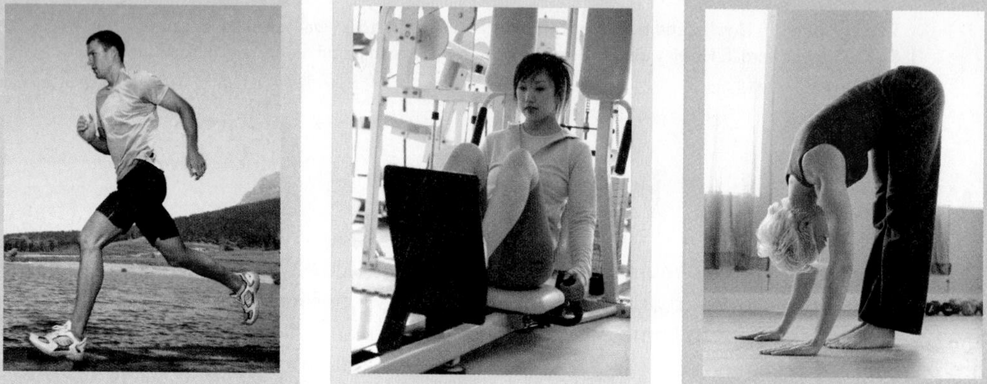

FIGURE 11.2 The FITT Principle Applied to the Health-Related Components of Fitness

Source: Adapted from "Position Stand on the Recommended Quantity and Quality of Exercise for Developing and Maintaining Cardiorespiratory and Muscular Fitness, and Flexibility in Healthy Adults," *Medicine and Science in Sports and Exercise* 30, no. 6 (1998): 975–91. Copyright © 1998 American College of Sports Medicine.

the other components of fitness: muscular strength, muscular endurance, and flexibility. You can remember them with the acronym FITT, which stands for *frequency, intensity, time (duration),* and *type* of activity. **Figure 11.2** shows how the FITT principle can be applied to the different fitness components.

Determining Exercise Frequency To best improve your cardiovascular endurance, you will need to exercise vigorously at least 3 times a week. If you are a newcomer to exercise, you can still make improvements by doing less intense exercise but doing it more days a week, following the recommendations from the Centers for Disease Control and Prevention and the American College of Sports Medicine for moderate physical activity at least 5 days a week.

Determining Exercise Intensity There are several ways to measure exercise intensity. One of the main ways is using your **target heart rate zone.** To calculate target heart zone, start by subtracting your age from 220 to find your maximum heart rate. Your target heart zone is a certain range of this maximum heart rate. For moderate-intensity physical activity, you should work out at 50 to 70 percent of your maximum heart rate. Thus, if you are 20 years old, your 50 percent target heart zone would be:

$$(220 - 20) \times 0.50, \text{ or } 100 \text{ beats per minute (bpm)}$$

To determine 70 percent of a 20-year-old's maximum heart rate, you would use the following calculations:

$$(220 - 20) \times 0.70, \text{ or } 140 \text{ beats per minute}$$

target heart rate zone Calculated as a percentage of maximum heart rate (220 minus age); heart rate (pulse) is taken during aerobic exercise to check whether exercise intensity is at the desired level (e.g., 60 percent of maximum heart rate).

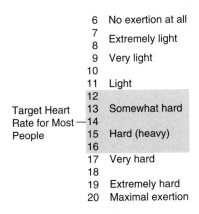

	6 No exertion at all
	7
	Extremely light
	8
	9 Very light
	10
	11 Light
	12
Target Heart	13 Somewhat hard
Rate for Most —	14
People	15 Hard (heavy)
	16
	17 Very hard
	18
	19 Extremely hard
	20 Maximal exertion

FIGURE 11.3 Rating of Perceived Exertion (RPE) Scale

Source: Borg-RPE-scale ® from G. Borg,(1998), *Borg's Perceived Exertion and Pain Scales.* Champaign, IL: Human Kinetics. © Gunnar Borg, 1970, 1985, 1994, 1998. Used with permission of Dr. G. Borg. For correct usage of the scale the exact design and instructions given in Borg's folders must be followed: The BORG-RPE SCALE ®, a method for measuring perceived exertion. © G. Borg, 1994, 2003. Order folders and scales from: Borg Products, Inc., "BPU," Joseph V. Myers III, 1579F, Monroe Drive, #416, Atlanta, GA 30324.

Thus, for a moderately intense cardiovascular workout, a 20-year-old would try to maintain aerobic exercise at an intensity of 100 to 140 beats per minute, or 50 to 70 percent of his or her maximum heart rate.

For more vigorous activities (e.g., running), aim for 70 to 85 percent of your maximum heart rate. People in poor physical condition should set a target heart rate between 40 and 50 percent of maximum and gradually increase the target rate in 5 percent increments.

Once you know your target heart zone, you can take your pulse to determine how close you are to this value during your workout. As you exercise, lightly place your index and middle fingers (don't use your thumb) on your radial artery (inside your wrist, on the thumb side). Using a watch or clock, take your pulse for 6 seconds, and multiply this number by 10 (just add a zero to your count) to get the number of beats per minute. Your pulse should be within a range of 5 beats per minute above or below your target heart rate. If necessary, adjust the pace or intensity of your workout to achieve your target heart rate.

Another way of determining intensity is to use the Borg rating of perceived exertion (RPE) scale **(Figure 11.3).** Perceived exertion is how hard you feel you are working, based on your heart rate, increased breathing rate, sweating, and muscle fatigue. This scale uses a rating from 6 (no exertion at all) to 20 (maximal exertion). This method corresponds to heart rate for most people. Experts agree that RPE ratings of 12 to 14 correspond to moderate-intensity activity and 15 to 17 for vigorous activity.

The easiest, but least scientific, method of measuring exercise intensity is the "talk test." If you are exercising moderately, you should be able to carry on a conversation

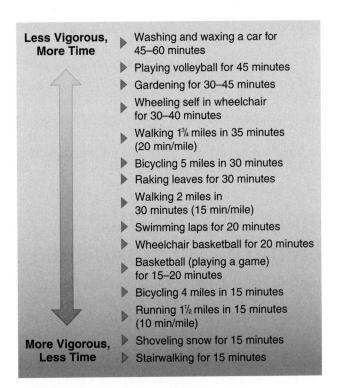

FIGURE 11.4 Levels of Physical Activity
A moderate amount of physical activity is roughly equivalent to physical activity that uses about 150 calories of energy per day, or 1,000 calories per week. Some activities can be performed at various intensities; the suggested durations correspond to expected intensity effort.

Source: Adapted from National Center for Chronic Disease Prevention and Health Promotion, *Physical Activity and Health: A Report of the Surgeon General* (Washington, DC: National Center for Chronic Disease Prevention and Health Promotion, 1996).

comfortably. If you are too out of breath to carry on a conversation, you are exercising vigorously.

Determining Exercise Duration Duration refers to the number of minutes of activity performed during any one session. Vigorous activities should be performed for at least 20 minutes at a time, and moderate activities for at least 30 minutes at a time.

The lower the intensity of your activity, the longer the duration you'll need to get the same caloric expenditure. The numbers of calories burned is higher for a person who weighs more than for someone who weighs less.[33] Aim to expend 300 to 500 calories per exercise session, with an eventual weekly goal of 1,500 to 2,000 calories. As you progress, add to your exercise load by increasing duration or intensity, but not both at the same time. From week to week, don't increase duration or intensity by more than 10 percent.

Many of the health benefits associated with cardio-respiratory fitness (such as lower blood pressure) may take several months to achieve; don't expect improvements overnight.[34] However, any physical activity of low to moderate intensity will benefit your overall health almost from the start **(Figure 11.4).**

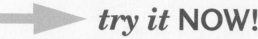

try it NOW!

Calculate your target heart rate zone. Use the formula in this chapter to calculate your maximum heart rate. Then, decide what intensity of exercise would best suit your fitness level—for example, 60, 70, or 80 percent of your maximum heart rate—and calculate your target heart rate zone. Next time you exercise, check your pulse periodically to see whether you are in your target zone.

Improving Muscular Strength and Endurance

To get a sense of what resistance training is about, do a resistance exercise. Start by holding your right arm straight down by your side, then turn your hand palm up and bring it up toward your shoulder. That's a resistance exercise: using a muscle, your biceps, to move a resistance, in this case just the weight of your hand—not very much resistance. Resistance training usually involves more weight or tension than this. Free weights, such as dumbbells and barbells, and all sorts of tension-producing machines are usually part of resistance training. It's not just bodybuilding that uses this type of exercise, either: fitness programs and many sports employ resistance training to improve strength and endurance. Also, resistance exercises are an integral part of rehabilitation programs to help patients recover from muscle and joint injury. Many college students are incorporating strengthening exercises into their physical fitness program. In a recent survey, 38 percent of college aged men and 26 percent of women reported doing exercises to strengthen or tone muscles at least 3 times a week.[35]

Strength and Endurance

In the field of resistance training, **muscular strength** refers to the amount of force a muscle or group of muscles is capable of exerting. The most common way to assess strength in a resistance exercise program is to measure the

one repetition maximum (1 RM), which is the maximum amount of weight a person can move one time (and no more) in a particular exercise. For example, 1 RM for the simple exercise done at the beginning of this section is the maximum weight you can lift to your shoulder one time. To calculate your maximum, begin with a weight that you can lift easily. Rest for 2 to 3 minutes between lifts, and then add 5 to 10 pounds of weight until you can no longer complete a successful lift. This muscle strength assessment is a good way to help create an effective weight-training program and monitor progress.

Muscular endurance is the ability of muscle to exert force repeatedly without fatiguing. If you can perform the exercise described earlier holding a 5-pound weight in your hand and lifting 10 times, you will have greater endurance than someone who attempts that same exercise but is able to lift the weight only seven times. There are two categories of muscle endurance. The first is static muscular endurance, or a force that is held as long as possible. An example of static abdominal endurance would be a measure of how long you can hold a double leg lift. The second is dynamic muscular endurance, or maximum repetitions completed at a determined rate. Timed sit-up or push-up tests are examples of dynamic muscle endurance (see the Assess Yourself box on page 326).

Principles of Strength Development

An effective **resistance exercise program** involves three key principles: tension, overload, and specificity of training.[36]

The Tension Principle The key to developing strength is to create tension within a muscle or group of muscles. Tension is created by resistance, provided by weights such as barbells or dumbbells, specially designed machines, or the weight of the body.

The Overload Principle The overload principle is the most important of our three key principles. Overload doesn't mean forcing a muscle or group of muscles to do too much, which could result in injuries. Rather, overload in resistance training requires muscles to do more than they are used to doing. Everyone begins a resistance-training program with an initial level of strength. To become stronger, you must regularly create a degree of tension in your muscles that is greater than you are accustomed to. This overload will cause your muscles to adapt to a new level. As your muscles respond to a regular program of overloading by getting larger, they become stronger.

Resistance-training exercises cause microscopic damage (tears) to muscle fibers, and the rebuilding process that increases the size and capacity of the muscle takes 24 to 48 hours. Thus, resistance-training exercise programs should

---

muscular strength The amount of force that a muscle is capable of exerting.

one repetition maximum (1 RM) The amount of weight or resistance that can be lifted or moved once, but not twice; a common measure of strength.

muscular endurance A muscle's ability to exert force repeatedly without fatiguing.

resistance exercise program A regular program of exercises designed to improve muscular strength and endurance in the major muscle groups.

include at least one day of rest and recovery between workouts before you overload the same muscles again.

The Specificity-of-Training Principle
According to the specificity principle, the effects of resistance exercise training are specific to the muscles being exercised. Only the muscle or muscle group that you exercise responds to the demands placed on it. For example, if you regularly do curls, the muscles involved—your biceps—will become larger and stronger, but the other muscles in your body won't change. It is important to note that if you exercise only certain muscle groups, you may put opposing muscle groups at increased risk for injury. For example, overworking your quadriceps muscles but neglecting your hamstrings can put you at risk for a hamstring muscle pull or strain.

Gender Differences in Weight Training

The results of resistance training in men and women are quite different. Women normally don't develop muscles to the same extent that men do. The main reason for this difference is that men and women have different levels of the hormone testosterone in their blood. Before puberty, testosterone levels are similar for both boys and girls. During adolescence, testosterone levels in boys increase dramatically (about tenfold) whereas testosterone levels in girls remain unchanged. Muscles will become larger (**hypertrophy**) as a result of resistance-training exercise, but typically this change is less dramatic in women because of their lower testosterone levels. To enhance muscle bulk, some bodybuilders (both men and women) take synthetic hormones (anabolic steroids) that mimic the effects of testosterone. However, using anabolic steroids is a dangerous and illegal practice (see Chapter 7).

Types of Muscle Activity

In the past, the term *contraction* was used to define the tension a muscle produces as it shortens. Because tension develops as muscles contract, the term *muscle action* is a better descriptor. Skeletal muscle actions fall into three different categories: isometric, concentric, and eccentric.[37] In **isometric muscle action** force is produced through tension and muscle contraction, not through movement. A **concentric muscle action** causes joint movement and a production of force while the muscle shortens. The empty-hand curl we did at the beginning of this section is a concentric exercise, with joint movement occurring at the elbow. In general, concentric muscle actions produce movement in a direction opposite to the downward pull of gravity.[38]

Eccentric muscle action describes the ability of a muscle to produce force while lengthening. Typically, eccentric muscle actions occur when movement is in the same direction as the pull of gravity. Once you've brought a weight up during a curl, lowering your hand and the weight back to their original position is an eccentric muscle action.

Methods of Providing Resistance

What types of exercises can I do to improve my muscular strength?

There are four commonly used resistance exercise methods: body weight resistance and fixed, variable, and accommodating resistance devices.

Body Weight Resistance (Calisthenics)
Strength and endurance training don't have to rely on equipment. You can use your own body weight to develop skeletal muscle fitness. Calisthenics (such as pull-ups or push-ups) use part or all of your body weight to offer resistance during exercise. Although they are less effective than other resistance methods in developing large muscle mass and strength, calisthenics improve general muscular fitness and muscle tone and maintain a level of muscular strength.

Fixed Resistance
Fixed resistance exercises provide a constant amount of resistance throughout the full range of movement. Free weights, such as barbells and dumbbells, and some machines provide fixed resistance because their weight, or the amount of resistance, does not change during an exercise. Fixed resistance equipment has the potential to strengthen all the major muscle groups in the body.

There are several advantages of using free weights. First, free weights require more balance and coordination. Also, free weights tend to recruit more muscle groups for action and promote more activity of the joint and stabilizer muscles. From a financial perspective, free weights are relatively inexpensive and can provide a great muscle workout.

Variable Resistance
Variable resistance equipment alters the resistance a muscle encounters during a movement, so that the muscle's effort is more consistent throughout the full range of motion. Variable resistance equipment provides a more controlled motion and specifically isolates certain muscle groups, and it is often used for rehabilitation of muscle injuries. Some of these machines are expensive and too big to move easily, but others are affordable and more portable. Many forms of variable resistance devices are sold for home use.

---

hypertrophy   Increased size (girth) of a muscle.

isometric muscle action   Force produced without any resulting joint movement.

concentric muscle action   Force produced while the muscle is shortening.

eccentric muscle action   Force produced while the muscle is lengthening.

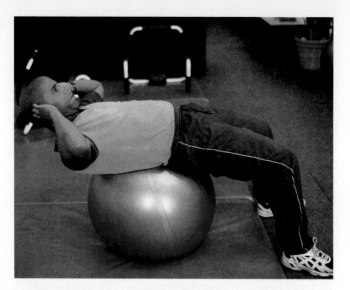
An exercise ball is one type of equipment that is excellent for increasing core body strength.

Accommodating Resistance Devices

Accommodating resistance devices, sometimes called isokinetic machines, maintain a constant speed through the range of motion. The exerciser performs at maximal level of effort while the device controls the speed of the exercise. The machine is set to a particular speed, and muscles being exercised must move at a rate faster than or equal to that speed to encounter resistance. These machines are often used in rehabilitation settings, but many health clubs have them, as well.

Core Strength Training

The body's core muscles are the foundation for movement. These muscles are the deep back and abdominal muscles that attach to the spine and pelvis. The contraction of these muscles provides the basis of support for movements of the upper and lower body and powerful movements of the extremities. A weak core increases your chances for poor posture, lower back pain, and muscle injuries. A strong core gives you a more stable center of gravity and a more stable platform for movements, thus reducing the chance of injury.

You can develop core strength by simple calisthenics, using fitness equipment such as a fitness ball, or taking an exercise class such as yoga or Pilates. Holding yourself in a plank, or "up" push-up, position and doing abdominal curl-ups are two examples of calisthenic exercises to increase core strength. Also, exercising with a fitness ball requires using core muscles for support.

Experts recommend doing core strengthening activities at least 3 times per week.[39] It's a good idea to get started with

flexibility The measure of the range of motion, or the amount of movement possible, at a particular joint.

the help of a professional (e.g., personal trainer or physical therapist), because body alignment and positioning are crucial.

Benefits of Strength Training

Does strength training offer any benefits beyond simply getting stronger? Indeed, regular strength training can reduce the occurrence of lower back pain and joint and muscle injuries. It can also postpone loss of muscle tissue due to aging and a sedentary lifestyle and help prevent osteoporosis.

Strength training enhances muscle definition and tone and improves personal appearance. This, in turn, enhances self-esteem. Strength training even has a hidden benefit: muscle tissue burns calories faster than most other tissues do, even when it is resting—so increasing your muscle mass can help you boost your metabolism and maintain a healthy weight.

Improving Flexibility
Stretching Exercises and Well-Being

Who would guess that improved flexibility can give you a sense of well-being, help you deal with stress better, and stop your joints from hurting as much as they used to? Stretching exercises are the main way to improve **flexibility,** a measure of the range of motion, or the amount of movement possible, at a particular joint. Improving the range of motion enhances efficiency, extent of movement, and posture. Today, stretching exercises are extremely popular, both because they are effective and because people can begin them at virtually any age and enjoy them for a lifetime. Flexibility exercises have been shown to be effective in reducing the incidence and severity of lower back problems and muscle or tendon injuries. Improved flexibility also means less tension and pressure on joints, resulting in less joint pain and joint deterioration.[40] See the Assess Yourself box on page 326 for one way to measure your own flexibility.

Flexibility is enhanced by the controlled stretching of muscles and muscle attachments that act on a particular joint. Each muscle involved in a stretching exercise is attached to our skeleton by tendons. The goal of stretching is to decrease the resistance of a muscle and its tendons to tension, that is, to reduce resistance to being stretched. Stretching exercises gradually result in greater flexibility. They involve stretching a muscle or group of muscles to a point of slight discomfort and holding that position for up to 30 seconds or more. For many people, a regular program of stretching exercises enhances psychological as well as physical well-being.

Types of Stretching Exercises

Static stretching techniques involve the slow, gradual stretching of muscles and their tendons, then holding them at a point. During this holding period—the stretch—participants may feel mild discomfort and a warm sensation in the stretched muscles. Static stretching exercises involve specialized tension receptors in our muscles. When done properly, these exercises slightly lessen the sensitivity of tension receptors, which allows the muscle to relax and be stretched to greater length.[41] The stretch is followed by a slow return to the starting position. As discussed in the next section, the physical aspect of yoga and tai chi is largely composed of static techniques, as are some of the exercises in Pilates programs.

Dynamic stretching is a technique that has recently been deemed an effective way of preparing muscles for intense aerobic activity, such as running, soccer, or dance.[42] Dynamic stretching technique involves moving parts of your body and gradually increasing reach, speed of movement, or both. This is not to be confused with the old stretching exercises, popular decades ago, that promoted bouncy, jerky movements. Dynamic stretching consists of controlled leg and arm swings that take you (gently!) to the limits of your range of motion. An example of dynamic stretching would be slow, controlled leg swings, arm swings, or torso twists.[43]

Yoga, Tai Chi, and Pilates

Three major styles of exercise that include stretching have become widely practiced in the United States and other Western countries: yoga, tai chi, and Pilates. All three emphasize a joining of mind and body as a result of intense concentration on breathing and body position. As mentioned earlier in the section on strength training, these styles of exercise are also an excellent way to improve core body strength.

Yoga One of the most popular fitness and static stretching activities, **yoga** originated in India about 5,000 years ago. Yoga blends the mental and physical aspects of exercise, a union of mind and body that participants find relaxing and satisfying. Done regularly, its combination of mental focus and physical effort improves flexibility, vitality, posture, agility, and coordination.

The practice of yoga focuses attention on controlled breathing as well as purely physical exercise. In addition to its mental dimensions, yoga incorporates a complex array of static stretching exercises expressed as postures (*asanas*). Over 200 postures exist, but only about 50 are commonly practiced. During a session, participants move to different asanas and hold them for 30 seconds or more. Yoga not only enhances flexibility, but also has the great advantage of being flexible itself. Asanas and combinations of asanas can be changed and adjusted for young and old and to accommodate

TABLE 11.2	Popular Yoga Styles

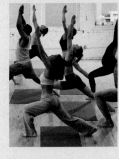

- **Iyengar yoga** focuses on precision and alignment in the poses. Standing poses are basic to this style and are often held longer than in other styles.
- **Ashtanga yoga** in its pure form is based on a specific flow of poses with an emphasis on strength and agility that creates internal heat. *Power yoga*, a style growing in popularity, is a derivative of ashtanga yoga.
- **Bikram yoga**, or hot yoga, is similar to power yoga but does not incorporate a specific flow of poses. Literally the hottest yoga going, it is performed in temperatures of 100°F, or even a bit higher. Proponents say that the heat increases the body's ability to move and stretch without injury.

people with physical limitations or disabilities. Asanas can also be combined to provide even conditioned athletes with challenging sessions.

A typical yoga session will move the spine and joints through their full range of motion. Yoga postures lengthen, strengthen, and balance musculature, leading to increased flexibility, stamina, and strength—and many people report a psychological sense of general well-being too. **Table 11.2** details three popular styles of yoga.

Tai chi **Tai chi** is an ancient Chinese form of exercise that, like yoga, combines stretching, balance, coordination, and meditation. It is designed to increase range of motion and flexibility while reducing muscular tension. Based on Chi Kung, a Taoist philosophy dedicated to spiritual growth and good health, tai chi was developed about AD 1000 by monks to defend themselves against bandits and warlords.

static stretching Techniques that gradually lengthen a muscle to an elongated position (to the point of discomfort) and hold that position for 10 to 30 seconds.

dynamic stretching Moving parts of your body in a gradual and controlled manner, taking you to the limits of your range of motion.

yoga A variety of Indian traditions geared toward self-discipline and the realization of unity; includes forms of exercise widely practiced in the West today that promote balance, coordination, flexibility, and meditation through postures and breathing exercises.

tai chi An ancient Chinese form of exercise, originally developed as a martial art, that promotes balance, coordination, flexibility, and stress reduction through a series of flowing postures and movements.

It involves a series of positions called *forms* that are performed continuously. Both yoga and tai chi are excellent for improving flexibility and muscular coordination.

Pilates Compared to yoga and tai chi, **Pilates** is the new kid on the exercise block. It was developed by Joseph Pilates, who came from Germany to New York City in 1926. Shortly after his arrival, he introduced his exercise methodology, which emphasizes flexibility, coordination, strength, and tone. Pilates combines stretching with movement against resistance, which is aided by devices such as tension springs or heavy rubber bands.

Pilates differs from yoga and tai chi because it includes a component designed to increase strength. The method consists of a sequence of carefully performed movements. Some are carried out on specially designed equipment, whereas others are performed on mats. Each exercise stretches and strengthens the muscles involved and has a specific breathing pattern associated with it. A Pilates class focuses on strengthening specific muscle groups, using equipment that provides resistance.

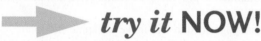

try it NOW!

Give yourself a break, and stretch. Stretching and improved flexibility are just as important in the classroom and library as they are in the gym. Sitting hunched over a pile of books for an extended period of time can be a pain in the neck! When studying, be sure to stretch every 20 minutes or so by doing shoulder rolls, shrugs, and neck stretches to help work out the kinks. These mini-stretch breaks will ease your muscles and your mind.

Body Composition

Body composition is the fourth and final component of a comprehensive fitness program. Body composition describes the relative proportions of lean tissue (muscle, bone, water, organs) and fat tissue in the body. Body composition parameters that can be influenced by regular physical activity include total body mass, fat mass, fat-free mass, and regional fat distribution. Aerobic activities that improve cardiovascular endurance also help improve body composition because they expend calories and contribute to weight loss and help with weight loss maintenance.

There are many ways to assess body composition. These range from simple (e.g., height–weight charts) to complex (e.g., underwater weighing). See the section on assessing fat levels in Chapter 10.

Pilates Exercise program developed by Joseph Pilates that combines stretching with movement against resistance, aided by devices such as tension springs and heavy rubber bands.

Creating Your Own Fitness Program

Identifying Your Fitness Goals

The first step in creating your fitness program is to identify your fitness goals. Do you want to improve your quality of life? Lose weight? Train for an upcoming 5K race? Think about a timeline for your goals. Do you want to be able to jog 3 miles before spring break? Hike across campus next semester with a heavy backpack and not be out of breath? Once you develop a specific goal, you can create a plan to help you achieve that goal.

When you become committed to regular physical activity and exercise, you will observe gradual improvements in your functional abilities and note progress toward your goals. Perhaps your most vital goal will be to become committed to fitness for the long haul—to establish a realistic schedule of diverse exercise activities that you can maintain and enjoy throughout your life.

Designing Your Program

How can I go about developing a fitness plan?

Now that you know the fundamentals of fitness, you can design your own personalized fitness program. There are several factors to consider that will boost your chances of successfully achieving your fitness goal. First, choose an activity that is appropriate for you. For example, don't plan on swimming if the pool is difficult to access. Choose activities that you like to do. If you hate to run, don't choose running as your exercise. Be creative in your activity choice; try something new! There are many different classes (e.g., salsa aerobics, boot camp classes) that can keep you motivated—and if you don't like one activity, you can always try another.

Your plan should include very specific ways to incorporate physical activity into your lifestyle. When will you exercise? For how long? At what intensity? How often? As you make specific goals for yourself, keep in mind the FITT principle and the recommendations in Figure 11.2 on page 328.

It is best to write out your exercise goals and plans and to put them in your daily planner as you would any other scheduled activity. Lack of time is the number-one reason given for not exercising. By looking at your weekly schedule, you can identify segments of time that work for you.

Reevaluate your fitness goal and action plan after 30 days. This time period should give you a good idea of whether or not the program is working for you. Make changes if necessary, and then make a plan to reevaluate after another 30-day period. See the **Skills for Behavior Change** box for more tips on starting and maintaining an exercise plan.

(Text continues on page 336.)

SKILLS FOR behavior change

ESTABLISHING AND MAINTAINING A SUCCESSFUL EXERCISE PROGRAM

STARTING AN EXERCISE ROUTINE

The most successful exercise program is one that is realistic and appropriate for your skill level and needs. Be realistic about the amount of time you will need to get into good physical condition. Perhaps the most significant factor early in an exercise program is personal comfort. Experiment and find an activity that you truly enjoy. Be open to exploring new activities and new exercise equipment.

- *Start slowly.* For the sedentary, first-time exerciser, any type and amount of physical activity will be a step in the right direction. If you are extremely overweight or out of condition, you might only be able to walk for 5 minutes at a time. Don't be discouraged; you're on your way!
- *Make only one life change at a time.* Success with one major behavioral change will encourage you to make other positive changes.
- *Set reasonable expectations for yourself and your fitness program.* Many people become exercise dropouts because their expectations were too high to begin with. Allow sufficient time to reach your fitness goals.
- *Choose a specific time to exercise, and stick with it.* Learning to establish priorities and keeping to a schedule are vital steps toward improved fitness. Experiment by exercising at different times of the day to learn what schedule works best for you.
- *Make exercise a positive habit.* Usually, if you are able to practice a desired activity for 3 weeks, you will be able to incorporate it into your lifestyle.
- *Keep a record of your progress.* Include various facts about your physical activities (duration, intensity), and chronicle your emotions and personal achievements as you progress.
- *Take lapses in stride.* Physical deconditioning—a decline in fitness level— occurs at about the same rate as physical conditioning. Renew your commitment to fitness, and restart your exercise program.

OVERCOMING COMMON OBSTACLES TO EXERCISE

There are many reasons why people do not exercise. These reasons range from personal ("I don't have time") to environmental ("I don't have a safe place"). You may be reluctant to start exercising if you are overweight or out of shape. Overcoming these barriers is an important part of starting and maintaining a regular exercise program.

What can I do to charge up my exercise routine and prevent boredom?

To evaluate your obstacles to physical activity, ask yourself what keeps you from being more active. Is it time? Do you lack a support group of family and friends to encourage your new plan? Is the gym or fitness center inconvenient, or do you lack money for a membership or equipment? Perhaps you're ready to begin but just can't get over that final hurdle of just getting started. Once you've evaluated why you don't move more, look at the chart below to determine how you can overcome your hurdle.

Obstacles to Physical Activity	Possible Solutions
Lack of time	■ Take a good look at your schedule. Can you find three 30-minute time slots in your week? ■ Multitask. Read while riding an exercise bike, or listen to lecture tapes while walking. ■ Add physical activity to your daily routine. Walk or ride your bike to work or shopping, organize school activities around physical activity, walk the dog. ■ Exercise during your lunch breaks or between classes. ■ Select activities that require minimal time, such as brisk walking or jogging.
Social influence	■ Invite family and friends to exercise with you. ■ Join a class to meet new people who share your exercise interests. ■ Explain the importance of exercise to people who may not support your efforts.
Lack of motivation/willpower/energy	■ Write your planned workout time in your schedule book. ■ Enlist the help of an exercise partner to make you accountable for working out. ■ Give yourself an incentive. ■ Schedule your workouts when you feel most energetic. ■ Remind yourself that exercise can give you more energy.
Lack of resources	■ Select an activity that requires minimal equipment, such as walking, jogging, jumping rope, or calisthenics. ■ Identify inexpensive resources on campus or in the community.

Source: National Center for Chronic Disease Prevention and Health Promotion, "Overcoming Barriers to Physical Activity" 2007, www.cdc.gov/nccdphp/dnpa/physical/life/overcome.htm.

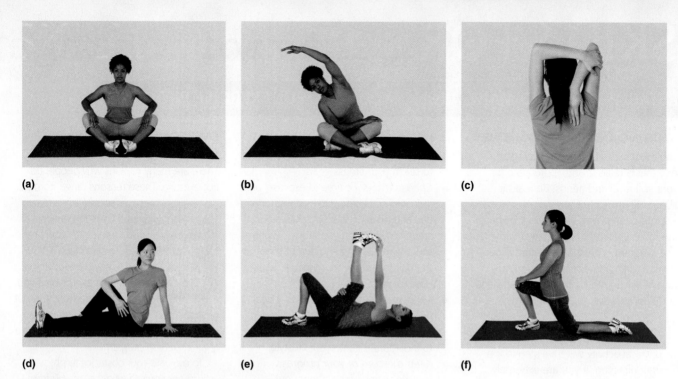

FIGURE 11.5 Stretching Exercises to Improve Flexibility
Use these stretches as part of your warm-up and cool-down. Hold each stretch for 10 to 30 seconds, and repeat four times for each limb. After only a few weeks of regular stretching, you'll begin to see more flexibility. **(a)** Stretching the inside of the thighs. **(b)** Stretching the upper arm and the side of the trunk. **(c)** Stretching the triceps. **(d)** Stretching the trunk and hip. **(e)** Stretching the hip, back of the thigh, and the calf. **(f)** Stretching the front of the thigh and the hip flexor.

Fitness Program Components

The amount and type of exercise required to yield beneficial results vary with the age and physical condition of the exerciser. Men over age 40 and women over age 50 should consult their physicians before beginning any fitness program.

Good fitness programs are designed to improve or maintain cardiorespiratory fitness, flexibility, muscular strength and endurance, and body composition. A comprehensive program could include a warm-up period of easy walking, followed by stretching activities to improve flexibility, then selected strength development exercises, followed by an aerobic activity for 20 minutes or more, and concluding with a cool-down period of gentle flexibility exercises.

Warming Up and Stretching
Warming up and stretching prepares your body for exercise and provides a transition from rest to physical activity. A 5-minute warm-up may consist of a 5-minute brisk walk to ease your cardiovascular system into the more vigorous activity and to increase blood flow to the exercising muscles. This 5-minute warm-up can increase the temperature and elasticity of muscles and connective tissue, making stretching more effective. Add 5 to 10 minutes of stretching to your fitness routine, and you'll be ready to go! **Figure 11.5** shows a selection of exercises that will stretch the major muscle groups of your body and can be used as a warm-up for other physical activities and exercise programs.

Resistance Training
When beginning a resistance-exercise program, always consider your age, fitness level, and personal goals. Strength-training exercises are done in a set, or a single series of multiple repetitions using the same resistance. For both men and women under the age of 50, the ACSM recommends working major muscle groups with at least one set of eight to ten different exercises 2 to 3 days per week.[44] Weight loads should be at a level to allow up to 8 to 12 repetitions. Beginners should use lighter weights and complete 10 to 15 repetitions. **Table 11.3** includes essential information on developing a resistance-training program. Remember, experts suggest allowing at least one day of rest and recovery between workouts of any specific muscle group.

Cardiorespiratory Training
You should spend the greatest proportion of exercise time developing cardiovascular fitness. Choose an aerobic activity you think you will like. Many people find cross training—alternate-day participation in two or more aerobic activities (such as jogging and swimming)—more enjoyable than long-term participation in only one activity. Cross training is also beneficial because it strengthens a variety of muscles, thus helping you avoid overuse injuries to muscles and joints.

Jogging, walking, cycling, rowing, step aerobics, and cross-country skiing are all excellent activities for developing cardiovascular fitness. Most colleges have recreation centers where students can use stair-climbing machines, stationary

TABLE 11.3 | **Resistance-Training Program Guidelines**

- Resistance training should be an integral part of an adult fitness program and be of sufficient intensity to enhance strength and muscular endurance and to maintain fat-free mass.
- Resistance training should be progressive, be individualized, and provide a stimulus (overload) to all major muscle groups in the body.
- The exercise sequence should include large- before small-muscle group exercises, multiple-joint exercises before single-joint exercises, and higher-intensity before lower-intensity exercises.
- Performing eight to ten exercises that train the major muscle groups 2 to 3 days per week is recommended.
- The amount of weight used and number of repetitions vary by individual's target goal, physical capacity, and training status.

Source: W. J. Kraemer et al., "American College of Sports Medicine Position Stand on Progression Models in Resistance Training for Healthy Adults," *Medicine and Science in Sports and Exercise* 3, no. 2 (2002): 364–80. Copyright © 2002 Lippincott, Williams, and Wilkins. Used with permission.

bicycles, treadmills, rowing machines, and ski-simulators. **Table 11.4** describes popular workout machines and provides tips for their use.

Cooling Down and Stretching
Just as you ease into a workout with a warm-up, you should slowly transition from activity to rest. At least 5 minutes of your workout should be devoted to a gradual slowdown, decreasing the intensity of your activity. For example, if you jog, walk briskly, then slowly, before stretching. Be sure to stretch the major muscle groups to help reduce the amount of soreness from exercise.

Choosing the Right Exercise Equipment

If you have a treadmill that you use as a clothes hanger or belong to a gym you haven't visited in months, you are not alone. Many people buy great equipment and don't get motivated to get moving, but others buy services and equipment that don't have a ghost's chance of being useful. Evaluate advertising claims for fitness products carefully **(Table 11.5).**

Popular and Practical Exercise Equipment

There are many useful exercise products that can help you take your exercise program to the next level. Here, we'll look at some of the most popular—and effective—equipment.

Heart Rate Monitors Fitness enthusiasts use heart rate monitors to become aware of their heart rate and training intensity and push performance higher. These monitors usually have a strap with a sensor for placing around the chest and a watchlike readout on the wrist. Monitors cost between $50 and $200 and can provide instant feedback about the intensity of your workouts. If you want a more technical way to measure heart rate than the fingers-to-the-wrist method, a heart rate monitor is for you.

Pedometers Pedometers offer features such as monitoring calories, counting number of steps, and keeping track of distance and speed. They are usually small and

TABLE 11.4	**Picking Your Workout Machine**	
Machine	**Advantages**	**Best Use**
Elliptical machine	This machine is designed for nonimpact cardiovascular exercise. Some machines are equipped with handles for arm action that improve the overall workout.	For machines without arm action, pump arms at your sides as you would if you were running. If the machine has arm handles, use resistance by pushing and pulling along with the handles.
Stair climber	This machine is a great low impact lower body workout and most can be adjusted from very easy to very difficult.	The degree of workout depends on working against your body weight, so stay upright and don't lean on the console. Try not to touch the handrails other than for balance. Keep your steps shallow (no deeper than 6 inches).
Stationary bike	This machine provides an excellent lower body workout. It is generally easy to use and most come with varied resistance programs. Recumbent bikes offer less strain on the back and knees.	Adjust the seat so your leg is almost fully extended when the pedal is at its lowest. Don't grip the handles too tightly or lean on the handlebars.
Treadmill	This machine offers a great lower body workout and improves cardiovascular fitness. It is relatively easy to use and burns more calories than bikes or a stair climber.	Most come with an emergency shut-off clip. Be sure to use this for safety. Start gradually and progress to either faster pace or increased incline. Arms should naturally swing at your sides.

Source: Copyright © 2006, S. Eyler, StarTrac Fitness. Used with permission.

easy to use, and they can help you figure out how far you've gone on your daily walk/run or measure how many steps you take on an average day. They can be an excellent motivator. Before you buy a pedometer, make sure it's simple to use and has an easy-to-read display. The unit should be accurate in its count when you wear it correctly—you may have to experiment with where to wear it. Distance accuracy depends on setting your stride length correctly. Some pedometers even come with a computer program to upload your step and distance records. Prices range from $20 to $100.

Exercise (Fitness) Balls Stabilizing yourself on a ball strengthens core muscles. If you sit on the ball and do arm or shoulder exercises, you work your abdominals as well as your arms and shoulders. High-quality balls are made of burst-resistant vinyl and are independently tested to withstand as much as 600 pounds while still retaining their shape and usefulness.

Choose a ball that is suited to both your weight and height. To determine whether the ball is right for you, sit on it. Your feet should be flat on the floor, your weight distributed evenly, and your knees at a 90-degree or slightly greater angle. Be sure to inflate the ball to the right height and use it properly, both for safety reasons and to ensure maximum workout results. Read the package carefully to be certain that if the ball is punctured, it will not drop you to the ground (high quality balls are designed to deflate slowly if punctured to minimize the risk of injury). Prices range from $25 to $50.

Balance Boards By doing strengthening moves on a balance board, your core muscles contract; thus you work your abs as well as other muscle groups. Athletes who regularly train with balance boards improve agility, reaction skills, and ankle strength. This greatly decreases the risk of ankle injury during play while improving coordination and overall athletic ability. For less-athletic types working out on a balance board can reduce your chances of tripping and falling in everyday life. The cost is $40 to $80.

Resistance Bands Resistance bands are usually rubber or elastic material with handles that can be used to work the muscles without weights. The bands can provide various ways to improve muscular endurance and strength, flexibility, and range of motion. They are lightweight and portable and can add variety to gym workouts. They are also compact and easy to pack when traveling. You can buy bands in varying degrees of resistance, depending on your fitness level or exercise goal, for $5 to $15.

 try it NOW!

Boost daily exercise today with small changes. For example, when you have a choice between elevator and stairs, choose the stairs. Walking up a few flights of stairs a day can be beneficial to your health, especially when you add the weight of a backpack or books. Walking stairs helps strengthen your legs, gets your heart pumping, and contributes to your daily activity level.

Fitness-Related Injuries

Overtraining is the most frequent cause of injuries associated with fitness activities and affects up to 20 percent of all athletes. Enthusiastic but out-of-shape beginners often injure themselves by doing too much too soon. Experienced athletes develop *overtraining syndrome* by engaging in systematic and progressive increases in training without getting enough rest and recovery time. Eventually, performance begins to decline, and training sessions become increasingly difficult. Adequate rest, good nutrition, and rehydration are important to sustain or improve fitness levels.

Pay attention to your body's warning signs. To avoid injuring a particular muscle group or body part, vary your fitness activities throughout the week to give muscles and joints a rest. Set appropriate short-term and long-term training goals. Establishing realistic but challenging fitness goals can help you stay motivated without overdoing it. Use common sense, and you're likely to remain injury-free.

Causes of Fitness-Related Injuries

There are two basic types of injuries stemming from fitness-related activities: overuse and traumatic. **Overuse injuries** are due to cumulative, day-after-day stresses placed on tendons, bones, and ligaments during exercise. These injuries occur most often in repetitive activities such as swimming, running, bicycling, and step aerobics. The forces that occur normally during physical activity are not enough to cause a ligament sprain or muscle strain, but when these forces are applied on a daily basis for weeks or months, they can result in an injury. Common sites of overuse injuries are the leg, knee, shoulder, and elbow joints.

Traumatic injuries occur suddenly and violently, typically by accident. Typical traumatic injuries are broken bones, torn ligaments and muscles, contusions, and lacerations. Some traumatic injuries occur quickly and are difficult to avoid—for example, spraining your ankle by landing on another person's foot after jumping up for a rebound in basketball. If your traumatic injury causes a noticeable loss of function and immediate pain or pain that does not go away after 30 minutes, consult a physician.

Preventing Injuries

Appropriate Footwear
Shoes are made to protect the foot from sport-specific movements. Proper footwear can decrease the likelihood of foot, knee, or back injuries.

When you purchase running shoes, look for several key components **(Figure 11.6).** Biomechanics research has revealed that running is a collision sport—with each stride, the runner's foot collides with the ground with a force three to five times the runner's body weight.[45] The force not absorbed by the running shoe is transmitted upward into the foot, leg, thigh, and back. Our bodies are able to absorb forces such as these but may be injured by the cumulative effect of repetitive impacts (such as running 40 miles per week). Therefore, the ability of running shoes to absorb shock is critical. Proper fit is also important.

Basketball, tennis, and other sport enthusiasts can also buy shoes specific to their sport. A cross-training shoe can be used for several different fitness activities by the novice or recreational athlete.

Appropriate Protective Equipment
Some activities require special protective equipment to reduce chances of injury. Eye injuries can occur in virtually all fitness-related activities, although some are more risky than others. As many as 90 percent of the eye injuries resulting from racquetball and squash could be prevented by wearing appropriate eye protection—for example, goggles with polycarbonate lenses.[46]

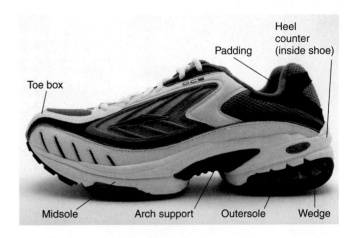

FIGURE 11.6 Anatomy of a Running Shoe
The midsole of your shoe is one of the most important factors in comfort. To evaluate the flexibility of the midsole, hold the shoe lengthwise between the index fingers of your right and left hands. When you push on both ends of the shoe, it should bend easily at the midsole. If the force exerted by your index fingers cannot bend the shoe, its midsole is probably too rigid and will be painful.

Nearly 100 million people in the United States ride bikes for pleasure, fitness, or competition. Wearing a helmet while bicycle riding is an important safety precaution. An estimated 45 to 88 percent of head injuries among cyclists can be prevented by wearing a helmet. The direct medical costs from cyclists' failure to wear helmets is $8.1 million a year.[47] Cyclists aren't the only ones who should be wearing helmets. People who skateboard, use kick-scooters, or snowboard should also wear helmets. Look for helmets that meet the standards established by the American National Standards Institute or the Snell Memorial Foundation.

 what do you THINK?

Given your activity level, what injuries do you risk on a regular basis? ■ What changes can you make in your equipment and clothing to reduce your risk?

Common Overuse Injuries

Three of the most common overuse injuries are plantar fasciitis, shin splints, and runner's knee.

Plantar Fasciitis *Plantar fasciitis* is an inflammation of the plantar fascia, a broad band of dense, inelastic tissue

overuse injuries Injuries that result from the cumulative effects of day-after-day stresses placed on tendons, muscles, and joints.

traumatic injuries Injuries that are accidental and occur suddenly and violently (such as fractured bones, ruptured tendons, and sprained ligaments).

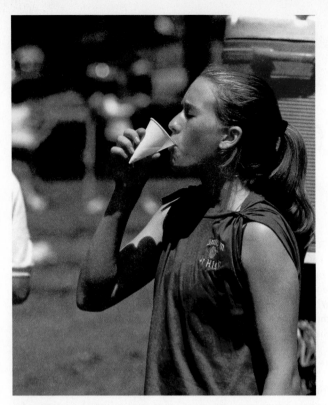

Avoiding dehydration is important when exercising in hot or cold weather, whether to avoid heat exhaustion, heatstroke, or hypothermia.

(fascia) that protects the nerves, blood vessels, and muscles of the foot from injury. Repetitive weight-bearing movements such as walking and running can inflame the plantar fascia. Common symptoms are pain and tenderness under the ball of the foot, at the heel, or at both locations.[48] This injury can often be prevented by regularly stretching the plantar fascia before and after exercise and by wearing athletic shoes with good arch support and shock absorbency. Stretch the plantar fascia by slowly pulling all five toes upward, holding for 10 to 15 seconds, and repeating this 3 to 5 times on each foot.

Shin Splints A general term for any pain that occurs below the knee and above the ankle is *shin splints*. This broad description includes more than 20 different medical conditions. Problems can be due to muscles, bones, or attachments from muscle to bone. Typically, there is pain and swelling along the middle of the shin in the soft tissues, not the bone.

Sedentary people who start a new weight-bearing exercise program are at the greatest risk for shin splints, though even well-conditioned aerobic exercisers who rapidly

increase their distance or pace may develop them. To help prevent shin splints, wear athletic shoes with good arch support and shock absorbency. Also, gradually increase training intensity and vary your routine. If the pain continues, see your physician. You may need to substitute a non–weight-bearing activity, such as swimming, during your recovery period.

Runner's Knee *Runner's knee* describes a series of problems involving the muscles, tendons, and ligaments around the knee. The main symptom of this kind of runner's knee is the pain experienced when downward pressure is applied to the kneecap after the knee is straightened fully. Symptoms include pain, swelling, redness, and tenderness around the kneecap.[49] If you have these symptoms, your physician will probably recommend that you stop running for a few weeks and reduce activities that compress the kneecap (for example, exercise on a stair-climbing machine or doing squats with heavy resistance) until you no longer feel any pain.

Treatment

First aid treatment for virtually all fitness-related injuries involves **RICE: r**est, **i**ce, **c**ompression, and **e**levation. *Rest,* the first component of this treatment, is required to avoid further irritation of the injured body part. *Ice* is applied to relieve pain and constrict the blood vessels to stop any internal or external bleeding. Never apply ice cubes, reusable gel ice packs, chemical cold packs, or other forms of cold directly to your skin. Instead, place a layer of wet toweling or elastic bandage between the ice and your skin. Ice should be applied to a new injury for approximately 20 minutes every hour for the first 24 to 72 hours. *Compression* of the injured body part can be accomplished with a 4- or 6-inch-wide elastic bandage; this applies indirect pressure to damaged blood vessels to help stop bleeding. Be careful, though, that the compression wrap not interfere with normal blood flow. Throbbing or pain in the hand or foot indicates that the compression wrap should be loosened. *Elevation* of the injured extremity above the level of your heart also helps to control internal or external bleeding by making the blood flow upward to reach the injured area.

Exercising in the Heat

Heat stress, which includes several potentially fatal illnesses resulting from excessive core body temperatures, should be a concern whenever you exercise in warm, humid weather. In these conditions, your body's rate of heat production can exceed its ability to cool itself.

You can help prevent heat stress by following certain precautions. First, proper acclimatization to hot and/or humid climates is essential. The process of heat acclimatization,

RICE Acronym for the standard first aid treatment for virtually all traumatic and overuse injuries: rest, ice, compression, and elevation.

which increases your body's cooling efficiency, requires about 10 to 14 days of gradually increasing activity in the hot environment. Second, avoid dehydration by replacing the fluids you lose during and after exercise. Third, wear clothing appropriate for your activity and the environment. And finally, use common sense—for example, on a day when the temperature is 85°F and the humidity is 80 percent, postpone your usual lunchtime run until the cool of evening.

The three different heat stress illnesses—heat cramps, heat exhaustion, and heatstroke—are progressive in severity. **Heat cramps** (heat-related muscle cramps), the least serious problem, can usually be prevented by warm-ups, adequate fluid replacement, and a diet that includes the electrolytes lost during sweating (sodium and potassium). **Heat exhaustion** is caused by excessive water loss resulting from prolonged exercise or work. Symptoms of heat exhaustion include nausea, headache, fatigue, dizziness and faintness, and, paradoxically, "goosebumps" and chills. If you are suffering from heat exhaustion, your skin will be cool and moist. Heat exhaustion occurs when the body's cooling system falters and circulation slows. **Heatstroke,** often called *sunstroke,* is responsible for at least 240 deaths in the United States each year. This condition triggers a series of metabolic events that may result in irreversible injury or death.[50] Heatstroke occurs during vigorous exercise when the body's heat production significantly exceeds its cooling capacities. Body core temperature can rise from normal (98.6°F) to 105°F to 110°F within minutes after the body's cooling mechanism shuts down. Rapidly increasing core temperatures can cause brain damage, permanent disability, and death. Common signs of heatstroke are dry, hot, and usually red skin; very high body temperature; and rapid heart rate.

If you experience any of the symptoms mentioned here, stop exercising immediately, move to the shade or a cool spot to rest, and drink large amounts of cool fluids. Be aware that heat stress can also result from prolonged immersion in a sauna, hot tub, or steam bath or from performing activity in lots of heavy clothing and equipment, such as a football uniform.[51]

Exercising in the Cold

Exercising in cool weather can lead to **hypothermia,** a potentially fatal condition resulting from abnormally low body core temperature, which occurs when body heat is lost faster than it is produced. Temperatures need not be frigid for hypothermia to occur; it can also result from prolonged, vigorous exercise in 40°F to 50°F temperatures, particularly if there is rain, snow, or a strong wind.

In mild cases of hypothermia, as body core temperature drops from the normal 98.6°F to about 93.2°F, you will begin to shiver. Shivering—the involuntary contraction of nearly every muscle in the body—increases body temperature by using the heat given off by muscle activity. You may also experience cold hands and feet, poor judgment, apathy, and amnesia. Shivering ceases in most hypothermia victims as body core temperatures drop to between 87°F and 90°F, a sign that the body has lost its ability to generate heat. Death usually occurs at body core temperatures between 75°F and 80°F.[52] To prevent hypothermia, pay attention to weather conditions, dress in layers, avoid dehydration, and exercise with a friend.[53]

Preventing Cramps

Although most of us have experienced the quick, intense pain of muscle cramps, they are poorly understood. A cramp is an involuntary and forcibly contracted muscle that does not relax. Cramps in legs, feet, arms, abdomen, and along the rib cage are common. A cramp can last a few seconds to 15 minutes or longer. There are several theories about cramping. According to the overexertion theory, when a muscle gets tired, the numerous muscle fibers that comprise it fail to contract in a synchronized rhythm, probably because of overstimulation from the nerves that trigger the muscles to contract.[54] Other theories relate cramping to dehydration. Dehydration may occur simply if someone doesn't consume sufficient liquids to compensate for loss in urine and sweat. Even if dehydration is not the only cause, it is clearly a problem for those who exercise and perspire heavily. Drinking enough fluids before, during, and after activity is important.

If you get cramps, what should you do? Generally massage, stretching, putting pressure on the muscle that is cramping, and deep breathing are useful remedies.

heat cramps   Muscle cramps that occur during or following exercise in warm or hot weather.

heat exhaustion   A heat stress illness caused by significant dehydration resulting from exercise in warm or hot conditions; frequent precursor to heatstroke.

heatstroke   A deadly heat stress illness resulting from dehydration and overexertion in warm or hot conditions; can cause body core temperature to rise from normal to 105°F to 110°F in just a few minutes.

hypothermia   Potentially fatal condition caused by abnormally low body core temperature.

TAKING charge

Summary

- The physiological benefits of regular physical activity include reduced risk of heart attack, some cancers, hypertension, and diabetes; and improved blood profile, skeletal mass, weight control, immunity to disease, mental health and stress management, and physical fitness. Regular physical activity can also increase life span.

- It is recommended that every adult participate in moderate-intensity activities for 30 minutes at least 5 days a week. For improvements in cardiorespiratory fitness, you should work out aerobically for at least 20 minutes, a minimum of 3 days per week. Exercise intensity involves working out at target heart rate. The longer the exercise period, the more calories burned and the greater the improvement in cardiovascular fitness.

- Key principles for developing muscular strength and endurance are the tension principle, the overload principle, and the specificity-of-training principle. The different types of muscle actions include isometric, concentric, and eccentric. Resistance training programs include body weight resistance (calisthenics), fixed resistance, variable resistance, and accommodating resistance devices.

- Flexibility exercises should involve static stretching exercises performed in sets of two to four repetitions held for 15 to 30 seconds, at least 2 to 3 days a week.

- Planning a fitness program involves setting goals and designing a program to achieve these goals. A comprehensive program would include a warm-up period, stretching activities, strength development exercises, an aerobic activity, and a cool-down period.

- Fitness injuries generally are caused by overuse or trauma; the most common ones are plantar fasciitis, shin splints, and runner's knee. Proper footwear and equipment can help prevent injuries. Exercise in the heat or cold requires special precautions.

Chapter Review

1. The maximum volume of oxygen consumed by the muscles during exercise defines
   a. target heart rate.
   b. muscular strength.
   c. aerobic capacity.
   d. muscular endurance.

2. What is physical fitness?
   a. the ability to respond to routine physical demands
   b. having enough reserves after working out to cope with a sudden challenge
   c. both aerobic and muscular strength
   d. all of the above

3. Which type of cancer may be prevented by being physically active?
   a. skin
   b. lung
   c. colon
   d. liver

4. Flexibility is the range of motion around
   a. specific bones.
   b. specific joints.
   c. the hips and pelvis.
   d. the muscles.

5. The "talk test" measures
   a. exercise intensity.
   b. exercise duration.
   c. exercise frequency.
   d. metabolism.

6. An example of aerobic exercise is
   a. brisk walking.
   b. bench pressing weights.
   c. stretching exercises.
   d. yoga breathing.

7. Theresa wants to lower her ratio of fat weight to her total body weight. She wants to work on her
   a. flexibility.
   b. muscular endurance.
   c. muscular strength.
   d. body composition.

8. Miguel is a cross-country runner and is therefore able to sustain moderate-intensity, whole-body activity for an extended time. This ability relates to what component of physical fitness?
   a. flexibility
   b. body composition
   c. cardiorespiratory fitness
   d. muscular strength and endurance

9. Janice has been lifting 95 pounds while doing three sets of 10 leg curls. To become stronger, she began lifting 105 pounds while doing leg curls. What principle of strength development does this represent?
   a. tension principle
   b. overload principle
   c. flexibility principle
   d. specificity-of-training principle

10. Joel enjoys various types of fitness exercises. He alternates his training days with jogging, cycling, and step aerobics. This type of training is called
    a. cardiac fitness training.
    b. static training.
    c. cross training.
    d. multisport training.

Answers to these questions can be found on page A-1.

Questions for Discussion and Reflection

1. How do you define *physical fitness*? What are the key components of a physical fitness program? What might you need to consider when beginning a fitness program?
2. How would you determine the proper intensity and duration of an exercise program? How often should exercise sessions be scheduled?
3. Why is stretching vital to improving physical flexibility? Why is flexibility important in everyday activities?
4. Identify at least four physiological and psychological benefits of physical fitness. How would you promote these benefits to nonexercisers?
5. Describe the different types of resistance employed in an exercise program. What are the benefits of each type of resistance?
6. Your roommate has decided to start running first thing in the morning in an effort to lose weight, tone muscles, and improve cardiorespiratory fitness. What advice would you give to make sure your roommate gets off to a good start and doesn't get injured?
7. What key components would you include in a fitness program for yourself?

Accessing Your Health on the Internet

The following websites explore further topics and issues related to personal health. For links to the websites below, visit the Companion Website for *Health: The Basics*, Eighth Edition at www.aw-bc.com/donatelle.

1. *ACSM Online.* A link with the American College of Sports Medicine and all their resources. www.acsm.org
2. *American Council on Exercise.* Information on exercise and disease prevention. www.acefitness.org
3. *Centers for Disease Control and Prevention, National Center for Chronic Disease Prevention and Health Promotion, Division of Nutrition, Physical Activity and Obesity.* A resource for current information on exercise and health. www.cdc.gov/nccdphp/dnpa
4. *National Strength and Conditioning Association.* A resource for personal trainers and others interested in conditioning and fitness. www.nsca-lift.org
5. *President's Council of Physical Fitness and Sports.* Provides information on fitness programs. www.fitness.gov

Further Reading

Fahey, T. D. *Super Fitness for Sports, Conditioning, and Health.* Boston: Allyn & Bacon, 2000.

   A brief guide to developing fitness that emphasizes training techniques for improving sports performance.

National Center for Chronic Disease Prevention and Health Promotion. *Physical Activity and Health: A Report of the Surgeon General.* Washington, DC: Department of Health and Human Services, 1996.

   This report brings together the findings from medical research and fitness research to describe the benefits of regular physical activity, to discuss the status of inactivity in the United States, and to provide guidelines for change.

Powers, S., and S. Dodd. *Total Fitness and Wellness,* 5th ed. San Francisco: Benjamin Cummings, 2009.

   A complete guide to improving all areas of fitness, including being a smart health consumer and the links between nutrition and fitness.

Schlosberg, S. *The Ultimate Workout Log: An Exercise Diary for Everyone,* 3rd edition. Boston: Houghton Mifflin, 2005.

   A 6-month log that also provides fitness definitions, training tips, and motivational quotes.

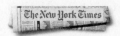

e-themes from *The New York Times*

For up-to-date articles about current health issues, visit
www.aw-bc.com/donatelle, select *Health: The Basics,* Eighth
Edition, Chapter 11, and click on "e-themes."

References

1. American College Health Association, *American College Health Association–National College Health Assessment: Reference Group Data Report, Fall 2006.* (Baltimore: American College Health Association, 2007).

2. Ibid.; National Center for Chronic Disease Prevention and Health Promotion, *Physical Activity for Everyone: The Importance of Physical Activity* (Atlanta: Centers for Disease Control and Prevention, 2007, www.cdc.gov/nccdphp/dnpa/physical/importance/index.htm.

3. American Heart Association, "Cardiovascular Disease Statistics," 2007, www.americanheart.org/presenter.jhtml?identifier=4478; Centers for Disease Control and Prevention, "Fact Sheet: Number of Americans with Diabetes Continues to Rise," 2005, www.cdc.gov/od/oc/media/pressrel/fs051026.htm.

4. National Center for Chronic Disease Prevention and Health Promotion, *Physical Activity for Everyone.*

5. U.S. Department of Health and Human Services, *Physical Activity and Health: A Report of the Surgeon General* (Atlanta: Centers for Disease Control, National Center for Chronic Disease Prevention and Health Promotion, 1996).

6. Ibid.

7. National Center for Chronic Disease Prevention and Health Promotion, "Nutrition and Physical Activity Recommendations," 2007, www.cdc.gov/nccdphp/dnpa/physical/recommendations/index.htm.

8. M. C. Lamarre and M. Pratt, "Physical Activity and Health Promotion," *Promotion and Education* 3 (2006): 4–5.

9. V. H. Heyward, *Advanced Fitness Assessment and Prescription,* 5th ed. (Champaign, IL: Human Kinetics, 2006).

10. X. Sui, M. J. Lamonte, and S. N. Blair, "Cardiorespiratory Fitness and Risk of Nonfatal Cardiovascular Disease in Women and Men with Hypertension," *American Journal of Hypertension* 20, no. 6 (2007): 608–15.

11. Heyward, *Advanced Fitness Assessment and Prescription,* 5th ed.

12. W. Wang et al., "A Longitudinal Study of Hypertension Risk Factors and Their Relation to Cardiovascular Disease," *Hypertension* 47 (2006): 403.

13. American College of Sports Medicine, *ACSM's Certification Review,* 2nd ed. (Philadelphia: Lippincott Williams & Wilkins, 2006).

14. American Stroke Association, "American Heart Association: Cholesterol," 2007, www.strokeassociation.org/presenter.jhtml?identifier=4488.

15. G. A. Colditz et al., "Physical Activity and Risk of Breast Cancer in Premenopausal Women," *British Journal of Cancer* 89, no. 5 (2003): 847–51; A. K. Samad et al., "A Meta-Analysis of the Association of Physical Activity with Risk of Colorectal Cancer," *Colorectal Disease* 7, no. 3 (2005): 204–13; L. Bernstein et al., "Lifetime Recreational Exercise Activity and Breast Cancer Risk Among Black and White Women," *Journal of the National Cancer Institute* 77, no. 22 (2005):1671–79.

16. American Institute for Cancer Research, "Physical Activity and Cancer Risk," 2005, www.aicr.org

17. K. J. Stewart et al., "Exercise Effects on Bone Mineral Density Relationships to Changes in Fitness and Fatness," *American Journal of Preventive Medicine* 28, no. 5 (2005): 453–60.

18. Ibid.

19. W. McArdle, F. Katch, and V. Katch, *Exercise Physiology,* 6th ed. (Philadelphia: Lippincott, Williams and Wilkins, 2006), 60–65.

20. J. Kruger, M. M. Yore, and W. H. Kohl, "Leisure Time Physical Activity Patterns by Weight Control Status: 1999–2002 NHANES," *Medicine and Science in Sports and Exercise* 39, no. 5 (2007): 788–95.

21. American College of Sports Medicine, "Exercise Recommendations: Guidelines for Physical Activity," 2001, www.acsm.org.

22. S. Lee et al., "Exercise without Weight Loss Is an Effective Strategy for Obesity Reduction in Obese Individuals with or without Type 2 Diabetes," *Journal of Applied Physiology* 99, no. 3 (2005): 1220–25.

23. G. Hu et al., "Epidemiological Studies of Exercise in Diabetes Prevention," *Applied Physiology, Nutrition, and Metabolism* 32, no. 3 (2007): 583–95; American Diabetes Association, "Diabetes Risk Test," 2004, www.diabetes.org/risk-test.jsp.

24. National Diabetes Information Clearinghouse, "Diabetes Prevention Program," NIH Publication no.06-5099, August 2006.

25. J. O. Hill et al., "Physical Activity and Managing Obesity and Type 2 Diabetes," *Nestle Nutrition Workshop Series: Clinical & Performance Program* 11 (2006): 183–91.

26. S. Carlsson et al., "Physical Activity and Mortality: Is the Association Explained by Genetic Selection?" *American Journal of Epidemiology,* May 10, 2007 e-publication; National Centers for Chronic Disease Prevention and Health Promotion, "Physical Activity and Health."

27. O. H. Franco et al., "Effects of Physical Activity on Life Expectancy with Cardiovascular Disease," *Archives of Internal Medicine* 165, no. 20 (2005): 2355–60.

28. J. Woods, "Physical Activity, Exercise, and Immune Function," *Brain, Behavior, and Immunity* 19, no. 5 (2005): 369–70; E. Quinn, "Exercise and Immunity," *Sports Medicine,* 2006, http://sportsmedicine.about.com/cs/exercisephysiology/a/aa100303a.htm.

29. E. Tollier et al., "Intense Training: Mucosal Immunity and Incidence of Respiratory Infections," *European Journal of Applied Physiology* 93, no. 4 (2005): 421–28.

30. D. C. Nieman et al., "Immune Response to a 30-Minute Walk," *Medicine and Science in Sports and Exercise* 37, no. 1 (2005): 57–62.

31. Ibid.

32. L. M. Hays, T. M. Damush, and D. O. Clark, "Relationships between Exercise Self-Definitions and Exercise Participation among Urban Women in Primary Care," *Journal of Cardiovascular Nursing* 20, no. 1 (2005): 9–17.

33. Centers for Disease Control and Prevention, "Calories Per Hour," 2006, www.cdc.gov/nccdphp/dnpa/spotlights/calories_per_hour_table.htm.

34. J. Gavin, *Life Fitness Coaching* (Champaign, IL: Human Kinetics, 2005).

35. American College Health Association, *American College Health Association–National College Health Assessment: Reference Group Executive Summary, Fall 2006* (Baltimore: American College Health Association, 2007).

36. American College of Sports Medicine, *Guidelines for Exercise Testing and Prescription,* 7th ed. (Philadelphia: Lippincott, Williams and Wilkins, 2005).

37. S. J. Fleck and W. I. Kraemer, *Designing Resistance Training Programs,* 3rd ed. (Champaign, IL: Human Kinetics, 2004).

38. D. C. Nieman, *Exercise Testing and Prescription,* 6th ed. (New York: McGraw-Hill, 2006).

39. Mayo Clinic, "Core Exercises: Beyond Your Average Abs Routine," October 6, 2005, www.mayoclinic.com/health/core-exercises/SM00071.

40. Arthritis Foundation, "Exercise and Arthritis," 2007, www.arthritis.org/exercise-intro.php; Arthritis Foundation, "Making Your Workout Well-Rounded," *Arthritis Today,* May 2007.

41. A. G. Nelson, J. Kokkonen, and J. M. McAlexander, *Stretching Anatomy* (Champaign, IL: Human Kinetics, 2006).

42. T. Little, "Effects of Differential Stretching Protocols During Warm-Ups on High Speed Motor Capacities of Professional Soccer Players," *Journal of Strength and Conditioning Research* 20, no. 1 (2006): 203–207.

43. Nelson, Kokkonen, and J. McAlexander, *Stretching Anatomy.*

44. American College of Sports Medicine, *ACSM's Certification Review,* 2nd ed.

45. U. G. Kersting and G. P Bruggemann, "Midsole Material-Related Force Control During Heel-Toe Running," *Research in Sports Medicine* 14, no. 1 (2006): 1–17.

46. American Optometric Association, "Sports-Related Eye Injuries," 2007, www.aoa.org/x7370.xml.

47. Bicycle Helmet Safety Institute, "Helmet-Related Statistics," 2007, www.helmets.org/stats.htm.

48. D. Richie, Jr., American Academy of Podiatric Sports Medicine, "Plantar Fasciitis: Treatment Pearls," 2007, www.aapsm.org/plantar_fasciitis.html.

49. S. Drozd, "Patellafemoral Pain Syndrome ("Runner's Knee")," *Runners' World,* 2006, www.runnersworld.com.

50. J. L. Glazer, "Management of Heat Stroke and Heat Exhaustion," *American Family Physician* 71, no. 11 (2005): 2141.

51. Ibid.

52. R. Curtis, *Outdoor Action Guide to Hypothermia and Cold Weather Injuries* (Atlanta: Centers for Disease Control and Prevention, 2006).

53. American Council on Exercise, *Exercising in the Cold, 2006* (Indianapolis: American Council on Exercise, 2006).

54. National Institutes of Health, Medline Plus, "Muscle Cramps," 2007, www.nlm.nih.gov/medlineplus/musclecramps.html.

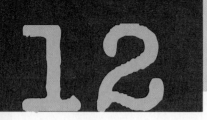

Cardiovascular Disease, Diabetes, and Cancer

REDUCING YOUR RISK

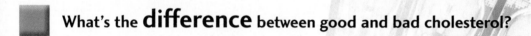

What's the **difference** between good and bad cholesterol?

Does cardiovascular **disease** run in families?

What can I do to reduce my **risk** for diabetes?

If I'm already a **smoker,** will quitting now reduce my risk of lung cancer?

Is a **tanning** booth safer than the sun?

OBJECTIVES

- Discuss the incidence, prevalence, and outcomes of cardiovascular disease in the United States, including its impact on society.
- Review major types of cardiovascular disease, controllable and uncontrollable risk factors, methods of prevention, and current strategies for diagnosis and treatment.
- Understand prediabetes, diabetes, and metabolic syndrome; their risk factors; and what you can do to reduce your risks of developing them.
- Explain what cancer is, and describe the different types of cancer, including the risks they pose to people at different ages and stages of life.
- Discuss cancer's risk factors, and outline strategies and recommendations for prevention, screening, and treatment.

In this chapter we consider three major health issues: cardiovascular disease, diabetes, and cancer. What do they have in common? Although these may seem to be different diseases, all of them pose serious health threats both in the United States and globally. All of them are responsible for significant rates of disability and death. Furthermore, often they develop over time as chronic health conditions, and many cases are related to lifestyle factors such as obesity, being sedentary, selected dietary factors, stress, smoking, or excessive alcohol consumption. The most important point they have in common is this: making healthy lifestyle choices now can significantly reduce your risk of developing any of them in the future. Among people who have a genetic predisposition to these diseases, lifestyle choices can delay their development and contribute to increased numbers of healthy years.

Cardiovascular Disease: An Epidemiological Overview

In 2007, nearly 80 million Americans—one out of every three adults—had some type of **cardiovascular disease (CVD),** the broad term used to describe diseases of the heart and blood vessels. Although numbers continue to increase, it's important to note that CVD has been the leading killer of U.S. adults in every year since 1900, with the exception of 1918, when a pandemic flu killed more people. We spend billions on research searching for prevention strategies, treatments and cures, and we have the most sophisticated media warnings and educational programs

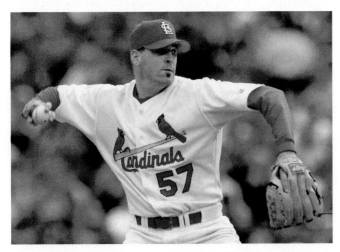

Cardiovascular disease can affect even the youngest and most fit people. Daryl Kile, a 33-year-old professional baseball player, died suddenly from atherosclerosis. It was discovered after his death that two of the main arteries in his heart were 80 to 90 percent blocked. His heart was also enlarged, weighing 20 percent more than normal.

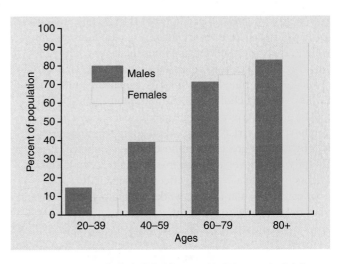

FIGURE 12.1 Prevalence of Cardiovascular Diseases in Adults Aged 20 and Older by Age and Sex

Source: American Heart Association, *Heart Disease and Stroke Statistics—2007 Update* (Dallas: American Heart Association, 2007). Reproduced by permission. © 2007 American Heart Association.

telling us what to do to avoid risks. Nevertheless, growing rates of obesity, hypertension, and diabetes contribute to the high incidence of CVD. Put into perspective, CVD claims more lives each year than the next four leading causes of death combined (cancer, chronic lower respiratory diseases, accidents, and diabetes), accounting for nearly 37 percent of all deaths in the United States.[1] Although we've made advances in diagnosis and in pharmaceutical and surgical treatments, CVD continues to pose a serious threat to the health of all Americans, no matter their age, socioeconomic status, or gender **(Figure 12.1).** Consider the following facts:[2]

- Over 147,000 Americans killed by CVD each year are under age 65.
- The probability at birth of eventually dying of CVD is 47 percent; of dying from cancer, 22 percent; from accidents, 3 percent; from diabetes, 2 percent; and from HIV, 0.7 percent.
- Among women, 1 in 30 deaths is from breast cancer; 1 in 2.6 is from CVD.
- If all forms of major CVD were eliminated, life expectancy would rise by almost 7 years; if all forms of cancer were eliminated, the gain would be 3 years.

The best defense against CVD is to prevent it from developing in the first place. How can you cut your risk? First, you need to take careful stock of just what your own risks are. From there, you need to take steps to reduce the risks that you can by changing certain behaviors. Controlling high blood pressure and reducing intake of saturated fats

cardiovascular disease (CVD) Disease of the heart and blood vessels.

and cholesterol are two examples of things you can do to lower your chances of heart attack. By maintaining your weight, exercising, decreasing your intake of sodium, not smoking, and changing your lifestyle to reduce stress, you can lower your blood pressure. You can also monitor the levels of fat and cholesterol in your blood and adjust your diet to prevent arteries from becoming blocked. Having combinations of risk factors seems to increase overall risk by a factor greater than those of the combined risks. Happily, the converse is also true: reducing several risk factors can have a dramatic effect. Understanding how your cardiovascular system works will help you understand your risk and how to reduce it.

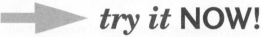
try it NOW!

Find out your risk of developing CVD! Right now, you can find out whether you are prone to CVD and take steps to modify your risk. The American Heart Association's Risk Assessment Tool is an easy online tool that can evaluate your risks and provide practical guidance to help you address and reduce those risks. Visit www.americanheart.org/presenter.jhtml? identifier=3003499, and click on "Learn Your Risk" to begin using the tool now.

Understanding the Cardiovascular System

The **cardiovascular system** is the network of organs and vessels through which blood flows as it carries oxygen and nutrients to all parts of the body. It includes the *heart, arteries, arterioles* (small arteries), and *capillaries* (minute blood vessels). It also includes *venules* (small veins) and *veins,* the blood vessels through which blood flows as it returns to the heart and lungs.

cardiovascular system A complex system consisting of the heart and blood vessels. It transports nutrients, oxygen, hormones, metabolic wastes, and enzymes throughout the body and regulates temperature, the water levels of cells, and the acidity levels of body components.

atria The two upper chambers of the heart, which receive blood.

ventricles The two lower chambers of the heart, which pump blood through the blood vessels.

arteries Vessels that carry blood away from the heart to other regions of the body.

The Heart: A Mighty Machine

The heart is a muscular, four-chambered pump, roughly the size of your fist. It is a highly efficient, extremely flexible organ that manages to contract 100,000 times each day and pumps the equivalent of 2,000 gallons of blood to all areas of the body. In a 70-year lifetime, an average human heart beats 2.5 billion times. This number is significantly higher for hearts that must work to keep people moving who are out of shape and overweight.

Under normal circumstances, the human body contains approximately 6 quarts of blood. This blood transports nutrients, oxygen, waste products, hormones, and enzymes throughout the body. Blood also aids in regulating body temperature, cellular water levels, and acidity levels of body components, and in aiding bodily defense against toxins and harmful microorganisms. An adequate blood supply is essential to health and well-being.

The heart has four chambers that work together to circulate blood constantly throughout the body (**Figure 12.2**). The two upper chambers of the heart, called **atria,** are large collecting chambers that receive blood from the rest of the body. The two lower chambers, known as **ventricles,** pump the blood out again. Small valves regulate the steady, rhythmic flow of blood between chambers and prevent inappropriate backwash. The *tricuspid valve* (located between the right atrium and the right ventricle), the *pulmonary valve* (between the right ventricle and the pulmonary artery), the *mitral valve* (between the left atrium and left ventricle), and the *aortic valve* (between the left ventricle and the aorta) permit blood to flow in only one direction.

Heart Function

Heart activity depends on a complex interaction of biochemical, physical, and neurological signals. Here are the basic steps involved in heart function:

1. Deoxygenated blood enters the right atrium after having been circulated through the body.

2. From the right atrium, blood moves to the right ventricle and is pumped through the pulmonary artery to the lungs, where it receives oxygen.

3. Oxygenated blood from the lungs then returns to the left atrium of the heart.

4. Blood from the left atrium moves into the left ventricle. The left ventricle pumps blood through the aorta to all body parts.

Various types of blood vessels are required for different parts of this process. **Arteries** carry blood away from the heart; all arteries carry oxygenated blood, *except* for pulmonary arteries, which carry deoxygenated blood to the lungs, where the blood picks up oxygen and gives off carbon dioxide. As the arteries branch off from the heart,

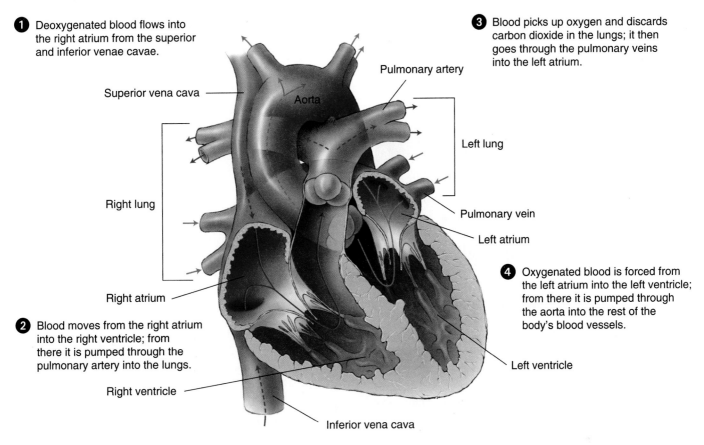

1 Deoxygenated blood flows into the right atrium from the superior and inferior venae cavae.

3 Blood picks up oxygen and discards carbon dioxide in the lungs; it then goes through the pulmonary veins into the left atrium.

Superior vena cava

Aorta

Pulmonary artery

Left lung

Right lung

Pulmonary vein

Left atrium

Right atrium

4 Oxygenated blood is forced from the left atrium into the left ventricle; from there it is pumped through the aorta into the rest of the body's blood vessels.

2 Blood moves from the right atrium into the right ventricle; from there it is pumped through the pulmonary artery into the lungs.

Left ventricle

Right ventricle

Inferior vena cava

FIGURE 12.2 Anatomy of the Heart

they divide into smaller blood vessels called **arterioles,** and then into even smaller blood vessels known as **capillaries.** Capillaries have thin walls that permit the exchange of oxygen, carbon dioxide, nutrients, and waste products with body cells. Carbon dioxide and other waste products are transported to the lungs and kidneys through **veins** and **venules** (small veins).

For the heart to function properly, the four chambers must beat in an organized manner. Your heartbeat is governed by an electrical impulse that directs the heart muscle to move when the impulse moves across it, which results in a sequential contraction of the four chambers. This signal starts in a small bundle of highly specialized cells, the **sinoatrial node (SA node),** located in the right atrium. The SA node serves as a natural pacemaker for the heart. People with a damaged SA node must often have a mechanical pacemaker implanted to ensure the smooth passage of blood through the sequential phases of the heartbeat.

The average adult heart at rest beats 70 to 80 times per minute, although a well-conditioned heart may beat only 50 to 60 times per minute to achieve the same results. When overly stressed, a heart may beat more than 200 times per minute. A healthy heart functions more efficiently and is less likely to suffer damage from overwork.

Types of Cardiovascular Disease

There are several types of cardiovascular disease **(Figure 12.3):**

- Atherosclerosis (fatty plaque buildup in the arteries)
- Coronary heart disease (CHD)
- Chest pain (angina pectoris)
- Irregular heartbeat (arrhythmia)
- Congestive heart failure (CHF)
- Congenital and rheumatic heart disease
- Stroke (cerebrovascular accident)

arterioles Branches of the arteries.

capillaries Minute blood vessels that branch out from the arterioles; their thin walls permit exchange of oxygen, carbon dioxide, nutrients, and waste products among body cells.

veins Vessels that carry blood back to the heart from other regions of the body.

venules Branches of the veins.

sinoatrial node (SA node) Cluster of electricity-generating cells that acts as a natural pacemaker for the heart.

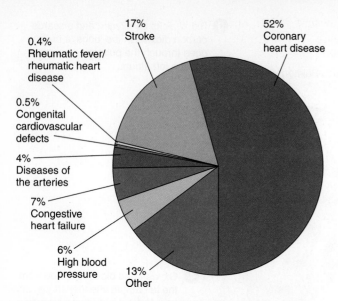

17% Stroke

0.4% Rheumatic fever/ rheumatic heart disease

52% Coronary heart disease

0.5% Congenital cardiovascular defects

4% Diseases of the arteries

7% Congestive heart failure

6% High blood pressure

13% Other

FIGURE 12.3 Percentage Breakdown of Deaths from Cardiovascular Disease in the United States

Source: From *Heart Disease and Stroke Statistics—2007 Update.* Reproduced with permission. © 2007, American Heart Association, Inc.

Methods of preventing and treating these diseases range from changes in diet and lifestyle to medications and surgery.

Atherosclerosis

Arteriosclerosis, thickening and hardening of arteries, is a condition that underlies many cardiovascular health problems and is believed to be the biggest contributor to disease burden globally. **Atherosclerosis** is actually a type of arteriosclerosis and is characterized by deposits of fatty substances, cholesterol, cellular waste products, calcium, and fibrin (a clotting material in the blood) in the inner lining of an artery. *Hyperlipidemia* (an abnormally high blood lipid level) is a key factor in this process, and the resulting buildup is referred to as **plaque.**

Often, atherosclerosis is called *coronary artery disease (CAD)* because of the resultant damage done to coronary arteries. According to current thinking, four factors are responsible for this damage: inflammation, elevated levels of cholesterol and triglycerides in the blood, high blood pressure, and tobacco smoke.[3]

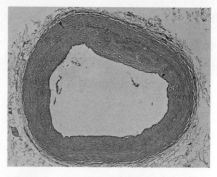

(a)

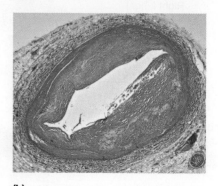

(b)

(a) Cross section of a normal coronary artery. **(b)** A coronary artery narrowed by plaque.

Inflammatory Risks New research has led many experts to believe that atherosclerosis is an *inflammatory* disease, and inflamed vessels are more prone to plaque formation.[4] What causes this inflammation in arterial walls? Although researchers aren't sure, there is evidence that a pathogen may be at the root of it. The most likely culprits are *Chlamydia pneumoniae* (a sexually transmitted infection), *Helicobacter pylori* (which causes stomach ulcers), *herpes simplex virus* (a virus to which the majority of Americans have been exposed by age 5), and *cytomegalovirus* (another herpes virus transmitted through body fluids and infecting most Americans before age 40).

During an inflammatory reaction, *C-reactive proteins (CRPs)* tend to be present at high levels. Many scientists believe the presence of these proteins may signal elevated risk for angina and heart attack. In the near future, CRP tests might be given as routinely as cholesterol screening tests for heart disease.

Researchers have recently discovered another substance that may signal increased risk for CVD: *homocysteine,* an amino acid normally present in the blood. When present at high levels, homocysteine may be related to higher risk of coronary heart disease, stroke, and peripheral vascular disease.[5] It is hypothesized that homocysteine works in much the same way as CRP, inflaming the inner lining of arteries and promoting fat deposits on the damaged walls and development of blood clots.

Folic acid and other B vitamins (such as B_6 and B_{12}) help break down homocysteine in the body; however, conclusive

---

arteriosclerosis A general term for thickening and hardening of the arteries.

atherosclerosis Condition characterized by deposits of fatty substances, cholesterol, cellular waste products, calcium, and fibrin in the inner lining of an artery.

plaque Buildup of deposits in the arteries.

evidence that folic acid reduces risk is not available, and authorities such as the American Heart Association do not currently recommend taking folic acid supplements to lower homocysteine levels and prevent CVD.[6] Other possible causes of inflammation include elevated low-density lipoproteins, free radicals caused by cigarette smoking, high blood pressure, and diabetes mellitus (see "Diabetes: Disabling, Deadly, and on the Rise," later in this chapter).

In an effort to combat the effects of inflammation, an explosive amount of research is being published to assess the potential role of anti-inflammatory drugs, such as aspirin, ibuprofen, statins, and a new generation of "super-aspirins" in CVD prevention.[7]

Metabolic Syndrome

A group of obesity-related health risk factors, **metabolic syndrome** dramatically increases the risk of heart disease and diabetes. Also known as syndrome X or MetS, metabolic syndrome is believed to increase the risk for atherosclerotic cardiovascular disease by as much as threefold. Affecting over 26 percent of adults or 50 million people, this disease has gained increasing attention worldwide.[8] Two of the main characteristics of metabolic syndrome are weight gain, particularly in the abdominal area, and insulin resistance, which means that cells don't work properly in handling blood glucose levels. Scientists indicate that when three or more of the following are present, the diagnosis is metabolic syndrome:

- Abdominal obesity (waist measurement of more than 40 inches in men or 35 in women)
- Elevated blood fat (triglycerides greater than 150)
- Low levels of "good" high density lipoprotein cholesterol (HDL): less than 40 in men and less than 50 in women
- Blood pressure greater than 130/85 mm Hg
- Elevated fasting glucose greater than 100 mg/dL (a sign of insulin resistance)

Coronary Heart Disease

Of all the major cardiovascular diseases, coronary heart disease (CHD) is the greatest killer, accounting for nearly one in five deaths in the United States. Of the nearly 1 million people who suffer a heart attack each year, over 38 percent will die from it.[9] A **myocardial infarction (MI),** or **heart attack,** involves an area of the heart that suffers permanent damage because its normal blood supply has been blocked. This condition is often brought on by a blood clot in a coronary artery or an atherosclerotic narrowing that blocks an artery. When blood does not flow readily, there is a corresponding decrease in oxygen flow. If the blockage is extremely minor, an otherwise healthy heart will adapt over time by enlarging existing blood vessels and growing new ones to reroute blood through other areas.

When heart blockage is more severe, however, the body is unable to adapt on its own, and outside lifesaving support is critical. The hour following a heart attack is the most crucial period—over 40 percent of heart attack victims die within

this time. See the **Skills for Behavior Change** box on page 352 to learn what to do in case of a heart attack.

Angina Pectoris

Atherosclerosis and other circulatory impairments often reduce the heart's blood and oxygen supply, a condition known as **ischemia.** People with ischemia often suffer from varying degrees of **angina pectoris,** or chest pain. In fact, an estimated 2.6 million men and 4.2 million women suffer mild to crushing forms of chest pain each day, many of whom take powerful medications to control their symptoms.[10] Symptoms may range from slight indigestion, to pain upon slight exertion, to a feeling that the heart is being crushed. Generally, the more serious the oxygen deprivation, the more severe the pain. Although angina pectoris is not a heart attack, it does indicate underlying heart disease.

Currently, there are several methods of treating angina. In mild cases, rest is critical. The most common treatments for more severe cases involve drugs that affect either the supply of blood to the heart muscle or the heart's demand for oxygen. Pain and discomfort are often relieved with *nitroglycerin,* a drug used to relax (dilate) veins, thereby reducing the amount of blood returning to the heart and thus lessening its workload. Patients whose angina is caused by spasms of the coronary arteries are often given drugs called *calcium channel blockers,* drugs that prevent calcium atoms from passing through coronary arteries and causing heart contractions. They also appear to reduce blood pressure and slow heart rate. *Beta blockers,* the other major type of drugs used to treat angina, control potential overactivity of the heart muscle.

Arrhythmias

Over 4 million Americans have experienced some type of **arrhythmia,** an irregularity in heart rhythm; about 480,400 of arrhythmia episodes have resulted in death.[11] A person who complains of a racing heart in the absence of exercise or anxiety may be experiencing *tachycardia,* the medical term for abnormally fast heartbeat. On the other end of the continuum is *bradycardia,* or abnormally slow heartbeat.

metabolic syndrome   A group of three or more characteristics, including abdominal obesity and high blood pressure, that can cause metabolic problems that raise CVD risk.

myocardial infarction (MI; heart attack)   A blockage of normal blood supply to an area in the heart.

ischemia   Reduced oxygen supply to a body part or organ.

angina pectoris   Chest pain occurring as a result of reduced oxygen flow to the heart.

arrhythmia   An irregularity in heartbeat.

SKILLS FOR behavior change

WHAT TO DO IN THE EVENT OF A HEART ATTACK

We tend to think of heart attacks as being like those shown on TV, in which someone clutches their chest in apparent pain and topples over, gasping for breath. Sometimes, heart attacks really are this obvious. However, for many people, the symptoms start out very slowly, with only mild pain or discomfort similar to heartburn or indigestion. Knowing how to spot both the subtle and more overt symptoms and acting promptly can mean the difference between life and death for you or your loved ones.

KNOW THE WARNING SIGNS OF A HEART ATTACK

- *Chest discomfort.* Most heart attacks involve discomfort in the center of the chest that lasts more than a few minutes or that goes away and comes back. It can feel like uncomfortable pressure, squeezing, fullness, or pain, and it can sometimes be mistaken for gaseous stomach or heartburn.
- *Discomfort in other areas of the upper body.* Symptoms can include pain or discomfort in one or both arms, the back, neck, jaw, or stomach. Sometimes it can radiate; other times it can come and go.

- *Shortness of breath.* This can occur with or without chest discomfort.
- *Other signs.* These may include breaking out in a cold sweat, nausea, or lightheadedness or dizziness.

For both men and women, the most common heart attack symptom is chest pain or discomfort. However, women are more likely than men to experience some of the other common symptoms, particularly shortness of breath, nausea/vomiting, and back or jaw pain. These symptoms often appear over several hours rather than minutes.

THE BOTTOM LINE: DON'T DELAY

When it comes to treating heart attacks, time is of the essence: 40 percent of heart attack victims die within the first hour of experiencing symptoms. Fast action can save lives and minimize permanent heart damage, so call 911 right away. Ambulance emergency medical staff can begin treatment as soon as they arrive and continue it on the way to the hospital. Patients with chest pain who arrive by ambulance usually get faster treatment, and they can benefit from new medications and treatments that, if given quickly, can make all the difference.

BE A HEART SAVER

If you're with someone who is showing signs of a heart attack and the warning signs last for 2 minutes or longer, act immediately. Expect a denial. It's normal for a person with chest discomfort to deny the possibility of anything as serious as a heart attack. Don't take no for an answer, however. Insist on taking prompt action. Call the emergency rescue service, or get to the nearest hospital emergency room that offers 24-hour emergency cardiac care. Know the signs of cardiac arrest: loss of responsiveness, no normal breathing, and no pulse. If you are with someone who goes into cardiac arrest, call 911 and immediately begin CPR (cardiopulmonary resuscitation).

You don't have to wait until an emergency to take action—sign up for a course in CPR, and learn the safe and proper techniques of mouth-to-mouth breathing and chest compression. The American Heart Association website provides information on the availability of CPR courses throughout the nation.

Source: From *Heart Attack, Stroke and Cardiac Arrest Warning Signs,* www.americanheart.org/presenter.jhtml?identifier=3053. Reprinted with permission. www.americanheart.org © 2007, American Heart Association, Inc.

When a heart goes into **fibrillation,** it beats in a sporadic, quivering pattern that results in extreme inefficiency in moving blood through the cardiovascular system. If untreated, fibrillation may be fatal.

Not all arrhythmias are life-threatening. In many instances, excessive caffeine or nicotine consumption can trigger an arrhythmia episode. However, severe cases may require drug therapy or external electrical stimulus to prevent serious complications.

Congestive Heart Failure

When the heart muscle is damaged or overworked and lacks the strength to keep blood circulating normally through the body, its chambers are often taxed to the limit. **Congestive heart failure (CHF)** affects over 5 million Americans and dramatically increases risk of premature death.[12] The heart muscle may be injured by a number of health conditions, including rheumatic fever, pneumonia, heart attack, or other cardiovascular problems. In some cases, the damage is due to radiation or chemotherapy treatments for cancer. These weakened muscles respond poorly, impairing blood flow out of the heart through the arteries. The return flow of blood through

fibrillation A sporadic, quivering pattern of heartbeat that results in extreme inefficiency in moving blood through the cardiovascular system.

congestive heart failure (CHF) An abnormal cardiovascular condition that reflects impaired cardiac pumping and blood flow; pooling blood leads to congestion in body tissues.

the veins begins to back up, causing congestion in body tissues. This pooling of blood enlarges the heart, makes it less efficient, and decreases the amount of blood that can be circulated. Fluid begins to accumulate in other body areas, such as the vessels in the legs, ankles, or lungs, where it can leak into surrounding tissues and cause swelling or difficulty in breathing.

Today, CHF is the single most frequent cause of hospitalization in the United States.[13] If untreated, it can be fatal. However, most cases respond well to treatment that includes *diuretics* ("water pills") to relieve fluid accumulation; drugs, such as *digitalis,* that increase the pumping action of the heart; and drugs called *vasodilators,* which expand blood vessels and decrease resistance, allowing blood to flow more easily and making the heart's work easier.

Congenital and Rheumatic Heart Disease

Approximately 1 out of every 125 children is born with some form of **congenital heart disease** (disease present at birth).[14] These forms may be relatively minor, such as slight *murmurs* (low-pitched sounds caused by turbulent blood flow through the heart) due to valve irregularities that some children outgrow. Other congenital problems involve serious complications in heart function that can be corrected only with surgery. Their underlying causes are unknown but may be related to hereditary factors; to maternal diseases, such as rubella, that occur during fetal development; or to chemical intake (particularly alcohol) by the mother during pregnancy. Because of advances in pediatric cardiology, the prognosis for children with congenital heart defects is better than ever.

Rheumatic heart disease can cause similar heart problems in children. It is attributed to rheumatic fever, an inflammatory disease that may affect many connective tissues of the body, especially those of the heart, joints, brain, or skin, and that is caused by an unresolved *streptococcal infection* of the throat (strep throat). In a small number of cases, this infection can lead to an immune response in which antibodies attack the heart as well as the bacteria. Many of the 82,000 annual operations on heart valves in the United States are related to rheumatic heart disease.[15]

Stroke

Like heart muscle, brain cells must have a continuous adequate supply of oxygen in order to survive. A **stroke** (also called a *cerebrovascular accident*) occurs when the blood supply to the brain is interrupted. Strokes may be caused by a clot that obstructs a blood vessel or an **aneurysm** (a weakening in a blood vessel that causes it to bulge and in severe cases burst, or *hemorrhage*). When any of these events occurs, oxygen deprivation kills brain cells, which do not have the capacity to heal or regenerate. Some strokes are mild and cause only temporary dizziness or slight weakness or numbness. More serious interruptions in blood flow may impair speech, memory, or motor control.

Other strokes affect parts of the brain that regulate heart and lung function and kill within minutes. According to the American Heart Association's latest statistics, every year nearly 6 million Americans suffer strokes, 157,000 of whom die as a result. Strokes cause countless levels of disability and suffering, and they account for 1 in 15 deaths, surpassed only by CHD and cancer.[16] About one in ten major strokes is preceded days, weeks, or months earlier by **transient ischemic attacks (TIAs),** brief interruptions of the blood supply to the brain that cause only temporary impairment. Symptoms of TIA include dizziness, particularly when first rising in the morning, weakness, temporary paralysis or numbness in the face or other regions, temporary memory loss, blurred vision, nausea, headache, slurred speech, or other unusual physiological reactions. TIAs are often indications of an impending major stroke.

Warning signs of stroke include the following:

- Sudden weakness or numbness of the face, arm, or leg on one side of the body
- Sudden dimness or loss of vision, particularly in only one eye
- Loss of speech, or trouble talking or understanding speech
- Sudden, severe headaches with no known cause
- Unexplained dizziness, unsteadiness, or sudden falls, especially with any of the previously listed symptoms

If you experience any of these symptoms, or if you are with someone who does, seek medical help *immediately.* The earlier treatment starts, the more effective it will be.

One of the greatest medical successes in recent years has been the decline in the fatality rates from strokes, a rate that has dropped by one-third in the United States since the 1980s and continues to fall. Improved diagnostic procedures, better surgical options, clot-busting drugs injected soon after a stroke has occurred, and acute care centers specializing in stroke treatment and rehabilitation have all been factors. Increased awareness of risk factors for stroke, especially high blood pressure, knowledge of warning signals, and an emphasis on prevention also have contributed. It is estimated that more than half of all strokes could be avoided if more people followed the recommended preventive standards.

---

congenital heart disease Heart disease that is present at birth.

rheumatic heart disease A heart disease caused by untreated streptococcal infection of the throat.

stroke A condition occurring when the brain is damaged by disrupted blood supply.

aneurysm A weakened blood vessel that may bulge under pressure and, in severe cases, burst.

transient ischemic attack (TIA) Brief interruption of the blood supply to the brain that causes only temporary impairment; often an indicator of impending major stroke.

Unfortunately, people who survive a stroke do not always make a full recovery. Some 50 to 70 percent of stroke survivors regain functional independence, but 15 to 30 percent are permanently disabled and require assistance. Today stroke is a leading cause of serious long-term disability and contributes a significant amount to Medicaid and Medicare expenses for older Americans, particularly women.

Reducing Your Risk for Cardiovascular Disease

 Factors that increase the risk for cardiovascular problems fall into two categories: those we can control and those we cannot. Fortunately, we can take steps to minimize many risk factors.

Risks You Can Control

Avoid Tobacco In spite of massive campaigns to educate us about the dangers of smoking, and in spite of increasing numbers of states and municipalities that have enacted policies to go "smoke-free," cigarette smoking remains the leading cause of preventable death in the United States, accounting for approximately one of every five deaths.[17] These statistics are particularly surprising given the fact that smoking rates have declined by 49 percent among people aged 18 and older since 1965.[18] The risk for cardiovascular disease is 70 percent greater for smokers than for nonsmokers. Smokers who have a heart attack are more likely to die suddenly (within one hour) than are nonsmokers. Evidence also indicates that chronic exposure to environmental tobacco smoke (ETS, or secondhand smoke) increases the risk of heart disease by as much as 30 percent, with over 35,000 nonsmokers dying from ETS exposure each year.[19]

How does smoking damage the heart? There are two plausible explanations. One is that nicotine increases heart rate, heart output, blood pressure, and oxygen use by heart muscles. Because the carbon monoxide in cigarette smoke displaces oxygen in heart tissue, the heart is forced to work harder to obtain sufficient oxygen. The other explanation is that chemicals in smoke damage and inflame the lining of the coronary arteries, allowing cholesterol and plaque to accumulate more easily. This additional buildup constricts the vessels, increasing blood pressure and forcing the heart to work harder.

When people stop smoking, regardless of how long or how much they've smoked, their risk of heart disease declines rapidly.[20] By 3 years after they quit, the risk of death from heart disease and stroke for people who had smoked a pack a day or less is almost the same as for people who have never smoked. Although the exact reasons are unknown, new findings from the Lung Health Study indicate that lung function improves more in women than in men after sustained smoking cessation.[21]

Cut Back on Saturated Fat and Cholesterol

Cholesterol is a soft, fatty, waxy substance found in the bloodstream and in your body cells. Although we hear only the bad things about it, in truth cholesterol plays an important role in the production of cell membranes and hormones and in other body functions. However, when it gets too high, risks for CVD escalate. Nearly 36 percent of adults in the United States aged 18 and above have been told they have high cholesterol, and vast numbers of others have never been tested yet probably have higher than normal levels. Less than half of people who should be on cholesterol-reducing medications are on them, and many who are on them are unable to reach their LDL and HDL goals.[22]

Just like the TV ads say, you get cholesterol from two primary sources—from your body (which involves genetic predisposition) and from food. Unfortunately, much of your cholesterol level is predetermined: 75 percent of blood cholesterol is produced by your liver and other cells, and the other 25 percent comes from the foods you eat. It's the 25 percent that you can control that may be the tipping point in determining your CVD risks.

Why all the fuss about fats and cholesterol? Diets high in saturated fat are known to raise cholesterol levels, send the body's blood-clotting system into high gear, and make the blood more viscous in just a few hours, increasing the risk of heart attack or stroke. Switching to a low-fat diet lowers the risk of clotting; even a 10 percent decrease in total cholesterol levels may result in an estimated 30 percent reduction in the incidence of heart disease.[23]

A fatty diet also increases the amount of cholesterol in the blood, contributing to atherosclerosis. In past years, cholesterol levels between 200 and 240 milligrams per 100 milliliters of blood (mg/dL) were considered normal. Recent research indicates that levels between 180 and 200 mg/dL are more desirable and that a level of 150 mg/dL would be even better in reducing CVD risk. People with multiple risk factors for CVD are advised to follow even more stringent guidelines.[24] See **Table 12.1** for recommended levels.

It isn't just the total cholesterol level that you should be concerned about. Cholesterol comes in two main varieties: **low-density lipoprotein (LDL)** and **high-density lipoprotein (HDL).** Low-density lipoprotein, often referred to as "bad" cholesterol, is believed to build up on artery walls. In contrast, high-density lipoprotein, or "good" cholesterol, appears to remove cholesterol from artery

What's the difference between good and bad cholesterol?

low-density lipoproteins (LDLs) Compounds that facilitate the transport of cholesterol in the blood to the body's cells and cause the cholesterol to build up on artery walls.

high-density lipoproteins (HDLs) Compounds that facilitate the transport of cholesterol in the blood to the liver for metabolism and elimination from the body.

walls, thus serving as a protector. In theory, if LDL levels get too high or HDL levels too low, cholesterol will accumulate inside arteries and lead to cardiovascular problems. Scientists now believe that there are other factors that may also increase CVD risk, such as lipoprotein-associated phospholipase A$_2$ (Lp-PLA$_2$), an enzyme that circulates in the blood and attaches to LDL. Lp-PLA$_2$ plays an important role in plaque accumulation and increased risk for stroke and coronary events, particularly in men. Studies suggest that the higher the Lp-PLA$_2$ level, the higher the risk of developing CVD.[25]

Triglycerides, another type of fat in the blood, also appear to promote atherosclerosis. As people get older, heavier, or both, their triglycerides and cholesterol levels tend to rise. Although some CVD patients have elevated triglyceride levels, a causal link between high triglyceride levels and CVD has yet to be established. It may be that high triglyceride levels do not directly cause atherosclerosis but, rather, are among the abnormalities that speed its development.

Current guidelines suggest that you should reduce consumption of saturated fat (which comes mostly from animal products) to less than 7 percent of your total daily caloric intake and minimize your consumption of *trans* fat, which is found in partially hydrogenated products such as margarine, fast foods, and packaged foods. By cutting your intake of saturated fats and *trans* fats, and consuming fewer than 200 milligrams per day of cholesterol, you can significantly reduce your risks. Although it is wise to cut back on saturated fat, be aware that some fat is necessary to overall health. (For a complete discussion of this topic, see Chapter 9.)

Monitor Your Cholesterol Levels

To get an accurate assessment of your total cholesterol and LDL and HDL levels, consider having a *lipoprotein analysis* done by a reputable health provider. In general, LDL is more closely associated with cardiovascular risk than is total cholesterol. However, most authorities agree that looking only at LDL ignores the positive effects of HDL. Perhaps the best method of evaluating risk is to examine the ratio of HDL to total cholesterol, or the percentage of HDL in total cholesterol.

The goal is to manage the ratio of HDL to total cholesterol by lowering LDL levels, raising HDL, or both. Of the more than 100 million Americans who need to worry about their cholesterol levels, almost half, particularly those at the low-to-moderate risk levels, should be able to reach their LDL and HDL goals through lifestyle changes alone. People who are at higher risk or those for whom lifestyle modifications are not effective may need to take cholesterol-lowering drugs while they continue modifying their lifestyle. Among the most commonly prescribed drugs are statins, which are very effective in reducing LDL levels. Folic acid and niacin drugs are often prescribed for people with low HDL and high triglyceride levels.

TABLE 12.1 | **Classification of LDL, Total, and HDL Cholesterol (mg/dl) and Recommended Levels for Adults**

LDL Cholesterol

<100	Optimal
100–129	Near optimal/above optimal
130–159	Borderline high
160–189	High
≥190	Very high

HDL Cholesterol

<40	Low
≥60	High

Total Cholesterol

<200	Desirable
200–239	Borderline high
≥240	High

Triglycerides

<150	Normal
150–199	Borderline high
200–499	High
≥500	Very high

Source: National Heart, Lung, and Blood Institute, *Third Report of the Expert Panel on Detection, Evaluation, and Treatment of High Blood Cholesterol in Adults.* (NIH Publication no. 05–3290), 2005, www.nhlbi.nih.gov/health/public/heart/chol/wyntk.htm.

Modify Other Dietary Habits

The National Heart, Lung, and Blood Institute (NHLBI) guidelines recommend the following dietary changes to reduce CVD risk:

- Consume 5 to 10 milligrams per day of soluble fiber from sources such as psyllium seeds, oat bran, fruits, vegetables, and legumes (see Chapter 9). Even this small dietary modification may result in a 5 percent drop in LDL levels.
- Consume about 2 grams per day of plant sterols or sterol derivatives from substances such as Benecol or Take Control margarine. These were the first widely available sources of sterols, but many other choices are available. This amount of plant sterols has the potential to reduce LDL by another 5 percent.

triglycerides The most common form of fat in the body; excess calories are converted into triglycerides and stored as body fat.

HEALTH headlines

Just when it seems most of your favorite treats carry health risks, there is new evidence that a class of antioxidants known as flavonoids, which are found in fruits, teas, red wine, and cocoa, may protect you from risks for cardiovascular diseases, diabetes, cancer, and other ailments. Sound too good to be true?

Consider results from these studies:

- At an international conference of the American Association for Cancer Research, reports of a study of 1,434 women with breast cancer and 1,440 healthy women supported a potential link between flavonoid intake and reduced risk for breast cancer. Women who consumed the most flavonoids had a 45 percent lower risk of breast cancer compared to those who consumed the least. Another study of 66,384 women reported that those women who consumed the most flavonoids had a lower risk of ovarian cancer than those who consumed the least flavonoids.

- Results of a 12-year study of 38,077 men with no prior history of CVD suggested that drinking 1 to 2 drinks per day, 3 to 4 days per week, decreased the risk of a heart attack by as much as 32 percent. In the same study, it was found that light alcohol consumption reduced the risk of stroke by 20 percent.

- A joint Norwegian–U.S. study of nearly 35,000 postmenopausal women reported that high dietary intake of several classes of flavonoids reduced the risk of mortality from cardiovascular disease and stroke by between 10 and 22 percent.

The reason for the effects observed in these studies is unclear. Some studies indicated that flavonoids impact CVD risk through an anti-inflammatory action. Other research suggests that the cancer-related health benefits come not from the flavonoids themselves, but from enzymes the body produces to metabolize and excrete the flavonoids. These enzymes may also act against mutagens and

carcinogens and inhibit tumor growth. Recently, however, a large review of studies indicated that flavonoids may not exert such strong or direct effects after all.

In spite of the promising nature of some of these studies, most experts warn that nondrinkers should not begin drinking to improve overall health. Likewise, balanced nutrition should not be abandoned for a daily chocolate bar. Until more research has established the nature and extent of these protective mechanisms, health experts continue to promote the "five a day" minimum consumption of fruits and vegetables and limited consumption of alcohol and chocolate.

Sources: S. B. Lotito and B. Frei, "Consumption of Flavoniod-Rich Foods and Increased Plasma Antioxidant Capacity in Humans: Cause, Consequence, or Epiphenomenon?" *Free Radical Biology and Medicine* 41 (2007): 1727–46; P. Lagiou, P. Szmitko, and V. Subodh, "Red Wine and Your Heart," *Circulation* 111 (2004). e10–e11; P. J. Mink et al., "Flavonoid Intake and Cardiovascular Disease Mortality: A Prospective Study in Postmenopause Women," *American Journal of Clinical Nutrition* 85 (2007): 895–909.

Maintain a Healthy Weight No question about it—body weight plays a role in CVD. Researchers are not sure whether high-fat, high-sugar, high-calorie diets are a direct risk for CVD or whether they invite risk by causing obesity, which strains the heart, forcing it to push blood through the many miles of capillaries that supply each pound of fat. A heart that has to continuously move blood through an overabundance of vessels may become damaged.

Overweight people are more likely to develop heart disease and stroke even if they have no other risk factors. If you're heavy, losing even 5 to 10 pounds can make a significant difference. This is especially true if you're an "apple" (thicker around your upper body and waist) rather than a "pear" (thicker around your hips and thighs). See Chapter 10 for tips on weight management.

Exercise Regularly Inactivity is a clear risk factor for CVD.[26] The good news is that you do not have to be an exercise fanatic to reduce your risk. Even modest levels of

low-intensity physical activity—walking, gardening, house-work, dancing—are beneficial if done regularly and over the long term. Exercise can increase HDL, lower triglycerides, and reduce coronary risks in several ways. For more information on the health benefits of exercise, see Chapter 11.

Control Diabetes Research underscores the unique CVD risks for people with diabetes. Diabetics who have taken insulin for a number of years have a greater chance of developing CVD. In fact, CVD is the leading cause of death among diabetic patients. Because overweight people have a higher risk for diabetes, distinguishing between the effects of the two conditions is difficult. People with diabetes also tend to have elevated blood fat levels, increased atherosclerosis, and a tendency toward deterioration of small blood vessels, particularly in the eyes and extremities. However, through a prescribed regimen of diet, exercise, and medication, they can control much of their increased risk for CVD (see the section on diabetes, later in this chapter).

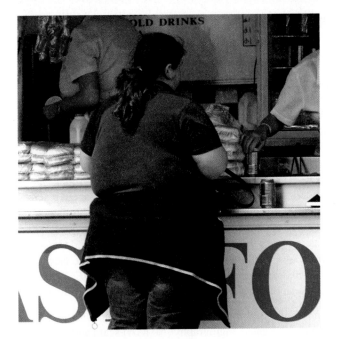

Excessive body weight increases the risk of developing CVD. Weight management should be a primary goal for CVD prevention.

	Systolic Reading (mm Hg)		Diastolic Reading (mm Hg)
TABLE 12.2	**Blood Pressure Classifications**		
Classification			
Normal	<120	and	<80
Prehypertension	120–139	or	80–89
Hypertension			
Stage 1	140–159	or	90–99
Stage 2	≥160	or	≥100

Note: If systolic and diastolic readings fall into different categories, treatment is determined by the highest category. Readings are based on the average of two or more properly measured, seated readings on each of two or more health care provider visits.
Source: National Heart, Lung, and Blood Institute, *The Seventh Report of the Joint National Committee on Prevention, Detection, Evaluation, and Treatment of High Blood Pressure* (NIH Publication no. 03-5233) (Bethesda, MD: National Institutes of Health, revised June 2005).

Control Your Blood Pressure Hypertension

refers to sustained high blood pressure. In general, the higher your blood pressure, the greater your risk for CVD. Hypertension is known as the "silent killer" because it usually has no symptoms. Its prevalence has increased by over 30 percent in the last 10 years; today 65 million adults in the United States have blood pressure above the recommended level.[27]

Blood pressure is measured in two parts and is expressed as a fraction—for example, 110/80, or "110 over 80." Both values are measured in *millimeters of mercury* (mm Hg). The first number refers to **systolic pressure,** or the pressure being applied to the walls of the arteries when the heart contracts, pumping blood to the rest of the body. The second value is **diastolic pressure,** or the pressure applied to the walls of the arteries during the heart's relaxation phase. During this phase, blood is reentering the chambers of the heart, preparing for the next heartbeat.

Normal blood pressure varies depending on weight, age, physical condition, gender, and race. Systolic blood pressure tends to increase with age, whereas diastolic blood pressure increases until age 55 and then declines. As a rule, men have a greater risk for high blood pressure than women until age 55, when their risks become about equal. After age 75, women are more likely to have high blood pressure than men.[28]

For the average person, 110/80 is a healthy blood pressure level. High blood pressure is usually diagnosed when systolic pressure is 140 or above. Diastolic pressure does not have to be high to indicate high blood pressure. When only systolic pressure is high, the condition is known as *isolated systolic hypertension (ISH),* the most

common form of high blood pressure in older Americans. See **Table 12.2** for a summary of blood pressure values and what they mean.

Treatment of hypertension can involve dietary changes (reducing sodium and calorie intake), weight loss (when appropriate), the use of diuretics and other medications (only when prescribed by a physician), regular exercise, and the practice of relaxation techniques and effective coping and communication skills.

Manage Stress Some scientists have noted a relationship

between CVD risk and a person's stress level, behavior habits, and socioeconomic status. These factors may influence established risk factors. For example, people under stress may start smoking or smoke more than they otherwise would. A large study funded by the National Heart, Lung, and Blood Institute found that impatience and hostility, two key components of the Type A behavior pattern, increase young adults' risk of developing high blood pressure. Other related factors, such as competitiveness, depression, and anxiety, did not appear to increase risk. The research was the first to study these factors as a group rather than individually and has clear implications for prevention.[29]

hypertension Sustained elevated blood pressure.

systolic pressure The upper number in the fraction that measures blood pressure, indicating pressure on the walls of the arteries when the heart contracts.

diastolic pressure The lower number in the fraction that measures blood pressure, indicating pressure on the walls of the arteries during the relaxation phase of heart activity.

Risks You Cannot Control

There are, unfortunately, some risk factors for CVD that we cannot prevent or control. The most important are these:

Does cardiovascular disease run in families?

- *Heredity.* A family history of heart disease appears to increase risk significantly. Whether the increase is due to genetics or environment is unresolved.
- *Age.* The risk for CVD increases with age for both sexes. Seventy-five percent of all heart attacks occur in people over age 65.
- *Gender.* Men are at greater risk for CVD until about age 60. Women under 35 have a fairly low risk unless they smoke or have high blood pressure, kidney problems, or diabetes. Hormonal factors appear to reduce risk for women, although after menopause or after estrogen levels are otherwise reduced (e.g., because of hysterectomy), women's LDL levels tend to go up, which increases their chances for CVD.
- *Race.* African Americans have a 45 percent greater risk for hypertension and thus a greater risk for CVD than whites. In addition, they are less likely to survive a heart attack.

New Weapons Against Heart Disease

The victim of a heart attack today has many options that were not available a generation ago. Medications can strengthen heartbeat, control arrhythmias, remove fluids in case of congestive heart failure, and relieve pain. New surgical procedures are saving many lives.

Techniques for Diagnosing Heart Disease

Several techniques are used to diagnose heart disease, including electrocardiogram, angiography, and positron

electrocardiogram (ECG)   A record of the electrical activity of the heart; may be measured during a stress test.

angiography   A technique for examining blockages in heart arteries.

positron emission tomography (PET)   Method for measuring heart activity by injecting a patient with a radioactive tracer that is scanned electronically to produce a three-dimensional image of the heart and arteries.

coronary bypass surgery   A surgical technique whereby a blood vessel is implanted to bypass a clogged coronary artery.

angioplasty   A technique in which a catheter with a balloon at the tip is inserted into a clogged artery; the balloon is inflated to flatten fatty deposits against artery walls, which allows blood to flow more freely. A stent is typically inserted to keep the artery open.

emission tomography scans. An **electrocardiogram (ECG)** is a record of the electrical activity of the heart. Patients may undergo a stress test, such as walking or running on a treadmill while their hearts are monitored. A more accurate method of testing for heart disease is **angiography** (often referred to as *cardiac catheterization*), in which a needle-thin tube called a *catheter* is threaded through heart arteries, a dye is injected, and an X-ray image is taken to discover which areas are blocked. A more recent and even more effective method of measuring heart activity is **positron emission tomography (PET),** which produces three-dimensional images of the heart as blood flows through it. During a PET scan, a patient receives an intravenous injection of a radioactive tracer and is then monitored at rest and during exercise. As the tracer decays, it emits positrons that are picked up by the scanner and transformed by a computer into color images of the heart. Newer *single-photon emission computed tomography (SPECT)* scans provide an even better view. Other tests include the following:

- *Radionuclide imaging* (includes thallium test, multinucleated gated angiography [MUGA] scan, and acute infarct scintigraphy). In these procedures, substances called radionuclides are injected into the bloodstream. Computer-generated pictures can then show them in the heart. These tests can show how well the heart muscle is supplied with blood, how well the heart's chambers are functioning, and which part of the heart has been damaged by a heart attack.
- *Magnetic resonance imaging (MRI).* This test uses powerful magnets to look inside the body. Computer-generated pictures can show the heart muscle and help physicians identify damage from a heart attack, diagnose congenital heart defects, and evaluate disease of larger blood vessels such as the aorta.
- *Ultrafast computed tomography (CT).* This is an especially fast form of X-ray imaging of the heart designed to evaluate bypass grafts, diagnose ventricular function, and measure calcium deposits.
- *Digital subtraction angiography (DSA).* This modified form of computer-aided imaging records pictures of the heart and its blood vessels.

Bypass Surgery versus Angioplasty

Coronary bypass surgery has helped many patients who suffered coronary blockages or heart attacks. In coronary bypass surgery, a blood vessel is taken from another site in the patient's body (usually the *saphenous vein* in the leg or the *internal mammary artery*) and implanted to "bypass" blocked arteries and transport blood. Bypass patients typically spend 4 to 7 days in the hospital to recuperate. Death rates are generally much lower at medical centers where surgical teams and intensive care teams see large numbers of patients.[30]

Another procedure, **angioplasty** (sometimes called *balloon angioplasty*), carries fewer risks and may be more effective than bypass surgery in selected cases. As in angiography, a thin catheter is threaded through blocked heart arteries. The catheter has a balloon at the tip, which is inflated to flatten fatty deposits against the artery walls, allowing blood to flow more freely. A *stent* (a meshlike tube) may be inserted to prop open the artery. In about 30 percent of patients, the treated arteries become clogged again within 6 months. Some surgeons argue that given this high rate of recurrence, bypass may be a more effective treatment. Today, newer forms of laser angioplasty and atherectomy, a procedure that removes plaque, are being done in several clinics.

Research suggests that in many instances, drug treatments may be just as effective in prolonging life as invasive surgical techniques, but it is critical that doctors prescribe an aggressive drug treatment program and that patients comply with it.

Aspirin for Heart Disease: Can It Help?

Research indicates that low doses of aspirin (80 milligrams daily or every other day) are beneficial to heart patients because of the drug's blood-thinning properties. Higher levels do not provide significantly more protection. Aspirin has even been advised as a preventive strategy for people with no current heart disease symptoms. However, major problems associated with chronic aspirin use are gastrointestinal intolerance and a tendency for some people to have difficulty with blood clotting, and these factors may outweigh aspirin's benefits in some cases. People taking aspirin face additional risks from emergency surgery or accidental bleeding. Aspirin should be taken as a preventative measure only if your physician recommends it.

Cardiac Rehabilitation

Every year, nearly 1 million people survive heart attacks. Over 7 million more have unstable angina, and about 650,000 undergo bypass surgery or angioplasty. Heart failure is the most common discharge diagnosis for hospitalized Medicare patients and the fourth most common diagnosis among all patients hospitalized in the United States. Most of these patients are eligible for cardiac rehabilitation (including exercise training and health education classes on good nutrition and CVD risk management), needing only a doctor's prescription for these services. However, many Americans do not have access to these programs. Even larger numbers are finding it difficult to afford them in light of skyrocketing costs for prescription drugs. Whereas some patients must choose between home health care and cardiac rehabilitation, others stay away from such programs because of cost, transportation, or other factors. Perhaps the biggest deterrent is fear that exercise may cause another attack. The benefits of cardiac rehabilitation (including increased stamina and strength and faster recovery), however, far outweigh the risks when these programs are run by certified health professionals.

what do you THINK?

With all the new diagnostic procedures, treatments, and differing philosophies about prevention and intervention techniques, how can health consumers ensure that they will get the best treatment? ■ Where can they go for information? ■ Why might patients need a health advocate who can help them get through the system?

Diabetes: Disabling, Deadly, and on the Rise

Diabetes is a serious, widespread, and costly chronic disease, affecting not just the 21 million Americans who live with it, but also their families and communities. Since 1980, diagnosed diabetes has increased over 50 percent among U.S. adults, giving it the dubious distinction of being the fastest growing chronic disease in American history.[31] One study by the Centers for Disease Control and Prevention indicated that diabetes seems to be increasing even more dramatically among younger adults—it is up by almost 70 percent among those in their thirties.[32]

What causes this serious disease? In healthy people, the *pancreas,* a powerful enzyme-producing organ, produces the hormone **insulin** in sufficient quantities to allow the body to use or store glucose (blood sugar). When the pancreas fails to produce enough insulin to regulate sugar metabolism or when the body fails to use insulin effectively, a disease known as **diabetes mellitus** occurs **(Figure 12.4).** Diabetics exhibit **hyperglycemia,** or elevated blood sugar levels, and high glucose levels in their urine. Other symptoms include excessive thirst, frequent urination, hunger, tendency to tire easily, wounds that heal slowly, numbness or tingling in the extremities, changes in vision, skin eruptions, and, in women, a tendency toward vaginal yeast infections. Of the 21 million people in the United States today who have diabetes, nearly 6 million are unaware of their condition.

The more serious form, *type 1 diabetes* (also known as insulin-dependent diabetes), is an autoimmune disease in which the immune system destroys the insulin-making beta cells. It most often appears during childhood or adolescence. People with type 1 diabetes typically must depend on insulin injections or infusions for the rest of their lives because insulin is not present in their bodies.

insulin A hormone produced by the pancreas; required by the body for the metabolism of carbohydrates.

diabetes mellitus A disease in which the pancreas fails to produce enough insulin or the body fails to use insulin effectively.

hyperglycemia Elevated blood sugar levels.

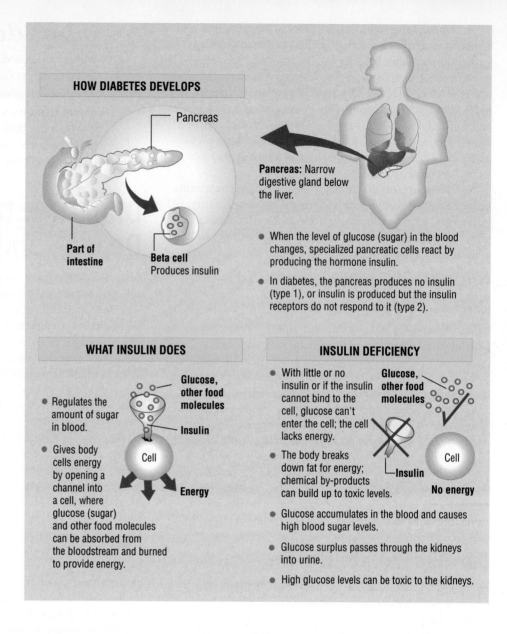

FIGURE 12.4 Diabetes: What It Is and How It Develops

Sources: Adaptation based on *Oregonian,* September 5, 2000, A6; *FDA Consumer* magazine; J. Mordis and W. Manis, *The Healing Handbook for Persons with Diabetes,* 3rd ed., 2000, www.umassmed.edu/HealingHandbook; L. Urdang, ed., *The Bantam Medical Dictionary,* 3rd ed. (New York: Bantam, 2000); American Medical Association, *American Medical Association Family Medical Guide,* 4th ed. (New York: Wiley, 2004); research by Jutta Scheibe.

HOW DIABETES DEVELOPS

Pancreas

Part of intestine

Beta cell
Produces insulin

Pancreas: Narrow digestive gland below the liver.

- When the level of glucose (sugar) in the blood changes, specialized pancreatic cells react by producing the hormone insulin.

- In diabetes, the pancreas produces no insulin (type 1), or insulin is produced but the insulin receptors do not respond to it (type 2).

WHAT INSULIN DOES

Glucose, other food molecules

Insulin

Cell

Energy

- Regulates the amount of sugar in blood.

- Gives body cells energy by opening a channel into a cell, where glucose (sugar) and other food molecules can be absorbed from the bloodstream and burned to provide energy.

INSULIN DEFICIENCY

- With little or no insulin or if the insulin cannot bind to the cell, glucose can't enter the cell; the cell lacks energy.

Glucose, other food molecules

Insulin

Cell

No energy

- The body breaks down fat for energy; chemical by-products can build up to toxic levels.

- Glucose accumulates in the blood and causes high blood sugar levels.

- Glucose surplus passes through the kidneys into urine.

- High glucose levels can be toxic to the kidneys.

In *type 2 diabetes* (non insulin-dependent diabetes), insulin production is deficient or the body is unable to utilize available insulin. Type 2 diabetes accounts for 90 to 95 percent of all diabetes cases and most often appears after age 40.[33] However, type 2 diabetes is now being diagnosed at younger ages, even among children and teens. This form of diabetes is typically linked to obesity and physical inactivity, both of which can be modified to control diabetes and improve health. If people with type 2 diabetes change their lifestyle, they may be able to avoid the need for oral medications or insulin indefinitely.

A third type of diabetes, *gestational diabetes,* can develop in a woman during pregnancy and affects 2 to 5 percent of all pregnant women. Although once believed to be only a transient event that disappeared after pregnancy, today experts realize that women with gestational diabetes have a significantly increased risk of progressing to type 2 diabetes within 5 to 10 years after giving birth.[34] This is particularly true for women who do not lose all of their gestational weight gain and for those who have additional pregnancies and weight "creep" with each subsequent one.

Understanding Risk Factors

Diabetes tends to run in families.[35] Being overweight, coupled with inactivity, dramatically increases the risk of type 2 diabetes. Older persons and mothers of babies weighing over 9 pounds also run an increased risk. Approximately 80 percent of all type 2 patients are overweight at the time of diagnosis. Weight loss, better nutrition, control of blood glucose levels, and regular exercise are important factors in lowering blood sugar and improving the efficiency of cellular use of insulin. These improvements can help prevent overwork of the pancreas and the development of diabetes. In fact, recent findings show that

What can I do to reduce my risk for diabetes?

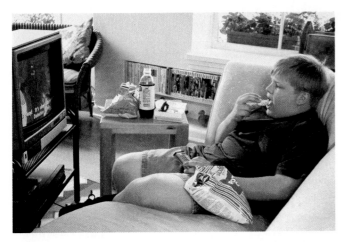

Unhealthy eating habits and a sedentary lifestyle can lead to type 2 diabetes even among children.

modest, consistent physical activity and a healthy diet can cut a person's risk of type 2 diabetes by a significant amount.[36] For unknown reasons, African Americans, Hispanics, and Native Americans have the highest rates of type 2 diabetes in the world—much higher than that of whites.[37]

Controlling Diabetes

Most physicians prescribe various oral medications for type 2 diabetes when patients are unable to control blood glucose with exercise and diet alone. For some type 2 diabetics, insulin may be necessary. Insulin is the prescribed treatment for type 1 diabetes. Recent breakthroughs in individual monitoring, implantable insulin monitors and pumps, and insulin inhalers have given many people with diabetes the opportunity to lead more normal lives. Some people with type 2 diabetes find that they can manage their diabetes effectively by losing weight, getting regular exercise, and eating foods that are rich in complex carbohydrates, low in sodium, and high in fiber.

Preventing Complications

Depending on the type and severity of the disease, diabetes can cause many complications and increase the severity of other existing conditions, including the following:[38]

- *Cardiovascular disease.* Heart disease and stroke cause about 65 percent of deaths among people with diabetes. More than 70 percent of people with diabetes have hypertension.
- *Eye disease and blindness.* Each year, 12,000 to 24,000 people become blind because of diabetic eye disease. In fact, it is the leading cause of new blindness in America today.
- *Kidney disease.* Each year almost 45,000 people with diabetes develop kidney failure; each year over 100,000 are in treatment for this condition.
- *Amputations.* Over 60 percent of nontraumatic amputations of lower limbs are due to diabetes. Foot care programs that include regular examinations and patient education could prevent up to 85 percent of these amputations.

- *Pregnancy complications.* Poorly controlled diabetes can cause major birth defects in 5 to 10 percent of all pregnancies and causes 15 to 20 percent of all spontaneous abortions.
- *Flu- and pneumonia-related deaths.* Each year, 10,000 to 30,000 people with diabetes die of complications from flu or pneumonia. They are roughly three times more likely to die of these complications than people without diabetes.

An Overview of Cancer

For Americans of all age groups, cancer continues to be the second leading cause of death, even though cancer-related mortality rates have declined over the last decade. Five-year survival rates (the relative rates for survival in persons who are living cancer-free 5 years after diagnosis) are up dramatically from the virtual death sentences of many cancers in the early 1900s and the 40 to 50 percent survival rates of the 1960s to 1970s. Today, of the approximately 1.5 million people diagnosed each year, about 66 percent will still be alive 5 years from now.[39] Many will be considered "cured," meaning that they have no subsequent cancer in their bodies 5 years after diagnosis and can expect to live a long and productive life. Some cancers have excellent prognosis for cure; others remain difficult to diagnose and treat because they are often not found until late in their progression. Survival rates for some cancers, such as pancreatic and liver, ovarian, and certain aggressive types of cancer, continue to be low.

What Is Cancer?

Cancer is the name given to a large group of diseases characterized by the uncontrolled growth and spread of abnormal cells. Think of a healthy cell as a small computer, programmed to operate in a particular fashion. Under normal conditions, healthy cells are protected by a powerful overseer, the immune system, as they perform their daily functions of growing, replicating, and repairing body organs. When something interrupts normal cell programming, however, uncontrolled growth and abnormal cellular development result in a **neoplasm,** a new growth of tissue serving no physiological function. This neoplasmic mass often forms a clumping of cells known as a **tumor.**

cancer A large group of diseases characterized by the uncontrolled growth and spread of abnormal cells.

neoplasm A new growth of tissue that serves no physiological function and results from uncontrolled, abnormal cellular development.

tumor A neoplasmic mass that grows more rapidly than surrounding tissue.

TABLE 12.3 — Probability of Developing Invasive Cancers over Selected Age Intervals by Sex, United States, 2001 to 2003*

		Birth to 39 (%)	40 to 59 (%)	60 to 69 (%)	70 and Older (%)	Birth to Death (%)
All sites†	Male	1.42 (1 in 70)	8.69 (1 in 12)	16.58 (1 in 6)	39.44 (1 in 3)	45.31 (1 in 2)
	Female	2.03 (1 in 49)	9.09 (1 in 11)	10.57 (1 in 9)	26.60 (1 in 4)	37.86 (1 in 3)
Urinary bladder‡	Male	0.02 (1 in 4381)	0.41 (1 in 241)	0.96 (1 in 105)	3.41 (1 in 29)	3.61 (1 in 28)
	Female	0.01 (1 in 9527)	0.13 (1 in 782)	0.26 (1 in 379)	0.96 (1 in 105)	1.14 (1 in 87)
Breast	Female	0.48 (1 in 210)	3.98 (1 in 25)	3.65 (1 in 27)	6.84 (1 in 15)	12.67 (1 in 8)
Colon and rectum	Male	0.07 (1 in 1342)	0.93 (1 in 107)	1.67 (1 in 60)	4.92 (1 in 20)	5.79 (1 in 17)
	Female	0.07 (1 in 1469)	0.73 (1 in 138)	1.16 (1 in 86)	4.45 (1 in 22)	5.37 (1 in 19)
Leukemia	Male	0.16 (1 in 640)	0.22 (1 in 452)	0.35 (1 in 286)	1.17 (1 in 86)	1.49 (1 in 67)
	Female	0.12 (1 in 820)	0.14 (1 in 694)	0.20 (1 in 491)	0.75 (1 in 132)	1.05 (1 in 95)
Lung and bronchus	Male	0.03 (1 in 3146)	1.09 (1 in 92)	2.61 (1 in 38)	6.76 (1 in 15)	8.02 (1 in 12)
	Female	0.04 (1 in 2779)	0.85 (1 in 117)	1.84 (1 in 54)	4.52 (1 in 22)	6.15 (1 in 16)
Melanoma of the skin	Male	0.13 (1 in 775)	0.53 (1 in 187)	0.56 (1 in 178)	1.32 (1 in 76)	2.04 (1 in 49)
	Female	0.21 (1 in 467)	0.42 (1 in 237)	0.29 (1 in 347)	0.62 (1 in 163)	1.38 (1 in 73)
Non-Hodgkin lymphoma	Male	0.14 (1 in 735)	0.45 (1 in 222)	0.57 (1 in 176)	1.56 (1 in 64)	2.14 (1 in 47)
	Female	0.08 (1 in 1200)	0.32 (1 in 313)	0.44 (1 in 229)	1.30 (1 in 77)	1.83 (1 in 55)
Prostate	Male	0.01 (1 in 10373)	2.59 (1 in 39)	7.03 (1 in 14)	13.83 (1 in 7)	17.12 (1 in 6)
Uterine cervix	Female	0.16 (1 in 631)	0.29 (1 in 346)	0.14 (1 in 695)	0.20 (1 in 512)	0.73 (1 in 138)
Uterine corpus	Female	0.06 (1 in 1652)	0.70 (1 in 142)	0.81 (1 in 124)	1.28 (1 in 78)	2.49 (1 in 40)

*For people free of cancer at beginning of age interval.

†All sites exclude basal and squamous cell skin cancers and in situ cancers except urinary bladder.

‡Includes invasive and in situ cancer cases.

Source: DevCan, Probability of Developing or Dying of Cancer Software, Version 6.1.0. Statistical Research and Applications Branch, National Cancer Institute, 2006, www.srab.cancer.gov/devcan.

Not all tumors are **malignant** (cancerous); in fact, most are **benign** (noncancerous). Benign tumors are generally harmless unless they grow to obstruct or crowd out normal tissues. A benign tumor of the brain, for instance, is life threatening when it grows enough to restrict blood flow and cause a stroke. The only way to determine whether a tumor is malignant is through **biopsy,** or microscopic examination of cell development.

Benign and malignant tumors differ in several key ways. Benign tumors generally consist of ordinary-looking cells enclosed in a fibrous shell or capsule that prevents their spreading to other body areas. Malignant tumors are usually not enclosed in a protective capsule and can therefore spread to other organs. This process, known as **metastasis,** makes some forms of cancer particularly aggressive in their ability to overcome bodily defenses. By the time they are diagnosed, malignant tumors have frequently metastasized throughout the body, making treatment extremely difficult. Unlike benign tumors, which merely expand to take over a given space, malignant cells invade surrounding tissue, emitting clawlike protrusions that disturb the RNA and DNA within normal cells. Disrupting these substances, which control cellular metabolism and reproduction, produces **mutant cells** that differ in form, quality, and function from normal cells.

How great is your own risk of cancer? **Table 12.3** helps put this into perspective. Age and gender have a great deal to do with who gets cancer and who does not. For example, women under age 39 have a relatively low rate of breast cancer (1 in 210), whereas women aged 60 and older face dramatic increases in risk of breast cancer, at 1 in 27.[40] However, cancer can strike anyone—even those for whom the risk is low. Many people would be surprised to learn that men can also develop breast cancer. In fact, 2,030 men developed breast cancer in 2007, and nearly 450 of them died, in part because of failure to recognize symptoms and seek prompt treatment.[41]

malignant Very dangerous or harmful; refers to a cancerous tumor.

benign Harmless; refers to a noncancerous tumor.

biopsy Microscopic examination of tissue to determine whether a cancer is present.

metastasis Process by which cancer spreads from one area to different areas of the body.

mutant cells Cells that differ in form, quality, or function from normal cells.

What Causes Cancer?

After decades of research, most cancer epidemiologists believe that cancers are, at least in theory, preventable and that many could be avoided by suitable choices in lifestyle and environment. Many specific causes of cancer are well documented, the most important of which are smoking, obesity, and a few viruses. However, wide global variations in common cancers, such as those of the breast, prostate, colon, and rectum, remain unexplained (**Figure 12.5**).

Most research supports the idea that cancer is caused by *environmental factors* (such as chemicals, radiation, viruses, and certain medical treatments), *lifestyle factors* (such as poor diet, inactivity, obesity, and alcohol consumption), and *internal factors* (such as hormones, immune conditions, and inherited mutations). Causal factors may act together or in sequence to promote cancer development.

Cellular Change/ Mutation Theories

One theory proposes that cancer results from spontaneous errors that occur during cell reproduction. Perhaps cells that are overworked or aged are more likely to break down, causing genetic errors that result in mutant cells.

Another theory suggests that cancer is caused by some external agent or agents that enter a normal cell and initiate the cancerous process. It is believed that 75 to 85 percent of all deaths from cancer are related to environmental factors. These include radiation, chemicals, hormonal drugs, immunosuppressant drugs (drugs that suppress the normal activity of the immune system), and other toxins. Such substances are considered possible **carcinogens** (cancer-causing agents); perhaps the most common carcinogen is the tar in cigarettes. The greater the dose or exposure to environmental hazards, the greater the risk of disease. People who are forced to work, live, and pass through areas that have high levels of environmental toxins may be at greater risk for several types of cancers.

A third theory emerged from research on certain viruses believed to cause tumors in animals. Scientists discovered **oncogenes,** suspected cancer-causing genes. Although oncogenes are typically dormant, scientists theorize that certain conditions such as age, stress, and exposure to carcinogens, viruses, and radiation may activate them. Once activated, they cause cells to grow and reproduce in an out-of-control manner. Scientists are uncertain whether only people who develop cancer have oncogenes or whether we all have genes that can become oncogenes under certain conditions.

Risks for Cancer—Lifestyle

Anyone can develop cancer; however, most cases affect adults beginning in middle age. In fact, nearly 76 percent of cancers are diagnosed at ages 55 and over. *Lifetime risk* refers to the probability that an

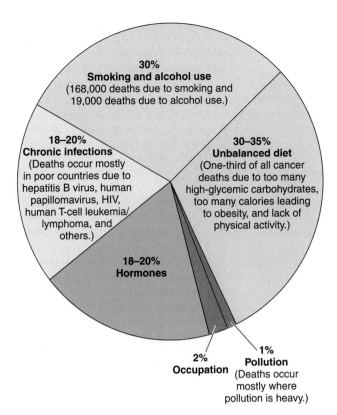

FIGURE 12.5 Factors Believed to Contribute to Global Causes of Cancer

Sources: S. Heacht et al., Public Session/Panel Discussion (Portland, OR: Linus Pauling Institute International Conference on Diet and Optimum Health, 2001); American Cancer Society, *Cancer Facts and Figures 2007* (Atlanta: American Cancer Society, 2007).

individual, over the course of a lifetime, will develop cancer or die from it. In the United States, men have a lifetime risk of about one in two; women have a lower risk of one in three.[42]

Relative risk is a measure of the strength of the relationship between risk factors and a particular cancer. Basically, relative risk compares your risk if you engage in certain known risk behaviors with that of someone who does not engage in such behaviors. For example, if you are a man and smoke, your chances of getting lung cancer are about 23 times greater than those of a nonsmoker.[43]

Over the years, researchers have found that people who engage in certain behaviors show a higher incidence of cancer. In particular, diet, sedentary lifestyle (and resultant obesity), consumption of alcohol or cigarettes, stress, and other lifestyle factors seem to play a role. **Table 12.4** summarizes the different types of cancers for which each of these factors has been shown to increase the relative risk of cancer development. Keep in mind that a high relative risk does not guarantee cause and effect. It merely indicates the likelihood of a particular risk factor being related to a particular outcome.

carcinogens Cancer-causing agents.

oncogenes Suspected cancer-causing genes.

TABLE 12.4	Lifestyle Risk Factors Contributing to Different Cancers
Lifestyle Risk Factor	**Increased Cancer Susceptibility**
Overweight/obesity	■ Breast cancer in postmenopausal women ■ Colon cancer ■ Thyroid cancer ■ Ovarian cancer ■ Cervical cancer ■ Prostate cancer ■ Endometrial cancer ■ Pancreatic cancer ■ Multiple myeloma ■ Hodgkin's disease ■ Cancer of the gallbladder ■ Adenocarcinoma of the esophagus ■ Cancer of the kidney
Sedentary lifestyle	■ Colon cancer ■ Breast cancer
Tobacco	■ Lung cancer ■ Cancers of the nasal cavity, lip, and oral cavity ■ Esophageal cancer ■ Pancreatic cancer ■ Uterine cancer ■ Cervical cancer ■ Cancer of the kidney ■ Bladder cancer ■ Stomach cancer ■ Cancer of the nasopharynx
Alcohol	■ Cancers of the mouth, pharynx, and larynx ■ Liver cancer ■ Esophageal cancer ■ Breast cancer

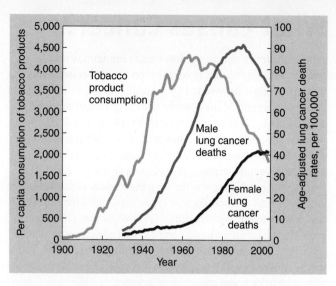

FIGURE 12.6 Tobacco Use and Lung Cancer Deaths in the United States, 1900–2003

A dramatic rise in lung cancer death rates echoed the rise in popularity of cigarettes and other tobacco products in the last century. After tobacco use and smoking rates began to decline in the 1980s, the lung cancer death rates began to decline as well.

Source: American Cancer Society, *Cancer Facts and Figures 2007* (Atlanta: American Cancer Society, 2007); U.S. Department of Agriculture, Tobacco Briefing Room, 2007, www.ers.usda.gov/Briefing/Tobacco.

Smoking and Cancer Risk

Of all the potential risk factors for cancer, smoking is among the greatest. In the United States, tobacco is responsible for nearly one in five deaths annually, accounting for at least 30 percent of all cancer deaths and 87 percent of all lung cancer deaths.[44]

In the last 20 years, lung cancer rates in Great Britain and the United States have shown a decline; however, lung cancer rates among men are still increasing in most developing countries and in Eastern Europe, where consumption of cigarettes remains high and is increasing in some areas. **Figure 12.6** demonstrates the correlation between smoking and lung cancer. See Chapter 8 for more on the risks of tobacco use.

Nutrition, Physical Activity, Obesity, and Cancer Risk

Mounting scientific evidence suggests that about one-third of the cancer deaths that occur in the United States each year may be due to additional lifestyle-related causes, such as diet and physical activity factors.[45] For people who don't use tobacco, dietary choices and physical activity are the most important modifiable determinants of cancer risk. Cancer is more common among people who are overweight and risk increases as obesity increases. Several studies indicate a relationship between a high body mass index (BMI) and death rates from cancers of the esophagus, colon, rectum, liver, stomach, kidney, and pancreas. Women with a high BMI have a higher mortality rate from breast, uterine, cervical, and ovarian cancers; men with a high BMI have higher death rates from prostate and stomach cancers. In a study of over 900,000 U.S. adults, 34 percent of all cancer deaths were attributable to overweight and obesity. Numerous other studies support this link.[46]

Risks for Cancer—Biological and Genetic Factors

Certain cancers, particularly those of the breast, stomach, colon, prostate, uterus, ovaries, and lungs, appear to run in families. For example, a woman runs a much higher risk of breast cancer if her mother or sisters (primary relatives) have had the disease, particularly at a young age. Hodgkin's disease and certain leukemias show similar familial patterns. Can we attribute these familial patterns to genetic susceptibility or to the fact that people in the same families experience similar environmental risks? To date, the research in this area is inconclusive. The complex interaction of hereditary predisposition, lifestyle, and environment on the development of cancer makes it impossible to determine a single cause.

Families with the following history are the most likely to have hereditary factors that increase their cancer risks:[47]

- Family members diagnosed with cancer at a younger age than usual for that cancer
- Three or more generations diagnosed with similar cancers
- Three or more cancers on the same side of the family
- Family members diagnosed with two or more different kinds of cancer, such as a woman who has had both breast and ovarian cancer.

It's important to note that even when different family members are diagnosed with the same cancer, it is not always due to an inherited problem. Biological sex also affects the likelihood of developing certain forms of cancer. However, although gender plays a role in certain cases of cancer, other variables such as lifestyle and occupational exposures are probably more significant.

Reproductive and Hormonal Risks for Cancer

The effects of reproductive factors on breast and cervical cancer have been well documented. Late menarche, early menopause, early first childbirth, and high parity (having many children) have been shown to reduce a woman's risk of breast cancer. Estrogen supplementation in the form of oral contraceptives or hormone replacement therapy increase the risk.[48]

Breast cancer is much more common in most Western countries than in developing countries. This is partly—perhaps largely—accounted for by dietary effects (consuming a diet high in calories and fat), combined with later first childbirth, having fewer children, shorter breast-feeding, higher obesity rates, and a longer life expectancy (people in developing countries may not live long enough to develop cancer).[49]

Risks for Cancer—Occupational and Environmental Factors

Overall, workplace hazards account for only a small percentage of all cancers. However, various substances are known to cause cancer when exposure levels are high or prolonged. One is asbestos, a fibrous material once widely used in the construction, insulation, and automobile industries. Nickel, chromate, and chemicals such as benzene, arsenic, and vinyl chloride have been shown definitively to be carcinogens for humans. Also, people who routinely work with certain dyes and radioactive substances may have increased risks for cancer. Working with coal tars, as in the mining profession, or with inhalants, as in the auto-painting business, is hazardous. So is working with herbicides and pesticides, although the evidence is inconclusive for low-dose exposures. Several federal and state agencies are responsible for monitoring such exposures and ensuring that businesses comply with standards designed to protect workers.

Radiation: Ionizing and Nonionizing Ionizing radiation (IR)—radiation from X rays, radon, cosmic rays, and ultraviolet radiation (primarily ultraviolet B, or UVB radiation)—is the only form of radiation proven to cause human cancer (see the section on skin cancer). Incidents such as the Chernobyl nuclear accident in the 1980s focused attention on the potential risks of ionizing radiation. Evidence that high-dose IR causes cancer comes from studies of atomic bomb survivors, patients receiving radiotherapy, and certain occupational groups (for example, uranium miners). Virtually any part of the body can be affected by IR, but bone marrow and the thyroid are particularly susceptible. Radon exposure in homes can increase lung cancer risk, especially in cigarette smokers. To reduce the risk of harmful effects, diagnostic medical and dental X rays are set at the lowest dose levels possible.

Although nonionizing radiation produced by radio waves, cell phones, microwaves, computer screens, televisions, electric blankets, and other products has been a topic of great concern in recent years, research has not demonstrated excess risk to date. People worry that cell phones, in particular, beam radiofrequency energy that can penetrate the brain's outer edge, raising questions about cancers of the head and neck, brain tumors, or leukemia. Most research, including the biggest ever study of the potential link between cancer and cell phone use, indicates that having an analog cell phone glued to your ear for hours may do little more than cause a sore ear and run up a hefty bill.[50] However, the National Cancer Institute (NCI) and the American Cancer Society (ACS) recommend that more research is necessary, particularly as phones switch from analog to digital signals and more and more people use wireless earbuds and other devices for longer periods of time.

Chemicals in Foods Among the food additives suspected of causing cancer is *sodium nitrate,* a chemical used to preserve and give color to red meat. The actual carcinogen is not sodium nitrate but *nitrosamines,* substances formed when the body digests sodium nitrate. Sodium nitrate has not been banned, primarily because it kills *Clostridium botulinum,* the bacterium that causes the highly virulent foodborne disease botulism. It should also be noted that the bacteria found in the human intestinal tract may contain more nitrates than a person could ever take in from eating cured meats or other nitrate-containing food products. Nonetheless, concern about the carcinogenic properties of nitrates has led to the introduction of meats that are free of nitrates or contain reduced levels of the substance.

Much of the concern about chemicals in foods centers on the possible harm caused by pesticide and herbicide residues. Although some of these chemicals cause cancer at high doses in experimental animals, the very low concentrations found in some foods are well within established government safety levels. Continued research regarding pesticide and herbicide use is essential, and scientists and consumer groups stress the importance of a balance between chemical use and the production of high-quality food products. Prevention efforts should focus on policies to protect consumers, develop low-chemical pesticides and herbicides, and reduce environmental pollution.

Risks for Cancer—Social and Psychological Factors

Many researchers claim that social and psychological factors play a major role in determining whether a person gets cancer. Stress has been implicated in increased susceptibility to several types of cancers. Although medical personnel are skeptical of overly simplistic solutions, we cannot rule out the possibility that negative emotional states contribute to illness.[51] People who are under chronic, severe stress or who suffer from depression or other persistent emotional problems show higher rates of cancer than their healthy counterparts. Sleep disturbances, diet, or a combination of factors may weaken the body's immune system, increasing susceptibility to cancer. Although psychological factors may play a part in cancer development, lifestyle habits such as tobacco use are far more important.

Infectious Diseases and Cancer

According to recent estimates, 17 percent of new cancers worldwide in 2006 were attributable to infection. Infections are thought to influence cancer development in several ways, most commonly through chronic inflammation, suppression of the immune system, or chronic stimulation.

Hepatitis B, Hepatitis C, and Liver Cancer

Viruses such as hepatitis B (HBV) and C (HCV) are believed to stimulate the growth of cancer cells in the liver because they are chronic diseases that inflame liver tissue. This may prime the liver for cancer or make it more hospitable for cancer development. Global increases in hepatitis B and C rates and concurrent rises in liver cancer rates seem to provide evidence of such an association.

Human Papillomavirus and Cervical Cancer

Nearly 100% of women with cervical cancer have evidence of human papillomavirus (HPV) infection, believed to be a major cause of cervical cancer. Fortunately, only a small percentage of HPV cases progress to cervical cancer.[52] Today, a new vaccine is available to help protect young women from becoming infected with HPV and developing cervical cancer. For more on this recent news, see the discussion of HPV in Chapter 13.

Risks for Cancer—Medical Factors

Some medical treatments increase a person's risk for cancer. One famous example is the prescription drug *diethylstilbestrol (DES)*, widely used from 1940 to 1960 to control problems with bleeding during pregnancy and reduce the risk of miscarriage. Not until the 1970s did the dangers of this drug become apparent. Although DES caused few side effects in the millions of women who took it, their daughters were found to have an increased risk for cancers of the repro-

ductive organs. Another example is the use of estrogen in treating menopausal symptoms. Estrogen use is now recognized to contribute to multiple cancer risks—and to provide fewer benefits than originally believed. Ironically, another medical factor is chemotherapy, which while being used to treat one cancer may increase the patient's risk of other forms of cancer.

 what do you THINK?

How do we determine whether a behavior or substance is a risk factor for a disease? ▪ Although a direct causal relationship between lung cancer and smoking has not been proved, the evidence supporting such a relationship is strong. Must a clearly established causal link exist before consumers are warned about risk? ▪ How does the consumer know what to believe?

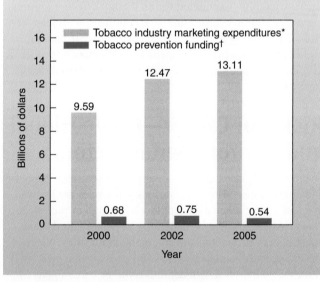

DID you KNOW?

In 2005, for every $1 spent in the United States on tobacco control efforts, the tobacco industry spent over $24 to promote its products. While industry marketing expenses continue to rise, tobacco control spending has declined to just $597.5 million in 2007.

*Marketing includes advertising and promotional expenditures.

†Tobacco prevention funding is by fiscal year totals based on estimates calculated by the Campaign for Tobacco-Free Kids.

Sources: Federal Trade Commission, *Federal Trade Commission Cigarette Report for 2004 and 2005* (Washington, DC: Federal Trade Commission, 2007); Campaign for Tobacco-Free Kids, *A Broken Promise to Our Children: The 1998 State Tobacco Settlement Eight Years Later* (Washington, DC: Campaign for Tobacco-Free Kids, 2006); American Cancer Society, *Cancer Prevention and Early Detection Facts and Figures 2007* (Atlanta: American Cancer Society, 2007).

Estimated New Cases*		Estimated Deaths	
Male	**Female**	**Male**	**Female**
Prostate 218,890 (29%)	Breast 178,480 (26%)	Lung & bronchus 89,510 (31%)	Lung & bronchus 70,880 (26%)
Lung & bronchus 114,760 (15%)	Lung & bronchus 98,620 (15%)	Prostate 27,050 (9%)	Breast 40,460 (15%)
Colon & rectum 79,130 (10%)	Colon & rectum 74,630 (11%)	Colon & rectum 26,000 (9%)	Colon & rectum 26,180 (10%)
Urinary bladder 50,040 (7%)	Uterine corpus 39,080 (6%)	Pancreas 16,840 (6%)	Pancreas 16,530 (6%)
Non-Hodgkin lymphoma 34,200 (4%)	Non-Hodgkin lymphoma 28,990 (4%)	Leukemia 12,320 (4%)	Ovary 15,280 (6%)
Melanoma of the skin 33,910 (4%)	Melanoma of the skin 26,030 (4%)	Liver & intrahepatic bile duct 11,280 (4%)	Leukemia 9,470 (4%)
Kidney & renal pelvis 31,590 (4%)	Thyroid 25,480 (4%)	Esophagus 10,900 (4%)	Non-Hodgkin lymphoma 9,060 (3%)
Leukemia 24,800 (3%)	Ovary 22,430 (3%)	Urinary bladder 9,630 (3%)	Uterine corpus 7,400 (3%)
Oral cavity and pharynx 24,180 (3%)	Kidney & renal pelvis 19,600 (3%)	Non-Hodgkin lymphoma 9,600 (3%)	Brain & other nervous system 5,590 (2%)
Pancreas 18,830 (2%)	Leukemia 19,440 (3%)	Kidney & renal pelvis 8,080 (3%)	Liver & intrahepatic bile duct 5,500 (2%)
All Sites 766,860 (100%)	**All Sites 678,060 (100%)**	**All Sites 289,550 (100%)**	**All Sites 270,100 (100%)**

*Excludes basal and squamous cell skin cancers and in situ carcinoma except urinary bladder.

FIGURE 12.7 Leading Sites of New Cancer Cases and Deaths, 2007 Estimates

Source: From *Cancer Facts and Figures 2007.* Copyright © 2007, American Cancer Society. Used with permission from American Cancer Society, Atlanta, GA.

Types of Cancers

As mentioned earlier, the term *cancer* refers not to a single disease, but to hundreds of different diseases. They are grouped into four broad categories based on the type of tissue from which the cancer arises:

- *Carcinomas.* Epithelial tissues (tissues covering body surfaces and lining most body cavities) are the most common sites for cancers. These cancers affect the outer layer of the skin and mouth as well as the mucous membranes. They metastasize through the circulatory or lymphatic system initially and form solid tumors.
- *Sarcomas.* Sarcomas occur in the mesodermal, or middle, layers of tissue—for example, in bones, muscles, and general connective tissue. They metastasize primarily via the blood in the early stages of disease. These cancers are less common but generally more virulent than carcinomas. They also form solid tumors.
- *Lymphomas.* Lymphomas develop in the lymphatic system—the infection-fighting regions of the body—and metastasize through the lymphatic system. Hodgkin's disease is an example. Lymphomas also form solid tumors.

- *Leukemias.* Cancer of the blood-forming parts of the body, particularly the bone marrow and spleen, is called leukemia. A nonsolid tumor, leukemia is characterized by an abnormal increase in the number of white blood cells.

Figure 12.7 shows the most common sites of cancer and the number of deaths annually from each type.

Lung Cancer

Lung cancer is the leading cause of cancer death for both men and women in the United States, killing an estimated 160,390 Americans in 2007, even as rates for men and women have decreased in recent decades as a result of declines in smoking and policies that prohibit smoking in public places.[53] Although reduction in smoking rates bodes well for cancer and CVD statistics, there is growing concern about the increasing number of youth, particularly young women, and persons of low income and low educational status who continue to pick up the habit.

Symptoms and Treatment Symptoms of lung cancer include a persistent cough, blood-streaked sputum, chest pain, and recurrent attacks of pneumonia or bronchi-

(Text continues on page 370.)

ASSESS *yourself*

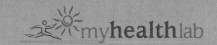

CANCER: UNDERSTANDING YOUR PERSONAL RISK

Fill out this assessment online at
www.aw-bc.com/myhealthlab or
www.aw-bc.com/donatelle.

Although you may be predisposed to some types of cancer because of genetic, biological, and/or environmental causes, there are many more that you may be able to prevent through lifestyle changes and risk reduction strategies. If you carefully assess your risks, you can then make behavior changes that may make you less susceptible to various cancers. The following questions will give you an indication of your susceptibility. Of course, no single instrument can serve as a complete risk assessment or diagnostic guide.

These questions merely serve as the basis for personal introspection and thoughtful planning about ways to reduce your risk.

Read each question, and circle the number corresponding to each yes or no. Be honest and accurate to get the most complete understanding of your cancer risks. You should not interpret individual scores for specific questions as a precise measure of relative risk, but the totals in each section give a general indication of your risk.

	Yes	No
SECTION 1: BREAST CANCER		
1. Do you check your breasts at least monthly using breast self-exam (BSE) procedures?	1	2
2. Do you look at your breasts in the mirror regularly, checking for any irregular indentations/lumps, discharge from the nipples, or other noticeable changes?	1	2
3. Has your mother, sister, or daughter been diagnosed with breast cancer?	2	1
4. Have you ever been pregnant?	1	2
5. Have you had a history of lumps or cysts in your breasts or underarm?	2	1

Total points _____

	Yes	No
SECTION 2: SKIN CANCER		
1. Do you spend a lot of time in the sun, either at work or at play?	2	1
2. Do you use sunscreens with an SPF rating of 15 or more when you are in the sun?	1	2
3. Do you use tanning beds or sun booths regularly to maintain a tan?	2	1
4. Do you examine your skin once a month, checking any moles or other irregularities, particularly in hard-to-see areas such as your back, genitals, neck, and under your hair?	1	2
5. Do you purchase and wear sunglasses that adequately filter out harmful sun rays?	1	2

Total points _____

	Yes	No
SECTION 3: CANCERS OF THE REPRODUCTIVE SYSTEM		
Men		
1. Do you examine your penis regularly for unusual bumps or growths?	1	2
2. Do you perform regular testicular self-examinations?	1	2
3. Do you have a family history of prostate or testicular cancer?	2	1
4. Do you practice safer sex and wear condoms with every sexual encounter?	1	2
5. Do you avoid exposure to harmful environmental hazards such as mercury, coal tars, benzene, chromate, and vinyl chloride?	1	2

Total points _____

	Yes	No
Women		
1. Do you have a regularly scheduled Pap test?	1	2
2. Have you been infected with the human papillomavirus, Epstein-Barr virus, or other viruses believed to increase cancer risk?	2	1
3. Has your mother, sister, or daughter been diagnosed with breast, cervical, endometrial, or ovarian cancer (particularly at a young age)?	2	1

	Yes	No
4. Do you practice safer sex and use condoms with every sexual encounter?	1	2
5. Are you obese, taking estrogen, and/or consuming a diet that is very high in saturated fats?	2	1

Total points _____

SECTION 4: CANCERS IN GENERAL

	Yes	No
1. Do you smoke cigarettes on most days of the week?	2	1
2. Do you consume a diet that is rich in fruits and vegetables?	1	2
3. Are you obese, and/or do you lead a primarily sedentary lifestyle?	2	1
4. Do you live in an area with high air pollution levels and/or work in a job where you are exposed to several chemicals on a regular basis?	2	1
5. Are you careful about the amount of animal fat in your diet, substituting olive oil or canola oil for animal fat whenever possible?	1	2
6. Do you limit your overall consumption of alcohol?	1	2
7. Do you eat foods rich in lycopene (such as tomatoes) and antioxidants?	1	2
8. Are you "body aware" and alert for changes in your body?	1	2
9. Do you have a family history of ulcers or of colorectal, stomach, or other digestive system cancers?	2	1
10. Do you avoid unnecessary exposure to radiation?	1	2

Total points _____

Analyzing Your Scores

Take a careful look at each question for which you received a score of 2. Are there any areas in which you received mostly 2s? Did you receive total points of 6 or higher in sections 1 to 3? Did you receive total points of 11 or higher in section 4? If so, you have at least one identifiable risk. The higher the score, the more risks you may have. However, rather than focusing just on your score, focus on which items you might change. Review the suggestions throughout this chapter, and list actions that you could take right now that might help you reduce your risk for these cancers.

MAKE it happen!

ASSESSMENT: The Assess Yourself activity above identifies certain behaviors that can contribute to increased cancer risks. If you have identified particular behaviors that may be putting you at risk, consider steps you can take to change these behaviors and improve your future health.

MAKING A CHANGE: To change your behavior, you need to develop a plan. Follow the steps below and complete your Behavior Change Contract to take action.

1. Evaluate your behavior, and identify patterns you are following and specific things you are doing. What can you change now? What can you change in the near future?

2. Select one pattern of behavior that you want to change.

3. Fill out the Behavior Change Contract found at the front of your book. It should include your long-term goals for change, your short-term goals, the rewards you'll give yourself for reaching these goals, potential obstacles along the way, and strategies for overcoming these obstacles. For each goal, list the small steps and specific actions that you will take.

4. Chart your progress in a journal. At the end of a week, consider how successful you were in following your plan.

(continued)

What helped you be successful? What made change more difficult? What will you do differently next week?

5. Revise your plan as needed. Are the short-term goals attainable? Are the rewards satisfying?

EXAMPLE: Keisha's assessment showed that although she was taking precautions to reduce her cancer risk in most areas, she was not doing what she should about her breast cancer risk. Her score in this area was 8 because she did not regularly examine her breasts, her mother had been diagnosed with breast cancer 2 years ago, and she had never been pregnant. Keisha decided she needed to learn how to examine her breasts and to make a plan to ensure she does

it every month. After studying this textbook's illustrations, she made an appointment with her gynecologist. While she was there, she asked the doctor to confirm that she was doing the examination correctly.

Next, Keisha decided that she would take the first 10 minutes of her morning once a month to do the exam and that she would give herself a reward for each month that she examined herself on schedule. On her way to campus after doing the exam, she would treat herself to a latte and a scone. After she stuck with her schedule for 6 months in a row, she would buy herself a new outfit. She also resolved to talk to her younger sister about the importance of the exam.

---

tis. Treatment depends on the type and stage of the cancer. Surgery, radiation therapy, and chemotherapy are all options. If the cancer is localized, surgery is usually the treatment of choice. If it has spread, surgery is combined with radiation and chemotherapy. Unfortunately, despite advances in medical technology, many people still are diagnosed at later stages, making treatment more difficult. Newer tests, such as low-dose CT scans, molecular markers in sputum and improved biopsy techniques, have helped improve diagnosis, but we still have a long way to go. In spite of improvements in diagnosis and treatment, the 5-year survival rates for lung cancer are only 16% for all stages and rise to 49% if diagnosed in the earliest stages.[54]

Prevention Smokers, especially those who have smoked for over 20 years, and people who have been exposed to industrial substances such as arsenic and asbestos or to radiation are at the highest risk for lung cancer. Exposure to secondhand cigarette smoke increases the risk for nonsmokers. Apparent increases in lung cancer among nonsmokers have caused increasing concern about the hazards of secondhand smoke, leading health advocates to argue vigorously for smoking bans.[55]

> **If I'm already a smoker, will quitting now reduce my risk of lung cancer?**

Researchers theorize that 90 percent of all lung cancers could be avoided if people did not smoke. Substantial improvements in overall prognosis have been noted in smokers who quit at the first signs of pre-

cancerous cellular changes and allowed their bronchial linings to return to normal.

Breast Cancer

In 2007, approximately 178,480 women and 2,030 men in the United States were diagnosed with invasive breast cancer for the first time. In addition, 62,030 new cases of in situ breast cancer, a more localized cancer, were diagnosed. About 40,460 women (and 450 men) died, making breast cancer the second leading cause of cancer death for women, even as rates continue to level off.[56]

Detection and Symptoms The earliest signs of breast cancer are usually observable on mammograms, often before lumps can be felt. However, mammograms are not foolproof. Hence, regular breast self-examination (BSE) is also important **(Figure 12.8).** Symptoms may include persistent breast changes, such as a lump in the breast or surrounding lymph nodes, thickening, dimpling, skin irritation, distortion, retraction or scaliness of the nipple, nipple discharge, or tenderness.

Risk Factors and Prevention The incidence of breast cancer increases with age. Although there are many possible risk factors, those that are well supported by research include family history of breast cancer, menstrual periods that started early and ended late in life, obesity after menopause, recent use of oral contraceptives or postmenopausal hormone

How to Examine Your Breasts

The best time for a woman to examine her breasts is when the breasts are not tender or swollen. Women who are pregnant, breast-feeding, or have breast implants can also choose to examine their breasts regularly.

1. Lie down and place your right arm behind your head. The exam is done while lying down, not standing up, because when lying down the breast tissue spreads evenly over the chest wall and it is as thin as possible, making it much easier to feel all the breast tissue.

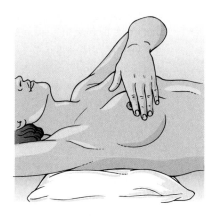

2. Use the finger pads of the three middle fingers on your left hand to feel for lumps in the right breast. Use overlapping dime-sized circular motions of the finger pads to feel the breast tissue.

3. Use three different levels of pressure to feel all the breast tissue. Light pressure is needed to feel the tissue closest to the skin; medium pressure to feel a little deeper; and firm pressure to feel the tissue closest to the chest and ribs. A firm ridge in the lower curve of each breast is normal. If you're not sure how hard to press, talk with your doctor or nurse. Use each pressure level to feel the breast tissue before moving on to the next spot.

4. Move around the breast in an up-and-down pattern, starting at an imaginary line drawn straight down your side from the underarm and moving across the breast to the middle of the chest bone. Be sure to check the entire breast area going down until you feel only ribs and up to the neck or collar bone (clavicle).

   There is some evidence to suggest that the up-and-down pattern (sometimes called the vertical pattern) is the most effective pattern for covering the entire breast without missing any breast tissue.

5. Repeat the exam on your left breast, using the finger pads of the right hand.

6. While standing in front of a mirror with your hands pressing firmly down on your hips, look at your breasts for any changes of size, shape, contour, or dimpling. (Pressing down on the hips contracts the chest wall muscles and enhances any breast changes.)

7. Examine each underarm while sitting up or standing and with your arm only slightly raised so you can easily feel in this area. (Raising your arm straight up tightens the tissue in this area and makes it difficult to examine.)

FIGURE 12.8 Breast Awareness and Self-Examination
Note that the American Cancer Society recommends the use of mammography and clinical breast exam in addition to self-examination.

Source: From "How to Examine Your Breast." Copyright © American Cancer Society. Reprinted by the permission of the American Cancer Society, Inc., from www.cancer.org.

therapy, never having children or having a first child after age 30, consuming two or more drinks of alcohol per day, and higher education and socioeconomic status.[57] Genes appear to account for approximately 5 to 10 percent of all cases of breast cancer. Screening for mutations in the *BRCA1* and *BRCA2* genes is recommended for women with a family history of breast cancer.

International differences in breast cancer incidence correlate with variations in diet, especially fat intake, although a causal role for these dietary factors has not been firmly established. Sudden weight gain has also been implicated. Research also shows that regular exercise, even some forms of recreational exercise, can reduce risk.[58]

Treatment Treatments range from a lumpectomy to radical mastectomy to various combinations of radiation or chemotherapy. Among nonsurgical options, promising results have been noted among women using *selective estrogen-receptor modulators (SERMs)* such as tamoxifen and raloxifene, particularly among women whose cancers appear to grow in response to estrogen. These drugs, as well as new *aromatase inhibitors,* work by blocking estrogen.[59]

Colon and Rectal Cancers

Colorectal cancers (cancers of the colon and rectum) continue to be the third most common cancer in both men and women, with over 153,760 cases diagnosed in 2007.[60] Although colon cancer rates have increased steadily in recent decades, many people are unaware of their risk.

Risk Factors Anyone can get colorectal cancer, but people who are over age 50, who are obese, who have a family history of colon and rectal cancer, a personal or family history of polyps (benign growths) in the colon or rectum, or inflammatory bowel problems such as colitis run an increased risk. Other possible risk factors include diets high in fat or low in fiber, smoking, sedentary lifestyle, high alcohol consumption, and low intake of fruits and vegetables.

Symptoms and Treatment In its early stages, colorectal cancer has no symptoms. Bleeding from the rectum, blood in the stool, and changes in bowel habits are the major warning signals. Because colorectal cancer tends to spread slowly, the prognosis is quite good if it is caught in the early stages. However, only 21 percent of all Americans over age 50

ARTIFICIAL TANS: SACRIFICING HEALTH FOR BEAUTY?

The media tell us that tan is "in." It's also a multibillion-dollar industry that pulls over 28 million Americans into over 25,000 tanning salons each year. High-profile actresses such as Eva Longoria "tan up" with professionally done "spray on" tans for awards ceremonies and weddings. Being tan is equated with being healthy, chic, and "hot," leading increasing numbers of men and women, particularly adolescent girls, to seek quick tans in packaged visits to tanning beds.

> **Is a tanning booth safer than the sun?**

Most tanning salon patrons incorrectly believe that tanning booths are safer than sitting in the sun. However, the truth is that there is no such thing as a safe tan from *any* source! A tan is visible evidence of skin damage—essentially tanning is your skin's response to injury. Every time you tan, whether in the sun or in a salon, you are exposing your skin to harmful UV light rays. Such exposure eventually thins the skin, making it less able to heal, as well as contributing to premature aging. The injury accumulated through years of tanning increases your risk for disfiguring forms of skin cancer, eye problems, and possible death from melanoma. Consider the following:

- Exposure to tanning beds before age 35 increases melanoma risk by 75 percent.
- People who use tanning beds are 2.5 times more likely to develop squamous cell carcinoma and 1.5 times more likely to develop basal cell carcinoma.
- New high-pressure sunlamps used in some salons emit doses of UV radiation that can be as much as 15 times that of the sun.
- Up to 90 percent of visible skin changes commonly blamed on aging are caused by the sun.

TANNING BOOTHS AND BEDS

Because of the many salons that are springing up across the country, the artificial tanning industry is difficult to monitor and regulate. Although a growing number of states require UV protective eyewear or have machine operators remain present during a client's session, tanning facilities sometimes fail to enforce regulations.

Dermatologists cite additional factors that make tanning in a salon as bad—or even worse—than sitting in the sun:

- Some tanning facilities do not calibrate the ultraviolet output of their tanning bulbs or ensure sufficient rotation of newer and older bulbs, which can lead to more or less exposure than you paid for.
- Tanning facility patrons often try for a total body tan. The buttocks and genitalia are particularly sensitive to UV radiation and are prone to developing skin cancer.
- Shared tanning booths and beds pose significant hygiene risks. Anytime you come in contact with body secretions from others, you run the risk of an infectious disease. Don't assume that those little colored water sprayers used to "clean" the inside of the beds are sufficient to kill organisms. The busier the facility, the more likely you are to come into contact with germs that could make you ill.

---

have had the most basic screening test—the fecal occult blood test—in the last 5 years, and only 33 percent have had a colonoscopy during the same time period. Colonoscopy or barium enemas are recommended screening tests for at-risk populations and everybody over age 50. Treatment often consists of radiation or surgery. Chemotherapy, although not used extensively in the past, is today a possibility.

Prevention Regular exercise, a diet with lots of fruits and plant-origin foods, a healthy weight, and moderation in alcohol consumption appear to be among the most promising prevention strategies. New research suggests that aspirin-like drugs, postmenopausal hormones, folic acid, calcium supplements, selenium, and vitamin E may also help.

malignant melanoma A virulent cancer of the melanocytes (pigment-producing cells) of the skin.

Skin Cancer

If you are one of the millions of people each year who try to get a "healthy tan," think again. Early signs of sun damage (photodamage) include sunburn, tanning, and increased freckling. This damage is cumulative, and it is followed by wrinkling, premature aging and age spots, cataracts and other forms of eye damage, sagging of the skin, and the most serious consequence: skin cancer.

Skin cancer is the most common form of cancer in the United States today, affecting over 1 million people every year (one in five of all adults). In 2007, an estimated 10,850 people died of skin cancer (8,110 from melanoma and 2,740 from other forms of skin cancer). **Malignant melanoma,** the deadliest form of skin cancer, is beginning to occur at a much higher rate in women under age 40. In fact, the highly virulent malignant melanoma has become the most frequent cancer in women aged 25 to 29 and runs second only to breast cancer in women aged 30 to 34.[61]

SUNLESS TANNERS AND BRONZERS

Although spray-on and lotion sunless tanners and bronzers are in vogue, there is no clear definition of the nature of these products, and even less protection for consumers because there are no enforceable regulations governing their use. The Skin Cancer Foundation posts a list of products that have earned their "Seal of Recommendation" on their site, www.skincancer.org.

Typically, *sunless tanners* refer to products that provide a tanned appearance without exposure to the sun or UV radiation and lasting for several days. *Bronzers* include a variety of products that allow you to achieve a temporary tan via tinted lotions or powders that wash off readily. Neither product has any ability to protect your skin from the damaging rays of the sun.

One ingredient commonly used in sunless tanners is the color additive dihydroxyacetone (DHA). DHA interacts with the dead surface cells in the outermost layer of the skin to darken skin color. DHA has been approved by the FDA for use in coloring the skin since 1977 and has typically been sold in lotions and creams. Complaints from consumers have been lodged against these products, most of which cite rashes, coughing, sneezing, dizziness and fainting, probably due to some form of allergic reaction. DHA is restricted to external application, so if you choose to use DHA spray or lotion, be sure to protect your mouth, eyes, and nose from it.

TANNING PILLS

Some companies market pills that contain the color additive canthaxanthin. When large amounts of canthaxanthin are ingested, the substance can turn the skin a range of colors, from orange to brown. However, there are no tanning pills approved by the FDA, and canthaxanthin is approved for use only as a color additive in foods and oral medications, and only in small amounts. Tanning pills have been associated with health problems, including an eye disorder called canthaxanthin retinopathy, which is the formation of yellow deposits on the eye's retina. According to the American Academy of Dermatology,

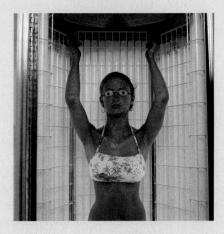

canthaxanthin has also been reported to cause liver injury and a severe itching condition called urticaria.

Sources: U.S. Food and Drug Administration, Center for Food Safety and Applied Science, CFSAN/Office of Cosmetics and Colors, "Sunless Tanners and Bronzers," October, 2006, www.cfsan.fda.gov/~dms/cos-tan4.html; S. Danoff-Berg and C. E. Mosher, "Prediction of Tanning Salon Use: Behavioral Alternatives for Enhancing Appearance, Relaxing and Socializing," *Journal of Health Psychology* 11, no. 3 (2006): 511–18; Skin Cancer Foundation, *2007 Skin Cancer Facts,* 2007, www.skincancer.org/skincancer-facts.php.

Risk Factors and Prevention Anyone who overexposes himself or herself without adequate protection is at risk for skin cancer. The risk is greatest for people who fit the following categories:

- Have fair skin; blonde, red, or light brown hair; blue, green, or gray eyes
- Always burn before tanning or burn easily and peel readily
- Don't tan easily but spend lots of time outdoors
- Have previously been treated for skin cancer or have a family history of skin cancer
- Use no or low-SPF sunscreens

Although sun exposure risks have been widely reported, over 60 percent of Americans 25 years and under report that they are "working on a tan" at some point during the year. Despite the red flag, why do people continue to tan? Recent research suggests a connection between high levels of ultraviolet light and endorphins. Those who tan in the sun or artificially may experience a short "high" for this reason, and tanning can become a type of addiction.

Preventing skin cancer is a matter of limiting exposure to harmful ultraviolet (UV) rays found in sunlight. What happens when you expose yourself to sunlight? Biologically, the skin responds to photodamage by increasing its thickness and the number of pigment cells (melanocytes), which produce the "tan" look. The skin's cells that ward off infection are also prone to photodamage, lowering the normal immune protection of our skin and priming it for cancer. Photodamage also causes wrinkling by impairing the elastic substances (collagens) that keep skin soft and pliable. See **Table 12.5** for practical tips on staying safe in the sun.

Detection, Symptoms, and Treatment Many people do not know what to look for when examining themselves for skin cancer. **Figure 12.9** shows examples of the three most prevalent types. Basal and squamous cell carcinomas can be a recurrent annoyance, showing up most commonly on the

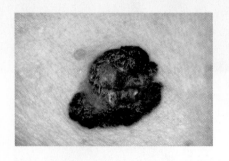
(a)

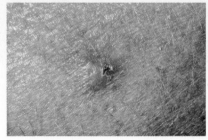
(b)

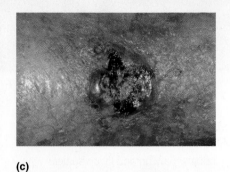
(c)

FIGURE 12.9 Types of Skin Cancers
Preventing skin cancer includes keeping a careful watch for any new pigmented growths and for changes to any moles. The ABCD warning signs of melanoma **(a)** include *asymmetrical* shapes, irregular *borders, color* variation, and an increase in *diameter.* Basal cell carcinoma **(b)** and squamous cell carcinoma **(c)** should be brought to your physician's attention but are not as deadly as melanoma.

face, ears, neck, arms, hands, and legs as warty bumps, colored spots, or scaly patches. Bleeding, itchiness, pain, or oozing are other symptoms of carcinomas. Surgery may be necessary to remove them, but they are seldom life-threatening.

In striking contrast is the insidious melanoma, an invasive killer that quickly spreads to regional organs and throughout the body, accounting for over 75 percent of all skin cancer deaths. Risks increase dramatically among whites after age 20.[62] Often, melanoma starts as a normal-looking mole but quickly develops abnormal characteristics. A simple *ABCD rule* outlines the warning signs of melanoma:

- *Asymmetry.* One half of the mole does not match the other half.
- *Border irregularity.* The edges are uneven, notched, or scalloped.
- *Color.* Pigmentation is not uniform. Melanomas may vary in color from tan to deeper brown, reddish black, black, or deep bluish black.
- *Diameter.* The diameter is greater than 6 millimeters (about the size of a pea).

If you notice any of these symptoms, consult a physician promptly.

Treatment of skin cancer depends on its seriousness. Surgery is performed in 90 percent of all cases. Radiation therapy, *electrodesiccation* (tissue destruction by heat), and *cryosurgery* (tissue destruction by freezing) are also common forms of treatment. For melanoma, treatment may involve surgical removal of the regional lymph nodes, radiation, or chemotherapy.

Prostate Cancer

Cancer of the prostate is the most common cancer in American men today, with the exception of skin cancer, and the second leading cause of cancer death in men, after lung cancer. In 2007, about 218,890 new cases of prostate cancer were diagnosed in the United States. About 1 man in 3 will be diagnosed with prostate cancer during his lifetime, but only 1 man in 33 will die of it.[63]

Symptoms The prostate is a muscular, walnut-sized gland that surrounds part of the urethra, the tube that

TABLE 12.5	Safe Sun Tips

- Avoid the sun, or seek shade, from 10:00 AM to 4:00 PM, when the sun's rays are strongest. Even on a cloudy day, up to 80 percent of the sun's rays can get through.
- Apply a sunscreen of SPF 15 or higher evenly to all uncovered skin before going outside. Look for a "broad-spectrum" sunscreen that protects against both UVA and UVB radiation. Check the label for how much time you should allow between applying the product and going outdoors. If the label does not specify, apply it 30 minutes before going outside. Ask a doctor before applying sunscreen to children under 6 months old.
- Remember to apply sunscreen to your eyelids, lips, nose, ears, neck, hands, and feet. If you don't have much hair, apply sunscreen to the top of your head, too.
- Reapply sunscreen often. The label will tell you how often you need to reapply it. If it isn't waterproof, reapply after swimming or if you are sweating a lot.

- Wear loose-fitting, light-colored clothing.
- Wear a wide-brimmed, light-colored hat to protect your head and face.
- Use sunglasses with 99 to 100 percent UV protection.
- Avoid artificial tanning methods such as sunlamps, tanning beds, tanning pills, and tanning makeup.
- Check your skin regularly for signs of skin cancer. Remember to look at the backs of your legs and the undersides of your arms. Check parts that are hard to see—such as your back, neck, and scalp—with a hand mirror. Look for changes in the size, shape, color, or feel of birthmarks, moles, and spots. If you find any changes or find sores that are not healing, see your doctor.

Sources: U.S. Food and Drug Administration, "Safer Sunning in Seven Steps," 2007, www.fda.gov/opacom/lowlit/sunsafty.html; Medline Plus, "Sun Exposure," 2007, www.nlm.nih.gov/medlineplus/sunexposure.html.

transports urine and sperm out of the body. As part of the male reproductive system, its primary function is to produce seminal fluid. Most symptoms of prostate cancer mimic signs of infection or an enlarged prostate. These may include weak or interrupted urine flow; difficulty starting or stopping urination; feeling the urge to urinate frequently; pain upon urination; blood in the urine; or pain in the low back, pelvis, or thighs. Many men have no symptoms in the early stages.

Prostate cancer may begin with a condition called prostatic intraephithelial neoplasia (PIN). In this condition, there are changes in the microscopic appearance of prostate gland cells, ranging from a bit different than normal to abnormal. PIN may appear in men in their twenties, and by the time men reach age 50, nearly 50 percent of men have these changes.

Risk Factors Factors that appear to increase the risk of prostate cancer include the following:[64]

- *Age.* Chances of developing prostate cancer increase dramatically with age. More than 70 percent of cancers are diagnosed in men over age 65.
- *Race.* African American men are 61 percent more likely to develop prostate cancer than white men and are much more likely to be diagnosed at an advanced stage. Prostate cancer is less common among Asian men and occurs at about the same rates among Hispanic men as it does among white men.
- *Nationality.* Prostate cancer is most common in North America and northwestern Europe and less common in Asia, Africa, Central America, and South America.
- *Family history.* Having a father or brother with prostate cancer more than doubles a man's risk of getting prostate cancer (interestingly, the risk is higher for men with an affected brother than it is for those with an affected father).
- *Diet.* Men in countries where the typical diet is high in fat have higher risks of prostate cancer than men in countries with lower-fat diets. Men who consume high levels of calcium also may be at greater risk, although studies have yet to confirm this.
- *Physical inactivity and overweight/obesity.* Regular physical activity and maintaining a healthy weight may help reduce the risk of prostate cancer.
- *Vasectomy.* Although there is concern among some groups that having a vasectomy, particularly before age 35, increases the risk of prostate cancer, most recent studies have not found this to be true.

Prevention and Treatment Eating more fruits and vegetables, particularly those containing lycopene, a pigment found in tomatoes and other red fruits, may lower the risk of prostate cancer. Some studies suggest that taking 50 milligrams (400 international units, or IU) of vitamin E and adequate amounts of selenium in your diet may reduce risk, whereas consuming high levels of vitamin A may increase risk. The best advice is to follow the dietary recommendations discussed in Chapter 9 and maintain a healthy weight.

Another important strategy is to get diagnostic tests on the schedule recommended by the American Cancer Society and the National Cancer Institute. Most health organizations do not recommend routine testing for men under age 40. Every man over age 40 should have an annual digital rectal prostate examination. The American Cancer Society recommends that men age 50 and over have an annual *prostate-specific antigen (PSA)* test.

Fortunately, 83 percent of all prostate cancers are detected while they are still in the local or regional stages, and they tend to progress slowly. Over the past 20 years, the survival rate for all stages combined has increased from 67 percent to 96 percent, largely because of earlier diagnosis and improved treatment.

Ovarian Cancer

Ovarian cancer is the fifth leading cause of cancer death for women, diagnosed in almost 22,430 women in 2007 and killing 15,280.[65] Ovarian cancer causes more deaths than any other cancer of the reproductive system because its insidious, often silent, course means women tend not to discover it until the cancer is at an advanced stage. Overall, 1-year survival rates are 76 percent, and 5-year suvival rates are 45 percent.

The most common symptom of ovarian cancer is enlargement of the abdomen. Women over 40 may experience persistent digestive disturbances, as well. Other symptoms include fatigue, pain during intercourse, unexplained weight loss, unexplained changes in bowel or bladder habits, and incontinence. However, many women have no early symptoms at all.

Risk factors for ovarian cancer include a family history of ovarian, breast, or colon cancer; never having been pregnant; taking fertility drugs; and genetic predisposition. The younger a woman is when she is diagnosed with ovarian cancer, the better her chances of survival. New diagnostic tests, including a blood test for the tumor marker, CA-125, can significantly improve chances of early diagnosis.[66]

Research shows that using birth control pills, adhering to a low-fat diet, having multiple children, and breast-feeding can all reduce risk of ovarian cancer. General prevention strategies such as focusing on diet, exercise, sleep, stress management, and weight control are good ideas to lower your risk for this and any of the diseases discussed in this chapter. To protect yourself, thorough annual pelvic examinations are important. Pap tests, although useful in detecting cervical cancer, do not reveal ovarian cancer. Women over age 40 should have a cancer-related checkup every year.

Cervical and Endometrial (Uterine) Cancer

Most uterine cancers develop in the body of the uterus, usually in the endometrium (lining). The rest develop in the cervix, located at the base of the uterus. In 2007, an estimated 11,150 new cases of cervical cancer and 39,080

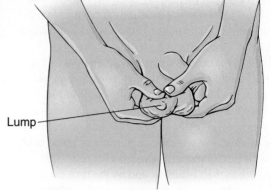

How to Examine Your Testicles

The best time to perform a testicular self-examination is after a warm shower or bath, when the testicles descend and the scrotal skin is relaxed.

1. Use a mirror to examine the scrotum for any visible swelling.

2. Using both hands, place the index and middle fingers of each hand on the underside of the testicle and the thumbs on top. Gently roll the testicle between the thumbs and fingers.

3. Identify the epididymis, the structure behind the testicle that carries sperm, so that you don't confuse it for a lump.

Lump

FIGURE 12.10 Testicular Self-Examination

cases of endometrial cancer were diagnosed in the United States.[67] The overall incidence of cervical and uterine cancer has been declining steadily over the past decade. This decline may be due to more regular screenings of younger women using the **Pap test,** a procedure in which cells taken from the cervical region are examined for abnormal cellular activity. Although Pap tests are very effective for detecting early-stage cervical cancer, they are less effective for detecting cancers of the uterine lining.

Risk factors for cervical cancer include early age at first intercourse, multiple sex partners, cigarette smoking, and certain sexually transmitted infections, including human papillomavirus (the cause of genital warts) and herpesvirus. For endometrial cancer, risk factors include age, endometrial hyperplasia, being overweight, diabetes, high blood pressure, a history of other cancers, race (white women are at higher risk), treatment with tamoxifen for breast cancer, and estrogen replacement therapy. Other factors also related to estrogen include having few or no children and entering menopause late in life.

Early warning signs of uterine cancer include bleeding outside the normal menstrual period or after menopause or persistent unusual vaginal discharge. These symptoms should be checked by a physician immediately.

Testicular Cancer

Testicular cancer is one of the most common types of solid tumors found in young adult men, affecting nearly 7,920 young men in 2007. Those between the ages of 15 and 35 are at greatest risk. There has been a steady increase in testicular cancer frequency over the past several years in this age group.[68] Although the cause of testicular cancer is unknown, several risk factors have been identified. Men with unde-

Pap test A procedure in which cells taken from the cervical region are examined for abnormal cellular activity.

scended testicles appear to be at greatest risk, and some studies indicate a genetic influence.

In general, testicular tumors first appear as an enlargement of the testis or thickening in testicular tissue. Because this enlargement is often painless, it is extremely important that all young men practice regular testicular self-examination **(Figure 12.10).**

One of the most remarkable testicular cancer stories is the survival of champion cyclist Lance Armstrong. Struck by an invasive form of testicular cancer that had spread to several parts of his body, including his brain, Armstrong and his indomitable spirit set a wonderful example of hope. Through a combination of superior medical care, exercise, and dietary and lifestyle changes, as well as a spiritual journey, Lance recovered from his cancer and went on to win the Tour de France seven consecutive times.

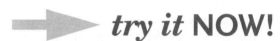

try it NOW!

Get in the habit of doing self-exams. The survival rate of breast and testicular cancer patients greatly increases with early detection. Make a commitment to perform a breast or testicular self-exam monthly. (See Figures 12.8 and 12.10 for instructions.) By knowing your body and detecting any abnormalities, you can take an active role in cancer prevention.

Pancreatic Cancer

The incidence of pancreatic cancer has increased substantially during the last 25 years to 37,170 cases in 2007.[69] It is now the fourth leading cause of cancer deaths for both men and women. Chronic inflammation of the pancreas (pancreatitis), obesity, physical inactivity, diabetes, cirrhosis, and a high-fat diet may contribute to its development. Smokers have double the risk of nonsmokers. Only 5 percent of patients live more than 5 years after diagnosis, usually

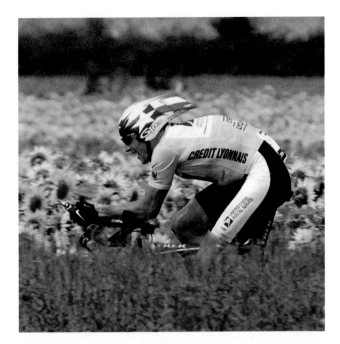

Lance Armstrong's battle with testicular cancer brought attention to a disease that strikes men who may consider themselves "too young" or "too healthy" to be at risk for cancer. His Lance Armstrong Foundation, with its "Live Strong" motto and trademark yellow wristbands, donates millions to cancer education, research, and advocacy.

because the disease is well advanced by the time there are any symptoms and it is diagnosed.

Leukemia

Leukemia is a cancer of the blood-forming tissues that leads to proliferation of millions of immature white blood cells. These abnormal cells crowd out normal white blood cells (which fight infection), platelets (which control hemorrhaging), and red blood cells (which carry oxygen to body cells). As a result, symptoms such as fatigue, paleness, weight loss, easy bruising, repeated infections, nosebleeds, and other forms of hemorrhaging occur.

Leukemia can be acute or chronic and can strike both sexes and all age groups. An estimated 44,240 new cases were diagnosed in the United States in 2007.[70] Chronic leukemia can develop over several months and have few symptoms. The 5-year survival rate for patients with chronic lymphocytic leukemia, one of the most common types, has risen to 74 percent.

Facing Cancer

Based on current rates, about 83 million people—or one in three of us now living—will eventually develop cancer. Despite these gloomy predictions, recent advancements in the diagnosis and treatment of many forms of cancer have reduced some of the fear and mystery that once surrounded this disease.

C	Change in bowel or bladder habits
A	A sore that does not heal
U	Unusual bleeding or discharge
T	Thickening or lump in the breast or elsewhere
I	Indigestion or difficulty in swallowing
O	Obvious change in wart or mole
N	Nagging cough or hoarseness

FIGURE 12.11 **CAUTION: Cancer's Seven Warning Signals**

Detecting Cancer

The earlier cancer is diagnosed, the better the prospect for survival. Make a realistic assessment of your own risk factors, and avoid the ones that you can control. Do you have a family history of cancer? If so, what types? Make sure you know which symptoms to watch for, and follow the recommendations for self-exams and medical checkups outlined in **Table 12.6.** Avoid known carcinogens—such as tobacco—and other environmental hazards. Eat a nutritious diet. Heeding the suggestions for primary prevention can significantly decrease your own risk for cancer.

Several high-tech tools to detect cancer have been developed. In **magnetic resonance imaging (MRI),** a huge electromagnet detects hidden tumors by mapping the vibrations of the various atoms in the body on a computer screen. The **computed tomography scan (CT scan)** uses X rays to examine parts of the body. In both of these painless, noninvasive procedures, cross-sectioned pictures can reveal a tumor's shape and location more accurately than can conventional X-ray images. *Prostatic ultrasound* (a rectal probe using ultrasonic waves to produce an image of the prostate) is being investigated as a means to increase the early detection of prostate cancer.

Figure 12.11 lists seven warning signals of cancer. If you notice any of these signals, and they don't appear to be related to anything else, see a doctor immediately.

New Hope in Cancer Treatments

Although cancer treatments have changed dramatically over the past 20 years, surgery, in which the tumor and surrounding

magnetic resonance imaging (MRI) A device that uses magnetic fields, radio waves, and computers to generate an image of internal tissues of the body for diagnostic purposes without the use of radiation.

computed tomography scan (CT scan) A scan by a machine that uses radiation to view internal organs not normally visible on X-ray images.

TABLE 12.6	Screening Guidelines for the Early Detection of Cancer in Asymptomatic People

Site	Recommendation
Cancer-related checkup	For individuals undergoing periodic health examinations, a cancer related checkup should include health counseling and, depending on a person's age, might include examination for cancers of the thyroid, oral cavity, skin, lymph nodes, testes, and ovaries, as well as for some nonmalignant diseases.
Breast	Women 40 and older should have an annual mammogram and an annual clinical breast exam (CBE) performed by a health care professional and should perform monthly breast self-examination (BSE). Ideally, the CBE should occur before the scheduled mammogram. Women aged 20–39 should have a clinical breast exam performed by a health care professional every 3 years. Women should know how their breasts normally feel and report any breast change promptly to their health care providers. Breast self-exam is an option for women starting in their twenties. Women at increased risk (e.g., with family history, genetic tendency, past breast cancer) should talk with their doctors about the benefits and limitations of starting mammography screening earlier, having additional tests (i.e., breast ultrasound and MRI), or having more frequent exams.
Colon and rectum	Beginning at age 50, men and women should follow one of the examination schedules below: ■ A fecal occult blood test (FOBT) every year, or a flexible sigmoidoscopy (FSIG) every 5 years, or both annual fecal occult blood test and flexible sigmoidoscopy every 5 years* ■ A double contrast barium enema every 5 to 10 years ■ A colonoscopy every 10 years
Prostate	The American Cancer Society recommends that both the prostate-specific antigen (PSA) blood test and the digital rectal examination be offered annually, beginning at age 50, to men who have a life expectancy of at least 10 more years. Men at high risk (African American men and men with a strong family history of one or more first-degree relatives diagnosed with prostate cancer at an early age) should begin testing at age 45. Information should be provided to patients about what is known and what is uncertain about the benefits and limitations of early detection and treatment of prostate cancer so that they can make an informed decision.
Uterus	■ **Cervix:** Screening should begin approximately 3 years after a woman begins having vaginal intercourse but no later than 21 years of age. Screening should be done every year with Pap tests or every 2 years using liquid-based tests. At or after age 30, women who have had three normal tests in a row may get screened every 2–3 years, unless they have certain risk factors, such as HIV infection or a weak immune system. Screening after total hysterectomy (with removal of the cervix) is not necessary unless the surgery was done as a treatment for cervical cancer. ■ **Endometrium:** The American Cancer Society recommends that all women be informed about the risks and symptoms of endometrial cancer and be strongly encouraged to report any unexpected bleeding or spotting to their physicians. Annual screening for endometrial cancer with endometrial biopsy beginning at age 35 should be offered to women with or at risk for hereditary nonpolyposis colon cancer (HNPCC).

*Combined testing is preferred over either annual FOBT or FSIG every 5 years alone. People who are at moderate or high risk for colorectal cancer should talk with a doctor about a different testing schedule.

Source: From *Cancer Facts and Figures 2007.* Copyright © 2007, American Cancer Society. Used with permission from American Cancer Society, Atlanta, GA.

tissue are removed, is still common. Today, treatments such as **radiotherapy** (the use of radiation) or **chemotherapy** (the use of drugs) to kill cancerous cells are also used.

Radiation works by destroying malignant cells or stopping cell growth. It is most effective in treating localized cancer masses. When cancer has spread throughout the body, it is necessary to use some form of chemotherapy. Whether used alone or in combination, radiotherapy and chemotherapy have side effects, including extreme nausea, nutritional deficiencies, hair loss, and general fatigue. In the process of killing malignant cells, some healthy cells are also destroyed. Long-term damage to the cardiovascular system and other body systems can be significant. Ongoing research promises to result in new drugs and treatments that are less toxic to normal cells.

Today, some researchers are targeting cancer as a genetic disease that is brought on by some form of mutation, either inherited or acquired. Promising treatments focus on stopping the cycle of these mutant cells, targeting toxins through monoclonal antibodies, and rousing the immune system to be more effective. Other areas of research include *immunotherapy,* which enhances the body's own disease-fighting mechanisms, *cancer-fighting vaccines* to combat abnormal cells, *gene therapy* to increase the patient's immune response, and various substances that block cancer-causing events along the *cancer pathway.* Another promising avenue of potential treatment is *stem cell research,* although controversy around the use of stem cells continues to slow research.

radiotherapy   Use of radiation to kill cancerous cells.

chemotherapy   Use of drugs to kill cancerous cells.

Cancer Survivors: Life after Cancer

Heightened public awareness and an improved prognosis have made the cancer experience less threatening and isolating than it once was. In fact, assistance for the cancer patient is more readily available than ever before. Cancer support groups, cancer information workshops, and low-cost medical consultation are just a few of the forms of assistance now offered in many communities. Groups have successfully lobbied the U.S. Congress to increase government funding for cancer research over the past decade. Increasing efforts in cancer research, improvements in diagnostic equipment, and advances in treatment provide hope for the future.

TAKING charge

Summary

- The cardiovascular system consists of the heart and circulatory system and is a carefully regulated, integrated network of vessels that supply the body with the nutrients and oxygen necessary to perform daily functions. Cardiovascular diseases include atherosclerosis, coronary heart disease, angina pectoris, arrhythmias, congestive heart failure, congenital and rheumatic heart disease, and stroke. These combine to make CVD the leading cause of death in the United States today.

- Many risk factors for CVD can be controlled, such as cigarette smoking, high blood cholesterol and triglyceride levels, hypertension, lack of exercise, a diet high in saturated fat, obesity, diabetes, and emotional stress. Some risk factors, such as age, gender, and heredity, cannot be controlled. Many of these factors have a compounded effect when combined.

- New methods developed for treating heart blockages include coronary bypass surgery and angioplasty. Drugs such as beta blockers and calcium channel blockers can reduce high blood pressure and treat other symptoms.

- Diabetes develops when the pancreas fails to produce enough insulin to regulate sugar metabolism or the cells are unable to adequately utilize the insulin that is present. The increase in the prevalence of diabetes is related to increases in obesity, sedentary lifestyle, and other factors.

- Cancer is a group of diseases characterized by uncontrolled growth and spread of abnormal cells. These cells may create tumors. Benign (noncancerous) tumors grow in size but do not spread; malignant (cancerous) tumors spread to other parts of the body.

- Lifestyle factors for cancer risk include smoking and obesity. Biological factors include inherited genes and gender. Components of the environment that may act as carcinogens include asbestos, radiation, preservatives, and pesticides. Infectious diseases that may lead to cancer include herpes, hepatitis, and human papillomavirus. Medical factors include certain drug therapies given for other conditions that may elevate the chance of cancer.

- There are many different types of cancer, each of which poses different risks, depending on a number of factors. Common cancers include lung, breast, colon and rectal, prostate, skin, testicular, ovarian, uterine, and pancreatic cancers, as well as leukemia.

- Early diagnosis improves cancer survival rate. Self-exams for breast, testicular, and skin cancer and knowledge of the seven warning signals of cancer aid early diagnosis. New types of cancer treatments include combinations of radiotherapy, chemotherapy, and immunotherapy.

Chapter Review

1. The function of the aorta is to
   a. return the blood from the lungs.
   b. pump the blood to the arteries in the rest of the body.
   c. pump blood to the lungs.
   d. return blood back to the heart.

2. Severe chest pain occurring as a result of reduced oxygen flow to the heart is called
   a. angina pectoris.
   b. arrhythmias.
   c. myocardial infarction.
   d. congestive heart failure.

3. Arteriosclerosis is more commonly referred to as
   a. hardening of the arteries.
   b. heart attack.
   c. high blood pressure.
   d. plaque.

4. A stroke results
   a. when a heart stops beating.
   b. when cardiopulmonary resuscitation has failed to revive the stopped heart.
   c. when blood to the brain has been blocked off.
   d. when the blood pressure rises too high.

5. The "bad" type of cholesterol found in the blood stream is known as
   a. high-density lipoprotein.
   b. low-density lipoprotein.
   c. total cholesterol.
   d. triglyceride.

6. Diabetes mellitus interferes with the body's ability to
   a. metabolize sugars.
   b. produce adrenaline.
   c. respond to saturated fats in the diet.
   d. all of the above.

7. The greatest number of cancer deaths for both men and women is caused by
   a. colorectal cancer.
   b. pancreatic cancer.
   c. lung cancer.
   d. stomach cancer.

8. The more serious, life-threatening type of skin cancer is
   a. basal cell.
   b. squamous cell.
   c. melanoma.
   d. lymphoma.

9. Suspected cancer-causing genes are called
   a. epigenes.
   b. oncogenes.
   c. primogenes.
   d. metastogenes.

10. The fecal occult blood test is the most basic screening test used for
   a. lung cancer.
   b. prostate cancer.
   c. cervical cancer.
   d. colorectal cancer.

Answers to these questions can be found on page A-1.

Questions for Discussion and Reflection

1. Trace the path of a drop of blood from the time it enters the vena cava until it reaches your little finger. Be sure to include the types of blood vessels involved.
2. List the different types of CVD. Compare and contrast their symptoms, risk factors, prevention, and treatment.
3. Discuss the role that exercise, stress management, dietary changes, medical checkups, sodium reduction, and other factors can play in reducing risk for CVD. What role may chronic infections play in CVD risk?
4. Describe some of the diagnostic and treatment alternatives for CVD. If you had a heart attack today, which treatment would you prefer? Explain why.
5. Describe the risk factors for diabetes and its symptoms and treatment. What is the difference between type 1 diabetes and type 2 diabetes?

6. List the likely causes of cancer. Do any of them put you at greater risk? What can you do to reduce your risk? What risk factors do you share with family members? With friends?
7. What are the symptoms of lung, breast, prostate, and testicular cancer? What can you do to reduce your risk of developing these cancers or increase your chances of surviving them?
8. Why are breast and testicular self-exams important for women and men? What could be the consequences of failing to do these exams regularly?
9. Discuss the seven warning signals of cancer. How soon should you seek treatment for any of the warning signs?

Accessing Your Health on the Internet

The following websites explore further topics and issues related to personal health. For links to the websites below, visit the Companion Website for *Health: The Basics,* Eighth Edition at www.aw-bc.com/donatelle.

1. *American Heart Association.* Home page for the leading private organization dedicated to heart health. This site provides information, statistics, and resources regarding cardiovascular care, including an opportunity to test your own risk for CVD. www.americanheart.org

2. *National Heart, Lung, and Blood Institute.* A valuable resource for information on all aspects of cardiovascular health and wellness. www.nhlbi.nih.gov
3. *American Diabetes Association.* Excellent resource for diabetes information. www.diabetes.org
4. *American Cancer Society.* Resources from the leading private organization dedicated to cancer prevention. This site provides information, statistics, and resources regarding cancer. www.cancer.org

5. *National Cancer Institute.* Check here for valuable information on clinical trials and the Physician Data Query (PDQ), a comprehensive database of cancer treatment information. www.cancer.gov

6. *Oncolink.* Sponsored by the Abramson Cancer Center of the University of Pennsylvania, this site seeks to educate cancer patients and their families by offering information on support services, cancer causes, screening, prevention, and common questions. www.oncolink.com

Further Reading

American Cancer Society. *A Breast Cancer Journey: Your Personal Guidebook,* 2nd ed. Atlanta: American Cancer Society, 2004.

Contains up-to-date information on treatments, medicines, reconstructive surgery, and complementary and alternative options. Also includes information for caregivers, family, and friends.

American Cancer Society. *Cancer Facts and Figures.* Atlanta: American Cancer Society, published annually.

A summary of major facts relating to cancer. Provides information on incidence, prevalence, symptomology, prevention, and treatment. Available through local divisions of the

American Cancer Society and online. Contains up-to-date information about the disease, medical options, and emotional support.

American Heart Association. *Heart Disease and Stroke Statistics.* Dallas: American Heart Association, published annually.

An annual overview providing facts and figures concerning CVD in the United States. Supplement provides key statistics about current trends and future directions in treatment and prevention. Available online.

Gersh, B., and M. Wood, eds. *The Mayo Clinic Heart Book.* New York: William Morrow, 2000.

Provides an overview of heart disease in America, including risk factors, trends, and options for patients.

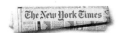

e-themes from *The New York Times*

For up-to-date articles about current health issues, visit www.aw-bc.com/donatelle, select *Health: The Basics,* Eighth Edition, Chapter 12, and click on "e-themes."

References

1. American Heart Association, *Heart Disease and Stroke Statistics—2007 Update* (Dallas: American Heart Association, 2007); Centers for Disease Control and Prevention, "Prevalence of Heart Disease—United States, 2005," *Morbidity and Mortality Weekly Report* 56, no. 6 (2007):113–18.

2. American Heart Association, *Heart Disease and Stroke Statistics—2007 Update.*

3. American Heart Association, *Heart Disease and Stroke Statistics—2007 Update;* C. Langenberg et al., "Cardiovascular Death and the Metabolic Syndrome: The Role of Adipose Signaling Hormones and Inflammatory Markers," *Diabetes Care* 29 (2006): 1363–69; J. de Jager et al., "Endothelial Dysfunctions and Low Grade Inflammation Explain Much of the Excess Mortality in Individuals with Type 2 Diabetes: The Hoorn Study," *Arteriosclerosis, Thrombosis, and Vascular Biology* 26 (2006): 1086–93; C. Meisinger et al., "Plasma Oxidized Low Density Lipoprotein: A Strong Predictor for Acute Coronary Heart Disease Events in Apparently Healthy Middle-Aged Men in the General Population," *Circulation* 112 (2005): 651–57.

4. Langenberg et al., "Cardiovascular Death and the Metabolic Syndrome"; de Jager et al., "Endothelial Dysfunctions and Low Grade Inflammation."

5. J. K. Victanen et al., "Homocysteine as a Risk Factor for CVD Mortality in Men with Other CVD Risk Factors: The Kuopio Ischemic Heart Risk Factor (KIHD) Study," *Journal of Internal Medicine* 257, no. 3 (2005): 209–317; American Heart Association, "Homocysteine, Folic Acid, and Cardiovascular Disease," 2007, www.americanheart.org.

6. American Heart Association, "Homocysteine, Folic Acid, and Cardiovascular Disease."

7. J. Berger et al., "Aspirin for the Primary Prevention of Cardiovascular Disease in Men and Women," *Journal of the American Medical Association* 295, no. 3 (2006): 306–13.

8. S. Mora et al., "Enhanced Risk Assessment in Asymptomatic Individuals with Exercise Testing and Framingham Risk Scores," *Circulation* 112, no. 11 (2005): 1566–72; G. Hu et al., "Prevalence of the Metabolic Syndrome and Its Relations to All-Cause and Cardiovascular Mortality in Non-Diabetic European Men and Women," *Archives of Internal Medicine* 164, no. 10 (2004): 1066–76; L. Girman et al., "An Exploratory Analysis of Criteria for the Metabolic Syndrome and Its Prediction of Cardiovascular Outcomes: The Hoorn Study," *American Journal of Epidemiology* 162, no. 5 (2005): 438–47; J. Ford et al., "Risks for All-Cause Mortality, Cardiovascular Diseases, and Diabetes Associated with the Metabolic Syndrome: A Summary of Evidence," *Diabetes Care* 28, no. 7 (2005): 1769–78; J. Bertrais et al., "Sedentary Behaviors, Physical Activity, and Metabolic Syndrome in Middle-Aged French Subjects," *Obesity Research* 13, no. 6 (2005): 936–44.

9. American Heart Association, *Heart Disease and Stroke Statistics— 2007 Update.*

10. Ibid.

11. Ibid.

12. Ibid.

13. Ibid.

14. Ibid.

15. Ibid.

16. Ibid.

17. Ibid.

18. National Center for Health Statistics, *Health, United States, 2006 with Chartbook on Trends in the Health of Americans* (Hyattsville, MD: National Center for Health Statistics, 2007).

19. American Heart Association, *Heart Disease and Stroke Statistics— 2007 Update.*

20. Ibid.

21. N. R. Anthonisen et al., for the Lung Health Study Research Group, "The Effects of a Smoking Cessation Intervention on 14.5 Year Mortality: A Randomized Controlled Trial," *Annals of Internal Medicine* 142 (2005): 223–39.

22. American Heart Association, *Heart Disease and Stroke Statistics— 2007 Update.*

23. B. Howard et al., "Low Fat Diet and Risk of Cardiovascular Disease," *Journal of the American Medical Association* 295, no. 6 (2006): 655–66; American Heart Association, *Heart Disease and Stroke Statistics—2007 Update.*

24. National Heart, Lung, and Blood Institute, *Third Report of the Expert Panel on Detection, Evaluation and Treatment of High Blood Cholesterol in Adults,* NIH Publication no. 05-3290, 2005, www.nhlbi.nih.gov/health/public/heart/chol/wyntk.htm; Centers for Disease Control and Prevention, Division for Heart Disease and Stroke Prevention. National Center for Chronic Disease Prevention and Health Promotion, "State Heart Disease and Stroke Prevention Programs Address High Blood Cholesterol," March 2007, www.cdc.gov/dhdsp/library/fs_state_cholesterol.htm.

25. C. A. Garza et al., "The Association between Lipoprotein-Associated Phospholipase A_2 and Cardiovascular Disease: A Systematic Review," *Mayo Clinic Proceedings* 82 (2007):159–65.

26. American Heart Association, *Heart Disease and Stroke Statistics— 2007 Update.*

27. Ibid.

28. Ibid.

29. L. L. Yan et al., "Psychosocial Factors and Risk of Hypertension," *Journal of the American Medical Association* 290, no. 16 (2003): 2138–48.

30. M. Eisenberg et al., "Outcomes and Cost of Coronary Artery Bypass Graft Surgery in the United States and Canada," *Archives of Internal Medicine* 165 (2005): 1506–13.

31. Centers for Disease Control and Prevention, *National Diabetes Fact Sheet: General Information and National Estimates on Diabetes in the United States, 2005* (Atlanta: U.S. Department of Health and Human Services, Centers for Disease Control and Prevention, 2005).

32. Ibid.

33. Ibid.

34. Ibid.

35. H. Brekke et al., "Long Term Effects of Lifestyle Intervention in Type 2 Diabetes Relatives," *Diabetes Research and Clinical Practice* 70 (2005): 225–34.

36. L. Azadbakaht et al., "Beneficial Effects of Dietary Approaches to Stop Hypertension Eating Plan on Features of the Metabolic Syndrome," *Diabetes Care* 28 (2005): 2823–31.

37. Centers for Disease Control and Prevention, *National Diabetes Fact Sheet.*

38. American Diabetes Association, "Complications of Diabetes in the United States," 2006, www.diabetes.org/diabetes-statistics/complications.jsp.

39. American Cancer Society, *Cancer Facts and Figures, 2007.* (Atlanta: American Cancer Society, 2007).

40. Ibid.

41. Ibid.

42. Ibid.

43. Ibid.

44. Ibid.

45. Ibid.

46. K. Rapp et al., "Obesity and Incidence of Cancer: A Large Cohort Study of Over 145,000 Adults in Austria," *British Journal of Cancer* 93, (2005):1062–67; S. Feedland, "Obesity and Prostate Cancer: A Growing Problem," *Clinical Cancer Research* 11, no. 19 (2005): 6763–66; R. MacInnis et al., "Body Size and Composition and Colon Cancer Risk in Women," *International Cancer Journal* 118 no. 6 (2005): 1496–1500; C. Samanic et al., "Relation of Body Mass Index to Cancer Risk in 362,552 Swedish Men," *Cancer Causes and Control* 17, no. 7 (2005): 10552–10600; M. McCullough et al., "Risk Factors for Fatal Breast Cancer in African American Women and White Women in a Large U.S. Prospective Cohort," *American Journal of Epidemiology* 162, no. 8 (2005): 734–42; P. Soliman et al., "Risk Factors for Young Premenopausal Women with Endometrial Cancer," *Obstetrics and Gynecology* 105 (2005): 575–80.

47. National Cancer Institute, "Cancer Risk: Understanding the Puzzle," May 2007, http://understandingrisk.cancer.gov.

48. P. Soliman et al., "Risk Factors for Young Premenopausal Women with Endometrial Cancer," *Obstetrics and Gynecology,* 105 (2005): 575–80.

49. B. Binkumar and A. Mathew, "Dietary Fat and Risk of Breast Cancer, *World Journal of Surgical Oncology,* 3 no. 45 (2005): 1477.

50. S. Joachim et al., "Cellular Telephone Use and Cancer Risk: Update of a Nationwide Danish Cohort" *Journal of the National Cancer Institute* 98, no. 23 (2006): 1707–13, DOI: 10.1093/jnci/djj46.

51. M. Bennett et al., "Humor and Laughter May Influence Health: Complementary Therapies and Humor in Clinical Population," *Evidence Based Complementary and Alternative Medicine* 3, no. 2 (2006):187–90.

52. American Cancer Society, "Overview: Cervical Cancer. What Causes Cancer of the Cervix?" 2006, www.cancer.org.

53. American Cancer Society, *Cancer Facts and Figures, 2007.*

54. Ibid.

55. H. A. Wakelee et al., "Lung Cancer Incidence in Never Smokers," *Journal of Clinical Oncology* 25, no. 5 (2007): 472–78.

56. American Cancer Society, *Cancer Facts and Figures, 2007.*

57. Ibid.

58. C. M. Dallal et al., "Long-Term Recreational Physical Activity and Risk of Invasive and In Situ Breast Cancer," *Archives of Internal Medicine* 167, no. 4 (2007): 408–15.

59. National Breast Cancer Organization, "Hormonal Therapy," 2007, www.y-me.org.

60. American Cancer Society, *Cancer Facts and Figures, 2007.*

61. Ibid.

62. Ibid.

63. Ibid.

64. Ibid.

65. Ibid.

66. Ibid.

67. Ibid.

68. National Cancer Institute, "Testicular Cancer," 2007, www.cancer.gov/cancertopics/types/testicular.

69. American Cancer Society, *Cancer Facts and Figures, 2007.*

70. Ibid.

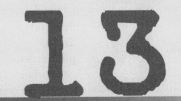

Infectious and Noninfectious Conditions

RISKS AND RESPONSIBILITIES

How does my body **fight** an infection?

Can I get a sexually transmitted **infection** from "outercourse"?

How is herpes **transmitted?**

What can I do for these killer **headaches?**

OBJECTIVES

- Explain how your immune system works to protect you and what you can do to boost its effectiveness.
- Describe the most common pathogens infecting humans today and the typical diseases each causes.
- Discuss the various sexually transmitted infections, their means of transmission, and actions that can be taken to prevent their spread.
- Discuss human immunodeficiency virus (HIV) and acquired immunodeficiency syndrome (AIDS), trends in infection and treatment, and the impact on special populations.
- Discuss noninfectious diseases, including asthma and lower back pain.

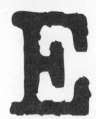very moment of every day, you are in contact with microscopic organisms that have the ability to cause illness or even death. These disease-causing agents, known as **pathogens,** are found in air and food and on nearly every object and person with whom you come in contact. New varieties of pathogens arise all the time, and scientific evidence indicates that many have existed for as long as there has been life on the planet. Fossil evidence shows that infections, cancer, heart disease, and a host of other ailments afflicted the earliest humans. At times, infectious diseases have wiped out whole groups of people through epidemics such as the Black Death, or bubonic plague, which killed up to one-third of the population of Europe in the 1300s. A **pandemic,** or global epidemic, of influenza killed more than 20 million people in 1918, and strains of tuberculosis and cholera continue to cause premature death throughout the world.

In spite of our best efforts to eradicate them, these diseases continue to be a menace, and new diseases emerge all the time. The news isn't all bad; even though we are bombarded by potential pathogenic threats, our immune systems are remarkably adept at protecting us. Millions of microorganisms live in and on our bodies all the time, usually in peaceful coexistence and to our mutual benefit. For people in good health and whose immune systems are functioning properly, these *endogenous organisms* are generally harmless; but, in sick people or those with weakened immune systems, these organisms can cause serious health problems.

Exogenous microorganisms are organisms that do not normally inhabit the body. When they do, however, they are apt to produce an infection and/or illness. The more easily these pathogens can gain a foothold in the body and sustain themselves, the more **virulent,** or aggressive, they may be in causing disease. By keeping your immune system strong, you will increase your ability to resist and fight off even the most virulent attacker.

The Process of Infection and Your Body's Defenses

Most diseases are **multifactorial diseases**—that is, they are caused by the interaction of several factors from inside and outside the person. For a disease to occur in a person, or host, the host must be *susceptible,* which means that the immune system

must be in a weakened condition; an agent capable of *transmitting* a disease must be present; and the environment must be *hospitable* to the pathogen in terms of temperature, light, moisture, and other requirements. Although all pathogens pose a threat if they take hold in your body, the chances that they will do so are actually quite small. First, they must overcome a number of effective barriers, many of which were established in your body before you were born.

Your Susceptibility to Disease

Factors You Cannot Control Unfortunately, some of the factors that make you susceptible to a certain disease are beyond your control. The following are the most common:

- *Heredity.* Perhaps the single greatest factor influencing disease risk is genetics. Being born into a family in which heart disease, cancer, or other illnesses are prevalent increases a person's risk. It is often unclear whether hereditary diseases are due to inherited genetic traits or to inherited insufficiencies in the immune system. Some believe that we may inherit even the quality of our immune system, so that some people are naturally "tougher" than others and more resilient to disease and infection.
- *Aging.* After age 40 we become more vulnerable to most chronic diseases. Moreover, as we age, our immune systems respond less efficiently to invading organisms, thus increasing risk for infection and illness. The very young are also at risk for many diseases, particularly if they are not vaccinated against them.
- *Environmental conditions.* Unsanitary conditions and the presence of drugs, chemicals, and hazardous pollutants and wastes in food and water probably have a great effect on our immune systems. A growing body of research points to changes in the environment (such as global warming) and natural disasters as significant contributors to increasing numbers of infectious diseases.[1]
- *Organism resistance.* Some organisms, such as the food-borne organism that causes *botulism* (a severe type of food poisoning), are particularly virulent, and even tiny amounts may make the most hardy of us ill. Other organisms have mutated and become resistant to the body's defenses as well as to medical treatments designed to protect against them. Still other, newer pathogens pose unique challenges that our bodily defenses are ill adapted to fight.

Factors You Can Control The good news is that we all have some degree of personal control over many risk factors for disease. Too much stress, inadequate nutrition, a low level of physical fitness, lack of sleep, misuse or abuse of legal and illegal substances, poor personal hygiene, high-risk behaviors, and other variables significantly increase the risk for a number of diseases. Fortunately, many of these are within our control, at least partly. **Table 13.1** lists actions you can take to keep your body's defenses healthy.

pathogen   A disease-causing agent.

pandemic   Global epidemic of a disease.

virulent   Strong enough to overcome host resistance and cause disease.

multifactorial disease   Disease caused by interactions of several factors.

TABLE 13.1	Bolstering Your Defenses
Eat for health	Follow established nutritional guidelines. Eat moderately, being sure to balance calories, getting enough protein, fats, carbohydrates, vitamins, and minerals. If you take supplements, buy high-quality ones, and avoid excessive doses.
Get adequate rest	Sleep really is the great elixir. Get whatever amount you need to feel refreshed and renewed when you wake in the morning.
Take time for calming and rejuvenating your mind and body	General indicators tell us that people who seek peace, harmony, and happiness, who practice mindfulness strategies, and who engage in relaxing and rejuvenating experiences are more resilient in times of illness. Meditation, yoga, mindfulness exercises, and other such activities can "quiet" the mind and body and may, in fact, help mobilize your immune system.
Avoid stress in your life	People who experience high levels of stress, or who have chaos and anger in their lives, tend also to have lower immune functioning. Stress can lead to a greater susceptibility for common infectious diseases and a decreased ability to battle infections.
Exercise regularly	Exercise can not only relax you but also reduce stressful body reactions, calm your spirit, and help mobilize your cells to do battle against infectious agents.
Get age-appropriate vaccinations	Review the vaccination schedule available in this chapter and at the CDC website, www.cdc.gov. Consider your risks, and whenever possible, opt for vaccinations designed to protect you from infectious agents.
Limit your exposure to pathogens	Hospitals, airplanes, airports, escalator and stair rails, grocery cart handles, and other commonly used and touched surfaces pose considerable risks to you if you touch them and don't wash your hands. Avoid people you know to be sick. If you want to help them, limit your exposure time, and wash your hands on arriving and leaving.
Wash your hands	The hands are the biggest single contributor to the spread of infectious diseases. Wash them, wash them often, and use warm water and a basic lubricating soap that helps wash organisms down the drain.
Don't overuse antibiotics	Overuse and misuse of antibiotics can allow organisms to adapt to them over time until they are no longer effective. If your doctor prescribes antibiotics for you, ask for the oldest or least strong drugs that will still work. Avoid the newer, more potent antibiotics that are easier to take and more powerful. Be sure to use the entire prescription, rather than stopping when your symptoms subside.
Don't abuse alcohol or other drugs	One of the surest ways to mess with your own immune system is to bring it down by taking drugs that may harm the system and, ultimately, make you more susceptible.

Routes of Transmission

Pathogens enter the body in several ways. They may be transmitted by *direct contact* between infected persons, such as during sexual relations, kissing, or touching, or by *indirect contact,* such as by touching an object the infected person has had contact with. **Table 13.2** lists common routes of transmission.

The hands are probably the greatest source of infectious disease transmission. You may also **autoinoculate** yourself, or transmit a pathogen from one part of your body to another. For example, you may touch a sore on your lip that is teeming with viral herpes and then transmit the virus to your eye when you scratch your itchy eyelid.

Your best friend may be the source of *animal-borne pathogens.* Dogs, cats, livestock, and wild animals can spread numerous diseases through their bites or feces or by carrying infected insects into living areas and transmitting diseases either directly or indirectly. Although *interspecies transmission* of diseases (diseases passed from humans to animals and vice versa) is rare, it does occur.

Physical and Chemical Defenses: Your Body Responds

Perhaps our single most critical early defense system is the skin. Layered to provide an intricate web of barriers, the skin allows few pathogens to enter. *Enzymes,* complex proteins manufactured by the body that appear in body secretions such as sweat, provide additional protection, destroying microorganisms on skin surfaces by producing inhospitable pH levels. In either case, microorganisms that flourish at a selected pH will be weakened or destroyed as these changes occur. Only when cracks or breaks occur in the skin can pathogens gain easy access to the body.

The internal linings of the body provide yet another protection. Mucous membranes in the respiratory tract and other

autoinoculate Transmit a pathogen from one part of your own body to another part.

TABLE 13.2 Routes of Disease Transmission

Mode of Transmission	Aspects of Transmission
Contact	Either *direct* (e.g., skin or sexual contact) or *indirect* (e.g., infected blood or body fluid)
Food- or waterborne	Eating or coming in contact with contaminated food or water or products passed through them
Airborne	Inhalation; droplet spread as through sneezing, coughing, or talking
Vectorborne	Transmitted by an animal, such as a mosquito, tick, snail, or bird, by means of its secretions, biting, or egg laying; transmission depends on how infectious the organism is
Perinatal	Similar to contact infection; happens in the uterus or as the baby passes through the birth canal

linings of the body trap and engulf invading organisms. *Cilia,* hairlike projections in the lungs and respiratory tract, sweep invaders toward body openings, where they are expelled. Tears, nasal secretions, ear wax, and other secretions found at body entrances contain enzymes designed to destroy or neutralize pathogens. Finally, any organism that manages to breach these initial lines of defense faces a formidable specialized network of defenses thrown up by the immune system.

The Immune System: Your Body Fights Back

How does my body fight an infection?

Immunity is a condition of being able to resist a particular disease by counteracting the substance that produces the disease. Any substance capable of triggering an immune response is called an **antigen.** An antigen can be a virus, a bacterium, a fungus, a parasite, a toxin, or a tissue or cell from another organism. When invaded by an antigen, the body responds by forming substances called **antibodies** that are matched to that specific antigen, much as a key is matched to a lock. Antibodies belong to a group of large molecules known as *immunoglobulins,* nine chemically distinct protein substances, each of which plays a role in neutralizing, setting up for destruction, or actually destroying antigens.

antigen Substance capable of triggering an immune response.

antibodies Substances produced by the body that are individually matched to specific antigens.

Once an antigen breaches the body's initial defenses, the body begins a process of antigen analysis. It considers the size and shape of the invader, verifies that the antigen is not part of the body itself, and then produces a specific antibody to destroy or weaken the antigen. This process, which is much more complex than described here, is part of a system called *humoral immune responses.* Humoral immunity is the body's major defense against many bacteria and the poisonous substances, called *toxins,* that they produce.

Cell-mediated immunity is characterized by the formation of a population of *lymphocytes* (specialized white blood cells) that can attack and destroy the foreign invader. These lymphocytes constitute the body's main defense against viruses, fungi, parasites, and some bacteria, and they are found in the blood, lymph nodes, bone marrow, and certain glands. Other key players in this immune response are *macrophages* (a type of phagocytic, or cell-eating, white blood cell).

Two forms of lymphocytes in particular, the *B lymphocytes* (B cells) and *T lymphocytes* (T cells), are involved in the immune response. They are named according to the area of the body in which they develop: most B cells are manufactured in the soft tissue of the hollow shafts of the long bones. T cells, in contrast, develop and multiply in the thymus, a multilobed organ that lies behind the breastbone.

T cells assist the immune system in several ways. *Regulatory T cells* help direct the activities of the immune system and assist other cells, particularly B cells, to produce antibodies. Dubbed "helper T cells," these cells are essential for activating B cells, other T cells, and macrophages. Another form of T cell, known as the *killer T cell* or *cytotoxic T cell,* directly attacks infected or malignant cells. Killer T cells enable the body to rid itself of cells that have been infected by viruses or transformed by cancer; they are also responsible for rejecting tissue and organ grafts. The third type of T cells, *suppressor T cells,* turns off or suppresses the activity of B cells, killer T cells, and macrophages. Suppressor T cells circulate in the bloodstream and lymphatic system, neutralizing or destroying antigens, enhancing the effects of the immune response, and helping to return the activated immune system to normal levels.

After a successful attack on a pathogen, some of the attacker T and B cells are preserved as *memory T and B cells,* enabling the body to recognize and respond quickly to subsequent attacks by the same kind of organism at a later time.

Once people have survived certain infectious diseases, they become immune to those diseases, meaning that in all probability they will not develop them again. Upon subsequent attack by the same disease-causing microorganisms, their memory T and B cells are quickly activated to come to their defense. **Figure 13.1** provides a summary of the immune response.

Autoimmune Diseases Although white blood cells and the antigen–antibody response generally work in our favor by neutralizing or destroying harmful antigens, the body sometimes makes a mistake and targets its own tissue as the enemy, builds up antibodies against that tissue, and

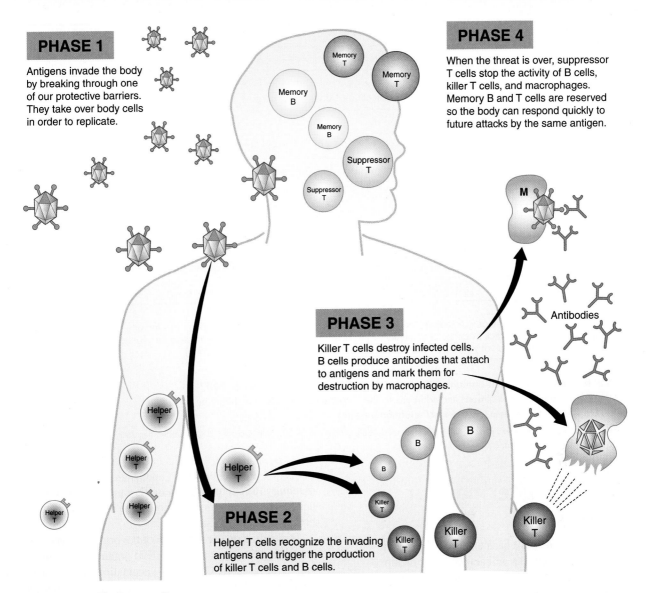

PHASE 1

Antigens invade the body by breaking through one of our protective barriers. They take over body cells in order to replicate.

PHASE 4

When the threat is over, suppressor T cells stop the activity of B cells, killer T cells, and macrophages. Memory B and T cells are reserved so the body can respond quickly to future attacks by the same antigen.

PHASE 3

Killer T cells destroy infected cells. B cells produce antibodies that attach to antigens and mark them for destruction by macrophages.

PHASE 2

Helper T cells recognize the invading antigens and trigger the production of killer T cells and B cells.

Memory T
Memory T
Memory B
Memory B
Suppressor T
Suppressor T
Helper T
Antibodies
M
B
B
Killer T
Killer T
Killer T
Killer T

FIGURE 13.1 The Immune Response

attempts to destroy it. This is known as *autoimmune disease* (*auto* means "self"). Common autoimmune disorders are rheumatoid arthritis, systemic lupus erythematosus (SLE), and myasthenia gravis.

In some cases, the antigen–antibody response completely fails to function. The result is a form of *immunodeficiency syndrome* such as that found in HIV and AIDS (see the section on HIV/AIDS in this chapter).

Fever

If an infection is localized, pus formation, redness, swelling, and irritation often occur. These symptoms indicate that the invading organisms are being fought systematically. Another indication is the development of a *fever,* or a rise in body temperature above the average norm of 98.6°F. Fever is frequently caused by toxins secreted by pathogens that interfere with the control of body temperature. Although extremely elevated

temperatures are harmful to the body, a mild fever is believed to act as a form of protection: raising body temperature by 1 or 2 degrees provides an environment that destroys some disease-causing organisms. A fever also stimulates the body to produce more white blood cells, which destroy more invaders.

Pain

Although you may not usually think of pain as a defense mechanism, it is a response to injury and plays a valuable role in the body's response to invasion. Pain tends to be the earliest sign that an injury has occurred and often causes the person to slow down or stop the activity that was aggravating the injury, thereby protecting against further damage. Because it is often one of the first warnings of disease, persistent pain should not be overlooked or masked with short-term pain relievers.

Vaccine	Age group		
	19–49 years	50–64 years	≥ 65 years
Tetanus, diphtheria, pertussis (Td/Tdap)	1-dose Td booster every 10 years		
	Substitute 1 dose of Tdap for Td		
Human papillomavirus (HPV)	3 doses (females)		
Measles, mumps, rubella (MMR)	1 or 2 doses	1 dose	
Varicella	2 doses (0, 4–8 weeks)	2 doses (0, 4–8 weeks)	
Influenza	1 dose annually	1 dose annually	
Pneumococcal (polysaccharide)	1–2 doses		1 dose
Hepatitis A	2 doses (0, 6–12 mos, or 0, 6–18 months)		
Hepatitis B	3 doses (0, 1–2, 4–6 months)		
Meningococcal	1 or more doses		

For all persons in this category who meet the age requirements and who lack evidence of immunity (e.g., lack documentation of vaccination or have no evidence of prior infection)

Recommended if some other risk factor is present (e.g., based on medical, occupational, lifestyle, or other indications)

FIGURE 13.2 Recommended Adult Immunization Schedule, by Vaccine and Age Group, 2007
Note that there are important explanations and additions to these recommendations that should be consulted by checking the latest schedule (available on the Centers for Disease Control and Prevention website).

Source: Centers for Disease Control and Prevention, "Recommended Adult Immunization Schedule, October 2006–September 2007," 2007, www.cdc.gov/vaccines/recs/schedules/adult-schedule.htm.

Vaccines: Bolstering Your Immunity

Recall that once people have been exposed to a specific pathogen, subsequent attacks will activate their memory T and B cells, thus giving them immunity. This is the principle on which **vaccination** is based.

A vaccine consists of killed or weakened versions of a disease-causing microorganism or an antigen that is similar to but less dangerous than the disease antigen. It is administered to stimulate the person's immune system to produce antibodies against future attacks—without actually causing the disease (or by causing a very minor case of it). Vaccines typically are given orally or by injection, and this form of artificial immunity is termed *artificially acquired active immunity,* in contrast to *naturally acquired active immunity* (which is obtained by exposure to antigens in the normal course of daily life) or *naturally acquired passive immunity* (as occurs when a mother passes immunity to her fetus via their shared blood supply or to an infant via breast milk).

Depending on the virulence of the organism, vaccines containing live, attenuated, or dead organisms are given for a variety of diseases. Childhood vaccinations are key, but so are adult vaccinations. **Figure 13.2** shows the recommended schedule for adult vaccinations.

Living with Allergies

An **allergy** occurs as part of the body's attempt to defend itself against a specific antigen or *allergen* by producing specific antibodies. When foreign pathogens such as bacteria or viruses invade the body, the body responds by producing antibodies to destroy these invading antigens. Under normal conditions, the production of antibodies is a positive element in the body's defense system. However, for unknown reasons, in some people the body overreacts by developing an overly elaborate protective mechanism against relatively harmless substances. The resulting *hypersensitivity reaction* to specific antigens in the environment is fairly common, as anyone who has awakened with a runny nose or itchy eyes will testify. Most commonly, these hypersensitivity, or allergic, responses occur as a reaction to environmental antigens such as molds, animal dander (hair and dead skin), pollen, ragweed, or dust. Once excessive antibodies to these antigens are produced, they trigger the

vaccination Inoculation with killed or weakened pathogens or similar, less dangerous antigens to prevent or lessen the effects of some disease.

allergy Hypersensitive reaction to a specific antigen or allergen in the environment, in which the body produces excessive antibodies to that antigen or allergen.

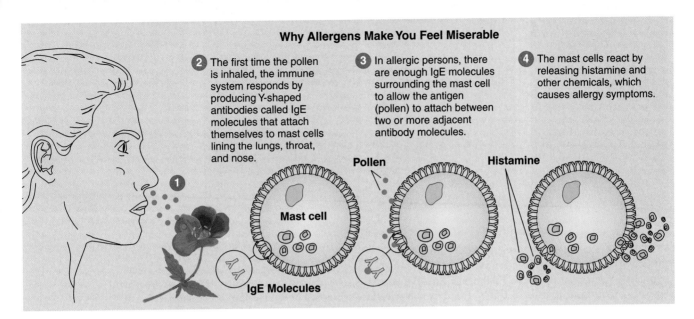

Why Allergens Make You Feel Miserable

2 The first time the pollen is inhaled, the immune system responds by producing Y-shaped antibodies called IgE molecules that attach themselves to mast cells lining the lungs, throat, and nose.

3 In allergic persons, there are enough IgE molecules surrounding the mast cell to allow the antigen (pollen) to attach between two or more adjacent antibody molecules.

4 The mast cells react by releasing histamine and other chemicals, which causes allergy symptoms.

Pollen

Histamine

Mast cell

IgE Molecules

FIGURE 13.3 Steps of an Allergic Response

release of **histamine,** a chemical substance that dilates blood vessels, increases mucous secretions, causes tissues to swell, and produces other allergy symptoms, particularly in the respiratory system (**Figure 13.3**). Many people take allergy shots to reduce the severity of their symptoms, with some success. In most cases, once the offending antigen has disappeared, allergy-prone people suffer few symptoms.

Food Allergies: New Problem for Many Over 20 percent of all Americans suffer from one form of allergy or another.[2] For increasing numbers of us, certain foods have become the enemy, prompting the new legislation, the Food Allergy Labeling and Consumer Protection Act (FALCPA), designed to make sure that we don't accidently eat something that causes an allergic reaction. Essentially, FALCPA covers the eight allergens that account for more than 90 percent of all documented food allergies in the United States: milk and other dairy products, eggs, fish, shellfish, tree nuts, peanuts, wheat, and soybeans.

In addition to labeling improvements, the food industry is responding by producing foods that are less likely to cause allergies in the first place. For example, millions of Americans are allergic to gluten, the protein found in wheat and related grains. As a result, gluten-free products are appearing daily on U.S. grocery shelves. As of 2008, gluten-free labeling is mandatory on food produced and sold in the United States.

Hay Fever **Hay fever,** or pollen allergies, is common throughout the world and is one of the most common chronic diseases in the United States. Hay fever attacks, which are characterized by sneezing and itchy, watery eyes and nose, make countless people miserable for weeks at a time every year. As with other allergies, hay fever results from an overzealous immune system, and it appears to run in families. Many trees, grasses, and weeds produce pollen that is associ-

ated with hay fever in some people. Avoiding the environmental triggers is the best way to prevent hay fever. If you can't prevent it, shots or antihistamines often provide relief.

Types of Pathogens and Diseases They Cause

We can categorize pathogenic microorganisms into six major types: bacteria, viruses, fungi, protozoa, parasitic worms, and prions. **Figure 13.4** shows examples of several of these pathogens.

Bacteria

Bacteria (singular: *bacterium*) are simple, single-celled microscopic organisms. There are three major types of bacteria, as classified by their shape: cocci, bacilli, and spirilla. Although there are several thousand known species of bacteria (and many thousands more that are unknown), just over

histamine Chemical substance that dilates blood vessels, increases mucous secretions, and produces other symptoms of allergies.

hay fever A chronic respiratory allergic disorder that is most prevalent when ragweed and flowers bloom.

bacteria (singular: *bacterium*) Simple, single-celled microscopic organisms. About 100 known species of bacteria cause disease in humans.

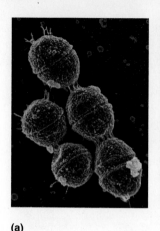
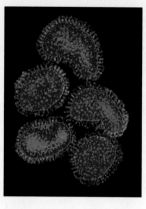
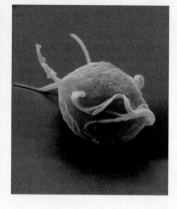
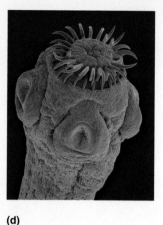

(a)   (b)   (c)   (d)

FIGURE 13.4 Examples of 4 Major Types of Pathogens.
(a) Color-enhanced scanning electron micrograph (SEM) of *Streptococcus* bacteria, magnified 40,000×. (b) Colored transmission electron micrograph (TEM) of influenza (flu) viruses, magnified 32,000×. (c) Color TEM of *Trichomonas vaginalis*, a protozoan, magnified 9,000×. (d) Color-enhanced SEM of the adult head (scolex) of a mammalian intestinal tapeworm, magnified 20×.

100 cause diseases in humans. In many cases, it is not the bacteria themselves that cause disease but rather the toxins that they produce. The following are the most common bacterial infections.

Staphylococcal Infections
Staphylococci are normally present on our skin at all times and usually cause few problems, but when there is a cut or break in the *epidermis,* or outer layer of the skin, staphylococci may enter and cause a localized infection. If you have ever suffered from acne, boils, styes (infections of the eyelids), or infected wounds, you have probably had a "staph" infection. Although most such infections are readily defeated by your immune system, resistant forms of staph bacteria are on the rise. These bacteria pose serious risks to people infected and must be treated with heavy doses of antibiotics. Some health experts worry that in time, our ability to kill staph organisms will be compromised as organisms grow stronger and our arsenal of agents to kill them dwindles. Keeping wounds clean and sterile is a crucial part of reducing the risk of staph infections.

At least one staph-caused disorder, **toxic shock syndrome (TSS),** is potentially fatal. To date, most cases of TSS have occurred in menstruating women or after surgery among both men and women. If you are a menstruating woman, you can reduce the likelihood of toxic shock syndrome by taking the following precautions: (1) avoid superabsorbent tampons, except during the heaviest menstrual flow; (2) change tampons at least every 4 hours; and (3) use pads at night instead of tampons.

Streptococcal Infections
At least five types of the **streptococcus** microorganism are known to cause bacterial infections. Group A streptococci (GAS) cause the most common diseases, such as streptococcal pharyngitis ("strep throat") and scarlet fever, which is often preceded by a sore throat.[3] Group B streptococci can cause illness in newborn babies, pregnant women, older adults, and adults with other illnesses such as diabetes or liver disease.[4] One particularly virulent group of GAS can lead to a disease known as *necrotizing faciitis* (often referred to as "flesh-eating strep"); a rare, but serious, disease that leads to death in about 30 percent of all cases, even with vigorous antibiotic treatment.[5]

Meningitis
Meningitis is an infection and inflammation of the *meninges,* the membranes that surround the brain and spinal cord. Some forms of bacterial meningitis are contagious and can be spread through contact with saliva, nasal discharge, feces, or respiratory and throat secretions. *Pneumococcal meningitis,* the most common form of meningitis, is the most dangerous form of bacterial meningitis. Approximately 6,000 cases of pneumococcal meningitis are reported in the United States each year. *Meningococcal meningitis,* a virulent form of meningitis, has risen dramatically on college campuses in recent years.[6] College students living in dormitories have a higher risk of contracting this disease than those who live off campus.

The signs of meningitis are sudden fever, severe headache, and a stiff neck, particularly causing difficulty touching your

staphylococcus   A round bacterium, usually found in clusters.

toxic shock syndrome (TSS)   A potentially life-threatening bacterial infection that is most common in menstruating women who use tampons.

streptococcus   A round bacterium, usually found in chain formation.

meningitis   An infection of the meninges, the membranes that surround the brain and spinal cord.

chin to your chest. Pneumococcal meningitis symptoms may include nausea and vomiting, confusion and disorientation, drowsiness, and poor appetite. Persons who are suspected of having meningitis should receive immediate, aggressive medical treatment. The infection can progress quickly, and early treatment is critical to the outcome. Vaccines are available for some types of meningitis.

Pneumonia

In the early twentieth century, **pneumonia** was a leading cause of death in the United States. This lung disease is characterized by chronic cough, chest pain, chills, high fever, fluid accumulation, and eventual respiratory failure. One of the most common forms of pneumonia is caused by bacterial infection and responds readily to antibiotic treatment in the early stages. Other forms are caused by viruses, chemicals, or other substances in the lungs and are more difficult to treat. Although medical advances have reduced the overall incidence of pneumonia, it continues to be a major threat in the United States and throughout the world. Vulnerable populations include the poor, older adults, and people already suffering from other illnesses.

Tuberculosis

A major killer in the United States in the early twentieth century, **tuberculosis (TB)** was largely controlled in America by 1950 as a result of improved sanitation, isolation of infected persons, and treatment with drugs such as *rifampin* or *isoniazid*. Though many health professionals assumed that TB had been conquered, that appears not to be the case. During the past 20 years, several factors have led to an epidemic rise in the disease: deteriorating social conditions, including overcrowding and poor sanitation; failure to isolate active cases of TB; a weakening of public health infrastructure, which has led to less funding for screening; and migration of TB to the United States through immigration and international travel. In 2006, there were 13,767 active cases of tuberculosis in the United States. It is estimated that one-third of the world's inhabitants (over 2 billion humans) carry the TB bacterium, *Mycobacterium tuberculosis,* and infection is spreading at the rate of 1 person per second. An estimated 15 million people live with active TB, and 2 million people die from it each year.[7]

Tuberculosis is caused by bacterial infiltration of the respiratory system that results in a chronic inflammatory reaction in the lungs. Airborne transmission via the respiratory tract is the primary and most efficient mode of transmitting TB. Symptoms include persistent coughing, weight loss, fever, and spitting up blood. Infected people can be contagious without actually showing any symptoms themselves and can transmit the disease while talking, coughing, sneezing, or singing. Fortunately, TB is fairly difficult to catch, and prolonged exposure, rather than single exposure, is the typical mode of infection. Treatments are effective for most nonresistant cases and usually include rest, careful infection-control procedures, and drugs to combat the infection.

Peptic Ulcers

An ulcer is a lesion or wound that forms in body tissue as a result of some irritant. A **peptic ulcer** is a chronic ulcer that occurs in the lining of the stomach or the section of the small intestine known as the *duodenum.* The lining of these organs becomes irritated, the protective covering of mucus is reduced, and the gastric acid begins to digest the dying tissue, just as it would a piece of food. Research indicates that most peptic ulcers result from infection by a common bacterium, *Helicobacter pylori.* The disorder, which affects more than 4 million Americans every year, generally responds to antibiotics.

Viruses

Viruses are the smallest known pathogens, approximately 1/500th the size of bacteria. More than 150 viruses are known to cause disease in humans, although their role in various cancers and chronic diseases is still unclear. Essentially, a virus consists of a protein structure that contains either *ribonucleic acid (RNA)* or *deoxyribonucleic acid (DNA).* Viruses are incapable of carrying out any life processes on their own. To reproduce, they must enter a cell of a host and exploit that cell to make copies of the virus, which are then released to infect other host cells.

Viral diseases can be difficult to treat because many viruses can withstand heat, formaldehyde, and large doses of radiation with little effect on their structure. Some viruses have **incubation periods** (the length of time required to develop fully and cause symptoms in their hosts) that last for years, which delays diagnosis. Drug treatment for viral infections is also limited. Drugs powerful enough to kill viruses generally kill the host cells too, although some medications block stages in viral reproduction without damaging host cells.

The Common Cold

Colds are responsible for more days lost from work and more uncomfortable days spent at work than any other ailment. Caused by any number of viruses (some experts claim there may be over 100 different

---

pneumonia Disease of the lungs characterized by chronic cough, chest pain, chills, high fever, and fluid accumulation; may be caused by bacteria, viruses, chemicals, or other substances.

tuberculosis (TB) A disease caused by bacterial infiltration of the respiratory system.

peptic ulcer Damage to the stomach or intestinal lining, usually caused by digestive juices; most ulcers result from infection by the bacterium *Helicobacter pylori.*

viruses Minute microbes consisting of DNA or RNA that live inside another cell and use the cell's resources to reproduce themselves.

incubation period The time between exposure to a disease and the appearance of symptoms.

viruses responsible), colds are **endemic** (always present to some degree) throughout the world. Current research indicates that otherwise healthy people carry cold viruses in their noses and throats most of the time. These viruses are held in check until the host's resistance is lowered. In the true sense of the word, it is possible to "catch" a cold—from the airborne droplets of another person's sneeze or from skin-to-skin or mucous membrane contact—although the hands are the greatest avenue for transmitting colds and other viruses. Contrary to common thinking, you won't "catch" a cold from getting a chill, but the chill may lower your immune system's resistance to the cold virus or other pathogens.

Influenza
In otherwise healthy people, **influenza,** or flu, is usually not life-threatening. However, in combination with disorders such as respiratory or heart disease or among people over age 65 or under age 5, the flu can be very serious. Little can be done to treat flu patients once the infection has become established.

To date, three major varieties of flu virus have been discovered, with many different strains existing within each variety. If you contract one form of influenza you may develop immunity to it, but you will not necessarily be immune to other forms of the disease. See **Figure 13.5** for tips on how to distinguish the flu from other illnesses.

Some vaccines have proven effective against certain strains of flu virus, but they are totally ineffective against others. In spite of minor risks, people over age 65, pregnant women, people with heart or lung disease, and people with certain other illnesses should be vaccinated. Flu shots take 2 to 3 weeks to become effective, so people at risk should get these shots in the fall before the flu season begins. Because the vaccine contains a weakened version of the live virus, people who receive the vaccine may pose a risk to anyone with a weakened immune system who is around them.[8]

Infectious Mononucleosis
Initial symptoms of **mononucleosis,** or "mono," include sore throat, fever, headache, nausea, chills, and pervasive weakness/fatigue. As the disease progresses, lymph nodes may enlarge, and other signs may appear, such as spleen enlargement, body rashes, aching joints, and jaundice (yellowing of the whites of the eyes and the skin).

endemic Describing a disease that is always present to some degree.

influenza A common viral disease of the respiratory tract.

mononucleosis A viral disease that causes pervasive fatigue and other long-lasting symptoms.

hepatitis A viral disease in which the liver becomes inflamed, producing symptoms such as fever, headache, and possibly jaundice.

Caused by the *Epstein-Barr virus,* mono is readily detected through a blood test. Because many viruses are caused by transmission of body fluids, many people once believed that young people contracted mono through kissing (hence its nickname, "the kissing disease"). However, mono is not highly contagious and does not appear to be easily spread through normal, everyday personal contact; kissing is actually not a common mode of transmission. Treatment of mono is often a lengthy process that involves bed rest, balanced nutrition, and medications.

Hepatitis
One of the most highly publicized viral diseases is **hepatitis,** a virally caused inflammation of the liver. Hepatitis symptoms include fever, headache, nausea, loss of appetite, skin rashes, pain in the upper right abdomen, dark yellow (with brownish tinge) urine, and jaundice. In some regions of the United States and among certain segments of the population, hepatitis has reached epidemic proportions. Internationally, viral hepatitis is a major contributor to liver disease and accounts for high morbidity and mortality. Currently, there are seven known forms, with hepatitis A, B, and C having the highest rate of incidence.

- *Hepatitis A (HAV).* HAV is contracted from eating food or drinking water contaminated with human excrement. Handlers of infected food, people who ingest seafood from contaminated water, and people who use contaminated needles are also at risk. Fortunately, individuals infected with hepatitis A do not become chronic carriers, and vaccines for HAV are available.[9]

- *Hepatitis B (HBV).* This disease is spread primarily through body fluids shared through unprotected sex, but it also is contracted through sharing needles when injecting drugs, needlesticks on the job, or, in the case of a newborn baby, from an infected mother. Although 30 percent of people who are infected have no symptoms, symptoms can include jaundice, fatigue, abdominal pain, loss of appetite, nausea and vomiting, and joint pain. HBV can lead to chronic liver disease or liver cancer. HBV infection has been on the decline, largely because of a vaccine for HBV that has been available since 1982 and is now available on most college campuses for a modest cost.[10] However, because the vaccine can be costly and is not widely available globally, over 350 million people worldwide are chronic carriers.[11] A combination series vaccine for HAV and HBV is also an option for certain high-risk populations, such as day care workers, health care workers, and people traveling to regions of the world where HAV or HBV is prevalent.

- *Hepatitis C (HCV).* HCV infections are on an epidemic rise in many regions of the world as resistant forms of the virus are emerging. Some cases can be traced to blood transfusions or organ transplants. Over 85 percent of people infected develop chronic infections, and if the infection is left untreated, the person may develop cirrhosis of the liver, liver cancer, or liver failure. Liver failure due to chronic hepatitis C is the leading cause of liver

SYMPTOMS	AIRBORNE ALLERGY	COLD	FLU
Fever	Never	Rare	Usual; high (100–102° F, occasionally higher, especially in children); lasts 3–4 days
Headache	Rare	Rare	Common
General aches and pains	Never	Slight	Usual; often severe
Fatigue, weakness	Sometimes	Sometimes	Usual; can last up to 2–3 weeks
Extreme exhaustion	Never	Never	Usual; at the beginning of the illness
Stuffy nose	Common	Common	Sometimes
Runny nose	Common	Common	Sometimes
Sneezing	Usual	Usual	Sometimes
Itchy eyes	Common	Rare	Never
Sore throat	Sometimes	Common	Sometimes
Chest discomfort, cough	Sometimes	Common; mild to moderate, hacking cough	Common; can become severe
Nausea, vomiting	Never	Rare	Sometimes
Duration	Weeks (for example, 6 weeks for ragweed or grass pollen seasons)	3–14 days	3–14 days; longer if complications develop
COMPLICATIONS	Sinus infection, asthma	Sinus infection, middle ear infection, asthma	Bronchitis, pneumonia; can be life-threatening
PREVENTION	Avoid those things that you are allergic to, such as pollen, house dust mites, mold, pet dander	Wash your hands often; avoid close contact with anyone with a cold	Annual vaccination; prescription antiviral medicines, avoid close contact with anyone with a flu
TREATMENT	Antihistamines, nasal steroids, decongestants	Antihistamines, decongestants, nonsteroidal anti-inflammatory medicines	Prescription antiviral medicines

FIGURE 13.5 Is It an Allergy, a Cold, or the Flu?

Source: Adapted from the National Institute of Allergy and Infectious Diseases, "Is It a Cold or an Allergy?" 2005, and "Is It a Cold or the Flu?" 2005, www.niaid.nih.gov.

transplants in the United States.[12] Currently, there is no vaccine for HCV, although efforts are underway to develop one.

In the United States, hepatitis continues to be a major threat in spite of a safe blood supply and massive efforts at education about hand washing (for HAV) and safer sex (primarily for HBV). Treatment of all forms of viral hepatitis is somewhat limited.

Measles Measles is a viral disorder that often affects young children. Symptoms, appearing about 10 days after exposure, include an itchy rash and a high fever. **Rubella**

(German measles) is a milder viral infection that is believed to be transmitted by inhalation, after which it multiplies in the upper respiratory tract and passes into the bloodstream. It causes a rash, especially on the upper

measles   A viral disease that produces symptoms including an itchy rash and a high fever.

rubella (German measles)   A milder form of measles that causes a rash and mild fever in children and may cause damage to a fetus or a newborn baby.

extremities. It usually runs its course in 3 to 4 days and is not generally a serious health threat. The major exceptions to this are newborns and pregnant women. Rubella can damage a fetus, particularly during the first trimester, by creating a condition known as *congenital rubella,* in which the infant may be born blind, deaf, cognitively impaired, or with heart defects. Immunization has reduced the incidence of both measles and rubella. Infections in children not immunized against measles can lead to fever-induced problems such as rheumatic heart disease, kidney damage, and neurological disorders.

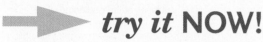 *try it* NOW!

Wash your hands to prevent infection. How can you clean your hands properly? Wet your hands with warm water, and lather up with soap; scrub your hands for about 20 seconds—try counting to 20 or saying the alphabet. Rinse well and dry your hands. Start following this basic procedure today whenever you use the bathroom, eat or prepare food, blow your nose, cough, or sneeze.

Other Pathogens

Fungi Our environment is inhabited by thousands of species of **fungi,** multicellular or unicellular organisms that obtain their food by infiltrating the bodies of other organisms, both living and dead. Many fungi are useful to humans, such as edible mushrooms, penicillin, and the yeast used in making bread, but some species of fungi can produce infections. *Candidiasis* (a vaginal yeast infection), athlete's foot, ringworm, and jock itch are examples of fungal diseases. With most fungal diseases, keeping the affected area clean and dry plus treating it with appropriate medications will generally bring prompt relief.

Protozoa **Protozoa** are microscopic, single-celled organisms that are generally associated with tropical diseases such as African sleeping sickness and malaria. Although these pathogens are prevalent in nonindustrialized countries, they are largely controlled in the United States. The most common

fungi A group of multicellular and unicellular organisms that obtain their food by infiltrating the bodies of other organisms, both living and dead; several microscopic varieties are pathogenic.

protozoa Microscopic single-celled organisms that can be pathogenic.

parasitic worms The largest of the pathogens, most of which are more a nuisance than a threat.

prion A recently identified self-replicating, protein-based pathogen.

protozoal disease in the United States is *trichomoniasis,* which we will discuss later in this chapter's section on sexually transmitted infections. A common waterborne protozoan disease in many regions of the country is *giardiasis.* People who drink or are exposed to the *Giardia* pathogen may suffer intestinal pain and discomfort weeks after infection. Protecting water supplies is the key to prevention.

Parasitic Worms **Parasitic worms** are the largest of the pathogens. Ranging in size from the small pinworms typically found in children to the relatively large tapeworms found in all warm-blooded animals, most parasitic worms are more a nuisance than a threat. Of special note today are the worm infestations associated with eating raw fish in sushi restaurants. Cooking fish and other foods to temperatures sufficient to kill the worms and their eggs can prevent this.

Prions A **prion** is a self-replicating, protein-based agent that can infect humans and other animals. One such prion is believed to be the underlying cause of spongiform diseases such as "mad cow disease."

Emerging and Resurgent Diseases

Although our immune systems are remarkably adept at responding to challenges, microbes and other pathogens appear to be gaining ground. Old scourges are back, and new ones are emerging. Within the past decade, rates for infectious diseases have rapidly increased, particularly for reemerging diseases such as tuberculosis. This trend can be attributed to a combination of overpopulation, inadequate health care systems, increasing poverty, extreme environmental degradation, and drug resistance.[13] As international travel increases (over 1 million people per day cross international boundaries), with germs transported from remote regions to huge urban centers within hours, the likelihood of infection by pathogens previously unknown on U.S. soil increases. Today's arsenal of antibiotics appears to be increasingly ineffective. Penicillin-resistant strains of diseases are on the rise as bacteria become able to outlast and outsmart even the best of our antibiotic weapons, and viruses are constantly mutating, making them potentially more lethal. See the **Health Headlines** box on page 396 for more on antibiotic resistance.

Tiny Invaders, Lethal Threats

"Mad Cow Disease" The American cattle industry is under new scrutiny, with confirmed U.S. cases of *bovine spongiform encephalopathy* (BSE, or "mad cow disease"). Evidence indicates that there is a relationship between ongoing outbreaks in Europe of BSE and a disease in humans known as *new variant Creutzfeldt-Jakob disease (nvCJD).*[14] Both disorders are invariably fatal brain diseases with unusually long incubation periods measured in years, and both are caused by unconventional transmittable agents known as prions.

BSE is thought to be transmitted when cows are fed slaughterhouse leftovers from sheep and other cows as a protein source. Failure to treat this protein by-product sufficiently to kill the BSE organism allows it to infect the cows, and the disease is believed to be transmitted to humans through the meat. The resultant variant of BSE in humans, nvCJD, is characterized by progressively worsening neurological damage and eventual death.

While scientists continue to investigate the presence of BSE in U.S. cattle, the United States Department of Agriculture (USDA) has cut back on its testing of beef cattle. USDA officials say that there is a very low risk to humans, amid bans on U.S. beef from countries around the world. To date, there have been no known human infections from U.S. beef. People living in the United States who have developed the disease are generally believed to have been infected during international travel.

West Nile Virus
Until 1999, few Americans had heard of *West Nile virus (WNV),* which is spread by the bite of an infected mosquito. Today, only Alaska and Hawaii remain free of the disease. During 2006 over 4,260 cases of WNV were reported, with over 119 deaths nationwide.[15]

Most people who become infected with West Nile virus will have mild symptoms or none at all. Rarely, WNV infection can result in severe and sometimes fatal illness. Symptoms include fever, headache, and body aches, often with skin rash and swollen lymph glands, and a form of encephalitis (inflammation of the brain). There is no vaccine or specific treatment for WNV, but avoiding mosquito bites is the best way to prevent it. Strategies to prevent mosquito bites include using a bug repellent with DEET (diethyl toluamide) and wearing long-sleeved clothing and long pants when outdoors; staying indoors during dawn, dusk and other peak mosquito feeding times; and removing any standing water sources around the home.

Ebola Hemorrhagic Fever
Another emerging disease, *Ebola hemorrhagic fever (Ebola HF)* is a severe, often fatal disease in humans and nonhuman primates (monkeys, gorillas, and chimpanzees). Researchers believe the Ebola virus is animal-borne and normally occurs in animal hosts that are native to the African continent.[16] The virus is spread via direct contact with blood or secretions and may also be airborne. With an incubation period of 2 to 21 days, the course of the disease is quick and characterized by fever, headache, joint and muscle aches, sore throat, and weakness, followed by diarrhea, vomiting, and stomach pain.[17] Fortunately, Ebola is not as prevalent worldwide as are many other diseases.

Severe Acute Respiratory Syndrome
Severe acute respiratory syndrome (SARS) is a viral respiratory illness that first emerged in Asia in 2003 and eventually infected over 8,000 people worldwide, with 774 deaths. SARS is thought to be spread by close personal contact with people who are infected, though research on other methods of transmission is ongoing. Symptoms of SARS include high fever, body aches, headache, diarrhea, and a cough. Eventually, this cough can progress to a pneumonia-like upper respiratory illness.[18]

Avian (Bird) Flu
Avian influenza is an infectious disease of birds. There has been considerable media flurry in the past few years over a strain of avian (bird) flu, H5N1, that is highly pathogenic and is capable of crossing the species barrier and causing severe illness in humans. This virulent flu strain began to emerge in bird populations throughout Asia, including domestic birds such as chickens and ducks, as early as 1997. By 2007, H5N1 bird flu had spread to birds in parts of western Europe, eastern Europe, Russia, and northern Africa.[19] Although the virus has yet to mutate into a form highly infectious to humans, outbreaks have occurred in rural areas of the world (where people often live in close proximity to poultry and other animals). As of July 2007, bird flu had caused 192 human deaths worldwide.[20]

Many health experts suggest that this virus, should it develop the ability to be transmissible between humans, is virulent enough to surpass the lethality of the influenza epidemics of 1918 and 1919, which swept the global community, causing millions of deaths. Thus far, the virus has infected only humans who have come in contact with infected birds; however, some scientists believe it is only a matter of time before the H5N1 strain will be readily passed from human to human.

The current spread of H5N1 throughout global bird populations has sparked international governments into action. Countries around the globe are working to develop strategic action plans and early warning systems, prevent the spread of disease, and create vaccines. However, developing countries are of great concern, because the same resources are not available to them. No vaccine is currently ready for production, and when it is ready, producing enough vaccine for an epidemic could present a challenge. Despite this, there are some promising treatments and tips for prevention. Antiviral medication, such as Tamiflu, can reduce the severity and duration of illness. Countries worldwide and the WHO are stockpiling these medications and developing plans for rapid distribution should an outbreak occur.

Escherichia coli O157:H7
Escherichia coli O157:H7 is one of over 170 types of *E. coli* bacteria that can infect humans. Most *E. coli* organisms are harmless and live in the intestines of healthy animals and humans; *E. coli* O157:H7, however, produces a lethal toxin and can cause severe illness or death.

HEALTH headlines

Imagine a world where people actually die from simple cuts or exposure to common household ailments such as the cold, minor burns and scrapes, or other seemingly innocent infections. According to the World Health Organization, "People of the world may only have a decade or two to make use of many of the medicines presently available to stop infectious diseases before antimicrobial resistance begins to be a major threat to health."

DRUG-RESISTANT INFECTIONS ARE ON THE RISE

Drug-resistant pathogens—those that are not killed or inhibited by antibiotics and other antimicrobial compounds—are on the rise globally:

- Strains of *Staphylococcus aureus* resistant to most antibiotics are endemic in many hospitals today. In some cities, 31 percent of staph infections are resistant, and in nursing homes as many as 71 percent of staph infections defy traditional antibiotic regimens.

- *Streptococcus pneumoniae* causes thousands of cases of meningitis and pneumonia and 7 million cases of ear infections in the United States each year. Currently, about 30 percent of these cases are resistant to penicillin, the primary drug for treatment. Many penicillin-resistant strains are also resistant to other antibiotics.

- An estimated 300 to 500 million people worldwide are infected with parasites that cause malaria, and an estimated 700,000 to 2.7 million people die each year from the disease. Resistance to chloroquine, once a widely used and highly effective treatment, is now found in most regions of the world, and other treatments are losing their effectiveness at alarming rates.

- Strains of *multidrug-resistant organisms (MDROs)* that defy our current arsenal of antibiotics have emerged over the last decade. Numbers of persons infected have risen dramatically throughout the world, prompting increased concern by health care professionals. Infection control units in hospitals and health care facilities are particularly concerned about outbreaks among patients whose immune systems are already compromised.

WHY IS ANTIMICROBIAL RESISTANCE GROWING?

Antibiotics typically wipe out bacteria that are susceptible to them. However, when used improperly, the antibiotics kill only the weak bacteria and leave the strongest versions to thrive and replicate. Because bacteria can swap genes with one another under the right conditions, hardy, drug-resistant germs can share their resistance mechanisms with other germs. Eventually, an entire colony of resistant bugs grows and passes on its resistance traits to new generations of bacteria.

Resistance commonly stems from incorrect use of antibiotics. For example, patients may begin an antibiotic regimen, start to feel better, and stop taking the drug to save money by using the drug another time. The surviving bacteria then build immunity to the drugs used to treat

---

E. coli O157:H7 can live in the intestines of healthy cattle and then contaminate food products at slaughterhouses. Eating ground beef that is rare or undercooked, drinking unpasteurized milk or juice, or swimming in sewage-contaminated water or public pools can cause infection through ingestion of feces that contain *E. coli.*

A symptom of infection is nonbloody diarrhea, usually 2 to 8 days after exposure; however, asymptomatic (symptom-free) cases have been noted. Children, older adults, and people whose immune systems have been weakened by other diseases are particularly vulnerable to serious side effects such as kidney failure.

Although *E. coli* organisms continue to pose threats to public health, strengthened regulations on the cooking of meat and regulation of chlorine levels in pools have helped. However, the 2006 *E. coli* outbreak linked to contaminated spinach has caused the USDA and others in the agriculture industry to consider new safety measures.

Bioterrorism: The New Global Threat

The idea of using infectious microorganisms as weapons is not new. In fact, during the seventeenth century wars, the English traded to Native Americans blankets impregnated with scabs from smallpox patients in hopes of spreading disease. The threat of delivering a lethal load of anthrax or other deadly microorganisms in the warheads of missiles or by a single person is a topic of much discussion among today's world leaders, particularly after the cases of anthrax delivered by mail following the September 11, 2001, terrorist attacks. For more information on what you can do to protect yourself from bioterrorism, see Chapter 4.

them. Also, doctors have overused antibiotics; the CDC estimates that one-third of the 150 million prescriptions written each year are unnecessary, resulting in bacterial strains that are tougher than the drugs used to fight them. Other factors may include the following:

- *Overuse of antibiotics in food production.* About 70 percent of antibiotic production today is used to treat sick animals and encourage growth in livestock and poultry. Farmed fish may be given antibiotics to fight off disease in controlled water areas. Although research is only in its infancy, many believe that ingesting meats, animal products, and fish that are rich in antibiotics may contribute to antibiotic resistance in humans.
- *Antibacterial soaps and other cleaning products.* Just how much these products contribute to overall resistance is also in question; as with antibiotics, the germs these products do not kill may become stronger than before.

REDUCING THE RISK OF ANTIMICROBIAL RESISTANCE

What can be done to slow the growth of resistant organisms? Individual and community actions include the following:

- Enact policies that severely restrict the use of antibiotics, growth hormones, and other products in our food supply.
- Buy foods and products that are antibiotic-free. This means requiring labeling of all foods in which antibiotics have been used in any stage of processing.
- Motivate people to take medications as prescribed and to finish all medications: killing the bugs the first time, all the time.
- Encourage doctors to prescribe antibiotics only when absolutely necessary, and encourage patients not to pressure their doctors to prescribe antibiotics for all ailments.
- Educate consumers about the fact that not all germs are inherently bad and that exposure to many of them

helps our immune systems develop arsenals capable of fighting pathogens.

- Educate people that washing their hands with a good flow of water and regular soap for at least 20 seconds is better than using antibacterial soaps.
- Choose hand soaps, bath soaps, dishwashing detergents, and household cleaners that are NOT "antibacterial."
- Encourage pharmaceutical companies to develop, test, and market new classes of antibiotics to keep up with growing resistance.

Sources: Centers for Disease Control and Prevention, "A Public Health Action Plan to Fight Microbial Resistance," 2007, www.cdc.gov/drugresistance/actionplan/index.htm; National Institute of Allergy and Infectious Diseases, "The Problem of Antimicrobial Resistance," 2006, www.niaid.nih.gov/factsheets/antimicro.htm; National Center for Infectious Diseases, "Malaria Fact Sheet," 2007, www.cdc.gov/malaria/facts.htm; World Health Organization, "Anti-Microbial Resistance," www.who.int; Centers for Disease Control and Prevention, "About Antibiotic Resistance," 2006, www.cdc.gov/drugresistance/community.

Sexually Transmitted Infections

Sexually transmitted infections (STIs) have been with us since our earliest recorded days on Earth. Today, there are more than 20 known types of STIs. Once referred to as *venereal diseases* and then *sexually transmitted diseases,* the current terminology is more reflective of the number and types of these communicable diseases. More virulent strains and antibiotic-resistant forms spell trouble in the days ahead.

Sexually transmitted infections affect men and women of all backgrounds and socioeconomic levels. In the United States alone, an estimated 19 million new cases of STIs are reported each year.[21] More than 65 million people are currently living with an incurable STI.[22]

Early symptoms of an STI are often mild and unrecognizable **(Figure 13.6).** Left untreated, some of these infections can have grave consequences, such as sterility, blindness, central nervous system destruction, disfigurement, and even death. Infants born to mothers carrying the organisms for these infections are at risk for a variety of health problems.

As with many communicable diseases, much of the pain, suffering, and anguish associated with STIs can be eliminated through education, responsible action, simple preventive strategies, and prompt treatment. Although STIs can happen to anyone, you can avoid them if you take appropriate precautions when you decide to engage in a sexual relationship.

sexually transmitted infections (STIs) Infectious diseases transmitted through some form of intimate, usually sexual, contact.

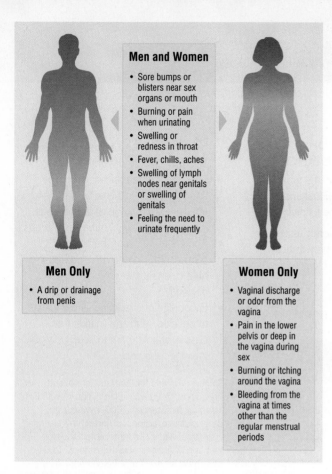

Men and Women
- Sore bumps or blisters near sex organs or mouth
- Burning or pain when urinating
- Swelling or redness in throat
- Fever, chills, aches
- Swelling of lymph nodes near genitals or swelling of genitals
- Feeling the need to urinate frequently

Men Only
- A drip or drainage from penis

Women Only
- Vaginal discharge or odor from the vagina
- Pain in the lower pelvis or deep in the vagina during sex
- Burning or itching around the vagina
- Bleeding from the vagina at times other than the regular menstrual periods

FIGURE 13.6 Signs or Symptoms of Sexually Trasmitted Infection
In their early stages, many STIs may be asymptomatic or have such mild symptoms that they are easy to overlook.

Possible Causes: What's Your Risk?

Several reasons have been proposed to explain the present high rates of STIs. The first relates to the moral and social stigma associated with these infections. Shame and embarrassment often keep infected people from seeking treatment. Unfortunately, they usually continue to be sexually active, thereby infecting unsuspecting partners. People who are uncomfortable discussing sexual issues may also be less likely to use and ask their partners to use condoms to protect against STIs and pregnancy.

Another reason proposed for the STI epidemic is our culture's casual attitude about sex. Bombarded by media hype that glamorizes easy sex, many people take sexual partners without considering the consequences. Generally, the more sexual partners a person has, the greater the risk for contracting an STI. Evaluate your own attitude and beliefs about STIs by completing the **Assess Yourself** box on page 400.

Ignorance—about the infections, their symptoms, and the fact that someone can be asymptomatic but still infected—is

also a factor. A person who is infected but asymptomatic can unknowingly spread an STI to an unsuspecting partner, who may, in turn, ignore or misinterpret any symptoms. By the time either partner seeks medical help, he or she may have infected several others. In addition, many people mistakenly believe that certain sexual practices—oral sex, for example—carry no risk for STIs. In fact, oral sex practices among young adults may be responsible for increases in herpes and other STIs.

Routes of Transmission

Can I get a sexually transmitted infection from "outercourse"?

STIs are generally spread through some form of intimate sexual contact. Sexual intercourse, oral–genital contact, hand–genital contact, and anal intercourse are the most common modes of transmission. Less likely, but still possible modes of transmission include mouth to mouth contact, or contact with fluids from body sores that may be spread by the hands. Although each STI is a different infection caused by a different pathogen, all STI pathogens prefer dark, moist places, especially the mucous membranes lining the reproductive organs. Most of them are susceptible to light, excess heat, cold, and dryness, and many die quickly on exposure to air. Like other communicable infections, STIs have both pathogen-specific incubation periods and periods of time during which transmission is most likely, called *periods of communicability*. Practicing the following behaviors will help you protect yourself and reduce your risk:

- Avoid casual sexual partners. Ideally, have sex only if you are in a long-term, mutually monogamous relationship with someone who is equally committed to the relationship and who has tested negative for STIs.
- Avoid unprotected sexual activity involving the exchange of blood, semen, or vaginal secretions with people whose present or past behaviors put them at risk for infection. Postpone sexual involvement until you are assured that he or she is not infected.
- Practice safer sex by using latex condoms. Remember, however, that condoms do not provide 100 percent safety. Avoid injury to body tissue during sexual activity. Some STIs can enter the bloodstream through microscopic tears in anal or vaginal tissues.
- Avoid unprotected oral sex or any sexual activity in which semen, blood, or vaginal secretions could penetrate mucous membranes through breaks in the membrane. Always use a condom or a dental dam during oral sex.
- Avoid using drugs (including alcohol) that may dull your senses and affect your ability to take responsible precautions with potential sex partners.
- If you are worried about your own STI status, have yourself tested. Don't risk infecting others.

Chlamydia

Chlamydia, a disease that often presents no symptoms, tops the list of the most commonly reported sexually transmitted infections in the United States. Chlamydia infects about 2.8 million people annually in the United States, the majority of them women.[23] Public health officials believe that the actual number of cases is probably higher because these figures represent only those cases reported. College students account for over 10 percent of infections, and these numbers seem to be increasing yearly.

In men, early symptoms may include painful and difficult urination, frequent urination, and a watery, puslike discharge from the penis. Symptoms in women may include a yellowish discharge, spotting between periods, and occasional spotting after intercourse. However, many chlamydia victims display no symptoms and therefore do not seek help until the disease has done secondary damage. Women are especially likely to be asymptomatic; over 70 percent do not realize they have the disease until secondary damage occurs.

The secondary damage resulting from chlamydia is serious in both genders. Men can suffer injury to the prostate gland, seminal vesicles, and bulbourethral glands as well as arthritis-like symptoms and inflammatory damage to the blood vessels and heart. In women, chlamydia-related inflammation can injure the cervix or fallopian tubes, causing sterility, and damage the inner pelvic structure, leading to pelvic inflammatory disease (PID). If an infected woman becomes pregnant, she has a high risk for miscarriage and stillbirth. Chlamydia may also be responsible for one type of *conjunctivitis,* an eye infection that affects not only adults but also infants, who can contract the disease from an infected mother during delivery. Untreated conjunctivitis can cause blindness.

If detected early, chlamydia is easily treatable with antibiotics. Unfortunately, chlamydia tests are not a routine part of many health clinics' testing procedures. Usually a person must specifically request a chlamydia check.

Gonorrhea

Gonorrhea is one of the most common STIs in the United States, surpassed only by chlamydia in number of cases. The Centers for Disease Control and Prevention (CDC) estimates that there are over 700,000 cases per year, plus numbers that go unreported.[24] Caused by the bacterial pathogen *Neisseria gonorrhoeae,* gonorrhea primarily infects the linings of the urethra, genital tract, pharynx, and rectum. It may spread to the eyes or other body regions by the hands or through body fluids, typically during vaginal, oral, or anal sex. Most cases occur in individuals between the ages of 20 and 24.[25] In men, a typical symptom is a white, milky discharge from the penis accompanied by painful, burning urination 2 to 9 days after contact. However, about 20 percent of all men with gonorrhea are asymptomatic.

In women, the situation is just the opposite: only 20 percent experience any discharge, and few develop a burning sensation on urinating until much later in the course of the infection (if

ever). The organism can remain in the woman's vagina, cervix, uterus, or fallopian tubes for long periods with no apparent symptoms other than an occasional slight fever. Thus a woman can be unaware that she has been infected and that she is infecting her sexual partners.

If the infection is detected early, antibiotic treatment is generally effective. In a man, untreated gonorrhea may spread to the prostate, testicles, urinary tract, kidney, and bladder. Blockage of the vasa deferentia due to scar tissue may cause sterility. In some cases, the penis develops a painful curvature during erection. If the infection goes undetected in a woman, it can spread to the fallopian tubes and ovaries, causing sterility or, at the very least, severe inflammation and PID. The bacteria can also spread up the reproductive tract or, more rarely, through the blood and infect the joints, heart valves, or brain. If an infected woman becomes pregnant, the infection can cause conjunctivitis in her infant. To prevent this, physicians routinely administer silver nitrate or penicillin preparations to the eyes of newborn babies.

Pelvic Inflammatory Disease

Pelvic inflammatory disease (PID) is a term used to describe a number of infections of the uterus, fallopian tubes, and ovaries. Although PID often results from an untreated sexually transmitted infection, especially chlamydia or gonorrhea, it is not actually an STI.

Symptoms of PID vary but generally include lower abdominal pain, fever, unusual vaginal discharge, painful intercourse, painful urination, and irregular menstrual bleeding.[26] Risk factors include young age at first sexual intercourse, multiple sex partners, high frequency of sexual intercourse, and change of sexual partners within the past 30 days. Regular gynecological examinations and early treatment for STI symptoms reduce risk.

Syphilis

Syphilis is caused by a bacterium, *Treponema pallidum.* Because the bacterium is extremely delicate and dies readily on exposure to air, dryness, or cold, it is generally transferred through direct sexual contact. Typically, this means contact between sexual organs during intercourse, but in rare instances, the organism enters the body through a

(Text continues on page 402.)

chlamydia   Bacterially caused STI of the urogenital tract.

gonorrhea   Second most common STI in the United States; if untreated, may cause sterility.

pelvic inflammatory disease (PID)   Term used to describe various infections of the female reproductive tract.

syphilis   One of the most widespread STIs; characterized by distinct phases and potentially serious results.

ASSESS yourself

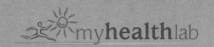

STI ATTITUDE AND BELIEF SCALE

Fill out this assessment online at
www.aw-bc.com/myhealthlab or
www.aw-bc.com/donatelle.

The following quiz will help you evaluate whether your beliefs and attitudes about STIs lead you to behaviors that increase your risk of infection. Indicate whether you believe the following items true or false by checking the corresponding box. Then consult the answer key that follows.

	True	False
1. You can usually tell whether someone is infected with an STI, especially HIV infection.	☐	☐
2. Chances are that if you haven't caught an STI by now, you probably have a natural immunity and won't get infected in the future.	☐	☐
3. A person who is successfully treated for an STI needn't worry about getting it again.	☐	☐
4. So long as you keep yourself fit and healthy, you needn't worry about STIs.	☐	☐
5. The best way for sexually active people to protect themselves from STIs is to practice safer sex.	☐	☐
6. The only way to catch an STI is to have sex with someone who has one.	☐	☐
7. Talking about STIs with a partner is so embarrassing that it's better not to raise the subject and instead hope the other person will.	☐	☐
8. STIs are mostly a problem for people who have numerous sex partners.	☐	☐
9. You don't need to worry about contracting an STI so long as you wash yourself thoroughly with soap and hot water immediately after sex.	☐	☐
10. You don't need to worry about AIDS if no one you know has ever come down with it.	☐	☐
11. When it comes to STIs, it's all in the cards. Either you're lucky or you're not.	☐	☐
12. The time to worry about STIs is when you come down with one.	☐	☐
13. As long as you avoid risky sexual practices, such as anal intercourse, you're pretty safe from STIs.	☐	☐
14. The time to talk about safer sex is before any sexual contact occurs.	☐	☐
15. A person needn't be concerned about an STI if the symptoms clear up on their own in a few weeks.	☐	☐

Scoring Key

1. *False.* While some STIs have telltale signs, such as the appearance of sores or blisters on the genitals or disagreeable genital odors, others do not. Several STIs, such as chlamydia, gonorrhea (especially in women), internal genital warts, and even HIV infection in its early stages cause few if any obvious signs or symptoms. You often cannot tell whether your partner is infected with an STI. Many of the nicest-looking and most well-groomed people carry STIs, often unknowingly. The only way to know whether a person is infected with HIV is by means of an HIV-antibody test.

2. *False.* If you practice unprotected sex and have not contracted an STI to this point, count your blessings. The thing about good luck is that it eventually runs out.

3. *False.* Sorry. Successful treatment does not render immunity against reinfection. You still need to take precautions to avoid reinfection, even if you have had an STI in the past and were successfully treated. If you answered "True" to this item, you're not alone. About one in five college students polled in a recent survey of more than 5,500 college students across Canada believed that a person who gets an STI cannot get it again.

4. *False.* Even people in prime physical condition can be felled by the tiniest of microbes that cause STIs. Physical fitness is no protection against these microscopic invaders.

5. *True.* If you are sexually active, practicing safer sex is the best protection against contracting an STI.

6. *False.* STIs can also be transmitted through nonsexual means, such as by sharing contaminated needles or, in some cases, through contact with disease-causing organisms on towels and bedsheets or even toilet seats.

7. *False.* Because of the social stigma attached to STIs, it's understandable that you may feel embarrassed about raising the subject with your partner. But don't let embarrassment prevent you from taking steps to protect your own and your partner's welfare.

8. *False.* Though it stands to reason that people who are sexually active with numerous partners stand a greater chance that one of their sexual partners will carry an STI,

all it takes is one infected partner to pass along an STI to you, even if he or she is the only partner you've had or even if the two of you had sex only once. STIs are a potential problem for anyone who is sexually active.

9. *False.* Though washing your genitals immediately after sex may have some limited protective value, it is no substitute for practicing safer sex.

10. *False.* You can never know whether you may be the first among your friends and acquaintances to become infected. Moreover, symptoms of HIV infection may not appear for years after initial infection with the virus, so you may have sexual contacts with people who are infected but don't know it and who are capable of passing along the virus to you. You in turn may then pass it along to others, whether or not you are aware of any symptoms.

11. *False.* Nonsense. While luck may play a part in determining whether you have sexual contact with an infected partner, you can significantly reduce your risk of contracting an STI.

12. *False.* The time to start thinking about STIs (thinking helps, but worrying only makes you more anxious than you need be) is now, not after you have contracted an infection. Some STIs, like herpes and AIDS, cannot be cured. The only real protection you have against them is prevention.

13. *False.* Any sexual contact between the genitals, or between the genitals and the anus, or between the mouth and genitals, is risky if one of the partners is infected with an STI.

14. *True.* Unfortunately, too many couples wait until they have commenced sexual relations to have "a talk." By then it

may already be too late to prevent the transmission of an STI. The time to talk is before any intimate sexual contact occurs.

15. *False.* Several STIs, notably syphilis, HIV infection, and herpes, may produce initial symptoms that clear up in a few weeks. But while the early symptoms may subside, the infection is still at work within the body and requires medical attention. Also, as noted previously, the infected person is capable of passing along the infection to others, regardless of whether noticeable symptoms were ever present.

Interpreting Your Score
First, add up the number of items you got right. The higher your score, the lower your risk. The lower your score, the greater your risk. A score of 13 correct or better may indicate that your attitudes toward STIs would probably decrease your risk of contracting them. Yet even one wrong response on this test may increase your risk of contracting an STI. You should also recognize that attitudes have little effect on behavior unless they are carried into action. Knowledge alone isn't sufficient to protect yourself from STIs. You need to ask yourself how you are going to put knowledge into action by changing your behavior to reduce your chances of contracting an STI.

Source: From Jeffrey S. Nevid with Fern Gotfried, *Choices: Sex in the Age of STDs*, 2nd ed., 10–13. © Copyright 1998/Pearson Education. Published by Allyn & Bacon, Boston, MA. Reprinted by permission of the publisher.

MAKE it happen!

ASSESSMENT: The Assess Yourself activity gave you the chance to consider your beliefs and attitudes about STIs and possible risks you may be facing. Now that you have considered these results, you can begin to change behaviors that may be putting you at risk.

MAKING A CHANGE: To change your behavior, you need to develop a plan. Follow these steps below and complete your Behavior Change Contract to take action.

1. Evaluate your behavior, and identify patterns and specific things you are doing. What can you change now? What can you change in the near future?

2. Select one pattern of behavior that you want to change.

3. Fill out the Behavior Change Contract found at the front of your book. It should include your long-term goals for change, your short-term goals, the rewards you'll give yourself for reaching these goals, potential obstacles along the way, and strategies for overcoming these obstacles. For each goal, list the small steps and specific actions that you will take.

4. Chart your progress in a journal. At the end of a week, consider how successful you were in following your plan. What helped you be successful? What made change more difficult? What will you do differently next week?

5. Revise your plan as needed. Are the short-term goals attainable? Are the rewards satisfying?

(continued)

EXAMPLE: Carlos had never thought that he was at risk for an STI. He dated only one woman at a time, and he had never had an STI himself. After he reviewed his answers to the self-assessment, however, he saw that there were several ways in which he was putting himself at risk.

He had thought that he would be able to tell whether someone was infected with an STI but the answer to question 1 informed him that, especially among women, some STIs show few if any obvious signs or symptoms. Carlos also believed that he was not at risk because he dated only one woman at a time, but the answer to question 8 pointed out that a person can pass on an STI that he or she contracted from a previous sex partner. Carlos decided it was time to take responsibility for his sexual activity. He had been on three dates with Sherry and felt things were progressing toward a more intimate stage; he wanted to

be sure that they discussed STIs before they put themselves at risk.

Carlos was nervous when he thought about talking to Sherry, so he wrote out a few ideas of ways to bring up the subject. This made him more confident that he would be able to talk honestly with Sherry. He also made sure that he had a supply of condoms, so there wouldn't be any reason not to practice safer sex. During their next date, Carlos asked Sherry whether they could have a serious conversation about the next step. When he told her that he wanted to talk about STIs, she told him that she was relieved that he had brought up the subject. She knew that she was healthy but hadn't been sure how to find out his status. Carlos was relieved that Sherry was as concerned about the issue as he was, and they were both glad that embarrassment had not prevented them from having this conversation.

break in the skin, through deep kissing in which body fluids are exchanged, or through some other transmission of body fluids.

Syphilis is called the "great imitator" because its symptoms resemble those of several other infections. Left untreated, syphilis generally progresses through several distinct stages. It should be noted, however, that some people experience no symptoms at all. Because the organism is bacterial, it is treated with antibiotics. The major obstacles to treatment are misdiagnosis of this "imitator" infection and lack of access to health care.

Primary Syphilis
The first stage of syphilis, particularly for men, is often characterized by the development of a *chancre* (pronounced "shank-er"), a sore located most frequently at the site of initial infection. Although painless, the dime-sized chancre is oozing with bacteria, ready to infect an unsuspecting partner. Usually it appears 3 to 4 weeks after initial infection.

In men, the site of the chancre tends to be the penis or scrotum because this is where the organism first enters the body. But if the infection was contracted through oral sex, the sore can appear in the mouth, throat, or other "first contact" area. In women, the site of infection is often internal, on the vaginal wall or high on the cervix. Because the chancre is not readily apparent, the likelihood of detection is not great. In both men and women, the chancre will completely disappear in 3 to 6 weeks.

Secondary Syphilis
A month to a year after the chancre disappears, secondary symptoms may appear,

including a rash or white patches on the skin or on the mucous membranes of the mouth, throat, or genitals. Hair loss may occur, lymph nodes may enlarge, and the victim may develop a slight fever or headache. In rare cases, sores develop around the mouth or genitals. As during the active chancre phase, these sores contain infectious bacteria, and contact with them can spread the infection. Because symptoms vary so much and appear so much later than the sexual contact that caused them, the victim seldom connects the two. The infection thus often goes undetected even at this second stage. Symptoms typically disappear, leaving the person thinking that all is well.

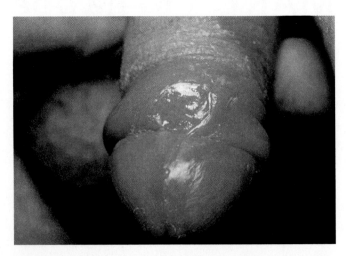

A chancre on the site of the initial infection is a symptom of primary syphilis.

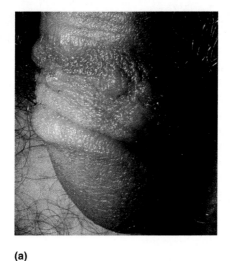

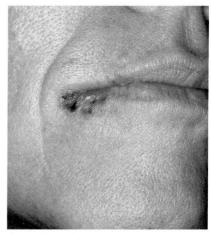

(a) Genital herpes is a highly contagious and incurable STI. It is characterized by recurring cycles of painful blisters on the genitalia. **(b)** Oral herpes, caused by the same virus as genital herpes, is extremely contagious and can cause painful sores and blisters around the mouth.

(a)   **(b)**

Latent Syphilis After the secondary stage, the syphilis bacteria begin to invade body organs. The infection now is rarely transmitted to others, except during pregnancy, when it can be passed to the fetus. The child will then be born with *congenital syphilis,* which can cause death or severe birth defects such as blindness, deafness, or disfigurement.

Late Syphilis Years after syphilis has entered the body, its effects become all too evident. Late-stage syphilis indications include heart and central nervous system damage, blindness, deafness, paralysis, premature senility, and, ultimately, dementia.

Herpes

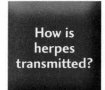

How is herpes transmitted?

Herpes is a general term for a family of infections characterized by sores or eruptions on the skin. Caused by herpesvirus, the herpes family of diseases is not transmitted exclusively by sexual contact. Kissing or sharing eating utensils can also exchange saliva and transmit the infection. Herpes infections range from mildly uncomfortable to extremely serious. **Genital herpes** is an infection caused by the herpes simplex virus (HSV) and affects over 45 million Americans aged 12 and older.[27]

There are two types of herpes simplex virus (HSV). Both herpes simplex types 1 and 2 can infect any area of the body, producing lesions (sores) in and around the vaginal area, on the penis, around the anal opening, on the buttocks or thighs, and around the mouth. For example, you may have a type 1 infection on your lip and transmit the HSV-1 organism to your partner's genitals during oral sex. Practically speaking, the resulting symptoms would be virtually the same as if you had transmitted the type 2 virus. Occasionally, sores appear on other parts of the body. HSV remains in certain nerve cells for life and can flare up, or cause symptoms, when the body's ability to maintain itself is weakened.[28]

The precursor phase of the infection is characterized by a burning sensation and redness at the site of infection. During this time, prescription medicines such as acyclovir and over-the-counter medications such as Abreva will often keep the disease from spreading. However, this phase of the disease is quickly followed by the second phase, in which a blister filled with a clear fluid containing the virus forms. If you pick at this blister or otherwise touch the site and spread this fluid with fingers, lipstick, lip balm, or other products, you can autoinoculate other body parts. Particularly dangerous is the possibility of spreading the infection to your eyes, for a herpes lesion on the eye can cause blindness.

Over a period of days, the unsightly blister will crust over, dry up, and disappear, and the virus will travel to the base of an affected nerve supplying the area and become dormant. Only when the victim becomes overly stressed, when diet and sleep are inadequate, when the immune system is overworked, or when excessive exposure to sunlight or other stressors occurs will the virus become reactivated (at the same site every time) and begin the blistering cycle all over again. These sores cast off (shed) viruses that can be highly infectious.

However, it is important to note that a herpes site can shed the virus even when no overt sore is present, particularly during the interval between the earliest symptoms and blistering. People may get genital herpes by having sexual contact with others who don't know they are infected or who are having outbreaks of herpes without any sores. A person with genital herpes can also infect a sexual partner during oral sex. The virus is spread only rarely, if at all, by touching objects such as a toilet seat or hot tub seat.[29]

Genital herpes is especially serious in pregnant women because the baby can be infected as it passes through the vagina during birth. Many physicians recommend cesarean deliveries for infected women. Additionally, women with a

genital herpes STI caused by the herpes simplex virus.

history of genital herpes appear to have a greater risk of developing cervical cancer.

Although there is no cure for herpes at present, certain drugs can reduce symptoms. Unfortunately, they seem to work only if the infection is confirmed during the first few hours after contact. The effectiveness of other treatments, such as L-lysine, is largely unsubstantiated. Over-the-counter medications such as Abreva may reduce the length of time you have sores/symptoms. Other drugs, such as famciclovir (FAMVIR), may reduce viral shedding between outbreaks. This means that if you have outbreaks, you may reduce risks to your sexual partners.[30] Although lip balms and cold-sore medications may provide temporary anesthetic relief, remember that rubbing anything on a herpes blister can spread herpes-laden fluids to other body parts. The following tips can help you prevent contracting herpes.

- If you know that you have frequent cold sores (caused by HSV-1), be extremely careful when kissing another person or sharing their drink glasses or utensils. Never kiss or let yourself be kissed by anyone with sores on their lips or nostrils. Don't share lipstick, lip balm, or other lip products.
- If you have questionable sores or lesions, seek medical help at once. Don't touch other parts of your body after touching your own cold sores or genital sores. Many people unknowingly spread herpes to their eyes, nose, or other areas by their hands.
- If you have herpes, reduce your risk of an outbreak by avoiding excessive stress, sunlight, or whatever else appears to trigger an episode.
- Use a condom or dental dam during oral sex. In spite of what many people mistakenly believe, oral sex is not safer than intercourse when it comes to transmitting herpes. Only about one in six Americans currently has HSV-2; however, nearly 58 percent have HSV-1, usually appearing as cold sores on their mouths. Whether you contract either HSV-1 or HSV-2 on your genitals, the net results may be just as painful, just as long term, and just as infectious for future partners.[31]
- Wash your hands thoroughly with soap and water after any kind of sexual contact and after disposing of condoms. If possible gargle with a mouthwash after oral sex.

Genital Warts (Human Papillomavirus)

Genital warts (also known as *venereal warts* or *condylomas*) are caused by a group of viruses known as **human papillomavirus (HPV).** There are over 100 different types of HPV,

genital warts   Warts that appear in the genital area or the anus; caused by the human papillomavirus (HPV).

human papillomavirus (HPV)   A group of viruses that cause genital warts.

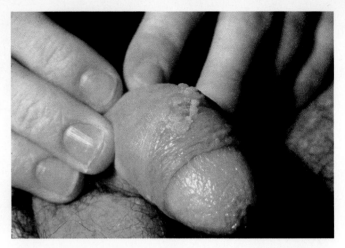

Genital warts are caused by the human papillomavirus and can be either full-blown or flat.

and more than 30 types are sexually transmitted. A person becomes infected when certain types of HPV penetrate the skin and mucous membranes of the genitals or anus through sexual contact. This is among the most common forms of STI, with 20 million Americans currently infected with genital HPV and approximately 6.2 million new cases each year.[32] Genital HPV appears to be relatively easy to catch. The typical incubation period is 6 to 8 weeks after contact. Many people have no symptoms, particularly if the warts are located inside the reproductive tract, whereas others may notice itchy bumps on the genitals. Genital warts are of two different types: (1) *full-blown genital warts,* which are noticeable as tiny bumps or growths; and (2) the much more prevalent *flat warts,* which are not usually visible to the naked eye.

Risks and Treatments of Genital Warts

Genital warts pose a significant risk for cervical cancer. They may lead to *dysplasia,* or changes in cells that may lead to a precancerous condition.

Exactly how HPV infection leads to cervical cancer is uncertain. It is known that within 5 years after infection, 30 percent of all HPV cases will progress to the precancerous stage. Of those cases that become precancerous and are left untreated, 70 percent will eventually result in actual cancer. In addition, HPV may pose a threat to a pregnant woman's unborn fetus if the fetus is exposed to the virus during birth. Cesarean deliveries may be considered in serious cases.

New research has also implicated HPV as a possible risk factor for coronary artery disease. It is hypothesized that HPV causes an inflammatory response in the artery walls, which makes cholesterol and plaque build up (see Chapter 12).

Genital warts can be treated with topical medications or be frozen with liquid nitrogen and then removed. Large warts may require surgical removal.

Human Papillomavirus Vaccination   In 2006,

a new vaccine to prevent HPV was approved by the FDA. The vaccine protects against the four types of HPV that lead to 70 percent of cervical cancers and 90 percent of genital warts. The vaccine is meant primarily for women aged 9 to 26 and is administered in a series of three shots over a 6-month period.[33]

Candidiasis (Moniliasis)

Unlike many STIs, which are caused by pathogens that come from outside the body, the yeastlike fungus *Candida albicans* normally inhabits the vaginal tract in most women. Only under certain conditions, in which the normal chemical balance of the vagina is disturbed, will these organisms multiply and cause the fungal disease **candidiasis.**

Symptoms of candidiasis, also sometimes called *moniliasis,* include severe itching and burning of the vagina and vulva, swelling of the vulva, and a white, cheesy vaginal discharge. These symptoms are collectively called *vaginitis,* or inflammation of the vagina. When this microbe infects the mouth, whitish patches form, and the condition is referred to as *thrush.* Thrush infection can also occur in men and is easily transmitted between sexual partners.

Antifungal drugs applied on the surface or by suppository usually cure candidiasis in just a few days. For approximately one out of ten affected women, however, nothing seems to work, and the infection returns again and again. Symptoms can be aggravated by contact of the vagina with soaps, douches, perfumed toilet paper, chlorinated water, and spermicides. Tight-fitting jeans and pantyhose can provide the combination of moisture and irritant the organism thrives on.

Trichomoniasis

Unlike many STIs, **trichomoniasis** is caused by a protozoan. Although as many as half of the men and women in the United States may carry this organism, most remain free of symptoms until their bodily defenses are weakened. Symptoms among women include a foamy, yellowish, unpleasant-smelling discharge accompanied by a burning sensation, itching, and painful urination. Most men with trichomoniasis do not have any symptoms, though some men experience irritation inside the penis, mild discharge, and a slight burning after urinating. Although usually transmitted by sexual contact, the "trich" organism can also be spread by toilet seats, wet towels, or other items that have discharged fluids on them. Treatment includes oral metronidazole, usually given to both sexual partners to avoid the possible "ping-pong" effect of repeated cross-infection typical of STIs.

Pubic Lice

Pubic lice, often called "crabs," are small parasitic insects that are usually transmitted during sexual contact. More annoying than dangerous, they move easily from partner to partner during sex. They have an affinity for pubic hair and attach themselves to the base of these hairs, where they deposit their eggs (nits). One to 2 weeks later, these nits

develop into adults that lay eggs and migrate to other body parts, thus perpetuating the cycle.

Treatment includes washing clothing, furniture, and linens that may harbor the eggs. It usually takes 2 to 3 weeks to kill all larval forms. Although sexual contact is the most common mode of transmission, you can "catch" pubic lice from lying on sheets or sitting on a toilet seat that an infected person has used.

General Urinary Tract Infections

Although *general urinary tract infections (UTIs)* can be caused by various factors, some forms are sexually transmitted. Anytime invading organisms enter the genital area, they can travel up the urethra and enter the bladder. Similarly, organisms normally living in the rectum, urethra, or bladder may travel to the sexual organs and eventually be transmitted to another person.

HIV/AIDS

Acquired immunodeficiency syndrome (AIDS) is a significant global health threat. Since 1981, when AIDS was first recognized, approximately 65 million people in the world have become infected with **human immunodeficiency virus (HIV),** the virus that causes AIDS.[34] At the end of 2006, there were approximately 39.5 million people living with HIV.[35]

Since 1981, there have been approximately 1.7 million people infected with HIV in the United States, and at least 550,000 have died.[36] The CDC estimated that in 2005, there were approximately 40,608 new AIDS cases diagnosed in the United States.[37]

A Shifting Epidemic

Initially, people with HIV were diagnosed as having AIDS only when they developed blood infections, the cancer known as Kaposi's sarcoma, or any of 21 other indicator

---

candidiasis   Yeastlike fungal disease often transmitted sexually. Also known as *moniliasis.*

trichomoniasis   Protozoan STI characterized by foamy, yellowish discharge and unpleasant odor.

pubic lice   Parasitic insects that can inhabit various body areas, especially the genitals.

acquired immunodeficiency syndrome (AIDS) Extremely virulent sexually transmitted disease that renders the immune system inoperative.

human immunodeficiency virus (HIV)   The slow-acting virus that causes AIDS.

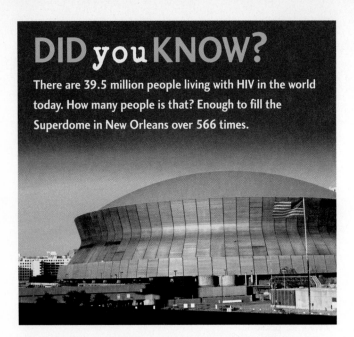

Source: UNAIDS, "A Global View of HIV Infection," 2006, www.unaids.org.

diseases, most of which were common in male AIDS patients. The CDC has expanded the indicator list to include pulmonary tuberculosis, recurrent pneumonia, and invasive cervical cancer. Perhaps the most significant indicator today is a drop in the level of the body's master immune cells, called CD4 cells, to one-fifth the level in a healthy person.

AIDS cases have been reported state by state throughout the United States since the early 1980s. Today, the CDC recommends that all states report HIV infections as well as AIDS. Because of medical advances in treatment and increasing numbers of HIV-infected persons who do not progress to AIDS, it is believed that AIDS incidence statistics may not provide a true picture of the epidemic, the long-term costs of treating HIV-infected individuals, and other key information. HIV incidence data also provide a better picture of infection trends. Currently, most states mandate that people who test positive for the HIV antibody be reported. Although there is significant pressure to mandate reporting in all states, there is controversy over implementing such a mandate. Many believe that if we require reporting of HIV-positive tests, people will refuse to be tested even if they suspect they are infected.

How HIV Is Transmitted

HIV typically enters one person's body when another person's infected body fluids (e.g., semen, vaginal secretions, blood) gain entry through a breach in body defenses. Mucous membranes of the genital organs and the anus provide the easiest route of entry. If there is a break in the mucous membranes (as can occur during sexual intercourse, particularly anal intercourse), the virus enters and begins to multiply. After initial infection, HIV multiplies rapidly, invading the

bloodstream and cerebrospinal fluid. It progressively destroys helper T cells (recall that these cells call the rest of the immune response to action), weakening the body's resistance to disease. The virus also changes the genetic structure of the cells it attacks. In response to this invasion, the body quickly begins to produce antibodies.

Despite some myths, HIV is not highly contagious. Studies of people living in households with an AIDS patient have turned up no documented cases of HIV infection through casual contact.[38] Other investigations provide overwhelming evidence that insect bites do not transmit HIV.

Engaging in High-Risk Behaviors
AIDS is not a disease of gay people or minority groups. People who engage in high-risk behaviors increase their risk for the disease; people who do not engage in these behaviors have minimal risk. The following activities are high-risk behaviors.

Exchange of Body Fluids
The greatest risk factor is the exchange of HIV-infected body fluids during vaginal or anal intercourse. Substantial research indicates that blood, semen, and vaginal secretions are the major fluids of concern. In rare instances the virus has been found in saliva, but most health officials state that saliva is a less significant risk than other shared body fluids. Even though these risks are well documented, millions of Americans report inconsistent safer sex practices, particularly when drugs or alcohol affect rational thinking.

Injecting Drugs
A significant percentage of AIDS cases in the United States result from sharing or using HIV-contaminated needles and syringes.[39] Though users of illegal drugs are commonly considered the only members of this category, others may also share needles—for example, people with diabetes who inject insulin or athletes who inject steroids. People who share needles and also engage in sexual activities with members of high-risk groups, such as those who exchange sex for drugs, increase their risks dramatically. Tattooing and piercing can also be risky (see the **Spotlight on Your Health** box).

Blood Transfusion Prior to 1985
A small group of people have become infected after receiving blood transfusions. In 1985, the Red Cross and other blood donation programs implemented a stringent testing program for all donated blood. Today, because of these massive screening efforts, the risk of receiving HIV-infected blood is almost nonexistent.

Mother-to-Child Transmission
Mother-to-child transmission occurs when an HIV-positive woman passes the virus to her baby. This can occur during pregnancy, during labor and delivery, or through breast-feeding. Without treatment, approximately 15 to 30 percent of babies born to HIV positive women will become infected with HIV during pregnancy and delivery, and a further 10 to 20 percent will become infected through breast-feeding.[40]

BODY PIERCING AND TATTOOING: RISKS TO HEALTH

A look around any college campus reveals many examples of the widespread trend of body piercing and tattooing, also known as "body art." Many people view the trend as a desire for self-expression, but whatever the reason, there is a booming business in both tattooing and body piercing.

However, health professionals cite several health concerns. The most common health-related problems associated with tattoos and body piercing include skin reactions, infections, allergic reactions, and scarring. Of even greater concern is the potential transmission of dangerous pathogens that any puncture of the human body exacerbates. The use of unsterile needles—which can cause serious infections and can transmit HIV, hepatitis B and C, tetanus, and a host of other diseases—poses a very real risk. Laws and policies regulating body piercing and tattooing vary greatly by state. Standards for safety usually include minimum age of use, standards of sanitation, use of aseptic techniques, sterilization of equipment, informed risks, instructions for skin care, record keeping, and recommendations for dealing with adverse reactions. Because of the lack of nationwide standards regulating this business and the potential for transmission of dangerous pathogens, anyone who receives a tattoo, body piercing, or permanent makeup tattoo cannot donate blood for 1 year.

Before deciding on a body artist to do your tattoo or piercing, you may want to watch the artist working on another client to evaluate the person's safety and skill. If you opt for tattooing or body piercing, remember to take the following safety precautions:

- Look for clean, well-lighted work areas, and inquire about sterilization procedures. Ask to see the autoclave used for sterilizing the instruments. Be wary of establishments that are reluctant to show you their autoclave or to discuss their sterilization procedures.
- Packaged, sterilized needles should be used only once and then discarded. A piercing gun should not be used, because it cannot be sterilized properly. Watch that the artist uses new needles and tubes from a sterile package before your procedure begins. Ask to see the sterile confirmation logo on the bag itself.
- Immediately before piercing or tattooing, the body area should be carefully sterilized. The artist should wash his or her hands and put on new latex gloves for each procedue. Make sure the artist changes those gloves if he or she needs to touch anything else, such as the telephone, while working.
- Leftover tattoo ink should be discarded after each procedure. Do not allow the artist to reuse ink that has been used for other customers. Used needles should be disposed of in a "sharps" container, a plastic contaner with the biohazard symbol clearly marked on it.

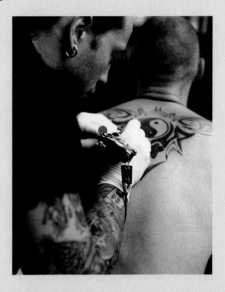

- Only jewelry made of noncorrosive metal, such as surgical stainless steel, niobium, or solid 14-karat gold, is safe for new piercing. Brass and nickel jewelry can cause allergic reactions.
- If any signs of pus, swelling, redness, or discoloration persist after a piercing, remove the piercing object, and contact a physician.

Sources: Mayo Clinic Staff, "Tattoos and Piercings: What to Know Beforehand," May Foundation for Medical Education and Research, 2007, www.mayoclinic.com/health/tattoos-and-piercings/MC00020; Center for Food Safety and Applied Nutrition, "Tattoos and Permanent Makeup," *Office of Cosmetics Fact Sheet*, 2006, www.cfsan.fda.gov/~dms/cos-204.html.

Women and AIDS

HIV is an equal-opportunity pathogen that can attack anyone—regardless of race, gender, sexual orientation, or socioeconomic status—who engages in high-risk behaviors. However, some groups seem to be at greater risk. Today women account for an increasing proportion of this epidemic. By 2005, women accounted for over 27 percent of newly reported AIDS cases in the United States. Among sexually active heterosexual teenagers, college students, and health care workers, nearly 60 percent of HIV cases are women.[41] Compounding the problems of women with HIV are serious deficiencies in our health and social service systems, including inadequate treatment for female drug addicts and lack of access to child care, health care, and social services for families headed by single women.

Women are four to ten times more likely than men to contract HIV through unprotected heterosexual intercourse with an infected partner **(Figure 13.7).** The vaginal area is more likely than the penis to incur microtears, and during sexual intercourse a woman is exposed to more semen than a man is to vaginal fluids. Women who have STIs are

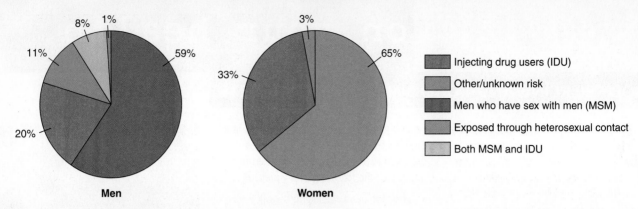

FIGURE 13.7 Sources of HIV Infection in Men and Women in the United States
Source: AVERT, "United States Statistics Summary," 2007, www.avert.org/statsum.htm.

more likely to be asymptomatic and therefore unaware they have a disease; preexisting STIs increase the risk of HIV transmission.[42]

Socioeconomic factors also correlate to a woman's likelihood to contract HIV. Women have been underrepresented in clinical trials for HIV treatment and prevention and may be less likely to seek medical treatment because of caregiving burdens, transportation problems, and lack of money. In some cultures, women are subordinate to men, especially in developing nations. This reduces women's decision-making power and ability to negotiate safer sex. These women are also more likely to be involved in nonconsensual sex or sex without condoms.

Symptoms of HIV/AIDS

A person may go for months or years after infection by HIV before any significant symptoms appear. The incubation time varies greatly from person to person. For adults who receive no medical treatment, it takes an average of 8 to 10 years for the virus to cause the slow, degenerative changes in the immune system that are characteristic of AIDS. During this time, the person may experience *opportunistic infections* (infections that gain a foothold when the immune system is not functioning effectively). Colds, sore throats, fever, tiredness, nausea, night sweats, and other generally non–life-threatening conditions commonly appear and are described as pre-AIDS symptoms. Some opportunistic infections, such as Kaposi's sarcoma and tuberculosis, are serious and potentially life-threatening. Research suggests that some very young children have shown the adult progression of AIDS.[43]

Testing for HIV Antibodies

Once antibodies have formed in reaction to HIV, a blood test known as the *ELISA* (enzyme-linked immunosorbent assay) may detect their presence. If sufficient antibodies are present, the test will be positive. When a person who previously tested *negative* (no HIV antibodies present) has a subsequent test that is *positive*, seroconversion is said to have occurred. In such a situation, the person would typically take another ELISA test, followed by a more precise test known as the *Western blot,* to confirm the presence of HIV antibodies.

It should be noted that these tests are not AIDS tests per se. Rather, they detect antibodies for HIV, indicating the presence of the virus in the person's system. Whether the person will develop AIDS depends to some extent on the strength of the immune system. Although we have made remarkable progress in prolonging the relatively symptom-free period between infection, HIV-positive status, and progression to symptomatic AIDS, it is important to note that a cure does not yet exist. The vast majority of infected people eventually develop some form of the disease.

As testing for HIV antibodies has improved, scientists have explored various ways of making it easier for individuals to be tested. Health officials distinguish between *reported* and *actual* cases of HIV infection because it is believed that many HIV-positive people avoid being tested. One reason is fear of knowing the truth. Another is the fear of recrimination from employers, insurance companies, and medical staff. However, early detection and reporting are important, because immediate treatment for someone in the early stages of HIV disease is critical.

what do you THINK?

Do you favor mandatory reporting of HIV and AIDS cases? ■ On the one hand, if you knew that your name and vital statistics would be "on file" if you tested positive for HIV, would you be less likely to take the HIV test? ■ On the other hand, do people who carry this contagious fatal disease have a responsibility to inform the general public and the health professionals who provide their care?

New Hope and Treatments

New drugs have slowed the progression from HIV to AIDS and have prolonged life expectancies for most AIDS patients. Current treatments combine selected drugs, especially protease inhibitors and reverse transcriptase inhibitors. *Protease inhibitors* (for example, amprenavir, ritonavir, and saquinavir) act to prevent the production of the virus in chronically infected cells that HIV has already invaded. Other drugs, such as AZT, ddI, ddC, d4T, and 3TC, inhibit the HIV enzyme *reverse transcriptase* before the virus has invaded the cell, thereby preventing the virus from infecting new cells.

All of the protease drugs seem to work best in combination with other therapies. These combination treatments are still quite experimental, and no combination has proven to be absolute for all people. As with other antiviral treatments, resistance to the drugs can develop. Individuals who already show resistance to AZT may not be able to use a protease-AZT combination, limiting their options for combination therapy.

Although these drugs provide new hope and longer survival rates for people living with HIV, it is important to maintain caution. We are still a long way from a cure. Apathy and carelessness may abound if too much confidence is placed in these treatments. Newer drugs that held much promise are becoming less effective as HIV develops resistance to them. Costs of taking multiple drugs are prohibitive, and side effects common. There is no cure. Furthermore, the number of people becoming HIV-infected each year has increased in some communities, meaning that we are still a long way from beating this disease. In fact, after years of declines in AIDS diagnoses due to new drug treatments, AIDS diagnoses have recently been on the rise.[44]

Preventing HIV Infection

Although scientists have been working on a variety of HIV vaccine trials, none is currently available.[45] The only way to prevent HIV infection is to avoid risky behaviors. HIV infection and AIDS are not uncontrollable conditions. You can reduce your risk by the choices you make in sexual behaviors and by taking responsibility for your own health and the health of your loved ones.

Unfortunately, the message has not gotten through to many Americans. They assume that because they are heterosexual, do not inject illegal drugs, and do not have sex with sex workers, they are not at risk. They couldn't be more wrong. Anyone who engages in unprotected sex is at risk, especially sex with a partner who has engaged in other high-risk behaviors. Sex with multiple partners is the greatest threat. You can't determine the presence of HIV by looking at a person; you can't tell by questioning the person, unless he or she has been tested recently, is HIV-negative, and is giving an honest answer. So what should you do?

Of course, the simplest answer is abstinence. If you don't exchange body fluids, you won't get the disease. As a second line of defense, if you decide to be intimate, the next best option is to use a condom. However, in spite of all the educa-

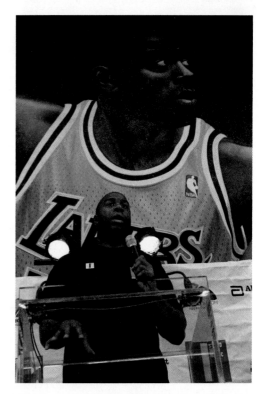

After publicly disclosing his HIV-positive status in 1991, former L.A. Laker star Earvin "Magic" Johnson became the first openly HIV-positive basketball player in the NBA. In 2006, his Magic Johnson Foundation launched the Campaign to End Black HIV/AIDS to address the alarming prevalence and rise of HIV among African Americans.

tional campaigns, surveys consistently indicate that most college students throw caution to the wind if they think they "know" someone—and they have unprotected sex. The **Skills for Behavior Change** box on page 410 presents ways to talk to your sexual partner about protecting yourselves from HIV and other STIs.

Noninfectious Diseases

Typically, when we think of major noninfectious ailments, we think of "killer" diseases such as cancer and heart disease. Clearly, these diseases make up the major portion of life-threatening diseases—accounting for nearly two-thirds of all deaths (see Chapter 12). Although these diseases capture much media attention, other chronic conditions can also cause pain, suffering, and disability. Fortunately, most of them can be prevented or their symptoms relieved.

Generally, noninfectious diseases are not transmitted by a pathogen or by any form of personal contact. Lifestyle and personal health habits are often implicated as underlying causes. Healthy changes in lifestyle and public health efforts aimed at research, prevention, and control can minimize the effects of these diseases.

SKILLS FOR behavior change

COMMUNICATING IN AN UNSAFE SEXUAL WORLD

At no time in your life is it more important to communicate openly than when you are considering an intimate relationship. Remember that you can't tell whether someone has an STI. The following will help you to communicate about potential risks.

- You have a responsibility to your partner to disclose your own STI and HIV status. You also have a responsibility to yourself to stay healthy. Ask about your partner's STI and HIV status. Suggest going through the testing together as a means of sharing something important.
- Be direct, honest, and determined in talking about sex before you become involved. Do not act silly or evasive. Get to the point, ask clear questions, and do not be put off in receiving a response. A person who does not care enough to talk about sex probably does not care enough to take responsibility for his or her actions.
- Discuss the issues without sounding defensive or accusatory. Develop a personal comfort level with the subject prior to raising the issue with your partner. Be prepared with complete information, and articulate your feelings clearly. Reassure your partner that your

reasons for desiring abstinence or safer sex arise from respect and not distrust.

- Encourage your partner to be honest and to share feelings. This will not happen overnight. If you have never had a serious conversation with this person before you get into an intimate situation, you cannot expect honesty and openness when the lights go out.
- Analyze your own beliefs and values ahead of time. Know where you will draw the line on certain actions, and be very clear with your partner about what you expect. If you believe that using a condom is necessary, make sure you communicate this.
- Decide what you will do if your partner does not agree with you. Anticipate potential objections or excuses, and prepare your responses accordingly.
- Discuss what "having sex" means to your sexual partner. Sometimes people vary in what they think "sex" really is. Oral sex and other non-monogamous relationships with others may also put you at risk. Set boundaries for protecting one another, even if you think certain "open" relationships are okay.
- Discuss the significance of monogamy in your partner's relationships. Decide early how important this relationship is

to you and how much you are willing to work at arriving at an acceptable compromise on lifestyle.

ONLINE DATING AND SUPPORT FOR PEOPLE WITH STIs

Even the most careful individuals run some risk of getting STIs. For those who contract one of these highly stigmatized diseases, their future may never be quite the same. However, support groups abound online, on campuses, and in communities to provide emotional support and educational resources. People with STIs not only can reach out to others struggling with similar problems through support groups, but also access new, Internet-based dating and other social services that are dedicated to infected people. Chat lines, interactive discussion groups, dating services and a whole host of venues are available for people who have STIs. Persons with STIs need not feel alone. Have herpes? Rather than struggling with "telling" a prospective partner about your problem, you can meet people who have similar issues online, in a format where stigma and rejection are gone. As with any online dating or networking service, be cautious about providing personal information when using these sites.

Chronic Lung Diseases

Chronic lung diseases pose a serious and significant threat to Americans today. Collectively, they have become the fourth leading cause of death.[46] Most sufferers live with a condition known as chronic *dyspnea* uncomfortable breathlessness even with mild exertion.[47] Chronic lung disease can result in major disability and lack of function as the lungs fill with

mucus, become susceptible to bacterial or viral infections, or cause acute stress on the heart as they struggle to get valuable oxygen. Over time, many of these underlying conditions lead to hospitalization and possible death.

Chronic Obstructive Pulmonary Diseases

Chronic obstructive pulmonary diseases (COPDs) include bronchitis, emphysema, and asthma. Eighty to 90 percent of persons with COPD have a history of smoking.[48] In addition to smokers, people who have been exposed to dust, fumes, or gases that irritate the lungs over time or in one big dose may be particularly vulnerable.

chronic obstructive pulmonary diseases (COPDs) A collection of chronic lung diseases including asthma, emphysema, and chronic bronchitis.

Bronchitis **Bronchitis** refers to an inflammation of the lining of the bronchial tubes. These tubes, the bronchi, connect the windpipe with the lungs. When the bronchi become inflamed or infected, less air is able to flow from the lungs, and heavy mucus begins to form. Acute bronchitis is the most common of the bronchial diseases, and symptoms often improve in a week or two.

When the symptoms of bronchitis last for at least 3 months of the year in two consecutive years, this may be the more serious form, *chronic bronchitis*. In some cases, this chronic inflammation and irritation of the lungs may lead to other chronic respiratory problems, such as asthma or emphysema. Over 9 million Americans suffer from chronic bronchitis.[49]

Emphysema Over 3.5 million Americans suffer from **emphysema,** which involves the gradual destruction of the **alveoli** (tiny air sacs) of the lungs.[50] As the alveoli are destroyed, the affected person finds it more and more difficult to exhale, struggling to take in a fresh supply of air before the air held in the lungs has been expended. The chest cavity gradually begins to expand, producing a barrel-shaped chest. For more on emphysema and smoking, see Chapter 8.

Asthma **Asthma** is a long-term, chronic inflammatory disorder that blocks air flow into and out of the lungs. Asthma causes tiny airways in the lung to overreact with spasms in response to certain triggers. Symptoms include wheezing, difficulty breathing, shortness of breath, and coughing spasms. Although most asthma attacks are mild and non–life-threatening, they can trigger bronchospasms (contractions of the bronchial tubes in the lungs) that are so severe that, without rapid treatment, death may occur. Between attacks, most people have few symptoms.

Asthma falls into two distinctly different types. *Intrinsic* or *nonallergic asthma* may be triggered by anything except an allergy—for example, smoke inhalation, chest infection, stress, laughter, exercise, or cold air. The more common form of asthma, known as *extrinsic* or *allergic asthma*, is typically associated with allergic triggers; it tends to run in families and develop in childhood. Often by adulthood, a person has few episodes, or the disorder completely goes away.

Asthma can occur at any age, but it is most likely to occur in children between infancy and age 5 and in adults before age 40. Other risk factors include having one or both parents affected, a history of respiratory infections in childhood, low birth weight, obesity, and gastroesophageal reflux disease. In childhood, asthma strikes more boys than girls; in adulthood, it strikes more women than men. The asthma rate is 50 percent higher among African Americans than whites, and four times as many African Americans die of asthma than do whites.[51] Midwesterners appear to be more prone to asthma than people from other areas of the country. In the last decade, asthma rates have risen dramatically, particularly among inner-city children.[52]

Relaxation techniques appear to help some asthma sufferers. Drugs may be necessary for serious cases. Determining whether a specific allergen provokes asthma attacks, taking steps to reduce exposure, avoiding triggers such as certain types of exercise or stress, and finding the most effective medications are big steps in asthma prevention and control. Numerous new drugs are available that cause fewer side effects than older medications.

Sleep Apnea

Sleep apnea is believed to affect more than 18 million Americans, or 1 in every 15 persons.[53] This condition is characterized by periodic episodes during sleep when breathing stops almost completely for 10 seconds or longer. Over time, sleep apnea can lead to high blood pressure, irregular heartbeats, heart attack, accidents, depression, and stroke.

There are two major types of sleep apnea: central and obstructive. *Central sleep apnea* occurs when the brain fails to tell the breathing muscles to initiate breathing. Abuse of alcohol and other medications can cause this condition. *Obstructive sleep apnea*, which is the more common form, occurs when air cannot move into and out of a person's nose or mouth, even though the body tries to breathe. What causes sleep apnea? Typically, obstructive apnea occurs when a person's throat muscles and tongue relax during sleep and block the airways.[54] People who are overweight or obese often have more tissue to flap or sag, making their risk of apnea greater.

It is a common misperception that breathing always stops entirely during the apnea phases of sleep. Often, breathing continues and the chest rises and falls, but the level of air that is exchanged is minimal. When the body doesn't get enough oxygen, the heart races, blood pressure goes up, body chemistry may change, and a host of other subtle and not so subtle events occur. Most importantly, as oxygen saturation levels in the blood fall, the body's autonomic nervous system moves to protect the body and signals it to breathe, often with a sudden gasp of breath. This response may wake a person, causing sufferers to rarely reach deep sleep and to wake up feeling tired and unwell. This restless sleeping pattern is often one of the first symptoms of a person with sleep apnea.

---

bronchitis Inflammation of the lining of the bronchial tubes.

emphysema A respiratory disease in which the alveoli become distended or ruptured and are no longer functional.

alveoli Tiny air sacs of the lungs where gas exchange occurs (oxygen enters the body and carbon dioxide is removed).

asthma A chronic respiratory disease characterized by attacks of wheezing, shortness of breath, and coughing spasms.

sleep apnea Disorder in which a person has numerous episodes of breathing stoppage during a night's sleep.

If diagnosed, there are several options available for treatment, the most common of which is a *continuous positive airway pressure (CPAP)* device, which consists of an airflow device, long tube, and mask. Persons with sleep apnea wear this mask during sleep, which forces air into the nose to keep the airway open. Snoring and sleep disturbances generally stop with the use of this machine. There are also surgical, laser, and other techniques for treating sleep apnea, but the results of these treatments are mixed. In people who have weight problems, losing weight often reduces the number and severity of apnea events; however, because many apnea patients have a hereditary predisposition to loose skin in the throat area without being obese, weight loss does not always solve the problem.

Neurological Disorders

Headaches

What can I do for these killer headaches?

Almost all of us have experienced at least one major headache. In fact, more than 80 percent of women and 65 percent of men experience headaches on a regular basis.[55] Over 90 percent of all headaches are of three major types: tension headaches, migraines, and cluster headaches.

Tension Headaches Tension headaches, also referred to as *muscular contraction headaches,* are generally caused by muscle contractions or tension in the neck or head. This tension may be caused by actual strain placed on neck or head muscles due to overuse, to holding static positions for long periods, or to tension triggered by stress. Other possible triggers include red wine, lack of sleep, fasting, and menstruation. Relaxation, hot water treatment, and massage are holistic treatments. Aspirin, ibuprofen, acetaminophen, and naproxen sodium remain the old standby treatments for pain relief.

Migraine Headaches More than 29 million Americans—three times more women than men—suffer from **migraine,** a type of headache that often has severe, debilitating symptoms. Usually migraine incidence peaks in young adulthood, people aged 20 to 45.[56] Migraines are often hereditary.

Symptoms vary greatly by individual, and attacks typically last anywhere from 4 to 72 hours, with distinct phases of symptoms. In about 15 percent of cases, migraines are preceded by a sensory warning sign known as an *aura,* such as flashes of light, flickering vision, blind spots tingling in arms or legs, or sensation of odor or taste. Sometimes nausea, vomiting, and extreme sensitivity to light and sound are present. Symptoms of migraine include excruciating pain behind or around one eye and usually on the same side of the head. In some people, there is sinus pain, neck pain, or an aura without headache.

The cause of migraines is unknown, but some research suggests they may occur when blood vessels dilate in the membrane that surrounds the brain. Critics of the blood vessel dilation theory question why only blood vessels of the head dilate in these situations. These researchers suggest that migraines originate in the cortex of the brain, where certain pain sensors are stimulated.

Historically, treatments have centered on reversing or preventing blood vessel dilation, with the most common treatment derived from the rye fungus *ergot.* Today, fast-acting ergot compounds are available by nasal spray, vastly increasing the speed of relief. However, ergot drugs have many side effects, the least of which may be that they are habit forming. Other drugs that are sometimes prescribed include lidocaine, a new group of drugs called triptans, and Imitrex, a drug tailor-made for migraines.

Cluster Headaches Fortunately, cluster headaches are among the more rare forms of headache, affecting fewer than 1 percent of people, usually men. Young adults in their twenties tend to be particularly susceptible.[57] Pain is often severe and has been described as "killer" or "suicidal" pain.[58] Usually these headaches cause stabbing pain on one side of the head, behind the eye, or in one defined spot. Other typical cluster headache characteristics include nasal discharge and tearing of the eye on the same side as the pain, a swollen or drooping eyelid and contracted pupil, congestion in the nostril on the affected side, flushing of the face on the affected side, and excessive sweating.

Cluster headaches can last for weeks and disappear quickly. However, more commonly they last for 40 to 90 minutes and often occur in the middle of the night, usually during REM sleep. Oxygen therapy, drugs, and even surgery have been used to treat severe cases.

Seizure Disorders

Approximately 2 million people in the United States suffer from **epilepsy** or some other form of seizure-related disorder (the word *epilepsy* derives from the Greek *epilepsia,* "seizure"). Each year, over 180,000 people in the United States will have a seizure for the first time, and it is estimated that 5 to 10 percent of the population will experience at least one seizure in their lives.[59] Seizure disorders are

migraine A condition characterized by localized headaches that possibly result from alternating dilation and constriction of blood vessels.

epilepsy A neurological disorder caused by abnormal electrical brain activity; can be accompanied by altered consciousness or convulsions.

generally caused by abnormal electrical activity in the brain and are characterized by loss of control of muscular activity and unconsciousness. Symptoms vary widely and can range from temporary confusion to major seizing.

Typically seizures fall into one of two categories. When they seem related to abnormal activity in just one region of the brain, they are classified as *partial*. When they involve all or most parts of the brain, they are *generalized*. About half of all cases of seizure disorder are of unknown origin. Possible causes include stroke, head injury, congenital abnormalities, injury or illness resulting in inflammation of the brain or spinal column, drug or chemical poisoning, tumors, nutritional deficiency, and heredity.

In most cases, people afflicted with seizure disorders can lead normal, seizure-free lives when under medical supervision. Public ignorance about these disorders is one of the most serious obstacles confronting people suffering from them. Improvements in medication and surgical interventions to reduce some causes of seizures are among the most promising treatments today.

Parkinson's Disease

Over 1.5 million Americans have **Parkinson's disease,** a chronic, slowly progressive neurological condition that typically strikes after age 50. Rates of Parkinson's disease have quadrupled in the past 30 years and may increase even more dramatically as more baby boomers pass age 60. Nearly 60,000 new cases are diagnosed each year.[60]

The hallmark of Parkinson's disease is a tremor, or "shaking palsy." Other symptoms are rigid or stiff muscles, slow movement, poor balance, shuffling steps, and slurred speech. The most common theories concerning its causes include familial predisposition, acceleration of age-related changes, and exposure to environmental toxins. Although Parkinson's disease is progressive and incurable, new drug therapies can keep symptoms under control, possibly for years. Surgical options such as brain tissue transplants and the use of fetal tissue stem cells or genetically engineered cell transplants have also provided promising results.

Multiple Sclerosis

Multiple sclerosis (MS) is a degenerative disease in which myelin, a fatty material that surrounds nerves and facilitates transmission of nerve impulses, breaks down and causes nerve malfunction. Multiple sclerosis typically appears between ages 15 and 50, and symptoms vary considerably by individual. Some people have periods of relapse (when symptoms flare up) and remissions (when symptoms are not present), and others have varying degrees of symptom severity. MS affects over 500,000 Americans.[61] Most MS patients have few flare-ups and can lead fairly normal lives. The cause of MS is unknown.

Digestion-Related Disorders

Lactose Intolerance

As many as 50 million Americans are unable to eat dairy products such as milk, cheese, ice cream, and other foods that the rest of us take for granted. These people suffer from **lactose intolerance,** which means that they have lost the ability to produce the digestive enzyme (lactase) that is necessary for the body to convert milk sugar (lactose) into glucose. That glass of milk becomes a source of stomach cramping, diarrhea, nausea, gas, and related symptoms. Once diagnosed, however, lactose intolerance can be treated by introducing low-lactose or lactose-free foods into the diet. Through trial and error, people usually find that they can tolerate one type of low-lactose food better than others. Someone who is lactose intolerant may need to experiment before settling into a diet that works.

Colitis and Irritable Bowel Syndrome

Ulcerative colitis is a disease of the large intestine in which the mucous membranes of the intestinal walls become inflamed. People with severe cases may have as many as 20 bouts of bloody diarrhea a day. Colitis can also produce severe stomach cramps, weight loss, nausea, sweating, and fever. Although some experts believe that colitis occurs more frequently in people with high stress levels, this theory is controversial. Hypersensitivity reactions to certain foods have also been considered as a possible cause. It is difficult to determine the cause of colitis because the disease goes into unexplained remission and then recurs without apparent reason. This pattern often continues over periods of years and may be related to the later development of colorectal cancer. Treatment focuses on relieving the symptoms by such methods as increasing fiber intake and taking anti-inflammatory drugs, steroids, and other medications to reduce inflammation and soothe irritated intestinal walls.

Parkinson's disease A chronic, progressive neurological condition that causes tremors and other symptoms.

multiple sclerosis (MS) A degenerative neurological disease in which myelin, an insulator of nerves, breaks down.

lactose intolerance Inability to produce lactase, an enzyme needed to convert milk sugar into glucose.

ulcerative colitis An inflammatory disorder that affects the mucous membranes of the large intestine, producing bloody diarrhea.

Irritable bowel syndrome (IBS), characterized by nausea, pain, gas, diarrhea, or cramps after eating certain foods or during unusual stress, commonly begins in early adulthood. Symptoms may vary from week to week and can fade for long periods of time, only to return. The cause is unknown, but researchers suspect that people with IBS have digestive systems that are overly sensitive to what they eat and drink, to stress, and to certain hormonal changes. Stress management, relaxation techniques, regular activity, and diet can control IBS in the vast majority of cases. Problems with diarrhea can be reduced by cutting down on fat and avoiding caffeine and excessive amounts of sorbitol, a sweetener found in dietetic foods and chewing gum. Constipation can be relieved by a gradual increase in fiber and increased fluid consumption. Some sufferers benefit from drugs that relax intestinal muscle or from antidepressant drugs and counseling to reduce stress.

Musculoskeletal Diseases

Arthritis: Many Types, Many Problems

Called "the nation's primary crippler," **arthritis** strikes one in five Americans, or over 46 million people.[62] There are over 100 types of arthritis diagnosed today, the most common of which are osteoarthritis, rheumatoid arthritis, gout, lupus, and fibromyalgia. Arthritis accounts for over 30 million lost workdays annually. The cost to the U.S. economy is over $128 billion per year in lost wages and productivity and untold amounts in hospital and nursing home services, prescriptions, and over-the-counter pain relief.[63] Unfortunately, as epidemic rates of obesity and sedentary lifestyle contribute to the development of arthritis, over 67 million Americans aged 18 and over will be diagnosed with the disease by 2030, a number that will have staggering consequences for our health care system.[64]

Osteoarthritis (OA), also known as *degenerative joint disease*, is a progressive deterioration of bones and joints that has been associated with the "wear and tear" theory of aging. Over 21 million Americans have OA.[65] Bones rub directly against each other, causing the pain, swelling, and limited movement characteristic of arthritis. Obesity, joint trauma, and repetitive joint usage all increase the risk and thus are important targets for prevention.

Over 80 percent of people with OA report that their activity has been limited as a result of the condition. Joint replacement and bone fusion are common surgical repair techniques. Anti-inflammatory drugs and pain relievers, applications of heat, mild exercise, and massage may relieve the pain.

Rheumatoid arthritis is an autoimmune disease involving chronic inflammation that most commonly appears between ages 20 and 45 and affects over 2.1 million Americans.[66] Symptoms include stiffness, pain, redness, and swelling of multiple joints (often including the hands and wrists) and can be gradually progressive or sporadic, with occasional unexplained remissions.

Treatment of rheumatoid arthritis is similar to that for osteoarthritis, emphasizing pain relief and improved functional mobility. Immunosuppressant drugs can reduce the inflammatory response.

Fibromyalgia

Fibromyalgia is a chronic, painful, rheumatoid-like disorder that affects 5 to 6 percent of the general population (nearly 4 million people) with bouts of muscle pain and extreme fatigue.[67] Persons with fibromyalgia experience an array of other symptoms, including headaches, dizziness, numbness and tingling, itching, fluid retention, chronic joint pain, abdominal or pelvic pain, and even occasional diarrhea. Suspected causes include sleep disturbances, stress, emotional distress, viruses, and autoimmune disorders; however, none has been proved in clinical trials. Because of fibromyalgia's multiple symptoms, it is usually diagnosed only after myriad tests have ruled out other disorders.

Systemic Lupus Erythematosus

Systemic lupus erythematosus (SLE, or lupus) is an autoimmune disease in which antibodies destroy or injure organs such as the kidneys, brain, and heart. The symptoms include sensitivity to sunlight, arthritis, kidney problems, anemia, aching muscles and joints, and multiple infections; they range from mild to severe and may disappear for periods of time. A butterfly-shaped rash covering the bridge of

---

irritable bowel syndrome (IBS) Nausea, pain, gas, or diarrhea caused by certain foods or stress.

arthritis Painful inflammatory disease of the joints.

osteoarthritis (OA) Progressive deterioration of bones and joints that has been associated with the wear-and-tear theory of aging.

rheumatoid arthritis An autoimmune inflammatory joint disease.

fibromyalgia A chronic rheumatoid-like disorder that can be highly painful and difficult to diagnose.

systemic lupus erythematosus (SLE, lupus) A disease in which the immune system attacks the body, producing antibodies that destroy or injure organs such as the kidneys, brain, and heart.

---

the nose and both cheeks is common. The disease affects 1 in 700 Caucasians and 1 in 250 African Americans; 90 percent of all victims are women who show initial symptoms between the ages of 15 and 45.[68] Extensive research has not yet found a cure for this sometimes fatal disease, although new studies suggest that there may be a genetic predisposition to it.

Lower Back Pain

Approximately 85 percent of all Americans will experience episodes of lower back pain (LBP) at some point. Some of these episodes result from muscular damage and are short-lived and acute; others may involve dislocations, fractures, or other problems with spinal vertebrae or discs, resulting in chronic pain or requiring surgery. Low back pain is epidemic throughout the world and the major cause of disability for people aged 20 to 45 in the United States, who suffer more frequently and severely from this problem than older people do.[69] Chapter 17 discusses massage therapy as a possible treatment for LBP.

Almost 90 percent of all back problems occur in the lumbar spine (lower back). You can avoid many problems by consciously maintaining good posture. Numerous studies have shown that wearing heavy backpacks, particularly among younger, school-aged children, can result in back pain. It is likely that carrying books and computers all day may also be a cause for concern among college students. Although no clear research has pointed this out, common sense suggests you use caution, making sure you purchase a good quality backpack that has straps to off-load some of the weight to your hips, rather than on your shoulders and back. Other things you can do to reduce risks of back pain include the following:

- Purchase a high-quality, supportive mattress, and avoid sleeping on your stomach.
- Avoid high-heeled shoes, which tilt the pelvis forward, and wear shoes with good arch support.
- Control your weight. Extra weight puts increased strain on knees, hips, and your back.
- Warm up and stretch before exercising or lifting heavy objects. When you lift, use your legs instead of your back.
- Buy a chair with good lumbar support for doing your work.
- Move your car seat forward so your knees are elevated slightly.
- Exercise regularly, particularly exercises that strengthen the abdominal muscles and stretch the back muscles.

Modern Maladies

During the past 20 years, several afflictions have surfaced that seem to be products of our time. Some of these health problems relate to specific groups of people, some

are due to technological advances, and others have not been explained.

Chronic Fatigue Syndrome

The diagnosis of **chronic fatigue syndrome (CFS)** depends on two major criteria and eight or more minor criteria. The major criteria are debilitating fatigue that persists for at least 6 months and the absence of other illnesses that could cause the symptoms. Minor criteria include headaches, fever, sore throat, painful lymph nodes, weakness, fatigue after exercise, sleep problems, and rapid onset of these symptoms. Treatment focuses on improved nutrition, rest, counseling for depression, judicious exercise, and development of a strong support network.

Despite extensive testing, no viral cause has been found. In the absence of a known pathogen, many researchers believe that the illness may have strong psychosocial roots.

Repetitive Stress Injuries

The Bureau of Labor Statistics estimates that 25 percent of all injuries in the labor force that result in lost work time are due to a **repetitive stress injury (RSI).** These are injuries to nerves, soft tissue, or joints that result from the physical stress of repeated motions.

One of the most common RSIs is **carpal tunnel syndrome.** Hours spent typing at the computer, flipping groceries through computerized scanners, or other jobs made simpler by technology can irritate the median nerve in the wrist, thus causing numbness, tingling, and pain in the fingers and hands. Risk of carpal tunnel syndrome can be reduced by proper placement of the keyboard, mouse, wrist pads, and other techniques. Better education and improvements in ergonomic workplace designs can eliminate many injuries of this nature.

chronic fatigue syndrome (CFS) A condition of unknown cause characterized by extreme fatigue that is not caused by other illness.

repetitive stress injury (RSI) An injury to nerves, soft tissue, or joints due to the physical stress of repeated motions.

carpal tunnel syndrome A common occupational injury in which the median nerve in the wrist becomes irritated, causing numbness, tingling, and pain in the fingers and hands.

TAKING charge

Summary

- Your body uses a number of defense systems to keep pathogens from invading. The skin is the body's major protection. The immune system creates antibodies to destroy antigens. Fever and pain play a role in defending the body. Vaccines bolster the body's immune system against specific diseases. Allergies are an overreaction of the body's natural defense system.

- The major pathogens are bacteria, viruses, fungi, protozoa, prions, and parasitic worms. Bacterial infections include staphylococcal infections, streptococcal infections, pneumonia, and tuberculosis. Major viral diseases include the common cold, influenza, mononucleosis, hepatitis, and measles. Emerging and resurgent diseases pose significant threats for future generations. Many factors contribute to these risks. Possible solutions focus on a public health approach to prevention.

- Sexually transmitted infections (STIs) are spread through intercourse, oral sex, anal sex, hand–genital contact, and sometimes mouth-to-mouth contact. Major STIs include chlamydia, gonorrhea, syphilis, herpes, genital warts, candidiasis, trichomoniasis, and pubic lice. Pelvic inflammatory disease (PID), although not an STI itself, is generally caused by STI. Sexual transmission may also be involved in some general urinary tract infections.

- Acquired immunodeficiency syndrome (AIDS) is caused by the human immunodeficiency virus (HIV). Globally, HIV/AIDS has become a major threat to the world's population. Anyone can get HIV by engaging in high-risk sexual activities that include exchange of body fluids, by having received a blood transfusion before 1985, and by injecting drugs (or having sex with someone who does). Women appear to be particularly susceptible to infection. You can cut your risk for AIDS by deciding not to engage in risky sexual activities.

- Chronic lung diseases include asthma, emphysema, and chronic bronchitis. Chronic obstructive pulmonary diseases (COPDs) are the fourth leading cause of death in the United States. Sleep apnea is another breathing-related condition increasing in prevalence.

- Neurological conditions include headaches, seizure disorders, Parkinson's disease, and multiple sclerosis. Headaches may be caused by a variety of factors, the most common of which are tension, dilation and/or rapid contraction of blood vessels in the brain, chemical influences on muscles and vessels that cause inflammation and pain, and underlying physiological and psychological disorders.

- Digestive conditions, such as colitis and irritable bowel syndrome, result from functional problems in various digestion-related organs or systems. Musculoskeletal diseases such as arthritis, fibromyalgia, systemic lupus erythematosus, and low back pain cause significant pain and disability in millions of people. Chronic fatigue syndrome (CFS) and repetitive stress injuries (RSIs, such as carpal tunnel syndrome) have emerged as major chronic maladies. CFS is associated with depression. Repetitive stress injuries are preventable by proper placement and usage of equipment.

Chapter Review

1. Which of the following is a *viral* disorder?
   a. measles
   b. pneumonia
   c. tuberculosis
   d. streptococcal infections

2. Acne, boils, and styes are types of
   a. viruses.
   b. fungi.
   c. staphylococcal infections.
   d. streptococcal infections.

3. If you are infected, which one of these STIs will remain in your body for life, regardless of treatment?
   a. chlamydia
   b. gonorrhea
   c. syphilis
   d. herpes

4. The most widespread sexually transmitted bacterium is
   a. gonorrhea.
   b. chlamydia.
   c. syphilis.
   d. chancroid.

5. Jennifer touched her viral herpes sore on her lip and then touched her eye. She ended up with herpesvirus in her eye as well. This is an example of
   a. acquired immunity.
   b. passive immunity.
   c. autoinoculation.
   d. self vaccination.

6. Which of the following is *not* a true statement about HIV?
   a. You can tell whether a potential sex partner has the virus by looking at the person.
   b. The virus can be spread through either semen or vaginal fluids.
   c. You cannot get HIV from a public restroom toilet seat.
   d. Unprotected anal sex increases risk of exposure to the HIV virus.

7. What is pelvic inflammatory disease (PID)?
   a. a sexually transmitted infection
   b. a type of urinary tract infection
   c. an infection of a woman's fallopian tubes or uterus
   d. a disease that both men and women can get

8. What degenerative disease involves the breakdown of myelin?
   a. epilepsy
   b. multiple sclerosis
   c. cerebral palsy
   d. Parkinson's disease

9. The gradual destruction of the alveoli in a smoker's lung will usually cause which respiratory condition?
   a. dyspnea
   b. bronchitis
   c. emphysema
   d. asthma

10. Which of the following conditions is the leading cause of employee sick time and lost productivity in the United States?
    a. low back pain
    b. the common cold
    c. asthma
    d. on-the-job injuries

Answers to these questions can be found on page A-1.

Questions for Discussion and Reflection

1. What are the major controllable risk factors for contracting infectious diseases? Using this knowledge, how would you change your current lifestyle to prevent such infection?
2. What is a pathogen? What are the similarities and differences between pathogens and antigens? Discuss uncontrollable and controllable risk factors that can threaten your health.
3. What are the six types of pathogens? What are the various means by which they can be transmitted? How have social conditions among the poor and homeless increased the risks for certain diseases, such as tuberculosis, influenza, and hepatitis? Why are these conditions a challenge to the efforts of public health officials?
4. Identify five STIs and their symptoms. How do they develop? What are their potential long-term effects?

5. Why are women more susceptible to HIV infection than men? What implication does this have for prevention, treatment, and research?
6. What are some of the major noninfectious chronic diseases affecting Americans today? Do you think there is a pattern in the types of diseases that we get? What are the common risk factors?
7. List common respiratory diseases affecting Americans. Which of these diseases has a genetic basis? An environmental basis? An individual basis? What, if anything, is being done to prevent, treat, and control each of these conditions?
8. What are the major disorders of the musculoskeletal system? Why do you think there aren't any cures? Describe the difference between osteoarthritis and rheumatoid arthritis.

Accessing Your Health on the Internet

The following websites explore further topics and issues related to personal health. For links to the websites below, visit the Companion Website for *Health: The Basics,* Eighth Edition at www.aw-bc.com/donatelle.

1. *American Academy of Allergy, Asthma, and Immunology.* Provides an overview of asthma and allergies. Offers interactive quizzes to test your knowledge and an ask-an-expert section. www.aaaai.org
2. *American Social Health Association.* Provides facts, support, resources, and referrals about sexually transmitted infections and diseases. www.ashastd.org

3. *Centers for Disease Control and Prevention (CDC).* Home page for the government agency dedicated to disease intervention and prevention, with links to all the latest data and publications put out by the CDC, including the *Morbidity and Mortality Weekly Report, HIV/AIDS Surveillance Report,* and the *Journal of Emerging Infectious Diseases.* Also provides access to Wonder, the CDC research database. www.cdc.gov
4. *National Center for Infectious Disease.* Up-to-date perspectives on infectious diseases of significance to the global community. www.cdc.gov/ncidod

5. *National Institute of Neurological Disorders and Stroke.* Many of the modern maladies result in chronic pain. This site provides up-to-date information to help you cope with pain-related difficulties. www.ninds.nih.gov
6. *San Francisco AIDS Foundation.* This community-based AIDS service organization focuses on ending the HIV/AIDS pandemic through education, services for AIDS patients, advocacy and public policy efforts, and global programs. www.sfaf.org
7. *World Health Organization (WHO).* Provides access to the latest information on world health issues, including infectious disease, and direct access to publications and fact sheets, with keywords to help users find topics of interest. www.who.int

Further Reading

Champeau, D., and R. Donatelle. *AIDS and STIs: A Global Perspective.* Englewood Cliffs, NJ: Prentice Hall, 2006.

> *An overview of issues, trends, and ethics surrounding the global pandemic of HIV/AIDS and STIs.*

Chin, J., ed. *Control of Communicable Diseases Manual,* 18th ed. Washington, DC: American Public Health Association, 2006.

> *Outstanding pocket reference for information on infectious diseases. Updated every 3 to 5 years to cover emerging diseases.*

Klatt, E. *Pathology of AIDS: Version 17.* Gainesville, FL: Florida State University Press, 2006.

> *Overview of AIDS risks, prevention, and control, as well as pathological development and historical basis.*

National Center for Health Statistics. *Morbidity and Mortality Weekly Report.* Published weekly. Available online at www.cdc.gov/mmwr.

> *Detailed government reports, usually published weekly, concerning mortality and morbidity data for the United States. Includes changes occurring in the rates of particular diseases and in health practices so that patterns and trends can be analyzed.*

Public Health Services, Centers for Disease Control and Prevention. *Chronic Disease News and Notes.* Washington, DC: U.S. Department of Health and Human Services.

> *Quarterly publication focusing on relevant chronic disease topics and issues.*

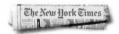

e-themes from *The New York Times*

For up-to-date articles about current health issues, visit www.aw-bc.com/donatelle, select *Health: The Basics*, Eighth Edition, Chapter 13, and click on "e-themes."

References

1. P. Wilkinson, "Infectious Diseases: Preparing for the Future," 2006, www.foresight.gov.uk.
2. National Institute of Allergy and Infectious Diseases, "Allergies: Fact Sheets and Brochures," 2007, www.niaid.nih.gov/publications/allergies.htm.
3. Centers for Disease Control and Prevention, "Group A Streptococcal Disease (GAS)," 2005, www.cdc.gov/ncidod/dbmd/diseaseinfo/groupastreptococcal_g.htm.
4. Centers for Disease Control and Prevention, Division of Bacterial and Mycotic Diseases, 2006, www.cdc.gov/ncidod/dbmd/index.htm.
5. Centers for Disease Control and Prevention, "Group A Streptococcal Disease (GAS)."
6. J. Tully et al., "Students May Have Higher Risk for Meningococcal Disease Than Other Adolescents," *British Medical Journal* 332 (2006): 1136–42.
7. Kaiser Family Foundation, "Global Health Report: Tuberculosis Overview," 2006, www.globalhealthreporting.org/tb.asp.
8. Centers for Disease Control and Prevention, *Preventing the Flu: Key Facts about Influenza Vaccine* (Atlanta: Centers for Disease Control and Prevention, 2007), www.cdc.gov/flu/protect/keyfacts.htm.
9. World Health Organization, "Immunization, Vaccines and Biologicals: Hepatitis A Vaccine," 2003, www.who.int/vaccines/en/hepatitisa.shtml.
10. *UroToday*, "Hepatitis B," 2006, www.urotoday.com/113/browse_categories/hepatitis_b/hepatitis_b.html.
11. Ibid.
12. National Center for Infectious Diseases, "Disease Burden from Hepatitis A, B, and C in the United States," 2006, www.cdc.gov/ncidod/diseases/hepatitis/resource/dz_burden.htm.
13. J. Ritterman, "Preventing Microbial Resistance: The Next Step," *The Permanente Journal* 10, no. 3 (2006): 22–24.
14. National Center for Infectious Diseases, "vCJD (Variant Creutzfeldt-Jakob Disease)," 2007, www.cdc.gov/ncidod/dvrd/vcjd/index.htm.
15. Centers for Disease Control and Prevention, Division of Vector-Borne Diseases, "West Nile Virus: Statistics, Surveillance, and Control," 2007, www.cdc.gov/ncidod/dvbid/westnile/surv&control.htm.
16. Centers for Disease Control and Prevention, "Special Pathogens Branch—Ebola Hemorrhagic Fever," 2006, www.cdc.gov/ncidod/dvrd/spb/mnpages/dispages/ebola.htm.
17. Ibid.

18. Centers for Disease Control and Prevention, "Severe Acute Respiratory Syndrome (SARS)," 2005, www.cdc.gov/ncidod/sars/.

19. World Health Organization, "Confirmed Human Cases of Avian Influenza A(H5N1)," 2007, www.who.int/csr/disease/avian_influenza/country/en.

20. Ibid.

21. Centers for Disease Control and Prevention, "Trends in Reportable Sexually Transmitted Diseases in the United States, 2005," 2006, www.cdc.gov/std/stats/trends2005.htm.

22. American Social Health Association, "STD/STI Statistics," 2006, www.ashastd.org/learn/learn_statistics.cfm.

23. Centers for Disease Control and Prevention, "Chlamydia—CDC Fact Sheet," 2006, www.cdc.gov/std/Chlamydia/STDFact-Chlamydia.htm.

24. Centers for Disease Control and Prevention, "Gonorrhea—CDC Fact Sheet," 2006, www.cdc.gov/std/Gonorrhea/STDFact-gonorrhea.htm.

25. U.S. National Library of Medicine, Medline Plus, "Gonorrhea," 2007, www.nlm.nih.gov/medlineplus/ency/article/007267.htm.

26. U.S. National Library of Medicine, Medline Plus, "Pelvic Inflammatory Disease (PID)," 2006, www.nlm.nih.gov/medlineplus/ency/article/000888.htm.

27. Centers for Disease Control and Prevention, "Genital Herpes—CDC Fact Sheet," 2006, www.cdc.gov/std/herpes/STDFact-Herpes.htm.

28. Ibid.

29. Ibid.

30. American Society for Microbiology, Fourth Annual Interscience Conference on Antimicrobial Agents and Chemotherapy. San Francisco. September 27–30, 2006; Centers for Disease Control and Prevention, "Genital Herpes—CDC Fact Sheet."

31. F. Xu, "Genital Herpes Virus Rate Drops," *Journal of the American Medical Association* 296 (2006): 964–73.

32. National Institutes of Health, National Institute of Allergy and Infectious Diseases, "Human Papillomavirus and Genital Warts," 2007, www3.niaid.nih.gov/healthscience/healthtopics/human_papillomavirus/overview.htm.

33. Centers for Disease Control and Prevention, Sexually Transmitted Diseases, "HPV Vaccine Questions and Answers," 2006, www.cdc.gov/std/hpv/STDFact-HPV-vaccine.htm.

34. UNAIDS, "Global Facts and Figures, 2006," 2006, http://data.unaids.org/pub/GlobalReport/2006/200605-FS_globalfactsfigures_en.pdf.

35. World Health Organization, "Global AIDS Epidemic Continues to Grow," 2006, www.who.int/hiv/mediacentre/news62/en/index.html; AVERT, "Worldwide HIV & AIDS Statistics," 2007, www.avert.org/worldstats.htm.

36. Kaiser Family Foundation, "HIV/AIDS Policy Fact Sheet," July 2007, www.kff.org/hivaids/upload/3029–071.pdf.

37. Centers for Disease Control and Prevention, "HIV/AIDS Statistics and Surveillance: Basic Statistics," 2007, www.cdc.gov/hiv/topics/surveillance/basic.htm.

38. San Francisco AIDS Foundation, "How HIV Is Spread," 2006, www.sfaf.org/aids101/transmission.html; National Institute of Allergy and Infectious Diseases, "HIV Infection and AIDS: An Overview—NIAID Fact Sheets," 2005, www.niaid.nih.gov/factsheets/hivinf.htm.

39. AVERT, "United States Statistics Summary," 2007, www.avert.org/statsum.htm.

40. Centers for Disease Control and Prevention, "Global HIV/AIDS: Preventing Mother to Child Transmission," 2005, www.cdc.gov/nchstp/od/GAP/pa_pmtct.htm; Centers for Disease Control and Prevention, "HIV/AIDS: Questions and Answers," 2007, www.cdc.gov/hiv/resources/qa/index.htm; AVERT, "Preventing Mother to Child Transmission of HIV," 2007, www.avert.org/motherchild.htm.

41. National Institute of Allergy and Infectious Disease, "HIV Infection in Women—NIAID Fact Sheet," 2006, www.niaid.nih.gov.

42. Centers for Disease Control and Prevention, "HIV/AIDS: Questions and Answers," 2007, www.cdc.gov/hiv/resources/qa/index.htm.

43. National Institute of Allergy and Infectious Diseases, "HIV Infection in Infants and Children—NIAID Fact Sheets," 2004, www.niaid.nih.gov.

44. Kaiser Family Foundation, "HIV/AIDS Policy Fact Sheet," July 2007, www.kff.org/hivaids/upload/3029-071.pdf.

45. Centers for Disease Control and Prevention, "HIV/AIDS: Research," 2007, www.cdc.gov/hiv/topics/research/index.htm#vaccine.

46. National Center for Health Statistics, *Health, United States, 2006, with Chartbook on Trends in the Health of Americans* (Hyattsville, MD: National Center for Health Statistics, 2007).

47. American Lung Association, "Results from the National Health Interview Survey, 1998–2004," 2006, www.lungusa.org; American Lung Association Epidemiology and Statistics Unit, "Trends in Chronic Bronchitis and Emphysema Morbidity and Mortality," 2005, www.lungusa.org.

48. American Lung Association, "Results from the National Health Interview Survey, 1998–2004."

49. National Center for Health Statistics, FASTSTATS, "Bronchitis," 2007, www.cdc.gov/nchs/fastats/brnchtis.htm.

50. National Center for Health Statistics, FASTSTATS, "Emphysema," 2007, www.cdc.gov/nchs/fastats/emphysema.htm.

51. American Lung Association, "Trends in Asthma Morbidity and Mortality, 2006," 2006, www.lungusa.org/site/pp.asp?c=dvLUK9OOE&b=33347.

52. Ibid.

53. Sleep Disorders Guide, "Sleep Apnea Statistics," 2007, www.sleepdisordersguide.com/sleepapnea/sleep-apnea-statistics.html.

54. National Sleep Foundation, "What Is Sleep Apnea?" 2007, www.sleepfoundation.org; American Sleep Apnea Association, "Information about Sleep Apnea," 2007, www.sleepapnea.org/geninfo.html.

55. National Headache Foundation, "Headache Topic Sheets," 2007, www.headaches.org/consumer/topicsheets/consumertopics.html.

56. Ibid.

57. Ibid.

58. National Headache Foundation, "Cluster: The Killer Headache," *NHF Headlines* 157 (July/August 2007), http://headaches.org/consumer/headlines/Issue157_cond.htm.

59. Epilepsy Foundation, "About Epilepsy," 2006, www.epilepsyfoundation.org/answerplace/ABOUTepilepsy.cfm.

60. National Parkinson Foundation, "Parkinson Primer," 2007, www.parkinson.org.

61. Multiple Sclerosis Foundation, "Frequently Asked Questions," 2007, www.msfacts.org/info_faq.php; S. Courtney, *All About Multiple Sclerosis* 3rd ed. (Cherry Hill, NJ: Multiple Sclerosis Association of America, 2006).

62. J. M. Hootman and C. G. Helmick, "Projections of U.S. Prevalence of Arthritis and Associated Activity Limitations," *Arthritis & Rheumatism* 54, no. 1 (2006): 226–29.

63. "National and State Medical Expenditures and Lost Earnings Attributable to Arthritis and Other Rheumatic Conditions—United States, 2003," *Morbidity and Mortality Weekly Report* 56, no. 1 (2007): 4–7.

64. Hootman and Helmick, "Projections of U.S. Prevalence of Arthritis."

65. Ibid.

66. Ibid.

67. Ibid.

68. Lupus Foundation of America, "Statistics," 2007, www.lupus.org.

69. National Institute of Neurological Disorders and Stroke, "Low Back Pain Fact Sheet," 2007, www.ninds.nih.gov/disorders/backpain/detail_backpain.htm.

Complementary and Alternative Medicine

NEW CHOICES AND RESPONSIBILITIES FOR HEALTHWISE CONSUMERS

Why are so many people using **alternative** medicine?

How do **acupuncture** needles work?

Do **herbal** remedies have any risks or side effects?

Will **echinacea** teas and cough drops cure my cold?

How do I evaluate **alternative** medical resources for reliability?

OBJECTIVES

- Describe complementary and alternative medicine (CAM), and identify its typical domains.
- Explain major types of complementary and alternative medicine providers and common treatments they offer.
- Discuss the various types of complementary and alternative medicines used today, who is most likely to use them, their patterns of use, and their potential benefits and risks.
- Understand how to evaluate testimonials and claims related to complementary and alternative products, services, and practitioners to ensure that you are getting accurate information and safe treatment.
- Summarize the challenges and opportunities related to complementary and alternative medicine in ensuring our health and wellness.

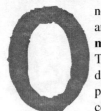One of the newest movements toward self-care and health promotion focuses on **complementary and alternative medicine (CAM)**. These therapies are defined as a group of diverse medical and health care systems, practices, and products that are not currently considered part of conventional medicine.[1] Various products and services offer today's consumers a new range of health choices and an opportunity for greater control over our own health care.

Complementary and Alternative Medicine: What Is It and Who Uses It?

Although often used interchangeably when referring to therapies, there is a distinction between the terms *complementary* and *alternative*. **Complementary medicine** is used *together with* conventional medicine, as part of the modern integrative-medicine approach. An example of complementary medicine is to use massage therapy along with prescription medicine to treat anxiety.[2] **Alternative medicine** has traditionally been used *in place of* conventional medicine, such as following a special diet or herbal remedy to treat cancer instead of using radiation, surgery, or other conventional treatments. However, as some alternative medical approaches have gained scientific credibility, they are used along with conventional treatment.[3] A survey conducted by the National Center for Complementary and Alternative Medicine (NCCAM) revealed that 36 percent of adults used some form of CAM within the past 12 months, and almost 50 percent reported having used CAM at some time.[4] When prayer specifically for health reasons is included in the definition of CAM, those numbers rise to 62 percent and 74 percent, respectively.[5]

Complementary and alternative therapies vary widely in terms of nature of treatment, extent of therapy, and types of problems for which they offer help. Typically, CAM therapies are compared with conventional medicine. Conventional medicine is practiced by holders of MD (medical doctor) or DO (doctor of osteopathy) degrees and by allied health professionals, such as physical therapists, psychologists, and registered nurses (see Chapter 16). Other terms for conventional medicine include *allopathy, Western, mainstream, orthodox,* and *biomedicine.* In general, practitioners of allopathic medicine treat disease by using remedies that include pharmaceutical drugs or surgery, have graduated from U.S.-sanctioned schools of medicine or nursing, or are licensed practitioners recognized by the American Medical Association (AMA), American Nurses Association (ANA), or other certification board. Some conventional medical practitioners are also CAM practitioners.

The list of practices that are considered CAM changes continually as therapies become accepted as "mainstream." In general, CAM therapies serve as alternatives to an allopathic system—the conventional Western system of medicine described in more detail in Chapter 16—that some people regard as too invasive, too high-tech, and too toxic in terms of laboratory-produced medications. CAM therapies incorporate a **holistic** approach to medicine that focuses on treating both the mind and the whole body, rather than just an isolated part of the body. Often CAM users seek what they perceive as a more natural, gentle approach to healing. Other CAM patients distrust the traditional medical approach and believe that alternative practices will give them greater control over their own health care. CAM therapies can vary based on whether they have been scientifically studied and whether those studies have shown them to be beneficial. Research has shown that many types of CAM, including acupuncture and massage therapy, are beneficial in treating conditions such as chronic back pain and cancer.[6]

Complementary and Alternative Medicine in the United States Today

Why are so many people using alternative medicine?

A survey of over 31,000 Americans revealed that 36 percent of adults use some form of CAM.[7] Why do so many people seek alternative therapy? Distinct patterns of who uses CAM emerge from this survey:

- More women than men
- People with higher educational levels
- People who had been hospitalized in the past year
- Former smokers (compared with current smokers or those who have never smoked)
- People with back, neck, head, or joint aches or other painful conditions
- People with gastrointestinal disorders or sleeping problems

Figure 14.1 summarizes the reasons respondents to the NCCAM survey stated for deciding to use CAM.

complementary and alternative medicine (CAM) Forms of treatment distinct from traditional allopathic medicine that until recently were neither taught widely in U.S. medical schools nor generally available in U.S. hospitals.

complementary medicine Treatment used in conjunction with conventional medicine.

alternative medicine Treatment used in place of conventional medicine.

holistic Term referring to treatment of both the mind and body.

Alternative Medical Systems

Alternative (whole) medical systems are built on specific systems of theory and practice. There are many alternative systems of medicine that have been practiced by various cultures throughout the world. Some have evolved from centuries-old practices, such as traditional Chinese medicine and Ayurveda, which are at the root of much of our CAM thinking today. Other alternative medical systems include homeopathy and naturopathy.

Traditional Chinese Medicine

Traditional Chinese medicine (TCM) emphasizes the proper balance or disturbances of *qi* (pronounced "chi"), or vital energy in health and disease, respectively. Diagnosis is based on personal history, observation of the body (especially the tongue), palpation, and pulse diagnosis, an elaborate procedure requiring considerable skill and experience by the practitioner. Techniques such as acupuncture, herbal medicine, massage, and *qigong* (a form of energy therapy) are among the TCM approaches to health and healing. These are discussed in more detail later in this chapter.

Ayurveda

Ayurveda (or Ayurvedic medicine) relates to the "science of life," an alternative medical system that began and evolved over thousands of years in India. Ayurveda seeks to integrate and balance the body, mind, and spirit and to restore harmony in the individual.[8] Ayurvedic practitioners use various techniques, including questioning, observing, touching patients, and classifying patients into one of three body types, or *doshas*, before establishing a treatment plan.[9] The goals of Ayurvedic treatment are to eliminate impurities in the body and reduce symptoms. Dietary modification and herbal remedies drawn from the vast botanical wealth of the Indian subcontinent are common. Treatments may also include animal and mineral ingredients, powdered gemstones, yoga, stretching, meditation, massage, steam baths, exposure to the sun, and controlled breathing.[10]

Training of Ayurvedic practitioners varies. There is no national standard for certifying or training Ayurvedic practitioners, although professional groups are working toward licensure. To find out more about the effectiveness of this medical system or any of its various modalities, visit the NCCAM Web pages.

Homeopathy

Homeopathic medicine is an unconventional Western system based on the principle that "like cures like." In other words, the same substance that in large doses produces the symp-

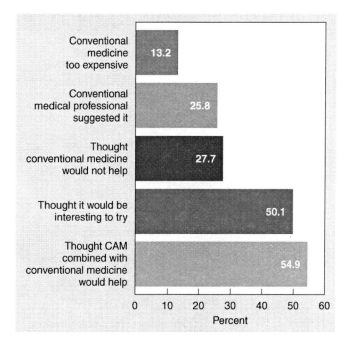

FIGURE 14.1 Reasons Adults in the United States Use CAM
Survey respondents who reported having used CAM were asked to describe why they used it. People could select more than one reason.
Source: P. Barnes et al., "Complementary and Alternative Medicine Use Among Adults: United States, 2002," *CDC Advance Data Report* no. 343, May 27, 2004, http://nccam.nih.gov/news/camstats.htm.

toms of an illness will in very small doses cure the illness. It was developed in the late 1700s by Samuel Hahnemann, a German physician, as an approach to medicine that was not as harsh as other treatments of the time, such as bloodletting and blistering.[11] Homeopathic physicians use herbal medicine, minerals, and chemicals in extremely diluted forms to kill infectious agents or ward off illnesses that are caused by more potent forms or doses of those substances. Homeopathic

---

alternative (whole) medical systems   Complete systems of theory and practice that involve several CAM domains.

traditional Chinese medicine (TCM)   Whole medical system that originated in China; based on the concepts of balancing *qi* and the forces of *yin* and *yang*. Practices of acupuncture, massage, meditation, and herbs used to aid healing and restore balance.

qi   Element of traditional Chinese medicine that refers to the vital energy force that courses through the body.

Ayurveda (Ayurvedic medicine)   A method of treatment derived largely from ancient India, in which practitioners diagnose by observation and touch and then assign a largely dietary treatment laced with herbal medicines.

homeopathic medicine   Unconventional Western system of medicine based on the principle that "like cures like."

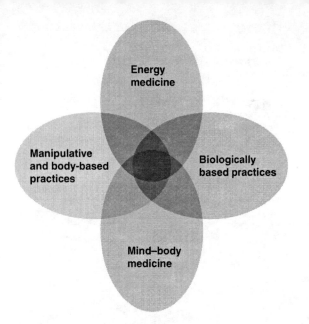

FIGURE 14.2 The Domains of Complementary and Alternative Medicine

training varies considerably and is offered through diploma programs, certificate programs, short courses, and correspondence courses. Laws that detail requirements to practice vary from state to state.

Naturopathy

Naturopathic medicine views disease as a manifestation of an alteration in the processes by which the body naturally heals itself. Disease results from the body's effort to ward off impurities and harmful substances from the environment. Naturopathic physicians emphasize restoring health rather than curing disease. They employ an array of healing practices, including diet and clinical nutrition; homeopathy; acupuncture; herbal medicine; hydrotherapy (the use of water in a range of temperatures and methods of application); spinal and soft-tissue manipulation; physical therapies involving electric currents, ultrasound, and light therapy; therapeutic counseling; and pharmacology. Several major naturopathic schools in the

---

naturopathic medicine System of medicine that attempts to restore natural processes of the body and promote healing through natural means.

manipulative and body-based practices Treatments involving manipulation or movement of one or more body parts.

energy medicine Therapies using energy fields, such as magnetic fields or biofields.

mind–body medicine Techniques designed to enhance the mind's ability to affect bodily function and symptoms.

biologically based practices Treatments using substances found in nature, such as herbs, special diets, or vitamin megadoses.

United States and Canada provide training, conferring the *naturopathic doctor (ND)* degree on students who have completed a 4-year graduate program that emphasizes humanistically oriented family medicine.

Other Alternative Medical Systems

Although these medical philosophies and patterns of treatment have exerted great influence on populations worldwide, other medical traditions are also noteworthy. Native American, Aboriginal, African, Middle Eastern, and South American cultures also have their own unique alternative systems. Surveys outside the United States indicate high CAM use in Italy, France, Denmark, Finland, and Australia, in addition to most Asian cultures.[12]

As the number of alternative therapists grows and systems become intertwined, so do the number of options available to consumers. Before considering any treatments, wise consumers will consult the most reliable resources to thoroughly evaluate risks, the scientific basis of claimed benefits, and any contraindications to using the CAM product or service. Avoid practitioners who promote their treatments as a cure-all for every health problem or who seem to promise remedies for ailments that have thus far defied the best scientific efforts of mainstream medicine. In short, apply the same strategies to researching CAM as you would to choosing allopathic care (see Chapter 16). See the **Skills for Behavior Change** box on page 486 for detailed information on choosing a CAM practitioner.

Major Domains of Complementary and Alternative Medicine

The United States government has created the National Center for Complementary and Alternative Medicine (NCCAM) within the National Institutes of Health (NIH) to provide a mechanism for reliable information about CAM practices. The NCCAM serves as a clearinghouse for CAM information and a focal point for research initiatives, policy development, and general recommendations. It has grouped the many varieties of CAM into four domains of practice **(Figure 14.2)**, recognizing that some domains may overlap:

- **Manipulative and body-based practices** are based on manipulation or movement of one or more body parts.
- **Energy medicine** involves the use of energy fields, such as magnetic fields or biofields (energy fields that some people believe surround and penetrate the body).
- **Mind–body medicine** uses a variety of techniques to enhance the mind's ability to affect bodily function and symptoms.
- **Biologically based practices** use substances found in nature, such as herbs, special diets, or vitamins (in doses outside those used in conventional medicine).

Manipulative and Body-Based Practices

Manipulative and body-based practices include methods that are based on manipulation and/or movement of the body. For example, chiropractors focus on the relationship between the body's structures (primarily the spine) and function and on how that relationship affects the preservation and restoration of health. Chiropractors use manipulation as a key therapy.[13]

Chiropractic Medicine

Chiropractic medicine has been practiced for more than 100 years. A century ago, allopathic medicine and chiropractic medicine were in direct competition. Today, however, many health care organizations work closely with chiropractors, and many insurance companies will pay for chiropractic treatment, particularly if recommended by a medical doctor. More than 20 million Americans now visit chiropractors each year.

Chiropractic medicine is based on the idea that a life-giving energy flows through the spine by way of the nervous system. If the spine is subluxated (partly misaligned or dislocated), that force is disrupted. Chiropractors use a variety of techniques to manipulate the spine back into proper alignment so the life-giving energy can flow unimpeded. It has been established that their treatment can be effective for back pain, neck pain, and headaches.

The average chiropractic training program requires 4 years of intensive courses in biochemistry, anatomy, physiology, diagnostics, pathology, nutrition, and related topics, combined with hands-on clinical training. Many chiropractors continue their training to obtain specialized certification, for instance, in neurology, geriatrics, or pediatrics. There are currently 15 accredited programs and 2 chiropractic institutions in the United States. Most state boards require 2 years of undergraduate education, and more states are requiring a bachelor's degree in addition to the doctor of chiropractic degree for licensure. The practice of chiropractic is licensed and regulated in all 50 states.[14]

You should investigate and question a chiropractor as carefully as you would any medical doctor. As with many health professionals, you may note vast differences in technique among specialists. It is recommended that you choose a chiropractor who follows standard chiropractic regimens for treating musculoskeletal conditions.

Massage Therapy

Massage therapy is defined as soft-tissue manipulation by trained therapists for healing purposes.[15] References to massage have been found in ancient writings from many cultures, including those of ancient Greece, ancient Rome, Japan, China, Egypt, and the Indian subcontinent.[16] Today, massage therapy is used as a means of treating painful conditions, including lower back pain;

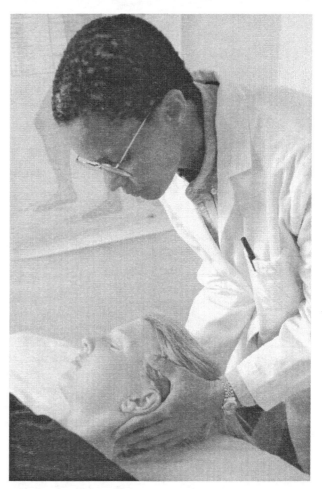

A chiropractor treats a patient by using a variety of techniques to manipulate the spine into proper alignment.

relaxing tired and overworked muscles; reducing stress and anxiety; rehabilitating sports injuries; and promoting general health.[17] This is accomplished by manipulating soft tissues to improve the body's circulation and to remove waste products from the muscles. There are many different types of massage therapy; the following are some of the more popular:[18]

- *Swedish massage* uses long strokes, kneading, and friction on the muscles and moves the joints to aid flexibility.
- *Deep tissue massage* uses patterns of strokes and deep finger pressure on parts of the body where muscles are tight or knotted, focusing on layers of muscle deep under the skin.
- *Trigger point massage* (also called *pressure point massage*) uses a variety of strokes but applies deeper, more focused pressure on myofascial trigger points—"knots" that can form in the muscles, are painful when pressed, and cause symptoms elsewhere in the body as well.
- *Shiatsu massage* uses varying, rhythmic pressure from the fingers on parts of the body that are believed to be important for the flow of vital energy.

chiropractic medicine   Medical system that emphasizes manipulation of the spine to allow proper energy flow.

SKILLS FOR behavior change

SELECTING A COMPLEMENTARY OR ALTERNATIVE MEDICINE PROVIDER

Selecting a CAM practitioner—or any health care provider—can be difficult. Although these recommendations apply to CAM, you should also consider them when selecting any health care product or service. Before starting a CAM therapy or choosing a practitioner, talk with your primary health care provider(s) and others who are knowledgeable about CAM. If they dismiss the therapy, ask why. Check their explanations with other sources to see whether their insights are confirmed.

FINDING A PRACTITIONER

- Ask your physician or other health professionals to recommend or refer you to a CAM therapist, or consult people you trust who have used CAM. They may have recommendations based on experience.
- Check with your insurers to see whether the cost of CAM therapy will be covered. If it is covered, ask your carrier for a list of approved CAM providers.
- Contact a professional organization for the type of practitioner you are seeking. Often they have standards of practice and websites or publications that list recommended providers. If there is a regulatory or licensing board for this specialty, verify that your practitioner has the proper credentials.

INTERVIEWING A PRACTITIONER

- Make a list of your options, and gather information about each before making your first visit. Ask about providers' credentials and experience.
- Ask whether it is possible to have a brief consultation in person or over the phone before agreeing to treatment.
- Write down questions to ask at your first visit. You may want to bring a friend or family member who can help you ask questions and note answers.
- Bring medical information with you, including any tests you've had, information about your health history, surgical history, allergies, and any medications (including prescription, over-the-counter, and herbal or other supplements).
- Ask whether there are health conditions in which the practitioner specializes and how frequently he or she treats patients with conditions like yours.
- Ask whether there is any research supporting the use of this treatment for your condition.
- Is the provider supportive of conventional as well as CAM treatments? Does he or she have a good relationship with conventional practitioners to give referrals to them?

- How many patients per day does the provider see, and how much time is spent with each one?
- What are the charges and payment options? What percentage of the payment might you have to pay out of pocket?
- During and after the consultation, assess the interaction and how you felt about the practitioner.

INVESTIGATING THE RECOMMENDED TREATMENT

Ask your CAM practitioner:

- What benefits, risks, and side effects can I expect from this therapy? Do the benefits outweigh the risks?
- Will I need to buy any special equipment or take any special supplements?
- How long will I need to undergo the therapy? How often will my progress or plan of treatment be assessed?
- Will this therapy interfere with any conventional medicine treatments?
- If there are problems, where would I be referred for further treatment?
- What is the history of success in treating this type of condition for someone of my age and health status?

Source: National Center for Complementary and Alternative Medicine, "Selecting a CAM Practitioner," NCCAM Publication no. D346, 2007, http://nccam.nih.gov/health/practitioner/index.htm.

Other varieties include massage of specific body parts, such as the feet or fingers, application of hot rocks, water massage, or other techniques.

There are about 1,300 massage therapy schools, college programs, and training programs in the United States. The course of study typically covers subjects such as anatomy and physiology; kinesiology; therapeutic evaluation; massage techniques; first aid; business, ethical, and legal issues; and hands-on practice. These educational programs vary in respect to length, quality, and whether they are accredited. Many require 500 hours of training, which is the same number of hours that many states require for certification. Some therapists also pursue specialty or advanced training.

Massage therapists work in an array of settings both private and public: private offices, studios, hospitals, nursing homes, fitness centers, and sports medicine facilities, for example.[19]

Body Work

Body work actually consists of several forms of exercise. The *Feldenkrais method* is a system of movements, floor exercises, and body work designed to retrain the central nervous system to find new pathways around areas of blockage or damage. It is gentle and effective in rehabilitating trauma victims. *Rolfing,* a more invasive form of body work, aims to restructure the musculoskeletal system by working on patterns of tension

MAKING A STATEMENT ABOUT MASSAGE

Massage has been credited with alleviating a wide variety of aches and pains, from migraines and carpal tunnel syndrome to anxiety and low back pain. In particular, massage has been looked at as a useful treatment for low back pain. More than 100 million Americans suffer from low back pain and spend nearly $25 billion a year in search of relief. In the Centers for Disease Control and Prevention's 30th annual report on the health status of the nation, *Health, United States, 2006,* low back pain was the most commonly reported type of pain, the most common cause of job-related disability, and a leading contributor to missed work and reduced productivity.

Medication may still be the most common way to treat low back pain, but increasing evidence suggests it is neither the most effective nor the safest treatment method. The need for more effective solutions to low back pain has led many health care organizations to increase research for alternative treatments such as massage therapy. A number of studies have indicated that massage is highly beneficial for people with chronic low back pain. For example, a recent study in the *Annals of Internal Medicine* showed that massage therapy produced better results and reduced the need for painkillers by 36 percent when compared to other therapies, including acupuncture and spinal modification. With 39 million American adults per year getting massages, and 30 percent of those adults using massage therapy for medical purposes, recent American Massage Therapy Association (AMTA) consumer surveys continue to show that massage therapy is a growing trend.

As evidence that massage therapy is increasingly on the minds of the public, the AMTA reports that 9 million more people discussed massage therapy with their health care provider in 2006 than in 2001. Moreover, almost twice as many doctors recommended massage therapy to their patients in 2006 than in 2001. When patients inquire about massage therapy, physicians are more likely to recommend it (59 percent), and nearly half of all chiropractors (48 percent) and physical therapists (47 percent) also recommended massage.

Although many people are coming to believe massage is not just a luxury but a medical necessity, Medicare and Medicaid have not yet supported insurance coverage for massage as a remedy for low back pain, and many insurance companies offer only limited coverage of massage therapy. To address this issue, AMTA and the Integrative Healthcare Policy Consortium (IHPC) have proposed that the National Institutes of Health (NIH) hold a consensus conference on the use of massage for low back pain. Through this conference, which is expected to occur in the next 2 years, the AMTA hopes to elicit a federal statement declaring that massage is effective for low back pain. Historically, the conference panel's findings have triggered Medicare and Medicaid reimbursement policies, which, in turn, have expanded insurance coverage policies. If the conference goal is reached, the AMTA anticipates that massage for low back pain will be widely accepted by the health care community.

Despite lingering pessimism from some in the conventional medical community, an

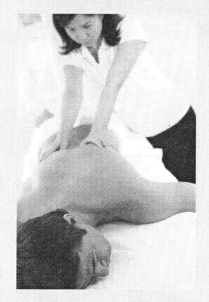

impressive 25 million more Americans each year are getting a massage today than they did 10 years ago, according to the 2006 AMTA study. Because massage therapy, as with most CAM care, is paid for by the patients themselves, it is not accessible to all Americans. Only those who can afford the out-of-pocket costs have access to broader choices in their health care. Massage patients, massage therapists, and affiliated health care organizations remain hopeful that the NIH consensus conference will convince the health care community and insurance providers of the benefits of massage therapy—a treatment that already provides much needed relief to millions of Americans.

Source: Adapted from M. Vivo, "Making a Statement About Massage," *Massage Today* 7, no. 2 (2007), www.massagetoday.com/mpacms/mt/article.php?id=13538.

---

held in deep tissue. The therapist applies firm—sometimes painful—pressure to different areas of the body. Rolfing can release repressed emotions as well as dissipate muscle tension. *Shiatsu* is a traditional healing art from Japan that applies firm finger pressure to specified points on the body and is intended to increase the circulation of vital energy. *Trager bodywork* employs gentle, shaking motions of the patient's limbs in a rhythmic fashion to induce states of deep, pleasant relaxation.[20]

Energy Medicine

Energy therapies focus either on energy fields thought to originate with the body (biofields) or on fields from other sources (electromagnetic fields). Biofield therapies are intended to affect energy fields said to surround and penetrate the human body. The existence of these fields has not been experimentally proven. Some forms of energy therapy manipulate biofields by

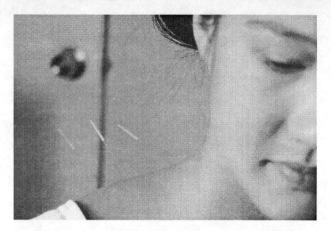

Acupuncture has been found to be effective in treating many problems but should always be performed by a licensed practitioner.

Acupuncture and Acupressure

Acupuncture, one of the oldest forms of traditional Chinese medicine (and one of the most popular among Americans), is sought for a wide variety of health conditions, including musculoskeletal dysfunction, mood enhancement, and wellness promotion. It describes a family of procedures that involve stimulating anatomical points of the body with a series of nee-

How do acupuncture needles work?

dles. The placement and manipulation of acupuncture needles is based on traditional Chinese theories of life-force energy (*qi*) flow through *meridians,* or energy pathways, in the body. Following acupuncture, most respondents and participants in clinical studies report high satisfaction with the treatment, improved quality of life, improvement in or cure of the condition, and reduced reliance on prescription drugs and surgery. In particular, results have been promising in the treatment of nausea associated with chemotherapy, dental pain, and knee pain.[25] Some Western researchers believe that acupuncture may work through stimulating or repressing the autonomic nervous system.[26]

Acupuncturists in the United States are state licensed, and each state has specific requirements regarding training programs. Most acupuncturists have either completed a 2- to 3-year postgraduate program to obtain a master of traditional Oriental medicine (MTOM) degree or have attended a shorter certification program in North America or Asia. Some licensed MDs and chiropractors have trained in acupuncture and obtained certification to use this treatment.

Acupressure is similar to acupuncture but does not use needles. Instead, the practitioner applies pressure to points critical to balancing *yin* and *yang,* the two Chinese principles that interact to influence overall harmony (health) of the body. Practitioners must have the same basic training and understanding of energy pathways as do acupuncturists.

applying pressure and/or manipulating the body by placing the hands in, or through, these fields.[21]

Popular examples of biofield therapy include *qigong, reiki,* and *therapeutic touch. Qigong,* a component of traditional Chinese medicine, combines movement, meditation, and regulation of breathing to enhance the flow of vital energy (*qi*), improve blood circulation, and enhance immune function.[22] *Reiki,* whose name derives from the Japanese word representing "universal life energy," is based on the belief that by channeling spiritual energy through the practitioner, the spirit is healed, and it in turn heals the physical body.[23] *Therapeutic touch* derives from the ancient technique of "laying on" of hands and is based on the premise that the healing force of the therapist brings about the patient's recovery and that healing is promoted when the body's energies are in balance. By passing the hands over the body, the healers identify bodily imbalances.[24]

Bioelectromagnetic-based therapies involve the unconventional use of electromagnetic fields—such as pulsed fields, magnetic fields, or alternating current or direct current fields—to treat asthma, cancer, pain, migraines, and other conditions. There is little scientific documentation to support claims for energy field techniques at this point. However, two derivatives of energy medicine have gained much wider acceptance in recent years: acupuncture and acupressure.

Mind–Body Medicine

Mind–body medicine employs a variety of techniques designed to facilitate the mind's capacity to affect bodily function and symptoms. Many therapies fall under this category, but some areas, such as biofeedback and cognitive-behavioral techniques, have been so well investigated that they are no longer considered alternative. However, meditation, yoga, tai chi, certain uses of hypnosis, dance, music and art therapy, prayer and mental healing, and several others are still categorized as complementary and alternative. See Chapter 11 for more on yoga and tai chi; see Chapters 2 and 3 for more on spirituality and the mind–body connection.

Psychoneuroimmunology

As discussed in Chapter 3, **psychoneuroimmunology (PNI)** is a relatively new field of study. It is defined as the "interaction of consciousness (*psycho*), brain and central nervous system

acupuncture Branch of traditional Chinese medicine that uses the insertion of long, thin needles to affect flow of energy (*qi*) along pathways (meridians) within the body.

acupressure Branch of traditional Chinese medicine, related to acupuncture. Uses application of pressure to selected body points to balance energy.

psychoneuroimmunology (PNI) Use of stress management and other techniques to enhance the function of the immune system.

(*neuro*), and the body's defense against external infection and internal aberrant cell division (*immunology*)."[27] A number of researchers have postulated that excessive stress and maladaptive coping can lead to immune system dysfunction and can increase the risk of disease. Scientists are exploring ways in which relaxation, biofeedback, meditation, yoga, laughter, exercise, and activities that involve either conscious or unconscious mind "quieting" may counteract negative stressors.

A classic study of PNI and mind–body health attempted to assess the effects of relaxation and coping techniques on the immune system by studying nursing home patients. Participants were divided into three groups: those who were taught relaxation techniques, those who were provided with abundant social contact, and those who received no special techniques or contact. After 1 month, immune system function greatly improved in participants who received stress management therapy as compared to the other groups.[28] Several studies have shown promising positive effects of mind–body techniques that encourage relaxation and other stress-reduction strategies for people with cancer or other health problems.[29]

Biologically Based Practices

Biologically based therapy is perhaps one of the most controversial domains of CAM practice because of the sheer number of options available and the many claims made about their supposedly magic effects. Many of these claims have not been thoroughly investigated, and regulation of this aspect of CAM has been slow in coming. Biologically based practices include natural and biologically based treatments, interventions, and products, many of which overlap with conventional medicine's use of dietary supplements. The U.S. Food and Drug Administration (FDA) defines a dietary supplement as a "product (other than tobacco) that is intended to supplement or add to the diet; contains one or more dietary ingredients (including vitamins, minerals, herbs or other botanicals, amino acids, or other substances that increase total dietary intake); and that is intended to be taken by mouth as a pill, capsule, tablet, or liquid; and is labeled on the front panel as being a dietary supplement."[30] Included are *herbal remedies, special dietary supplements, individual biological therapies,* and *functional foods* (see Chapter 9).[31] Typically, people take these supplements and remedies—often without guidance from any CAM practitioner—to improve health, prevent disease, or enhance mood.

Herbal Remedies

Largely derived from Ayurvedic and traditional Chinese medicine, herbal medications are widely available in the United States. Fueled by mass advertising and promoted as part of multiple vitamin and mineral regimens by major drug manufacturers, herbal supplements represent the hottest trend in the health market.

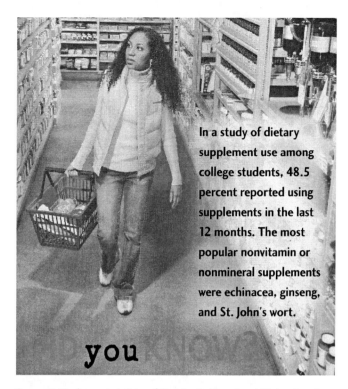

In a study of dietary supplement use among college students, 48.5 percent reported using supplements in the last 12 months. The most popular nonvitamin or nonmineral supplements were echinacea, ginseng, and St. John's wort.

Source: H. Newberry et al., "Use of Nonvitamin, Nonmineral Dietary Supplements among College Students," *Journal of American College Health* 50, no. 3 (2001): 123–29.

Herbal remedies are not to be taken lightly. Just because something is natural does not necessarily mean that it is safe. For example, in recent years, the FDA has warned that certain herbal products containing kava may be associated with severe liver damage.[32] Even rigorously tested products can be risky. Many plants are poisonous, and some can be toxic if ingested in high doses. Others may be dangerous when combined with prescription or over-the-counter drugs, or they could disrupt the normal action of the drugs.[33] Properly trained herbalists and homeopaths have received graduate-level training in special programs such as herbal nutrition or traditional Chinese medicine. These practitioners have been trained in diagnosis; in mixing herbs, titrations, and dosages; and in the follow-up care of patients.

> Do herbal remedies have any risks or side effects?

Herbal remedies come in several different forms. **Tinctures** (extracts of fresh or dried plants) usually contain a high percentage of grain alcohol to prevent spoilage and are among the best herbal options. Freeze-dried extracts are very stable and offer good value for your money. Standardized extracts, often available in pill or capsule form, are also among the more reliable forms of herbal preparations.

In general, herbal medicines tend to be milder than chemical drugs and produce their effects more slowly; they also

tinctures Herbal extracts usually combined with grain alcohol to prevent spoilage.

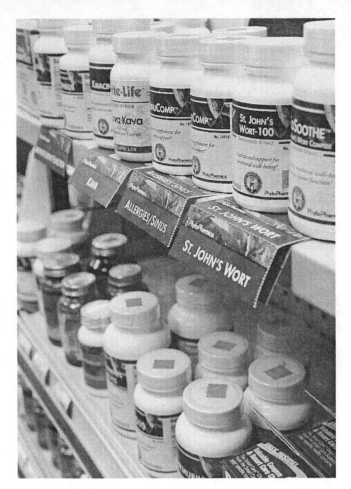

Buying herbal supplements can be confusing because so many brands exist and their manufacture is not strictly regulated for potency and quality.

are much less likely to cause toxicity because they are diluted rather than concentrated forms of drugs. But diluted or not, herbals are still drugs. No matter how natural they are, herbs still contain many of the same chemicals as synthetic prescription drugs. Too much of any herb, particularly one from nonstandardized extracts, can cause problems. Some herbs and specific dietary supplements can interact with prescription drugs or cause unusual side effects.

The following discussion gives an overview of some of the most common herbal supplements on the market.

Ginkgo Biloba

Ginkgo biloba is an extract from the leaves of a deciduous tree that lives up to 1,000 years. Chinese herbal medicine has used ginkgo leaves and seeds for medicinal purposes for centuries.[34] Today, ginkgo leaf extracts are widely prescribed in many countries and gaining in popularity.

Gingko biloba is said to have many benefits and is used to treat depression, impotence, premenstrual syndrome, diseases of the eye (such as retinopathy and macular degeneration), and general vascular disease. Though there is no definitive verdict on the benefits of gingko, numerous studies have been carried out for a variety of conditions. Some promising results have been seen for Alzheimer's disease and dementia, and research continues to determine the effect on its ability to enhance memory, reduce the incidence of cardiovascular disease, and decrease the rate of premature death. NCCAM is also looking at potential interactions between ginkgo and prescription drugs.[35]

Most nutritional experts and physicians recommend that people who are considering using ginkgo take a 40-milligram tablet three times a day for a month or so to determine whether there is any improvement. If there is none, continuing to take this supplement is largely unwarranted. It has been shown to cause gastric irritation, headache, nausea, dizziness, and allergic reactions. Also, remember that disturbing memory loss or difficulty thinking, regardless of age, should be discussed with a physician to determine underlying causes. Gingko should not be taken by people who are taking blood thinners or are otherwise at risk for bleeding.

Today, much of what we know about ginkgo biloba remains controversial, even though extensive research on its effects has been conducted. Until the results of these tests are available, consumers should use caution in any use of ginkgo.

St. John's Wort

The bright yellow, star-shaped flowers of St. John's wort (SJW) have a rich and varied history in Europe, Asia, and Africa. In the United States, SJW grows in abundance in northern California and southern Oregon and is also called *klammath weed*.

Today, SJW enjoys global popularity. It is the favored therapy for depression in a number of countries, including Germany, actually surpassing most standard antidepressants as the first mode of treatment for clinical depression. Research into the herb has yielded mixed results: some studies have indicated it is more effective than a placebo and has fewer side effects than prescription antidepressants, whereas others have found no effect on depression at all.[36]

NCCAM has published the following summary points about SJW:[37]

- There is some scientific evidence that St. John's wort is useful for treating mild to moderate depression. However, two large studies, one sponsored by NCCAM, showed that the herb was no more effective than placebo in treating major depression of moderate severity.
- Research shows that St. John's wort interacts with some drugs, including antidepressants, anticoagulants, and birth control pills.
- It is important to remember that St. John's wort is not a proven therapy for depression. If depression is not adequately treated, it can become severe. Anyone who may have depression should see a health care provider. There are effective, proven therapies available.

Like other plants, SJW contains a number of different chemicals, many of which are not clearly understood. The herb also has several side effects. Most are more bothersome than severe and range from slight gastrointestinal upset to fatigue, dry mouth, anxiety, sexual dysfunction, dizziness, skin rashes, and itching. Some people develop extreme sensitivity to sunlight.

Due to conflicting news about SJW, consumers should proceed with caution. Because the herb is sold in the United

States as a dietary supplement, not a drug, it has not been regulated by the FDA, and rigorous testing has not been done (see Chapter 7 for further information on the FDA's role in approving prescription and over-the-counter drugs). Anyone suffering from clinical depression should be under a physician's and psychologist's care. In addition, SJW should never be taken in combination with prescription antidepressants. When combined with other serotonin-enhancing drugs, such as Prozac and other selective serotonin reuptake inhibitors (SSRIs), SJW may result in serotonin overload, leading to tremors, agitation, or convulsions. SJW also should not be used by pregnant women or women who are nursing, by young children, or by the frail elderly, because the safety margins have not been established.[38]

Echinacea Echinacea, or the *purple coneflower,* is found primarily in the Midwest and prairie regions of the United States. Two of the nine species of *Echinacea* in the United States are now on the federal endangered species list, a cause of growing concern for many environmentalists as the herb's popularity has grown. Believed to be used extensively by Native Americans for centuries, echinacea eventually gained widespread acceptance in the United States before being shipped to Europe, where its use grew gradually over the eighteenth and nineteenth centuries.

Today, echinacea is the best-selling herb in the United States and is widely used throughout most of the world. It is said to stimulate the immune system and increase the effectiveness of the white blood cells that attack bacteria and viruses. Many people believe it to be helpful in preventing and treating the symptoms of a cold or flu.

Will echinacea teas and cough drops cure my cold?

However, echinacea remains controversial. Many studies in Europe have provided preliminary evidence of its effectiveness, but a 2005 controlled study in the United States indicated that echinacea is no more effective than a placebo in preventing or treating a cold.[39] As with many herbal treatments, little valid research has been conducted on the benefits and risks of echinacea. Because it can affect the immune system, people with autoimmune diseases such as arthritis should not take it. Other people who should avoid echinacea include pregnant women, people with diabetes or multiple sclerosis, and anyone allergic to the daisy family of plants.[40] Some studies have also raised concerns about increased risks for people who take echinacea before organ transplants.[41]

Ginseng Grown commercially throughout North America, ginseng is much prized for its reported sexual restorative value. It is believed that ginseng affects the pituitary gland, increasing resistance to stress, affecting metabolism, aiding skin and muscle tone, and providing the hormonal balance necessary for a healthy sex life. Other purported benefits include improvement in endurance, muscle strength, recovery from exercise, oxygen metabolism during exercise, auditory and visual reaction time, and mental concentration. To date, these benefits have not been scientifically validated.[42]

However, studies have raised questions about the appropriate dosages. Because the potency of plants varies considerably, dosage is difficult to control, and side effects are fairly common. Noteworthy side effects of high doses of ginseng include nervousness, insomnia, high blood pressure, headaches, skin eruptions, chest pain, depression, and abnormal vaginal bleeding.[43]

Green Tea Although some studies have shown promising links between consumption of green and white tea and cancer prevention, recent research questions the ability of tea to significantly reduce the risk of breast, lung, or prostate cancers.[44] At the same time, other research suggests that drinking two to three cups of green tea per day may reduce the risk of heart attack and hypertension and bolster immune function.[45] Some scientists suspect that green tea may boost heart health because it contains high levels of flavonoids (see the Health Headlines box on flavonoids in Chapter 12). These plant compounds, which are also found in fruits, vegetables, and red wine, are thought to promote health by combating oxidation, a process in which cell-damaging free radicals accumulate. Oxidative damage can be caused by outside factors, such as cigarette smoking, or by factors on the cellular level. Oxidation is suspected to increase the risk of heart disease, stroke, and several other diseases. Although the possibilities are promising, more research on the role of green tea must be conducted to determine whether its perceived benefits are actually due to the tea or to some other characteristic that tea drinkers have in common.

Ephedra (Ma Huang) An herbal ingredient formerly found in many weight loss and fitness supplements, ephedra's active ingredient is ephedrine, which is similar to amphetamine. Comprehensive research has found that ephedra has only limited effects on weight loss and athletic performance, but numerous adverse effects, including heart attack, stroke, and death. Other side effects such as heart palpitations, psychiatric problems, upper gastrointestinal effects, tremor, and insomnia were also noted.[46] In 2004, the FDA banned the sale of all supplements containing ephedra. These products are no longer legally available for sale in the United States.

Special Supplements

Not all the supplements on the market today are directly derived from plant sources. In recent years, there have been increasing reports in the media on the health benefits of various vitamins, minerals, amino acids, and other specific biological compounds.

When taken to increase work output or the potential for it, dietary supplements are labeled as **ergogenic aids.**

ergogenic aids Special dietary supplements taken to increase strength, energy, and the ability to work.

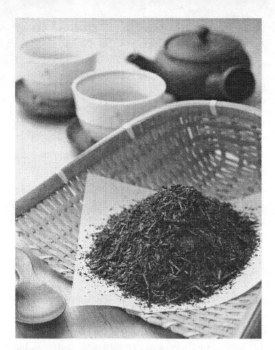

Green tea has become popular in recent years for its antioxidant properties and for its purported value in preventing cancer.

Examples include bee pollen, caffeine, glycine, carnitine, lecithin, brewer's yeast, and gelatin. In recent years, a new generation of performance-enhancing ergogenic aids has hit the market. Many of these claim to increase muscular strength and performance, boost energy, and enhance resistance to disease.

Muscle Enhancers Androstenedione ("andro"), a substance that is found naturally in meat and some plants and is also produced in the human body by the adrenal glands and gonads, is a precursor to the human hormone testosterone. In other words, the body converts andro directly into testosterone, which enables an athlete to train harder and recover more quickly. Andro has a chemical structure similar to that of anabolic steroids. When taken over time and in sufficient quantities, andro may increase the risk of serious medical conditions. Andro is no longer available over the counter.

Creatine is a naturally occurring compound found primarily in skeletal muscle that helps to optimize the muscles' energy levels. In recent years, the use of creatine supplements has increased dramatically because of claims that it increases muscle energy and allows a person to work harder with less muscle fatigue and to build muscle mass with less effort. Reports of creatine's benefits, however, appear exag-

gerated. Over one-third of people taking creatine are unable to absorb it into their muscles and thus achieve no benefit. Side effects include muscle cramping, muscle strains, and possible liver and kidney damage.[47]

Glucosamine Glucosamine is a substance produced by the body that plays a key role in the growth and development of cartilage. When present in sufficient amounts, it stimulates the manufacture of substances necessary for proper joint function and joint repair. It is manufactured commercially and sold under a variety of different names, usually glucosamine sulfate.

Glucosamine has been shown to be effective for treating osteoarthritis and for related degenerative joint diseases and appears to relieve swelling and decrease pain. Unlike many other herbal supplements, glucosamine sulfate has a good safety record with few noteworthy side effects. However, questions about its effectiveness have arisen in recent years. Although results of meta-analysis reviews and industry-sponsored research have shown glucosamine sulfate to be moderately effective, smaller independent studies have shown no significant benefits. The results of a large study, the Glucosamine Arthritis Intervention Trial, indicate that a combination of glucosamine and chondroitin sulfate appear to alleviate moderate to severe pain associated with osteoarthritis of the knee.[48]

SAMe SAMe (pronounced "Sammy") is the nickname for S-adenosyl-L-methionine, a compound produced biochemically in all humans to help perform some 40 functions in the body, ranging from bone preservation (hence its purported osteoarthritis benefits) to DNA replication.

SAMe has been reported to have a significant effect on mild to moderate depression without many of the side effects of prescription medications, such as sexual dysfunction, weight gain, and sleep disturbance. Scientists speculate that SAMe somehow affects brain levels of the neurotransmitters noradrenaline, serotonin, and possibly dopamine, all of which are related to the human stress response and the origins of depression in the body. Questions still remain over how much SAMe a person should take, in what form it should be administered, and whether there are long-term side effects such as liver toxicity or cancer.[49]

Antioxidants Although covered in depth in Chapter 9, it should be noted here that vitamins and minerals known to be antioxidants are among the most sought-after supplements on the market. Primary antioxidants include beta-carotene, selenium, vitamin C, and vitamin E. **Table 14.1** lists some other popular supplements with their associated risks and benefits.

Foods as Healing Agents

In Chapter 9, we discussed *functional foods*—foods or supplements designed to improve some aspect of physical or mental functioning. Sometimes referred to as **nutraceuticals**

nutraceuticals Term often used interchangeably with *functional foods*; refers to the combined nutritional and pharmaceutical benefit derived through use of foods or food supplements.

TABLE 14.1 Common Herbal, Vitamin, and Mineral Supplements: Benefits versus Risks

Supplement	Claims of Benefits	Potential Risks
Chondroitin (protein found in animal cartilage)	Improves osteoporosis and arthritis by improving cartilage function	Fewer benefits than glucosamine; benefits still unproven
Dehydroepiandrosterone (DHEA) (hormone)	Fights aging, boosts immunity, strengthens bones, and improves brain functioning	No antiaging benefits proven; could increase cancer risk and lead to liver damage, even when taken briefly
Dieter's teas, (e.g., herbal blends containing senna, aloe, rhubarb root, buckthorn, cascara, or castor oil)	Act as laxatives	Can disrupt potassium levels and cause heart arrhythmias; linked to diarrhea, vomiting, chronic constipation, fainting
Flaxseed (herb)	Used as a laxative and for hot flashes and breast pain; flaxseed oil is used for different conditions, including arthritis; both flaxseed and flaxseed oil have been used for high cholesterol levels and in an effort to prevent cancer	Delays absorption of medicine
Vitamin E (vitamin)	Antioxidant effect; reduces risk of heart disease; better chance of survival after heart attack	High-doses cause bleeding when taking blood thinners
Kava (herb)	Relaxation; relief of anxiety, insomnia, and menopausal symptoms; sometimes used topically as a numbing agent	Increases the effect of alcohol and other drugs; causes drowsiness; associated with severe liver damage
L-Carnitine (amino acid derivative)	Improves metabolism in heart muscle, purported to increase fat-burning enzymes; also used to combat fatigue and aging	Nausea, vomiting, abdominal cramps, diarrhea, "fishy" body odor; more rarely, muscle weakness in uremic patients and seizures in patients with seizure disorders; interacts with some medications
Licorice root (herb)	Reduces inflammation; used for stomach ulcers, bronchitis, and sore throat, as well as infections caused by viruses	Speeds potassium loss; may contribute to high blood pressure
Melatonin (hormone)	Used to regulate circadian rhythms and sleep patterns and to treat insomnia; claims of antiaging benefits	May cause nausea, headaches, dizziness, blood vessel constriction; possibly a danger for people with high blood pressure or other cardiovascular problems; no scientific support for antiaging claims.
Valerian (herb)	Relaxation; used for sleep disorders and anxiety; also used for headaches, depression, irregular heartbeat, and trembling	Mild side effects, such as headaches, dizziness, upset stomach, and tiredness the morning after use
Zinc (mineral)	Supports immune system; used to lessen duration and severity of cold symptoms; aids wound healing	Excessive intake associated with reduced immune function, reduced levels of high-density lipoproteins ("good" cholesterol)

Source: Office of Dietary Supplements, National Institutes of Health, "Dietary Supplement Fact Sheets," 2007, http://ods.od.nih.gov/ Health_Information/Information_About_Individual_Dietary_Supplements.aspx; National Center for Complementary and Alternative Medicine, "Herbs at a Glance," 2007, http://nccam.nih.gov/health/herbsataglance.htm.

for their combined nutritional and pharmaceutical benefit, several are believed to work in much the same way as pharmaceutical drugs in making a person well or bolstering the immune system.

The following are some of the most common healthful foods and their purported benefits:[50]

- *Plant sterol.* Can lower "bad" (LDL) cholesterol.
- *Oat fiber.* Can lower LDL cholesterol; serves as a natural soother of nerves; stabilizes blood sugar levels.
- *Sunflower.* Can lower risk of heart disease; may prevent angina.

- *Soy protein.* May lower heart disease risk by reducing LDL cholesterol and triglycerides.
- *Garlic.* Lowers cholesterol and reduces clotting tendency of blood; lowers blood pressure; may serve as form of antibiotic.
- *Ginger.* May prevent motion sickness, stomach pain, and stomach upset; discourages blood clots; may relieve rheumatism.
- *Yogurt.* Yogurt that is labeled "Live Active Culture" contains active, friendly bacteria that can fight off infections.

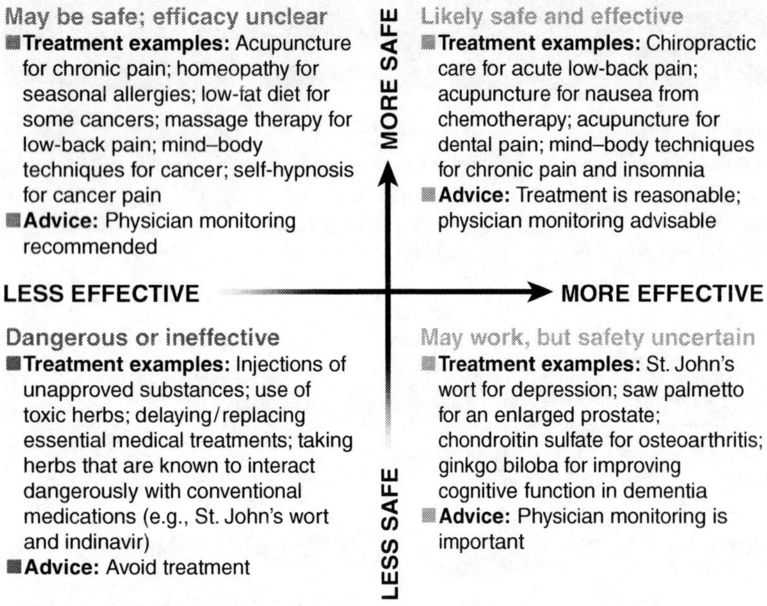

FIGURE 14.3 Assessing the Risks and Benefits of CAM Treatments

Medical experts devised this chart to gauge the potential liability of recommending alternative treatments, but by categorizing treatments according to their relative safety and effectiveness, it can also help patients and consumers make appropriate choices.

Source: M. H. Cohen and D. M. Eisenberg, "Potential Physician Malpractice Liability Associated with Complementary and Integrative Medical Therapies," *Annals of Internal Medicine* 136, no. 8 (2002): 596–603. Copyright © 2002 American College of Physicians. Used with permission.

May be safe; efficacy unclear
- **Treatment examples:** Acupuncture for chronic pain; homeopathy for seasonal allergies; low-fat diet for some cancers; massage therapy for low-back pain; mind–body techniques for cancer; self-hypnosis for cancer pain
- **Advice:** Physician monitoring recommended

Likely safe and effective
- **Treatment examples:** Chiropractic care for acute low-back pain; acupuncture for nausea from chemotherapy; acupuncture for dental pain; mind–body techniques for chronic pain and insomnia
- **Advice:** Treatment is reasonable; physician monitoring advisable

MORE SAFE / LESS SAFE / LESS EFFECTIVE / MORE EFFECTIVE

Dangerous or ineffective
- **Treatment examples:** Injections of unapproved substances; use of toxic herbs; delaying/replacing essential medical treatments; taking herbs that are known to interact dangerously with conventional medications (e.g., St. John's wort and indinavir)
- **Advice:** Avoid treatment

May work, but safety uncertain
- **Treatment examples:** St. John's wort for depression; saw palmetto for an enlarged prostate; chondroitin sulfate for osteoarthritis; ginkgo biloba for improving cognitive function in dementia
- **Advice:** Physician monitoring is important

Protecting Consumers and Regulating Claims

Although many CAM procedures and products appear promising, be aware that most of them are not currently regulated in the United States as strictly as are food, drugs, and Western medical procdures. Supplement regulation in particular is in sharp contrast to nations such as Germany, where the government holds companies to strict standards for ingredients and manufacturing. In the United States, new FDA regulatory controls are just starting to take place. While FDA regulations of supplements are being phased in and until other regulations of CAM are in place, it is important to have as much information as possible to make a smart decision when evaluating CAM options (**Figure 14.3**). Evaluate your supplement savvy with the **Assess Yourself** exercise on page 496.

Strategies to Protect Supplement Consumers' Health

The burgeoning popularity of herbal supplements and nutraceuticals concerns many scientists. Though some alternative therapies, such as acupuncture, have been widely studied, there is little quality research to support the many claims that are made for nutraceuticals. Two good places to start your own research if you are considering the use of herbal supplements or functional foods are the websites for NCCAM (http://nccam.nih.gov) and the Cochrane Collaboration's review on complementary and alternative medicine (www.cochrane.org).

As mentioned in Chapter 9, herbal supplements and functional foods can currently be sold without FDA approval. This raises issues of consumer safety to new lev-

els. Even when products are dispensed by CAM practitioners, the situation can be risky. Unfortunately, some unskilled and untrained people, who do not fully understand the potential chemical interactions of their preparations, are treating patients.

Consumer groups, scientists, and government officials are calling for action. Pressure has mounted to establish consistent standards for herbal supplements and functional foods similar to those used in Germany and other countries. Many scientists have advocated a more stringent FDA approval process for supplements sold in the United States. As a result, the FDA has instituted new regulations to oversee the manufacture of dietary supplements, including herbal supplements. These new regulations require manufacturers to evaluate the identity, purity, strength, and composition of the supplements to ensure they contain what the label claims. However, these regulations are in the process of being phased in by June 2010,[51] and many supplements are currently not tested. The official public standards-setting authority for all medicines, supplements, and other health care products manufactured and sold in the United States is the U.S. Pharmacopeia, which currently tests select products, including herbal supplements, to comply with safety and purity standards. Products that meet these standards display a "USP Dietary Supplement Verified" seal.[52]

Looking to Science for More Answers

Even as CAM treatments gain credibility, this credibility must be tempered with good science. The NCCAM has established research centers at universities and other institutions throughout the United States, where many clinical trials are being conducted.[53] Numerous other studies into alternative treatments such as acupuncture, green tea, fish oil, flaxseed, shark cartilage, and others are taking place across the United States. One of the most promising aspects of this research is the enthusiastic support of professionals who have the training and laboratory expertise to evaluate the efficacy of market-driven claims.

what do you THINK?

Why do you think the government has not acted more aggressively to regulate herbal and other dietary supplements? ■ Why are many CAM treatments not covered under typical insurance plans?

Healthy Living in the New Millennium

Clearly, CAM appears to serve a very real need for consumers. But while consumers are making the adjustment to CAM in record numbers, members of the health care delivery system seem slow to act. Although progress has been noted, there is still a long way to go before CAM therapies become fully accepted in mainstream medical practice.

Enlisting Support from Insurers and Providers

More and more insurers are hiring alternative practitioners or covering alternative care, at least to some degree. This is especially true as criticisms of managed care increase and government agencies get involved.

Today, nearly all health insurance providers cover at least one form of CAM, with acupuncture and massage therapy the most common. The changing nature of HMOs and health care insurers makes it impossible to determine exactly how many companies cover CAM therapies today. In spite of this progress, many patients will continue to pay out-of-pocket for alternative therapies until the scientific evidence supporting these alternative medical care choices is impossible to ignore. What is known is that the numbers are increasing despite a reimbursement system that is biased in favor of traditional treatments.

Support from professional organizations, such as the American Medical Association, is also increasing as more physician training programs require or offer electives in alternative treatment modalities. In many cases, medical schools are educating a new generation of medical doctors to be better prepared to advise patients about the pros and cons of alternative treatments and how to follow integrative practices. Although alternative medicine is becoming increasingly integrated into today's health care programs and plans, there is still a long way to go. As we learn more, we will be better able to apply both traditional and alternative care.

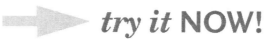

try it NOW!

What kinds of CAM resources are available to you? Check with your college's health clinic to find out what types of alternative therapies are offered. Acupuncture? Massage for back injuries? Chiropractor visits? Or, check with your health insurance provider to see what is covered. Ask what expenses you'll be responsible for and whether you are limited to a certain network of practitioners.

Self-Care: Protecting Yourself

Today we are faced with an exciting array of possible health choices. To help you make the best decisions, consider these pointers and refer to the **Consumer Health** box on page 498 on evaluating Internet resources.

■ Take charge of your health by being an informed consumer. Find out what scientific studies have been done on the safety and effectiveness of the CAM treatment in which you are interested. Consult only reliable sources—texts, journals, periodicals, and government resources. Start with the websites listed at the end of this and every chapter.

■ Remember that decisions about treatment should be made in consultation with your health care provider and should be based on your own condition and needs. If you use any CAM therapy, including herbal supplements, inform your primary health care provider. This is particularly important if you are thinking about replacing or augmenting your prescribed treatment with one or more supplements, are currently taking a prescription drug, have a chronic medical condition, are planning to have surgery, are pregnant or nursing, or are thinking about giving supplements to children or pets.

■ If you use a CAM therapy provided by a practitioner, such as acupuncture, choose the practitioner with care. Check with your insurer to see whether the services will be covered.

■ Remember that *natural* and *safe* are not necessarily synonyms. Many people have become seriously ill from seemingly harmless "natural" products. Be cautious about combining herbal medications, just as you should be cautious about combining other drugs. Seek help if you notice any unusual side effects.

■ Realize that no one is closely monitoring the purity of herbal supplements. Also recognize that dosage levels in many herbal products are in the process of getting regulated. Look for the word *standardized* or the "USP Dietary Supplement Verified" seal on any herbal product you buy, and look for reputable manufacturers. German manufacturers produce identical batches of herbal remedies as required by law.

As we enter a new era of medicine, more than ever you are being called on to take responsibility for what goes into your body. This means you must educate yourself. CAM can offer new avenues toward better health, but it is up to you to make sure that you are on the right path.

Fill out this assessment online at www.aw-bc.com/myhealthlab or www.aw-bc.com/donatelle.

Like millions of Americans, you may already be taking an herbal or nutritional supplement every day. Though supplements can often be beneficial, many people take them without knowing enough to ensure their safety and best results.

Take this quiz to assess your supplement savvy; indicate that you believe the following items are true or false by checking the corresponding box. Then consult the answer key that follows.

	True	False
1. If I don't eat a balanced, varied diet to get all the important nutrients my body needs, I may need to take a multivitamin.	☐	☐
2. Taking supplements is a good idea, because even if a product isn't helpful, it isn't likely to be harmful.	☐	☐
3. There isn't any difference between brand name and generic brand supplements.	☐	☐
4. Natural herbs and supplements are superior to synthetic supplements and worth the extra cost.	☐	☐
5. The term *natural* on a supplement package means that the product is healthful and safe.	☐	☐
6. The expiration dates on supplements are not important.	☐	☐
7. When buying supplements, I should choose those with the USP (United States Pharmacopeia) seal on their labels.	☐	☐
8. I should choose a vitamin-mineral combination limited to 100% of the Daily Value of each nutrient.	☐	☐
9. If I am a vegetarian who eliminates all animal products from my diet, I may need additional vitamin B_{12} and other nutrient supplements.	☐	☐
10. There is no reason for me to consult a physician before taking a supplement.	☐	☐
11. Any potentially dangerous supplement product is required to have cautionary information on the label.	☐	☐
12. A recall of a harmful product guarantees that all such harmful products will be immediately and completely removed from the marketplace.	☐	☐
13. Most adults do not get all the calcium they need to prevent osteoporosis from their diets alone.	☐	☐
14. If older people took a multivitamin with minerals each day, they could reduce the total number of days they are sick from infectious disease by 50 percent.	☐	☐
15. Fewer than 10 percent of Americans use dietary supplements.	☐	☐

Scoring Key

1. *True.* On average, fewer than 10 percent of Americans regularly meet the Recommended Dietary Allowances (RDAs) for most of the 18 vitamins and minerals for which RDAs have been established. Those who eat a balanced and varied diet that includes 2 cups of fruits and 2 1/2 cups of vegetables per day probably do not need vitamin supplements.

2. *False.* When consumed in high enough amounts, for a long enough time, or in combination with certain other substances, all chemicals can be toxic, including nutrients, plant components, and other biologically active ingredients.

3. *True.* Experts say that generic brands are just as effective, and they are usually cheaper.

4. *False.* There's no general difference between synthetic and natural supplements.

5. *False.* The term *natural* on labels is not well defined and is sometimes used ambiguously to imply unsubstantiated benefits or safety. For example, many weight-loss products claim to be "natural" or "herbal," but this doesn't necessarily make them safe. Their ingredients may interact with drugs or may be dangerous for people with certain medical conditions.

6. *False.* Supplements do have expiration dates, and it is important to check the expiration date and to look for supplements with an expiration date that's at least 1 year away.

7. *True.* The FDA regulations are in the process of being implemented, so the USP symbol is the best current way to tell whether the supplement has been tested and dissolves properly in the body.

8. *True.* The higher the dosage of certain vitamins and minerals, the more likely you are to have side effects or interactions with other medications you might be taking.

9. *True.* Fortified cereals are also a good source of vitamin B_{12} for vegetarians who consume no meats, eggs, or dairy products.

10. *False.* Supplements can interact with prescription medications, so telling your doctor what you intend to take can help him or her check for such interactions.

11. *False.* Dietary supplement manufacturers may not necessarily include warnings about potential adverse effects on the labels of their products. If consumers want to know about the safety of a specific dietary supplement, they should contact the manufacturer of that brand directly.

12. *False.* A product recall of a dietary supplement is voluntary, and although many manufacturers do their best, a recall does not necessarily remove all harmful products from the marketplace.

13. *True.* Because of the diet they choose, most American adults need to take a calcium supplement to get the recommended 1,000 to 1,200 mg of calcium daily.

14. *True.* Research has shown that regular use of a multivitamin with minerals by older people can significantly boost their immune function—and cut the number of days they are sick from infectious illness in half. This may be due to the fact that individuals over 65 may not absorb vitamins B_6 and B_{12} nutrients as well as the bodies of younger people and that older peoples' bodies do not manufacture as much vitamin D.

15. *False.* National surveys indicate that about half of all Americans use dietary supplements. Research shows that people who take supplements tend to have better diets and generally healthier habits than those who don't. They also tend to have higher levels of both education and income.

Interpreting Your Score

First, add up the number of items you got right. The higher your score, the better your knowledge of the potential risks and benefits of herbal and other dietary supplements. Any incorrect responses may indicate areas of supplement use that you need to learn more about to be an informed consumer. Ultimately, you are the one most responsible for your own health and safety, so think about ways to increase your awareness and understanding of the supplement products you consume.

Sources: D. Sinovic, "Choosing and Using Supplements," Meriter Healthy Living, Created for Wellness Library, 2006, http://meriter .staywellsolutionsonline.com/InteractiveTools/Quizzes/ 40,SupplementsVitaminsMQuiz; Council for Responsible Nutrition, "The Benefits of Nutritional Supplements Test Your Supplement Savvy," 2007, www.crnusa.org/benpdfs/CRN00benefits_quiz.pdf; U.S. Food and Drug Administration, Center for Food Safety and Applied Nutrition, "Tips For The Savvy Supplement User: Making Informed Decisions And Evaluating Information, 2002, www.cfsan.fda.gov/~dms/ ds-savvy.html.

MAKE it happen!

ASSESSMENT: The Assess Yourself activity gave you the chance to test your knowledge of health effects related to nutritional supplements. Now that you have reviewed your results, you can decide whether you need to consult your physician about taking supplements for health benefits.

MAKING A CHANGE: To change your behavior, you need to develop a plan. Follow these steps below and complete your Behavior Change Contract to take action.

1. Evaluate your behavior, and identify patterns and specific things you are doing. What can you change now? What can you change in the near future?

2. Select one pattern of behavior that you want to change.

3. Fill out the Behavior Change Contract found at the front of your book. It should include your long-term goals for change, your short-term goals, the rewards you'll give yourself for reaching these goals, potential obstacles along the way, and strategies for overcoming these obstacles. For each goal, list the small steps and specific actions that you will take.

4. Chart your progress in a journal. At the end of a week, consider how successful you were in following your plan. What helped you be successful? What made change more difficult? What will you do differently next week?

5. Revise your plan as needed. Are the short-term goals attainable? Are the rewards satisfying?

EXAMPLE: Andrea realized that she had little knowledge about the health benefits of natural supplements. She decided to keep track of her regular diet for a week and then evaluate the benefits of a multivitamin. She thought she was getting a balanced diet but was surprised to find that she was not getting the recommended amount of nutrients on a daily basis. She decided to consult her physician, who agreed that she could benefit from a multivitamin and also suggested she take a daily calcium supplement. With her doctor's approval, Andrea reviewed the chapter to find out how to select safe supplements. When she went shopping for the supplements, she looked for ones with the USP seal, carefully checked for the expiration date, and made sure the multivitamin did not exceed 100% of the RDA for the vitamins and minerals. She then read the label on how to safely take both the multivitamin and the calcium supplement. Her goal was to start taking both daily. When she is used to taking the multivitamin and calcium, Andrea is considering going back to her physician to discuss other natural supplements that might have health benefits for her.

EVALUATING COMPLEMENTARY AND ALTERNATIVE MEDICINE RESOURCES ON THE WEB

Planning to research CAM information online? The National Center for Complementary and Alternative Medicine recommends that you ask these questions about any website you visit.

1. *Who runs this site?* Any good health-related website should be clear about who is responsible for the site and its information, with the name of the site's sponsor and a link to its home page on every major page of the site.

2. *Who pays for the site?* How does the site pay for its existence? The source

> **How do I evaluate alternative medical resources for reliability?**

of its funding should be clearly stated or readily apparent. For example, Web addresses ending in ".gov" denote a federal government–sponsored site. Does the site sell advertising? Is it sponsored by a drug company? The source of funding can affect what content is chosen, how the information is presented, and what the site owners want to accomplish.

3. *What is the purpose of the site?* This question is related to who owns and pays for the site. An "About This Site" link appears on many sites; if it's there, use it. The purpose of the site should be clearly stated and should help you evaluate the trustworthiness of the information.

4. *Where does the information come from?* Many health and medical sites post information collected from other websites or sources. If the person or organization in charge of the site did not create the information, the

original source should be clearly identified.

5. *What is the basis of the information?* The site should describe the evidence that the material is based on. Medical facts and figures should have references (such as articles in medical journals). Also, opinions or advice should be clearly set apart from information that is evidence-based (that is, information based on research results).

6. *How is the information selected?* Is there an editorial board listed for the site? Do people with excellent professional and scientific qualifications review the material before it is posted?

7. *How current is the information?* Websites should be reviewed and updated on a regular basis. It is particularly important that medical information be current. The most recent update or review date should be clearly posted. Even if the information has not changed, you want to know whether the site owners have reviewed it recently to ensure that it is still valid.

8. *How does the site choose links to other sites?* Some websites take a conservative approach and don't link to any other sites. Some link to any site that asks—or pays—for a link. Others link only to sites that have met certain criteria.

9. *What information about you does the site collect, and why?* Websites routinely track the paths visitors take through their sites to determine which pages are being used. However, many health websites ask for you to "subscribe" or "become a member." In

some cases, the purpose of this request may be to collect a user fee or select information for you that is relevant to your concerns. In all cases, complying with this request will give the site personal information about you. Any credible health site asking for this kind of information should tell you exactly what will and will not be done with it. Many commercial sites sell data about their users to other companies—information such as what percentage of their users are women with breast cancer, for example. In some cases they may collect and reuse information that is "personally identifiable," such as your zip code, gender, and birth date. Be certain that you read and understand any privacy policy or similar language on the site, and don't sign up for anything that you do not fully understand.

10. *How does the site manage interactions with visitors?* There should always be a way for you to contact the site owner if you run across problems or have questions or feedback. If the site hosts chatrooms or other online discussion areas, it should tell visitors what the terms of using this service are. Is it moderated? If so, by whom, and why? It is always a good idea to spend time reading the discussion without joining in, so that you feel comfortable with the environment before becoming a participant.

Source: National Center for Complementary and Alternative Medicine, "Ten Things to Know about Evaluating Medical Resources on the Web," NCCAM Publication No. D337, 2006, http://nccam.nih.gov/health/webresources.

TAKING charge

Summary

- The National Center for Complementary and Alternative Medicine (NCCAM) groups complementary and alternative medicine (CAM) practices into four major domains: manipulative and body-based methods, energy medicine, mind–body medicine, and biologically based practices. Several alternative medical systems, including Ayurveda, traditional Chinese medicine, homeopathy, and naturopathy cut across all of these domains.

- Throughout the world people are choosing complementary and alternative medicine options in increasing numbers. Much of the influence of these CAM strategies may be traced to other cultures, particularly those that are part of traditional Chinese medicine, such as acupuncture, or Ayurvedic medicine, such as yoga.

- Herbal remedies include ginkgo biloba, St. John's wort, echinacea, ginseng, and green tea. Special supplements include muscle enhancers, ginseng, glucosamine, SAMe, and antioxidants. A number of functional foods may also serve as healing agents.

- Though many positive effects are associated with CAM, there are also many risks. As a consumer, you must be aware of the risks and check reputable sources to ensure that you are not being lured by false claims and promises.

- Health in the new millennium provides an interesting assortment of choices for health care consumers. By enlisting the support of health care professionals and health care services and by making informed decisions, you will reap positive rewards in your quest for health enhancement in the days ahead.

Chapter Review

1. Which of the following treatments is based on soft-tissue manipulation by trained therapists for healing purposes?
   a. acupuncture
   b. reiki
   c. psychoneuroimmunology
   d. massage therapy

2. What type of practitioner diagnoses by observation and touch and assigns patients to one of three body types?
   a. chiropractic practitioner
   b. naturopathic practitioner
   c. Ayurvedic practitioner
   d. homeopathic practitioner

3. The alternative system of medicine based on the principle that "like cures like" is
   a. naturopathic medicine.
   b. homeopathic medicine.
   c. Ayurvedic medicine.
   d. chiropractic medicine.

4. Chiropractic treatment is based on the theory that diseases can be caused by
   a. misalignment of the bones.
   b. poor eating habits.
   c. taking too many drugs.
   d. muscle atrophy.

5. The use of techniques to improve the psychoneuro-immunology of the human body is called
   a. acupressure.
   b. mind–body medicine.
   c. reiki.
   d. body work.

6. What alternative medicine system places equal emphasis on body, mind, and spirit and strives to restore the innate harmony of the individual?
   a. Ayurvedic medicine
   b. homeopathic medicine
   c. naturopathic medicine
   d. traditional Chinese medicine

7. What is the best-selling herbal remedy in health and natural food stores in the United States?
   a. green tea
   b. ginkgo biloba
   c. St. John's wort
   d. echinacea

8. Plant sterol, oat fiber, sunflower, and soy protein are examples of
   a. antioxidants.
   b. ergogenic aids.
   c. nutraceuticals.
   d. phytomedicines.

9. The energy therapy derived from the ancient technique of "laying on" of hands is
   a. reiki.
   b. qigong.
   c. therapeutic touch.
   d. acupressure.

10. The food that may fight motion sickness, stomach pain, and stomach upset and that discourages blood clots is
    a. garlic.
    b. ginger.
    c. sunflower.
    d. oat fiber.

Answers for these questions can be found on page A-1.

Questions for Discussion and Reflection

1. What are some of the potential benefits and risks of CAM? Why do you think these practices and products are becoming so popular?
2. What are the major domains of CAM treatments? Have you tried any of them? Would you feel comfortable trying any new ones? Why or why not?
3. What are the major herbal remedies? Special supplements? What are some of the risks and benefits associated with each?
4. What can you do to ensure that you are receiving accurate information regarding CAM treatments or medicines? Which federal agency oversees CAM in the United States?
5. What is being done in the United States to ensure continued growth of CAM?

Accessing Your Health on the Internet

The following websites explore further topics and issues related to personal health. For links to the websites below, visit the Companion Website for *Health: The Basics,* Eighth Edition at www.aw-bc.com/donatelle.

1 *National Center for Complementary and Alternative Medicine (NCCAM).* A division of the National Institutes of Health dedicated to providing the latest information on complementary and alternative practices, including NCCAM-funded centers of research on alternative medicine. http://nccam.nih.gov

2 *ClinicalTrials.gov.* Includes the latest information on CAM research and clinical trials. Search for results from NCCAM and complementary and alternative medicine. http://clinicaltrials.gov

3 *Acupuncture.com.* Provides resources for consumers regarding traditional Asian therapies; geared to students and practitioners. www.acupuncture.com

4 *National Institutes of Health, Office of Dietary Supplements.* An excellent resource for information on dietary supplements. Includes access to CARDS (Computer Access to Research on Dietary Supplements), a database of federally funded research projects pertaining to dietary supplements. http://dietary-supplements .info.nih.gov

Further Reading

Cuellar, N. *Conversations in Complementary and Alternative Medicine: Insights and Perspectives from a Leading Practitioner.* Sudbury, MA: Jones and Bartlett, 2006.

Based on interviews with 27 leading experts in CAM, including acupuncturists, chiropractors, massage therapists, and herbalists. Includes questions about practice, education, and research.

Rakel, D. *Complementary Medicine in Practice.* Sudbury, MA: Jones and Bartlett, 2006.

Evidence-based overview of common CAM therapies, particularly those supported by research and accepted by physicians and consumers.

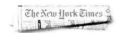

e-themes from *The New York Times*

For up-to-date articles about current health issues, visit
www.aw-bc.com/donatelle, select *Health: The Basics*, Eighth
Edition, Chapter 17, and click on "e-themes."

References

1. National Center for Complementary and Alternative Medicine, "What Is CAM?" 2007, http://nccam.nih.gov/health/whatiscam.
2. Mayo Clinic Staff, "Complementary and Alternative Medicine: What Is It?" Mayo Clinic, 2005, www.mayoclinic.com/health/alternative-medicine/PN00001.
3. H. A. Tindle et al., "Complementary and Alternative Medicine Used Widely by One Third of U.S. Adults Remains Unchanged from 1997," *Alternative Therapies in Health and Medicine* 11, no. 1 (2005): 42–49; National Institutes of Medicine, Board on Health Promotion and Disease Prevention, *Complementary and Alternative Medicine in the U.S.—2005* (Washington, DC: National Academies Press, 2005).
4. P. Barnes et al., "Complementary and Alternative Medicine Use Among Adults: United States, 2002," *CDC Advance Data Report* no. 343, May 27, 2004, http://nccam.nih.gov/news/camstats.htm.
5. Ibid.
6. J. Tsao, "Effectiveness of Massage Therapy for Chronic, Non-malignant Pain: A Review," *Evidence Based Complementary and Alternative Medicine* 4, no. 2 (2007): 165–79; American Medical Student Association, "EDCAM: CAM and Medical Education Report," 2007, www.amsa.org/humed/CAM/mededreport.cfm; National Cancer Institute, "Acupuncture: Human/Clinical Studies," 2007, www.cancer.gov/cancertopics/pdq/cam/acupuncture/HealthProfessional/page5.
7. Tindle et al., "Complementary and Alternative Medicine."
8. National Center for Complementary and Alternative Medicine, "A Closer Look at Ayurvedic Medicine," *CAM at the NIH: Focus on Complementary and Alternative Medicine* 12, no. 4 (2006), http://nccam.nih.gov/news/newsletter/2006_winter/ayurveda.htm.
9. National Center for Complementary and Alternative Medicine, "What Is Ayurvedic Medicine?" NCCAM Publication no. D287, 2007, http://nccam.nih.gov/health/ayurveda.
10. Ibid.
11. National Center for Complementary and Alternative Medicine, "Questions and Answers about Homeopathy," NCCAM Publication no. D183, 2003, http://nccam.nih.gov/health/homeopathy.
12. British Medical Association, "Complementary Medicine: New Approaches to Good Practice," 2006, www.bma.org.uk; P. DeSmet, "Herbal Medicine in Europe—Releasing Regulatory Standard," *New England Journal of Medicine*, 352 (2005) 1176–78; D. Sibbritt et al., "A Longitudinal Analysis of Mid-Age Women's Use of CAM in Australia," *Women's Health*, 40 (2004): 41–56.
13. National Center for Complementary and Alternative Medicine, "About Chiropractic and Its Use in Treating Low-Back Pain," NCCAM Publication no. D196, 2003, http://nccam.nih.gov/health/chiropractic.
14. Bureau of Labor Statistics, *U.S. Department of Labor, Occupational Outlook Handbook 2006–07 Edition*, "Chiropractors," 2006, www.bls.gov/oco/ocos071.htm.
15. Tsao, "Effectiveness of Massage Therapy."
16. National Center for Complementary and Alternative Medicine, "Massage Therapy as CAM," NCCAM Publication no. D327, 2006, http://nccam.nih.gov/health/massage.
17. Mayo Clinic Staff, "Massage: A Relaxing Method to Relieve Stress and Pain" Mayo Clinic, 2006, www.mayoclinic.com/health/massage/SA00082; National Center for Complementary and Alternative Medicine, "Massage Therapy as CAM."
18. National Center for Complementary and Alternative Medicine, "Massage Therapy as CAM."
19. Bureau of Labor Statistics, *U.S. Department of Labor, Occupational Outlook Handbook 2006–07 Edition*, "Massage Therapists," 2006, www.bls.gov/oco/ocos295.htm.
20. National Center for Complementary and Alternative Medicine, "Manipulative and Body Based Practices: An Overview," NCCAM Publication no. D238, 2007, http://nccam.nih.gov/health/backgrounds/manipulative.htm; United States Trager Association, "The Trager Approach," 2007, www.trager-us.org/the_trager_approach.html.
21. National Center for Complementary and Alternative Medicine, "Energy Medicine: An Overview," NCCAM Publication no. D235, 2007, http://nccam.nih.gov/health/backgrounds/energymed.htm.
22. Ibid.
23. Ibid.
24. Ibid.
25. National Institutes of Health Consensus Panel, "Acupuncture: National Institutes of Health Consensus Development Panel Statement," 2006, http://consensus.nih.gov; B. Berman et al., "Effectiveness of Acupuncture as Adjunct Therapy in Osteoarthritis of the Knee: A Randomized, Controlled Trial," *Annals of Internal Medicine* 141, no. 12 (2004): 901–10; C. Karels et al., "Treatment of Arm, Neck and Shoulder Complaints," *Spine* 31, no. 17 (2006): E584-E589.
26. National Center for Complementary and Alternative Medicine, "Acupuncture," NCCAM Publication no. D003, 2004, http://nccam.nih.gov/health/acupuncture.
27. K. Pelletier and D. Herzing, "Psychoneuroimmunology: Toward a Mind–Body Model, *Advances* 5, no. 1 (1988): 27–56, as cited in B. Seaward, *Managing Stress*, 5th ed. (Sudbury, MA: Jones and Bartlett, 2006), 51.
28. J. Robins et al., "Research in Psychoneuroimmunology: Tai Chi as a Stress Management Approach for Individuals with HIV Disease," *Applied Nursing Research* 19, no. 1 (2006): 2–9; M. Opp et al., "Sleep and Psychoneuroimmunology," *Neurology Clinician* 24, no. 3 (2006): 493–506; A. Starkweather et al., "Immune Function, Pain and Psychological Stress in Patients Undergoing Spinal Surgery," *Spine* 31, no. 18 (2006): E641-E647.
29. National Center for Complementary and Alternative Medicine, "Mind-Body Medicine: An Overview," NCCAM Publication no. D239, 2007, http://nccam.nih.gov/health/backgrounds/mindbody.htm.
30. Office of Dietary Supplements, National Institutes of Health, "Dietary Supplements: Background Information," 2006, http://ods.od.nih.gov/factsheets/dietarysupplements.asp.
31. National Center for Complementary and Alternative Medicine, "Biologically Based Practices: An Overview," NCCAM Publication no. D237, 2007, http://nccam.nih.gov/health/backgrounds/biobasedprac.htm.

32. National Center for Complementary and Alternative Medicine, "Consumer Advisory: Kava Linked to Liver Damage," modified July 2007, http://nccam.nih.gov/health/alerts/kava.

33. E. Ernst, "Herbal Remedies for Anxiety: A Systematic Review of Controlled Clinical Trials," *Phytomedicine* 13, no. 3 (2006): 205–208.

34. University of Maryland Medical Center, "Ginkgo Biloba," 2006, www.umm.edu/altmed/articles/ginkgo-biloba-000247.htm.

35. National Center for Complementary and Alternative Medicine, "Herbs at a Glance: Ginkgo," NCCAM Publication no. D290, 2005, http://nccam.nih.gov/health/ginkgo.

36. National Center for Complementary and Alternative Medicine, "St. John's Wort (*Hypericum perforatum*) and the Treatment of Depression," NCCAM Publication no. D005, 2004, http://nccam.nih.gov/health/stjohnswort/sjwataglance.htm.

37. Ibid.

38. Ibid.

39. R. Turner et al., "An Evaluation of Echinacea in Experimental Rhinovirus Infections," *New England Journal of Medicine* 353, no. 4 (2005): 341–48.

40. University of Maryland Medical Center, "Echinacea," 2006, www.umm.edu/altmed/articles/echinacea-000239.htm.

41. Ibid.

42. T. Palisin at al., "Ginseng: Is It in the Root?" *Current Sports Medicine Report* 5, no. 4 (2006): 210–14.

43. Ibid.

44. U.S. Food and Drug Administration, "FDA Issues Information for Consumers about Claims for Green Tea and Certain Cancers," 2005, www.fda.gov/bbs/topics/NEWS/2005/NEW01197.html.

45. C. Cabrera et al., "Beneficial Effects of Green Tea: A Review," *Journal of American College Nutrition* 25, no. 2 (2006): 79–99.

46. Mayo Clinic Staff, "Ephedra (*Ephedra sinica*/Ma huang)" Mayo Clinic, 2006, Mayo Clinic, www.mayoclinic.com/health/ephedra/NS_patient-ephedra.

47. Natural Standard Research Collaboration, "Creatine," Medline Plus, www.nlm.nih.gov/medlineplus/druginfo/natural/patient-creatine.html.

48. D. Clegg et al., "Glucosamine, Chondriotin Sulfate and the Two in Combination for Painful Knee Osteoarthritis," *New England Journal of Medicine* 354 (2006): 795–808.

49. PDRhealth, "S-Adenosyl-L-Methionine (SAMe)," 2007, www.pdrhealth.com/drug_info/nmdrugprofiles/nutsupdrugs/sad_0231.shtml.

50. International Foods Information Council, "Functional Foods Backgrounder," 2006, www.ific.org/nutrition/functional/index.cfm; The George Mateljan Foundation, "Ginger," 2007, www.whfoods.org/ genpage.php?tname=foodspice&dbid=72.

51. C. Paddock, "FDA Tightens Up Dietary Supplement Manufacturing and Labeling," *Medical News Today,* June 26, 2007, www.medicalnewstoday.com/articles/75250.php.

52. Mayo Clinic Staff, "Herbal Supplements: What to Know Before You Buy," Mayo Clinic, 2007, www.mayoclinic.com/health/herbal-supplements/SA00044/rss=1.

53. National Center for Complementary and Alternative Medicine, "What Is CAM?"

Caring for Older Adults

Older women far outnumber older men in American society, and the discrepancy increases with age. Because women live 7 years longer than men do on average, older women are more likely to live alone. Further, they are more likely to experience poverty and to have multiple chronic health problems, a situation referred to as **comorbidity.** Consequently, more women than men are likely to need assistance from children, other relatives, friends, and neighbors.

Women usually have been the primary caregivers for older Americans, often for their ailing husbands. Research also indicates that women spend more hours than men do (38 hours versus 27 hours per week) in caregiving activities and perform a wider range of services. Regardless of the time spent, caregiving is a difficult and stressful experience for both women and men. *Respite care,* or care that is given by someone who relieves the primary caregiver, should be available to ease the burden. As the population ages and more older adults require care, it will become even more important to support caregivers' health and well-being.

Understanding Death

Death eventually comes to everyone, but if you live life to the fullest and learn as much about end-of-life issues as you can, you will be better able to accept the inevitable. To cope effectively with dying, we must address the needs of people facing life's final transition. Let's begin by investigating what death means, at least in medical terms.

Defining Death

Dying is the process of decline in body functions that results in the death of an organism. **Death** can be defined as the "final cessation of the vital functions" and also refers to a state in which these functions are "incapable of being restored."[20] This definition has become more significant as medical advances make it increasingly possible to postpone death.

Legal and ethical issues led to the Uniform Determination of Death Act in 1981. This act, which has been adopted by several states, reads as follows: "An individual who has sustained either (1) irreversible cessation of circulatory and respiratory functions, or (2) irreversible cessation of all functions of the entire brain, including the brainstem, is dead. A determination of death must be made in accordance with accepted medical standards."[21]

The concept of **brain death,** defined as the irreversible cessation of all functions of the entire brainstem, has gained increasing credence. As defined by the Ad Hoc Committee of the Harvard Medical School, brain death occurs when the following criteria are met:[22]

- Unreceptivity and unresponsiveness—that is, no response even to painful stimuli
- No movement for a continuous hour after observation by a physician, and no breathing after 3 minutes off a respirator

- No reflexes, including brainstem reflexes; fixed and dilated pupils
- A "flat" electroencephalogram (EEG, which monitors electrical activity of the brain) for at least 10 minutes
- All of these tests repeated at least 24 hours later with no change
- Certainty that hypothermia (extreme loss of body heat) and depression of the central nervous system caused by use of drugs such as barbiturates are not responsible for these conditions

The Harvard report provides useful guidelines; however, the definition of *death* and all its ramifications continue to concern us.

what do you THINK?

Why is there so much concern over the definition of death? ■ How does modern technology complicate the understanding of when death occurs?

Denying Death

Attitudes toward death tend to fall on a continuum. At one end of the continuum, death is viewed as the mortal enemy of humankind. Both medical science and certain religions have promoted this idea. At the other end of the continuum, death is accepted and even welcomed. For people whose attitudes fall at this end, death is a passage to a better state of being. Most of us, however, perceive ourselves to be in the middle of this continuum. From this perspective, death is a bewildering mystery that elicits fear and apprehension while profoundly influencing beliefs and actions throughout life. See the **Assess Yourself** box on page 430 to evaluate your own level of anxiety about death.

In the United States, a high level of discomfort is associated with death and dying. We may avoid speaking about death to limit our own discomfort. Those who deny death tend to

- Avoid people who are grieving after the death of a loved one so they won't have to talk about it.
- Fail to validate a dying person's frightening situation by talking to the person as though nothing were wrong.

(Text continues on page AA-4.)

---

comorbidity The presence of a number of diseases at the same time.

dying The process of decline in body functions, resulting in the death of an organism.

death The permanent ending of all vital functions.

brain death The irreversible cessation of all functions of the entire brainstem.

ASSESS yourself

DEATH-RELATED ANXIETY SCALE

Fill out this assessment online at
www.aw-bc.com/MyHealthLab or
www.aw-bc.com/donatelle.

How anxious or accepting are you about the prospect of your death?
Indicate how well each statement describes your attitude.

		Not True at All	Mainly Not True	Not Sure	Somewhat True	Very True
1.	I tend not to be very brave in crisis situations.	0	1	2	3	4
2.	I am an unusually anxious person.	0	1	2	3	4
3.	I am something of a hypochondriac and am perhaps obsessively worried about infections.	0	1	2	3	4
4.	I have never had a semi-mystical, spiritual, out-of-body, near-death, or "peak" experience.	0	1	2	3	4
5.	I tend to be unusually frightened in planes at takeoff and landing.	0	1	2	3	4
6.	I do not have a particular religion or philosophy that helps me to face dying.	0	1	2	3	4
7.	I do not believe in any form of survival of the soul after death.	0	1	2	3	4
8.	Personally, I would give a lot to be immortal in this body.	0	1	2	3	4
9.	I am very much a city person and not really close to nature.	0	1	2	3	4
10.	Anxiety about death spoils the quality of my life.	0	1	2	3	4
11.	I am superstitious that preparing for dying might hasten my death.	0	1	2	3	4
12.	I don't like the way some of my relatives died and fear that my death could be like theirs.	0	1	2	3	4
13.	My actual experience of friends dying has been wholly negative.	0	1	2	3	4
14.	I would feel easier being with a dying relative if he or she had not been told he or she was dying.	0	1	2	3	4
15.	I have fears of dying alone without friends around me.	0	1	2	3	4
16.	I have fears of dying slowly.	0	1	2	3	4
17.	I have fears of dying suddenly.	0	1	2	3	4
18.	I have fears of dying before my time or while my children are still young.	0	1	2	3	4
19.	I have fears of dying before fulfilling my potential and fully using my talents.	0	1	2	3	4
20.	I have fears of dying without adequately having expressed my love to those I am close to.	0	1	2	3	4
21.	I have fears of dying before having really experienced much *joie de vivre*.	0	1	2	3	4
22.	I have fears of what may or may not happen after death.	0	1	2	3	4
23.	I have fears of what could happen to my family after my death.	0	1	2	3	4
24.	I have fears of dying in a hospital or an institution.	0	1	2	3	4
25.	I have fears of those caring for me feeling overwhelmed by the strain of it.	0	1	2	3	4

	Not True at All	Mainly Not True	Not Sure	Somewhat True	Very True
26. I have fears of not getting help with euthanasia when the time comes.	0	1	2	3	4
27. I have fears of being given unofficial and unwanted euthanasia.	0	1	2	3	4
28. I have fears of getting insufficient pain control while dying.	0	1	2	3	4
29. I have fears of being overmedicated and unconscious while dying.	0	1	2	3	4
30. I have fears of being declared dead when not really dead or being buried alive.	0	1	2	3	4
31. I have fears of getting confused at death or not being able to follow my spiritual practices.	0	1	2	3	4
32. I have fears of what may happen to my body after death.	0	1	2	3	4
33. I have fears of an Alzheimer's-type mental degeneration near death.	0	1	2	3	4
34. Overall I would say that I am unusually anxious about death and dying.	0	1	2	3	4

Total points _____

Interpreting Your Score

Add up your scores. If you are extremely anxious (scoring 65 or more), you might consider counseling or therapy; if you are unusually anxious (scoring between 40 and 64), you might want to find a method of meditation, philosophy, or spiritual practice to help experience, explore, and accept your feelings about death. Average anxiety is a score under 40. Continue to work toward developing a thoughtful and open ability to consider your own death in time.

MAKE it happen!

ASSESSMENT: The Assess Yourself activity above encouraged you to explore your death-related anxiety. How anxious are you? Do you want to reduce your fears and increase your acceptance of this inevitable part of life?
MAKING A CHANGE: To change your behavior, you need to develop a plan. Follow these steps below and complete your Behavior Change Contract to take action.

1. Evaluate your behavior and identify patterns and specific things you are doing. What can you change now? What can you change in the near future?

2. Select one pattern of behavior that you want to change.

3. Fill out the Behavior Change Contract found at the front of your book. It should include your long-term goals for change, your short-term goals, the rewards you'll give yourself for reaching these goals, potential obstacles along the way, and strategies for overcoming these obstacles. For each goal, list the small steps and specific actions that you will take.

4. Chart your progress in a journal. At the end of a week, consider how successful you were in following your plan. What helped you be successful? What made change more difficult? What will you do differently next week?

5. Revise your plan as needed: Are the short-term goals attainable? Are the rewards satisfying?

(continued)

EXAMPLE: Peter's score of 60 points on the self-assessment indicated that he was unusually anxious about death. The experience of his grandmother's death had been a very difficult one. He was only 6 years old at the time of her death, and no one in his family discussed it with him. He visited her once in the hospital and witnessed an argument between his parents and her doctors over the steps that should be taken to prolong her life.

Peter decided that one way to feel more in control and less anxious about death would be to learn about advance directives. He went to a low-cost legal clinic near campus and asked for information. There, he was given a sample directive to discuss with his parents and his physician. It listed various medical procedures for him to indicate which he did and did not want taken.

Peter also decided to fill out an organ donation card. He wanted to be sure his parents knew what he wanted done after his death, and he believed that donating any needed body parts was a worthy and fulfilling decision.

- Substitute euphemisms for the word *death* (for example, "passing away," "kicking the bucket," "no longer with us," "going to heaven," or "going to a better place").
- Give false reassurances to dying people by saying things like, "Everything is going to be okay."
- Shut off conversation about death by silencing people who are trying to talk about it.
- Avoid touching people who are dying.

Recent years have shown a greater effort on the part of the American public to mourn openly, as is indicated in part by roadside memorials placed at the sites of violent or unexpected deaths. Although these are fairly new additions to the American landscape, these memorials have long been popular in other parts of the world, particularly in predominantly Catholic countries.[23]

The Process of Dying

Dying is a complex process that includes physical, intellectual, social, spiritual, and emotional dimensions. Now that we have examined the physical indicators of death, we must consider the emotional aspects of dying and "social death."

Coping Emotionally with Death

Science and medicine have enabled us to understand many changes throughout the life span, but they have not fully explained the nature of death. This may explain why the transition from life to death evokes so much mystery and emotion. Although emotional reactions to dying vary, many people share similar experiences during this process. Terms such as *tasks*, *stages*, and *phases* have been used in models that have been developed to understand the process of dying.

thanatology   The study of death and dying.

Kübler-Ross and the Stages of Dying Much of our knowledge about reactions to dying stems from the work of Elisabeth Kübler-Ross, a pioneer in **thanatology**, the study of death and dying. In 1969, Kübler-Ross published *On Death and Dying*, a sensitive analysis of the reactions of terminally ill patients. This pioneering work encouraged the development of death education as a discipline and prompted efforts to improve the care of dying patients. Kübler-Ross identified five psychological stages that people coping with death often experience:[24]

1. *Denial.* ("Not me: there must be a mistake.") A person intellectually accepts the impending death but rejects it emotionally and feels a sense of shock and disbelief. The patient is too confused and stunned to comprehend "not being" and thus rejects the idea.

2. *Anger.* ("Why me?") The person becomes angry at having to face death when others, including loved ones, are healthy and not threatened. The dying person perceives the situation as unfair or senseless and may be hostile to friends, family, physicians, or the world in general.

3. *Bargaining.* ("If I'm allowed to live, I promise . . .") This stage generally occurs at about the middle of the progression. The dying person may resolve to be a better person in return for an extension of life or may secretly pray for a short reprieve from death to experience a special event, such as a family wedding or birth.

4. *Depression.* ("It's really going to happen to me, and I can't do anything about it.") Depression eventually sets in as vitality diminishes and the person begins to experience symptoms with increasing frequency. The person's deteriorating condition becomes impossible for him or her to deny. Common feelings experienced in this stage include doom, loss, worthlessness, and guilt over the emotional suffering of loved ones and the arduous but seemingly futile efforts of caregivers.

5. *Acceptance.* ("I'm ready.") This is often the final stage. The patient stops battling with emotions and becomes

tired and weak. With acceptance, the person does not give up and become sullen or resentfully resigned to death but rather becomes passive. According to one dying person, the acceptance stage is "almost void of feelings . . . as if the pain had gone, the struggle is over, and there comes a time for the final rest before the long journey."[25]

Some of Kübler-Ross's contemporaries consider her stage theory too neat and orderly. Subsequent research has indicated that the experiences of dying people do not fit easily into specific stages, and patterns vary from person to person. Some people may never go through this process and instead remain emotionally calm; others may pass back and forth between the stages. Even if it is not accurate in all its particulars, however, Kübler-Ross's theory offers valuable insights for those seeking to understand or deal with the process of dying.

Corr's Coping Approach
Others have developed alternative models for understanding the ways in which we cope with death and significant losses. Charles Corr believes that there are unique challenges and responses for the dying person and those who love them.[26] He suggests four dimensions of coping with loss: *physical*—doing everything possible to make ourselves comfortable and minimize pain; *psychological*—living to the fullest, focusing on life accomplishments, and seeking satisfaction in daily activities; *social*—nurturing relationships, keeping loved ones involved, and sharing emotions; and *spiritual*—identifying what matters in life and reaffirming meaningful experiences.

Social Death

The need for recognition and appreciation within a social group is nearly universal. Loss of being valued or appreciated by others can lead to **social death,** a seemingly irreversible situation in which a person is not treated like an active member of society. Dramatic examples of social death include the exile of nonconformists from their native countries or the excommunication of dissident members of religious groups. More often, however, social death is inflicted by denying a person normal social interaction. Numerous studies indicate that people are treated differently when they are dying. The following common behaviors contribute to the social death that often isolates people who are terminally ill:[27]

- The dying person may be excluded from conversations or referred to as though he or she were already dead.
- Dying patients often are moved to terminal wards and given minimal care.
- Bereaved family members are avoided, often for extended periods, because friends and neighbors feel uncomfortable in the presence of grief.
- Medical personnel may make degrading comments about patients in their presence.

This decrease in meaningful social interaction often strips dying and bereaved people of their identity as valued members of society at a time when belonging is critical. Some

dying people choose not to speak of their inevitable fate in an attempt to make others feel more comfortable and thus preserve vital relationships.

Coping with Loss

The losses resulting from the death of a loved one are extremely difficult to cope with. The dying person, as well as close family and friends, frequently suffers emotionally and physically from the impending loss of critical relationships and roles.

Bereavement generally is defined as the loss or deprivation that a survivor experiences when a loved one dies. Because relationships vary in type and intensity, reactions to loss also vary. In the lives of the bereaved or of close survivors, the loss of loved ones leaves "holes." We can think of bereavement as the awareness of these holes. Time and courage are necessary to fill these spaces.

A special case of bereavement occurs in old age. Loss is an intrinsic part of growing old. The longer we live, the more losses we are likely to experience. They include physical, social, and emotional losses as our bodies deteriorate and more and more of our loved ones die. The theory of *bereavement overload* has been proposed to explain the effects of multiple losses and the accumulation of sorrow in the lives of some older people. This theory suggests that the gloomy outlook, disturbing behavior patterns, and apparent apathy that characterize these people may be related more to bereavement overload than to intrinsic physiological degeneration in old age.[28]

Grief is a state of mental distress that occurs in reaction to significant loss, including one's own impending death, the death of a loved one, or a quasi-death experience (a loss, such as the end of a relationship or job, that resembles death because it involves separation, grief, or change in personal identity). Grief reactions include any adjustments needed for one to make it through the day and may include changes in patterns of eating, sleeping, working, and even thinking.

When a person experiences a loss that cannot be openly acknowledged, publicly mourned, or socially supported, coping may be much more difficult. This type of grief is referred to as *disenfranchised grief.*[29] It may occur among people who miscarry, are developmentally disabled, or are close friends rather than blood relatives of the deceased. It may also include those relationships that are not socially approved, such as those between extramarital lovers or homosexual couples.

social death A seemingly irreversible situation in which a person is not treated like an active member of society.

bereavement The loss or deprivation experienced by a survivor when a loved one dies.

grief The state of mental distress that occurs in reaction to significant loss, including one's own impending death, the death of a loved one, or a quasi-death experience.

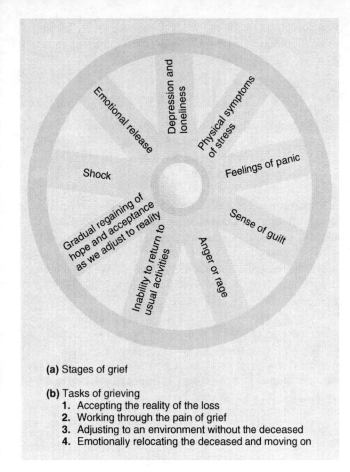

(a) Stages of grief

(b) Tasks of grieving
1. Accepting the reality of the loss
2. Working through the pain of grief
3. Adjusting to an environment without the deceased
4. Emotionally relocating the deceased and moving on

FIGURE 1 **The Stages and Tasks of Grief**
(a) People react differently to losses, but most eventually adjust. Generally, the stronger the social support system, the smoother the progression through the stages of grief. **(b)** Worden's developmental tasks associated with grief are another way to understand the grieving process.

The term *mourning* is often incorrectly equated with the term *grief*. As we have noted, *grief* refers to a wide variety of feelings and actions that occur in response to bereavement. **Mourning,** in contrast, refers to culturally prescribed and accepted time periods and behavior patterns for the expression of grief. In Judaism, for example, *sitting shiva* is a designated mourning period of 7 days that involves prescribed rituals and prayers. Depending on a person's relationship with the deceased, various other rituals may continue for up to a year.

Symptoms of grief vary in severity and duration, depending on the situation and the individual. However, the bereaved person can benefit from emotional and social support from

mourning The culturally prescribed behavior patterns for the expression of grief.

grief work The process of accepting the reality of a person's death and coping with memories of the deceased.

family, friends, clergy, employers, and traditional support organizations, including the medical community and the funeral industry. The larger and stronger the support system, the easier readjustment is likely to be.

What Is "Normal" Grief?

Grief responses vary widely from person to person but frequently include the following symptoms:

- Periodic waves of physical distress lasting from 20 minutes to an hour
- A feeling of tightness in the throat
- Choking and shortness of breath
- A frequent need to sigh
- Feelings of emptiness and muscular weakness
- Intense anxiety that is described as actually painful

Other common symptoms of grief include insomnia, memory lapses, loss of appetite, difficulty concentrating, a tendency to engage in repetitive or purposeless behavior, an "observer" sensation or feeling of unreality, difficulty in making decisions, lack of organization, excessive speech, social withdrawal or hostility, guilt feelings, and preoccupation with the image of the deceased. Susceptibility to disease increases with grief and may even be life-threatening in severe and enduring cases.

A bereaved person may suffer emotional pain and exhibit a variety of grief responses for many months after the death. The rate of the healing process depends on the amount and quality of grief work that a person does. **Grief work** is the process of integrating the reality of the loss into everyday life and learning to feel better. Often, the bereaved person must deliberately and systematically work at reducing denial and coping with the pain that results from memories of the deceased. This process takes time and requires emotional effort.

Worden's Model of Grieving Tasks

William Worden, a researcher into the death process, developed an active grieving model which suggests four developmental tasks to complete in the grief work process **(Figure 1):** [30]

1. *Accept the reality of the loss.* This task requires acknowledging and realizing that the person is dead. Traditional rituals, such as the funeral, help many bereaved people move toward acceptance.

2. *Work through the pain of grief.* It is necessary to acknowledge and work through the pain associated with loss, or it will manifest itself through other symptoms or behaviors.

3. *Adjust to an environment in which the deceased is missing.* The bereaved may feel lonely and uncertain about a new identity without the person who has died. This loss confronts them with the challenge of adjusting their own sense of self.

4. *Emotionally relocate the deceased and move on with life.* Individuals never lose memories of a significant relationship. They may need help in letting go of the emotional energy that used to be invested in the person who has died, finding an appropriate place for the deceased in their emotional lives.

Models of the grief process can be viewed as "generalized maps"—each theory is an attempt by an investigator to understand and guide grieving people through their pain. However, each individual will travel through grief at his or her own speed using an appropriate route.

? *what do you* THINK?

If you have experienced death among your family or friends, how did you grieve? ■ Did you accomplish Worden's tasks? ■ Does the model match your experience?

Life-and-Death Decision Making

Many complex—and often expensive—life-and-death decisions must be made during a highly distressing period in people's lives, when a loved one is dying. We will not attempt to present definitive answers to moral and philosophical questions about death; instead, we offer these topics for your consideration.

The Right to Die

Few people would object to a proposal for the right to a dignified death. Going beyond that concept, however, many people today believe that they should be allowed to die if their condition is terminal and their existence depends on mechanical life support devices or artificial feeding or hydration systems. Artificial life support techniques that may be legally refused in some states by competent patients include the following:

- Electrical or mechanical heart resuscitation
- Mechanical respiration by machine
- Nasogastric tube feedings
- Intravenous nutrition
- Gastrostomy (tube feeding directly into the stomach)
- Medications to treat life-threatening infections

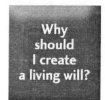
Why should I create a living will?

As long as a person is conscious and competent, he or she has the legal right to refuse treatment, even if this decision will hasten death. However, when a person is in a coma or otherwise incapable of speaking on his or her own behalf, medical personnel, family members,

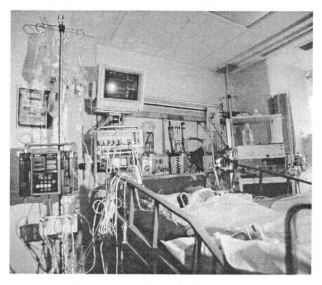

Sophisticated life-support technology allows a patient's life to be prolonged even in cases of terminal illness or mortal injury. It has also raised legal and moral questions for patients, their families, and health care professionals.

and administrative policy will dictate treatment. This issue has evolved into a battle involving personal freedom, legal rulings, health care administration policy, and physician responsibility. The living will and other advance directives were developed to assist in solving these conflicts.

Even young, apparently healthy people need a living will. Consider Terri Schiavo, who collapsed at age 26 from heart failure that led to irreversible brain damage. Schiavo, unable to survive without life support, never left any written guidelines about her wishes should she become incapacitated. After a 15-year legal battle between her parents, who wanted her to be kept alive, and her husband, who felt she should be allowed to die, the courts sided with her husband, and she was removed from life support.

In other instances, the wishes of people who had signed a living will (or other directive) indicating their desire not to receive artificial life support were not honored by their physician or medical institution. Many legal experts suggest that you take the following steps to ensure that your wishes are carried out:

1. *Be specific.* Complete an advance directive that permits you to make very specific choices about a variety of procedures, including cardiopulmonary resuscitation (CPR); being placed on a ventilator; being given food, water, or medication through tubes; being given pain medication; and organ donation. It is also essential to attach that document to a completed copy of the standard advance directive for your state.

2. *Get an agent.* You may want to also appoint a family member or friend to act as your agent, or *proxy,* by making out a form known as either a *durable power of attorney for health care* or a *health care proxy.*

SKILLS FOR Behavior Change

TALKING TO FRIENDS WHEN SOMEONE DIES

It's always hard to know just what to say and how to say it when talking with a grieving friend or relative. Here are some do's and don'ts.

How can I help a friend who has just experienced a loss?

DO

- Let your genuine concern and caring show; say you are sorry about their loss and about their pain.
- Be available to help with children or run errands.
- Allow them to express as much grief as they are feeling and are willing to share. Listen to them talk about the person who has died as much and as often as they want to.
- Encourage them to be patient with themselves and not to worry about things they should be doing.
- Talk about the special, endearing qualities of the person who has died.

- Reassure them that they did everything that they could, that the medical care given was the best, or whatever else you know to be true and positive about the care given.

DON'T

- Let your own sense of helplessness keep you from reaching out to a bereaved person.
- Avoid them because you are uncomfortable (this adds pain to an already painful experience).
- Say you know how they feel (unless you've suffered a similar loss, you probably don't).
- Say, "You ought to be feeling better by now," or anything else that implies a judgment about their feelings or actions.
- Change the subject when they mention the person who has died.
- Avoid mentioning the name of the deceased out of fear of reminding them of their pain.

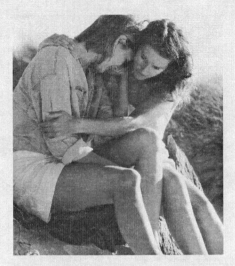

- Make any comments that suggest that the care given to the deceased at home, in the hospital, or wherever was inadequate. Bereaved people are already plagued by feelings of doubt and guilt.

Source: Interior Alzheimer's Society, "Do's and Don'ts of Helping Bereaved People," retrieved July 18, 2007, www.alzheimer-society.ca/grief4.htm.

---

3. *Discuss your wishes.* Discuss your preferences in detail with your proxy and your doctor. Going over the situations described in the form will give them a clear idea of just how much you are willing to endure to preserve your life.

4. *Deliver the directive.* Distribute several copies, not only to your doctor and your agent, but also to your lawyer and to immediate family members or a close friend. Make sure *someone* knows to bring a copy to the hospital in the event you are hospitalized.[31]

rational suicide The decision to kill oneself rather than endure constant pain and slow decay.

active euthanasia "Mercy killing," in which a person or organization knowingly acts to end the life of a terminally ill person.

passive euthanasia The intentional withholding of treatment that would prolong life.

Rational Suicide

Although exact numbers are not known, medical ethicists and specialists in forensic medicine (the study of legal issues in medicine) estimate that thousands of terminally ill people every year decide to kill themselves rather than endure constant pain and slow decay. This alternative to the extended dying process is known as **rational suicide.** To these people, the prospect of an undignified death is unacceptable. This issue has been complicated by advances in death prevention techniques that allow terminally ill patients to exist in an irreversible disease state for extended periods of time. Medical personnel, clergy, lawyers, and patients all must struggle with this ethical dilemma.

Euthanasia is often referred to as "mercy killing." The term **active euthanasia** refers to ending the life of a person (or animal) who is suffering greatly and has no chance of recovery. An example might be a physician-prescribed lethal injection. **Passive euthanasia** refers to the intentional withholding of treatment that would prolong life. Deciding not to place a person with massive brain trauma on life support is an example of passive euthanasia.

Dr. Jack Kevorkian, a physician in Michigan, started a one-person campaign to force the medical profession to review its position regarding physician-assisted death. Kevorkian assisted many terminally ill patients in dying and argued that the present situations in our society demand a shift in medical thinking and practice. He believes that acceptance of euthanasia, specifically physician-assisted death, is one of those changes.

Kevorkian's actions have led many to discuss the merits of physician-assisted suicide. According to public opinion polls, most Americans believe that suicide is morally wrong but are divided on whether physician-assisted suicide is morally acceptable. Roughly 70 percent of Americans believe doctors should be allowed to help end an incurably ill patient's life painlessly at the patient's request.[32]

Legalization of assisted suicide has been debated in many states across the nation. Currently, 38 states have enacted statues explicitly prohibiting assisted suicide, 4 states are undecided (meaning there are no statutes or case laws specifically prohibiting assisted suicide), and Oregon is the only state that allows physician-assisted suicide under certain circumstances, outlined in Oregon's Death with Dignity Act.[33]

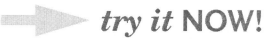 *try it* NOW!

You can never be too young to consider completing an advance directive. Right now, go to www.uslivingwillregistry.com/forms.shtm, select the state you live in, and print out your state's advance directive for health care form. Read through the form, and think about the health care decisions you would make to complete the form.

Making Final Arrangements

Caring for dying people and dealing with the practical and legal questions surrounding death can be difficult and painful. The problems of the dying person and the bereaved loved ones involve a wide variety of psychological, legal, social, spiritual, economic, and interpersonal issues.

Hospice Care: Positive Alternatives

Since the mid-1970s, **hospice** programs have grown from a mere handful to more than 2,500 and are available in nearly every community. Improving quality of care at the end of life is a top priority of the American Medical Association.

The primary goals of hospice programs are to relieve the dying person's pain; offer emotional support to the dying person and loved ones; and restore a sense of control to the dying person, family, and friends. Although home care with maximum involvement by loved ones is emphasized, hospice programs are directed by cooperating physicians; coordinated by specially trained nurses; and fortified with the skills of counselors, clergy, and trained volunteers. Hospice programs usually include the following characteristics.

1. Both the patient and family constitute the unit of care, because the physical, psychological, social, and spiritual problems of dying confront the family as well as the patient.

2. Emphasis is placed on symptom control, primarily the alleviation of pain. Curative treatments are curtailed as requested by the patient, but sound judgment must be applied to avoid a feeling of abandonment.

3. There is overall medical direction of the program, with all health care provided under the direction of a qualified physician.

4. Services are provided by an interdisciplinary team, because no one person can provide all the needed care.

5. Coverage is provided 24 hours a day, 7 days a week, with emphasis on the availability of medical and nursing skills.

6. Carefully selected and extensively trained volunteers who augment but do not replace staff service are an integral part of the health care team.

7. Care of the family extends through the bereavement period.

8. Patients are accepted on the basis of their health needs, not on their ability to pay.

Despite the growing number of people considering the hospice option, many people prefer to go to a hospital to die. Others choose to die at home, without the intervention of medical staff or life-prolonging equipment. Each dying person and his or her family should decide as early as possible what type of terminal care is most desirable and feasible. This will allow time for necessary emotional, physical, and financial preparations.

Pressures on Survivors

There are many decisions concerning the funeral ritual that can be burdensome for survivors, some of which must be made within 24 hours of a person's death. These decisions relate to the method and details of body disposal, the type of memorial service, display of the body, the site of burial or body disposition, the cost of funeral options, organ donation, ordering floral displays, contacting friends and relatives, planning for guests, choosing markers, gathering and submitting obituary information to newspapers, printing

hospice A concept of care for terminally ill patients designed to maximize quality of life.

```
UNIFORM DONOR CARD

I, _____, have spoken to my family
about organ and tissue donation. The following people have witnessed
my commitment to be a donor. I wish to donate the following:
☐ any needed organs and tissue
☐ only the following organs and tissue: _____

_____
Donor
Signature _____    Date _____
Witness _____
Witness _____
```

FIGURE 2 Sample Uniform Organ Donor Card

memorial folders, and many other details. In our society, people who make their own funeral arrangements can save their loved ones from having to deal with unnecessary problems.

Making Funeral Arrangements

Anthropological evidence indicates that all cultures throughout human history have developed some sort of funeral ritual. For this reason, social scientists agree that funerals assist survivors of the deceased in coping with their loss.

In the United States, with its diversity of religious, regional, and ethnic customs, funeral patterns vary. In some faiths, the deceased may be displayed to formalize last respects and increase social support for the bereaved. This part of the funeral ritual is referred to as a *wake* or *viewing*. The funeral service may be held in a church, in a funeral chapel, or at the burial site. Some people choose to replace the funeral service with a simple memorial service held within a few days of the burial. Social interaction associated with funeral and memorial services is valuable in helping survivors cope with their loss.

Common methods of body disposal include burial in the ground, entombment above ground in a mausoleum, cremation, and anatomical donation. Expenses vary according to

intestate   Dying without a will.

holographic will   A will written in the testator's own handwriting and unwitnessed.

testator   A person who leaves a will or testament at death.

the method chosen and the available options. It should be noted that if burial is selected, an additional charge may be assessed for a burial vault. Burial vaults—concrete or metal containers that hold the casket—are required by most cemeteries to limit settling of the gravesite as the casket disintegrates and collapses. The actual container for the remains is only one of many issues that must be dealt with when a person dies.

Organ Donation

In recent years, organ transplant techniques have become so refined, and the demand for transplant tissues and organs so great, that many people are being encouraged to donate these gifts of life upon death. Uniform donor cards are available through the U.S. Department of Health and Human Services, as well as many health care foundations and nonprofit organizations (**Figure 2**); donor information is printed on the backs of drivers' licenses; and many hospitals include the opportunity for organ donor registration in their admission procedures. Although some people are opposed to organ transplants and tissue donation, others experience personal fulfillment from knowing that their organs may extend and improve someone else's life after their own deaths.

Wills

The issue of inheritance is controversial in some families and should be resolved before the person dies to reduce conflict and needless expense. Unfortunately, many people are so intimidated by the thought of making a will that they never do so and die **intestate** (without a will). This is tragic, especially because the procedure for establishing a legal will is relatively simple and inexpensive. In addition, if you don't make a will before you die, the courts (as directed by state laws) will make a will for you. Legal issues, rather than your wishes, will preside. Furthermore, it usually takes longer to settle an estate when the person dies intestate.

In some cases, other types of wills may substitute for the traditional legal will. One alternative is the **holographic will,** which is written in the handwriting of the **testator** (person who leaves a will) and unwitnessed. However, be very cautious concerning any alternatives to legally written and witnessed wills, because they are not honored in all states. For example, holographic wills are contestable in court.

ANSWERS TO CHAPTER REVIEW QUESTIONS

Chapter 1

1. d; 2. b; 3. b; 4. c; 5. d;
6. a; 7. a; 8. a; 9. c; 10. c

Chapter 2

1. a; 2. b; 3. b; 4. d; 5. a;
6. c; 7. b; 8. b; 9. c; 10. b

Chapter 3

1. c; 2. c; 3. d; 4. d; 5. c;
6. d; 7. c; 8. c; 9. c; 10. b

Chapter 4

1. a; 2. a; 3. c; 4. d; 5. d;
6. c; 7. a; 8. c; 9. b; 10. a

Chapter 5

1. b; 2. b; 3. c; 4. c; 5. c;
6. c; 7. a; 8. d; 9. b; 10. b

Chapter 6

1. c; 2. d; 3. a; 4. c; 5. b;
6. a; 7. c; 8. d; 9. c; 10. a

Chapter 7

1. a; 2. c; 3. d; 4. c; 5. c;
6. c; 7. a; 8. a; 9. d; 10. b

Chapter 8

1. c; 2. c; 3. d; 4. b; 5. d;
6. a; 7. b; 8. d; 9. c; 10. d

Chapter 9

1. c; 2. a; 3. a; 4. b; 5. b;
6. a; 7. d; 8. b; 9. d; 10. c

Chapter 10

1. b; 2. c; 3. b; 4. b; 5. c;
6. c; 7. c; 8. a; 9. d; 10. b

Chapter 11

1. c; 2. d; 3. c; 4. b; 5. a;
6. a; 7. d; 8. c; 9. b; 10. c

Chapter 12

1. b; 2. a; 3. a; 4. c; 5. b;
6. a; 7. c; 8. c; 9. b; 10. d

Chapter 13

1. a; 2. c; 3. d; 4. b; 5. c;
6. a; 7. c; 8. b; 9. c; 10. b

Chapter 14

1. d; 2. b; 3. b; 4. a; 5. a;
6. a; 7. a; 8. c; 9. c; 10. d

Chapter 15

1. b; 2. c; 3. d; 4. a; 5. a;
6. d; 7. b; 8. b; 9. d; 10. c

Chapter 16

1. b; 2. a; 3. c; 4. d; 5. c;
6. a; 7. b; 8. b; 9. a; 10. b

Chapter 17

1. d; 2. c; 3. b; 4. a; 5. b;
6. a; 7. d; 8. c; 9. c; 10. b

Preventing Injuries and Providing Emergency Care

Preventing Injuries

Unintentional injuries are a major public health problem facing the United States today. On an average day, more than a million people suffer a nonfatal injury, and almost 100,000 people die each year as a result of unintentional injuries. Unintentional injuries are the fifth leading cause of death, after heart disease, cancer, stroke, and lung disease, and they are the leading cause of death for Americans under age 44.

Residential Safety

Injuries within the home typically are due to falls or burns. Some populations, such as older adults, are particularly vulnerable. However, older adults are not the only victims; each year, hundreds of children suffer severe burns or die from accidental fires, falls, and other home-based injuries.

Fall-Proof Your Home   Home falls are a common source of home injury. Take the following measures to prevent falls:

- Leave nothing lying around on the floor, and use rubberized mats or strips to fasten rugs to the floor.
- Train your pets to stay away from your feet.
- Install slip-proof mats, treads, or decals in showers and tubs and on the stairs.

Avoid Burns and Fires   To prevent the risk of fires and related injuries, follow these tips:

- Extinguish all cigarettes in ashtrays before bed, and never smoke in bed at any time!
- Set all lamps away from drapes, linens, and paper.
- Be cautious in the kitchen. Keep hotpads and kitchen cloths away from stove burners, avoid reaching over hot pans, and use caution when lighting barbecue grills.
- Keep candles under control and away from combustibles. Never leave candles unattended or burning while you sleep.
- Avoid overloading electrical circuits with appliances and cords. Older buildings are at particular risk for fire from such overloads.
- Have the proper fire extinguishers ready in case of fire. Test smoke detectors and replace batteries periodically.

Workplace Safety

American adults spend most of their waking hours on the job. Although most job situations are pleasant and productive, others pose physical and emotional hazards. Outdoor occupations show the highest fatality and injury rates. Highway crashes are the leading cause of on-the-job fatalities; most involve truck drivers. Sixteen percent of worker fatalities result from other types of transportation-related incidents, such as tractors and forklifts overturning in fields or warehouses, workers being struck by vehicles, aircraft and railway crashes, and water vehicles crashing or capsizing.

Although on-the-job deaths are rare enough to capture media attention, serious injuries and disabilities are more common. Injuries that cause the greatest number of lost-work days include carpal tunnel syndrome; hernia; amputation of a limb; fractures, sprains, and strains (often of the back); cuts or lacerations; and chemical burns. For example, nearly half of all workers with carpal tunnel syndrome miss 30 days or more of work each year. Because so many work injuries are due to repetitive motion, overexertion, or inappropriate motion, they are largely preventable through training and techniques designed to reduce employees' risks. For more information on back pain and repetitive stress injuries, see Chapter 13.

Vehicle Safety

The risk of dying in an automobile crash is related to age, and driving drunk is the single greatest risk for drivers. Young drivers (aged 16 to 24) have the highest death rate, owing to their inexperience and immaturity. Each year about 40,000 Americans die in automobile crashes, and another 1.9 million are disabled, 140,000 permanently. Most of these car crashes are avoidable. The best way to prevent crashes is to practice risk management driving and accident-avoidance techniques and to be aware of safety technology when purchasing a car.

Risk Management Driving   Risk management driving techniques, which help reduce chances of being involved in a collision, include the following:

- Don't drink and drive.
- Don't drive when you are tired or in a highly emotional or stressed state.
- Surround your car with a safety "bubble." The rear bumper of the car ahead of you should be 3 seconds away.

- Scan the road ahead of you and to both sides.
- Drive with your low-beam headlights on, *day and night*, to make your car more visible to other drivers.

Other important techniques include anticipating other drivers' actions, obeying all traffic laws, and using safety belts.

Accident-Avoidance Techniques   To avoid a serious accident, you may need to steer into another, less severe collision. Here are the American Automobile Association's (AAA) rules for accident avoidance:

- Generally, veer to the right.
- Steer—don't skid—off the road. (It is easy to roll a vehicle over if you swerve suddenly off the edge of the road.)
- If you have to hit a vehicle, hit one moving in the same direction as your own.
- If you have to hit a stationary object, try to hit a soft one (bushes, small trees) rather than a hard one (boulders, brick walls, giant trees).
- If you have to hit a hard object, hit it with a glancing blow.
- Avoid hitting pedestrians, motorcyclists, and bicyclists at all cost.

Safety Technology   How a car is equipped can mean the difference between life and death. The Insurance Institute for Highway Safety recommends that you look for the following features when purchasing a car:

- Does the car have airbags? Where and what kind? Remember, airbags do not eliminate the need to wear safety belts.
- Does the car have antilock brakes? Traction and stability control? Each of these can be the difference between life, crippling injury, or death.
- Does the car have impact-absorbing crumple zones?
- Are there strengthened passenger compartment side walls?
- Is there a strong roof support? (The center door post on four-door models gives you an extra roof pillar.)

In Case of Mechanical Breakdown   If your car breaks down, follow these steps:

- Get as far off the road as possible.
- Turn on your car's emergency flashers, and raise the hood. Set out flares or reflective triangles.
- Stay in the car until a law enforcement officer arrives. If others stop to help, ask them to contact the police, sheriff's office, or state patrol.

Safe Refueling   Gasoline is a flammable substance. Follow these guidelines from the Petroleum Equipment Institute any time you are filling up a car, truck or motorcycle:

- Turn off the engine while refueling.
- Do not reenter your vehicle during refueling.
- Do not use cell phones, laptops, or other battery-operated devices near fueling pumps; fire may result.

- In the event of fire due to static electricity, leave the nozzle in the tank, and back away from the vehicle. Notify the attendant immediately.
- Avoid prolonged breathing of gasoline vapors. Keep gasoline away from your eyes and skin; it can cause irritation. Never use it to wash your hands or as a cleaning solvent.
- If you are dispensing gasoline into a container or storing it, be sure the container is approved for such a use.
- Never siphon gasoline by mouth; it can be harmful or fatal if swallowed.

Pedestrian Safety

Each year, approximately 13 percent of all motor vehicle deaths involve pedestrians, and another 82,000 pedestrians are injured each year. The highest death rates involving pedestrians occur among the very young and older populations. Pedestrian injuries occur most frequently after dark, in urban settings, and primarily in intersections where pedestrians may walk or dart into traffic. It is not uncommon for alcohol to play a role in the death or injury of a pedestrian. How can you protect yourself from being injured? AAA offers the following suggestions for joggers and walkers:

- Carry or wear reflective material at night to help drivers see you.
- Cross only at crosswalks. Keep to the right in crosswalks.
- Before crossing, look both ways. Be sure the way is clear before you cross.
- Cross only on the proper signal.
- Watch for turning cars.
- Never enter the roadway from between parked cars.
- Where there is no sidewalk and it is necessary to walk in a roadway, walk on the left side, facing traffic.
- Don't wear headphones for a portable music player. These may interfere with your ability to hear sounds of motor vehicles.

Cycling Safety

Currently over 63 million Americans of all ages ride bicycles for transportation, recreation, and fitness. The Consumer Product Safety Commission reports about 800 deaths per year from cycling accidents. The biggest risk factors are failure to wear a helmet, being male, and riding after dark. Approximately 87 percent of fatal collisions were due to cyclists' errors, usually failure to yield at intersections. Alcohol also plays a significant role in bicycle deaths and injuries. Cyclists should consider the following suggestions.

- Wear a helmet. It should be approved by the American National Standards Institute (ANSI) or the Snell Memorial Foundation (SNELL). Wearing a helmet can reduce head injuries by 85 percent.
- Don't drink and ride.
- Respect traffic, and ride with the flow of traffic.

- Wear light, reflective clothing that is easily seen at night and during the day.
- Avoid riding after dark.
- Know and use proper hand signals.
- Keep your bicycle in good working condition.
- Use bike paths whenever possible.
- Stop at stop signs and traffic lights.

Water Safety

Drowning is the third most common cause of accidental death in the United States, according to the National Safety Council. About 85 percent of drowning victims are teenaged males, and many drowned swimmers are strong swimmers. Alcohol plays a significant role in many boat accidents and drownings. Never drink when operating a boat of any kind, and always wear a life preserver.

Most drownings occur in unorganized or unsupervised facilities, such as ponds or pools with no lifeguards present. Swimmers should take the following precautions:

- Don't drink alcohol before or while swimming.
- Don't enter the water unless you can swim at least 50 feet unassisted.
- Know your limitations; get out of the water when you start to feel even slightly fatigued.
- Never swim alone, even if you are a skilled swimmer. You never know what might happen.
- Never leave a child unattended, even in extremely shallow water.
- Before entering the water, check the depth. Most neck and back injuries result from diving into water that is too shallow.
- Never swim in muddy or dirty water that obstructs your view of the bottom.
- Never swim in a river with currents too swift for easy, relaxed swimming.

Providing Emergency Care

Ideally, first aid procedures should be performed only by someone who has received formal training from the American Red Cross or other reputable institution. If you do not have such training and are injured or with an injured person, contact a physician or call your local emergency medical service (EMS) by dialing 911 or your local emergency number. In life-threatening situations, however, you may need to begin first aid immediately and continue until help arrives. This section contains basic information for various emergency situations. Simply reading these directions, however, may not prepare you fully to handle these situations. For this reason, you may want to enroll in a first aid course.

Calling for Emergency Assistance

When calling for emergency assistance, be prepared to give exact details. Be clear and thorough, and do not panic. Never hang up until the dispatcher has informed you that he or she has all the information needed. Be ready to answer the following questions:

1. Where are you and the victim located? This is the most important information the EMS will need.
2. What is your phone number and name?
3. What has happened? Was there an accident, or is the victim ill?
4. How many people need help?
5. What is the nature of the emergency? What is the victim's apparent condition?
6. Are there any life-threatening situations that the EMS should know about (for example, fires, explosions, or fallen electrical lines)?
7. Is the victim wearing a medic-alert tag (a tag indicating a specific medical condition such as diabetes)?

Are You Liable?

According to the laws in most states, you are not required to administer first aid unless you have a special obligation to the victim. For example, parents must provide first aid for their children, and a lifeguard must provide aid to a swimmer.

Before administering first aid, you should obtain the victim's consent. If the victim refuses aid, you must respect that person's rights. However, you should make every reasonable effort to persuade the victim to accept your help. In emergency situations, consent is *implied* if the victim is unconscious. Once you begin to administer first aid, you are required by law to continue. You must remain with the victim until someone of equal or greater competence takes over.

Can you be held liable if you fail to provide adequate care or if the victim is further injured? To protect people who render first aid, most states have "Good Samaritan" laws. These laws grant immunity (protection from civil liability) if you act in good faith to provide care to the best of your ability, according to your level of training. Because these laws vary, you should become familiar with the Good Samaritan laws in your state.

When Someone Stops Breathing

If someone has stopped breathing, you should perform mouth-to-mouth resuscitation. This involves the following steps:

1. Check for responsiveness by gently tapping or shaking the victim. Ask loudly, "Are you OK?"
2. Call the local EMS for help (usually 911).
3. Gently roll the victim onto his or her back.

4. Open the airway by tilting the victim's head back, placing your hand nearest the victim's head on the victim's forehead, and applying backward pressure to tilt the head back and lift the chin.

5. Check for breathing (3 to 5 seconds): look, listen, and feel for breathing.

6. Give two slow breaths.
   - Keep the victim's head tilted back.
   - Pinch the victim's nose shut.
   - Seal your lips tightly around the victim's mouth.
   - Give two slow breaths, each lasting $1\frac{1}{2}$ to 2 seconds.

7. Check for pulse at side of neck; feel for pulse for 5 to 10 seconds.

8. Begin rescue breathing.
   - Keep the victim's head tilted back.
   - Pinch the victim's nose shut.
   - Give one breath every 5 to 6 seconds.
   - Look, listen, and feel for breathing between breaths.

9. Recheck pulse every minute.
   - Keep the victim's head tilted back.
   - Feel for pulse for 5 to 10 seconds.
   - If the victim has a pulse but is not breathing, continue rescue breathing. If there is no pulse, begin CPR.

There are some variations when performing this procedure on infants and children. For children aged 1 to 8, at step 8, give one slow breath every 4 seconds. For infants, you should not pinch the nose. Instead, seal your lips tightly around the infant's nose and mouth. Also for infants, at step 8 you should give one slow breath every 3 seconds.

If the victim has no pulse, cardiopulmonary resuscitation (CPR) should be performed. This technique involves a combination of artificial respiration and chest compressions. You should not perform CPR unless you have received training in it. You cannot learn CPR simply by reading directions, and without training, you could injure the victim further. The American Red Cross offers courses in mouth-to-mouth resuscitation and CPR as well as general first aid. If you have taken a CPR course in the past, you should be aware that certain changes have been made in the procedure. Consider taking a refresher course.

When Someone Is Choking

Choking occurs when an object obstructs the trachea (windpipe), thus preventing normal breathing. Failure to expel the object and restore breathing can lead to death within 6 minutes. The universal signal of distress related to choking is the clasping of the throat with one or both hands. Other signs of choking include not being able to talk and/or noisy and difficult breathing. If a victim can cough or speak, do not interfere. The most effective method for assisting choking victims is the Heimlich maneuver, which involves applying pressure to the victim's abdominal area to expel the foreign object. The Heimlich maneuver involves the following steps:

If the Victim Is Standing or Seated

1. Recognize that the victim is choking.

2. Wrap your arms around the victim's waist, making a fist with one hand.

3. Place the thumb side of the fist on the middle of the victim's abdomen, just above the navel and well below the tip of the sternum.

4. Cover your fist with your other hand.

5. Press your fist into victim's abdomen, with up to five quick upward thrusts.

6. After every five abdominal thrusts, check the victim and your technique.

7. If the victim becomes unconscious, gently lower him or her to the ground.

8. Try to clear the airway by using your finger to sweep the object from the victim's mouth or throat.

9. Give two rescue breaths. If the passage is still blocked and air will not go in, proceed with the Heimlich maneuver.

If the Victim Is Lying Down

1. Facing the person, kneel with your legs astride the victim's hips. Place the heel of one hand against the abdomen, slightly above the navel and well below the tip of the sternum. Put the other hand on top of the first hand.

2. Press inward and upward using both hands with up to five quick abdominal thrusts.

3. Repeat the following steps in this sequence until the airway becomes clear or the EMS arrives:
   a. Finger sweep.
   b. Give two rescue breaths.
   c. Do up to five abdominal thrusts.

Alcohol Poisoning

Alcohol overdose is considered a medical emergency when an irregular heartbeat or coma occurs. The two immediate causes of death in such cases are cardiac arrhythmia and respiratory depression. If a person is seriously uncoordinated and has possibly also taken a depressant, the risk of respiratory failure is serious enough to contact a physician. When dealing with someone who is drunk, remember these points:

1. Stay calm. Assess the situation.

2. Keep your distance. Before approaching or touching the person, explain what you intend to do.

3. Speak in a clear, firm, reassuring manner.

4. Keep the person still and comfortable.

5. Stay with the person if she or he is vomiting. When helping him or her to lie down, turn the head to the side to prevent it from falling back. This helps to keep the person from choking on vomit.

6. Monitor the person's breathing.

When Someone Is Bleeding

External Bleeding   Controlling external bleeding is an important part of emergency care, because the loss of one quart of blood or more threatens the person's survival. There are three major procedures to control external bleeding.

1. *Direct pressure.* The best method is to apply firm pressure by covering the wound with a sterile dressing, bandage, or clean cloth. Wearing disposable latex gloves or an equally protective barrier, apply pressure for 5 to 10 minutes to stop bleeding.

2. *Elevation.* Elevate the wounded section of the body to slow the bleeding. For example, raise a wounded arm or leg above the level of the victim's heart.

3. *Pressure points.* Pressure points are sites where an artery that is close to the body's surface lies directly over a bone. Pressing the artery against the bone can limit the flow of blood to the injury. This technique should be used only as a last resort when direct pressure and elevation have failed to stop bleeding.

Knowing where to apply pressure to stop bleeding is critical (see the figure). For serious wounds, seek medical attention immediately.

Internal Bleeding   Although internal bleeding may not be immediately obvious, you should be aware of the following signs and symptoms:

1. Symptoms of shock (discussed on page A-7)

2. Coughing up or vomiting blood

3. Bruises or contusions of the skin

4. Bruises on chest or fractured ribs

5. Black, tarlike stools

6. Abdominal discomfort or pain (rigidity or spasms)

In some cases, a person who has suffered an injury (such as a blow to the head, chest, or abdomen) that does not cause external bleeding may bleed internally. If you suspect internal bleeding, follow these steps:

1. Have the person lie on his or her back on a flat surface with knees bent.

2. Treat for shock. Keep the victim warm. Cover the person with a blanket, if possible.

3. Expect vomiting. If vomiting occurs, keep the victim on his or her side for drainage, to prevent inhalation of vomit, and to prevent expulsion of vomit from the stomach.

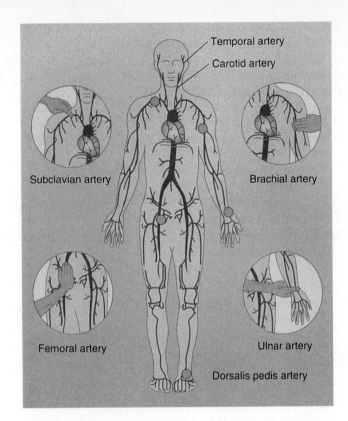

FIGURE A.1 Pressure Points
Pressure can be applied to these points to stop bleeding. However, unless absolutely necessary, avoid applying pressure to the carotid arteries, which supply blood to the brain. Never apply pressure to both carotid arteries at the same time.

4. Do *not* give the victim any medications or fluids.

5. Send someone to call for emergency medical help immediately.

Nosebleeds   To control a nosebleed, follow these steps:

1. Have the victim sit down and lean slightly forward to prevent blood from running into the throat. If you do not suspect a fracture, pinch the person's nose firmly closed using the thumb and forefinger. Keep the nose pinched for at least 5 minutes.

2. While the nose is pinched, apply a cold compress to the surrounding area.

3. If pinching does not work, gently pack the nostril with gauze or a clean strip of cloth. Do not use absorbent cotton, which will stick. Be sure that the ends of the gauze or cloth hang out so that it can be easily removed later. Once the nose is packed with gauze, pinch it closed again for another 5 minutes.

4. If the bleeding persists, seek medical attention.

Treatment for Burns

Minor Burns   For minor burns caused by fire or scalding water, apply running cold water or cold compresses for 20 to 30 minutes. Never put butter, grease, salt water, aloe vera, or topical burn ointments or sprays on burned skin. If the burned area is dirty, gently wash it with soap and water, and blot it dry with a sterile dressing.

Major Burns   For major burn injuries, call for help immediately. Wrap the victim in a clean, dry sheet. Do not clean the burns or try to remove any clothing attached to burned skin. Remove jewelry near the burned skin immediately, if possible. Keep the victim lying down and calm.

Chemical Burns   Remove clothing surrounding the burn. Wash skin that has been burned by chemicals by flushing with water for at least 20 minutes. Seek medical assistance as soon as possible.

Shock

Shock is a condition in which the cardiovascular system fails to provide sufficient blood circulation to all parts of the body. Victims of shock display the following symptoms:

- Dilated pupils
- Cool, moist skin
- Weak, rapid pulse
- Vomiting
- Delayed or unrelated responses to questions

All injuries result in some degree of shock. Therefore, treatment for shock should be given after every major injury. The following are basic steps for treating shock:

1. Have the victim lie flat with his or her feet elevated approximately 8 to 12 inches. (In the case of chest injuries, difficulty breathing, or severe pain, elevate the victim's head slightly if there is no sign of spinal injury.)
2. Keep the victim warm. If possible, wrap him or her in blankets or other material. Keep the victim calm and reassured.
3. Seek medical help.

Electrical Shock

Do not touch a victim of electrical shock until the power source has been turned off. Approach the scene carefully, avoiding any live wires or electrical power lines. Pay attention to the following:

1. If the victim is holding onto the live electrical wire, do not remove it unless the power has been shut off at the plug, circuit breaker, or fuse box.
2. Check the victim's breathing and pulse. Electrical current can paralyze the nerves and muscles that control breath-

ing and heartbeat. If necessary, give mouth-to-mouth resuscitation. If there is no pulse, CPR might be necessary. (Remember that only trained people should perform CPR.)
3. Keep the victim warm, and treat for shock. Once the person is breathing and stable, seek medical help or send someone else for help.

Poisoning

Of the 1 million cases of poisoning reported in the United States each year, about 75 percent occur in children under age 5, and the majority are caused by household products. Most cases of poisoning involving adults are attempted suicides or attempted murders.

You should keep emergency telephone numbers for the poison control center and the local EMS close at hand. Many people keep these numbers on labels on their telephones. Check the front of your telephone book for these numbers. Be prepared to give the following information when calling for help:

- What was ingested? Have the container of the product and the remaining contents ready so you can describe it. Bring the container with you to the emergency room.
- When was the substance taken?
- How much was taken?
- Has vomiting occurred? If the person has vomited, save a sample to take to the hospital.
- Are there any other symptoms?
- How long will it take to get to the nearest emergency room?

When caring for a person who has ingested poison, keep these basic principles in mind:

1. Maintain an open airway. Make sure the person is breathing.
2. Call the local poison control center. Follow their advice for neutralizing the poison.
3. If the poison control center or another medical authority advises you to induce vomiting, then do so.
4. If a corrosive or caustic (that is, acid or alkali) substance was swallowed, immediately dilute it by having the victim drink at least one or two 8-ounce glasses of cold water or milk.
5. Place the victim on his or her left side. This position will delay advancement of the poison into the small intestine, where absorption into the victim's circulatory system occurs more quickly.

Injuries of Joints, Muscles, and Bones

Sprains   Sprains result when ligaments and other tissues around a joint are stretched or torn. Take the following steps to treat sprains:

1. Elevate the injured joint to a comfortable position.

2. Apply an ice pack or cold compress to reduce pain and swelling.

3. Wrap the joint firmly with a roller bandage.

4. Check the fingers or toes periodically to ensure that blood circulation has not been obstructed. If the bandage is too tight, loosen it.

5. Keep the injured area elevated, and continue ice treatment for 24 hours.

6. Apply heat to the injury after 48 hours if there is no further swelling.

7. If pain and swelling continue or if a fracture is suspected, seek medical attention.

Fractures Any deformity of an injured body part usually indicates a fracture. A fracture is any break in a bone, including chips, cracks, splinters, and complete breaks. Minor fractures (such as hairline cracks) might be difficult to detect and might be confused with sprains. If there is doubt, treat the injury as a fracture until X-ray films have been taken.

Do not move the victim if a fracture of the neck or back is suspected; this could result in a spinal cord injury. If the victim must be moved, apply splints to immobilize the fracture (and thereby to prevent further damage) and to decrease pain. Following are some basic steps for treating fractures and applying splints to broken limbs:

1. If the person is bleeding, apply direct pressure above the site of the wound.

2. If a broken bone is exposed, do not try to move it back into the wound. This can cause contamination and further injury.

3. Do not try to straighten out a broken limb. Splint the limb as it lies.

4. The following materials are needed for splinting:
   - *Splint:* wooden board, pillow, or rolled up magazines and newspapers.
   - *Padding:* towels, blankets, socks, or cloth.
   - *Ties:* cloth, rope, or tape.

5. Place splints and padding above and below the joint. Never put padding directly over the break. Padding should protect bony areas and the soft tissue of the limb.

6. Tie splints and padding into place.

7. Check the tightness of the splints periodically. Pay attention to the skin color, temperature, and pulse below the fracture to make sure the blood flow is adequate.

8. Elevate the fracture and apply ice packs to prevent swelling and reduce pain.

Head Injuries

A head injury can result from an auto accident, a fall, an assault, or a blow from a blunt object. All head injuries can potentially lead to brain damage, which may result in cessation of breathing and pulse.

For Minor Head Injuries

1. For a minor bump on the head resulting in a bruise without bleeding, apply ice to decrease the swelling.

2. If there is bleeding, apply even, moderate pressure. Do not use excessive pressure; the skull may be fractured.

3. Observe the victim for a change in consciousness. Observe the size of pupils, including whether both pupils are dilated to the same degree, and note signs of inability to think clearly. Check for any signs of numbness or paralysis. Allow the victim to sleep, but wake him or her periodically to check for awareness.

For Severe Head Injuries

1. If the victim is unconscious, check the airway for breathing. If necessary, perform mouth-to-mouth resuscitation.

2. If the victim is breathing, check the pulse. If it is less than 55 or more than 125 beats per minute, the victim may be in danger.

3. Check for bleeding. If fluid is flowing from the ears or nose, do not stop it.

4. Do not remove any objects embedded in the victim's skull.

5. Cover the victim with blankets to maintain body temperature, but guard against overheating.

6. Seek medical help as soon as possible.

Temperature-Related Emergencies

Frostbite Frostbite is damage to body tissues caused by intense cold. Frostbite generally occurs at temperatures below 32°F. The body parts most likely to suffer frostbite are the toes, ears, fingers, nose, and cheeks. When skin is exposed to the cold, ice crystals form beneath the skin. Avoid rubbing frostbitten tissue, because the ice crystals can scrape and break blood vessels. To treat frostbite, follow these steps:

1. Bring the victim to a health facility as soon as possible.

2. Cover and protect the frostbitten area. If possible, apply a steady source of external warmth, such as a warm compress. The victim should avoid walking if the feet are frostbitten.

3. If the victim cannot be transported, warm the body part by immersing it in warm water (100°F to 105°F). Continue to warm until the frostbitten area is warm to the touch when removed from the bath. Do not allow the body part to

touch the sides or bottom of the water container. After warming, dry the body part gently and wrap it in bandages to protect from refreezing.

Hypothermia

Hypothermia Hypothermia is a condition of generalized cooling of the body, resulting from exposure to cold temperatures or immersion in cold water. It can occur at any temperature below 65°F and can be made more severe by wind chill and moisture. The following are key symptoms of hypothermia:

- Shivering
- Vague, slow, slurred speech
- Poor judgment
- A cool abdomen
- Lethargy, or extreme exhaustion
- Slowed breathing and heartbeat
- Numbness and loss of feeling in extremities

After contacting the EMS, take the following steps:

1. Get the victim out of the cold.

2. Keep the victim in a flat position. Do not raise the legs.

3. Squeeze as much water as possible from wet clothing, and layer dry clothing over wet clothing. Removing the clothing may jostle the victim and lead to other problems.

4. Give the victim warm drinks only if he or she is able to swallow. Do not give the victim alcohol or caffeinated beverages, and do not allow the victim to smoke.

5. Do not allow the victim to exercise.

Heatstroke Heatstroke, the most serious heat-related disorder, results from the failure of the brain's heat-regulating mechanism (the hypothalamus) to cool the body. The following are signs and symptoms of heatstroke:

- Rapid pulse
- Hot, dry, flushed skin (absence of sweating)
- Disorientation leading to unconsciousness
- High body temperature

Reduce body temperature as quickly as possible. Immerse the victim in a cool bath, lake, or stream. If there is no water nearby, loosen clothing, and use a fan to help lower the victim's body temperature.

Heat Exhaustion Heat exhaustion results from excessive loss of salt and water. The onset is gradual, with the following symptoms:

- Fatigue and weakness
- Anxiety
- Nausea
- Profuse sweating and clammy skin
- Normal body temperature

Move the victim to a cool place. Have the victim lie down flat, with feet elevated 8 to 12 inches. Replace lost fluids slowly and steadily. Sponge or fan the victim.

Heat Cramps Heat cramps result from excessive sweating, leading to an excessive loss of salt and water. Although heat cramps are the least serious heat-related emergency, they are the most painful. The symptoms include muscle cramps, usually starting in the arms and legs. To relieve symptoms, the victim should drink electrolyte-rich beverages or a light salt-water solution or eat salty foods.

First Aid Supplies

Every home, car, or boat should be supplied with a basic first aid kit. This kit should be stored in a convenient place, but kept out of the reach of children. Following is a list of supplies that should be included:

- Bandages, including triangular bandages (36 inches by 6 inches), butterfly bandages, a roller bandage, rolled white gauze bandages (2- and 3-inch widths), adhesive bandages
- Sterile gauze pads and absorbent pads
- Adhesive tape (2- and 3-inch widths)
- Cotton-tipped applicators
- Scissors
- Thermometer
- Antibiotic ointment
- Aspirin
- Calamine lotion
- Antiseptic cream or petroleum jelly
- Safety pins
- Tweezers
- Latex gloves
- Flashlight
- Paper cups
- Blanket

You cannot be prepared for every medical emergency. Yet these essential tools and a knowledge of basic first aid will help you cope with many emergency situations.

Behavior Change Contract

Complete the Assess Yourself questionnaire, and read the Skills for Behavior Change box describing the stages of change. After reviewing your results and considering the various factors that influence your decisions, choose a health behavior that you would like to change, starting this quarter or semester (see other side for a sample filled-in contract). Sign the contract at the bottom to affirm your commitment to making a healthy change, and ask a friend to witness it.

My behavior change will be:

_____

My long-term goal for this behavior change is:

_____

These are three obstacles to change (things that I am currently doing or situations that contribute to this behavior or make it harder to change):

1. _____

2. _____

3. _____

The strategies I will use to overcome these obstacles are:

1. _____

2. _____

3. _____

Resources I will use to help me change this behavior include:

a friend/partner/relative: _____

a school-based resource: _____

a community-based resource: _____

a book or reputable website: _____

In order to make my goal more attainable, I have devised these short-term goals:

short-term goal _____ target date _____ reward _____

short-term goal _____ target date _____ reward _____

short-term goal _____ target date _____ reward _____

When I make the long-term behavior change described above, my reward will be:

_____ target date _____

I intend to make the behavior change described above. I will use the strategies and rewards to achieve the goals that will contribute to a healthy behavior change.

Signed: _____ Witness: _____

Sample Behavior Change Contract

Complete the Assess Yourself questionnaire, and read the Skills for Behavior Change box describing the stages of change. After reviewing your results and considering the various factors that influence your decisions, choose a health behavior that you would like to change, starting this quarter or semester (see other side for a sample filled-in contract). Sign the contract at the bottom to affirm your commitment to making a healthy change, and ask a friend to witness it.

My behavior change will be:

To snack less on junk food and more on healthy foods.

My long-term goal for this behavior change is:

Eat junk food snacks no more than once a week

These are three obstacles to change (things that I am currently doing or situations that contribute to this behavior or make it harder to change):

1. *The grocery store is closed by the time I come home from school.*
2. *I get hungry between classes, and the vending machines only carry candy bars.*
3. *It's easier to order pizza or other snacks than to make a snack at home.*

The strategies I will use to overcome these obstacles are:

1. *I'll leave early for school once a week so I can stock up on healthy snacks in the morning.*
2. *I'll bring a piece of fruit or other healthy snack to eat between classes.*
3. *I'll learn some easy recipes for snacks to make at home.*

Resources I will use to help me change this behavior include:

a friend/partner/relative: *my roommates: I'll ask them to buy healthier snacks instead of chips when they do the shopping.*

a school-based resource: *the dining hall: I'll ask the manager to provide healthy foods we can take to eat between classes.*

a community-based resource: *the library: I'll check out some cookbooks to find easy snack ideas*

a book or reputable website: *the USDA nutrient database at www.nal.usda.gov/fnic: I'll use this site to make sure the foods I select are healthy choices*

In order to make my goal more attainable, I have devised these short-term goals:

short-term goal *Eat a healthy snack 3 times per week*   target date *September 15*   reward *new CD*

short-term goal *Learn to make a healthy snack*   target date *October 15*   reward *Concert ticket*

short-term goal *Eat a healthy snack 5 times per week*   target date *November 15*   reward *new shoes*

When I make the long-term behavior change described above, my reward will be:

ski lift tickets for winter break   target date *December 15*

I intend to make the behavior change described above. I will use the strategies and rewards to achieve the goals that will contribute to a healthy behavior change.

Signed: *Elizabeth King*   Witness: **Susan Baner**

PHOTO CREDITS

Chapter 1   p. 1 Getty Images; p. 2 Corbis; p. 14 (left) Scott Barbour/ Allsport; p. 14 (right) Richard Price/Getty Images; p. 15 Kirsty Wigglesworth/ Associated Press, PAMPC PA; p. 17 Rick Friedman/Corbis; p. 20 Randy M. Ury/Corbis; p. 21 Roy Morsch/Corbis; p. 26 Masterfile.

Chapter 2   p. 31 RubberBall/SuperStock; p. 37 Timothy Shonnard/Getty Images; p. 40 Nancy Sheehan Photography; p. 43 Rob Melnychuk/Getty Images; p. 46 Randy Faris/Corbis; p. 49 Andrew Errington/Getty Images; p. 50 Lawrence Manning/Corbis; p. 52 Corbis.

Chapter 3   p. 61 Spike Mafford/Photodisc; p. 65 Corbis; p. 68 Reuters/ Corbis; p. 72 Daniel Garcia/AFP/Getty Images; p. 74 Leland Bobbe/Getty Images; p. 76 Ulrike Welsch/PhotoEdit; p. 82 Corbis; p. 85 Chuck Savage/ Corbis.

Chapter 4   p. 90 Joshua Sheldon/Getty Images; p. 96 AP Wide World Photos; p. 98 Bill Aron/PhotoEdit; p. 102 AP/Wide World Photos; p. 106 William Thomas Cain/Getty Images; p. 109 Jonathan White/ iStockphoto.

Chapter 5   p. 116 Stockbyte/Getty Images; p. 118 Jose Luis Pelaez/Corbis; p. 127 Purestock/Getty Images; p. 131 Bruce Ayres/Getty Images; p. 134 Scott Wintrow/Getty Images; p. 142 Hans Zimmermann/Das Fotoarchiv/ Peter Arnold.

Chapter 6   p. 151 Nancy R. Cohen/Getty Images; p. 156 Corbis; p. 157 Dorling Kindersley; p. 158 (top) (a) Jules Selmes and Debi Treloar/Dorling Kindersley; p. 158 (bottom) FemCap, Inc., and Alfred Shihata, MD; p. 159 (top) Joel Gordon Photography/Design Conceptions; p. 159 (bottom) Allendale Pharmaceuticals, Inc.; p. 160 (left) Jonnie Miles/Getty Images; p. 160 (right) Tom Pantages/Phototake; p. 161 Reuters NewMedia/Corbis; p. 162 Joel Gordon/Joel Gordon Photography; p. 167 AP Wide World Photos; p. 171 Leland Bobbe/Getty Images; p. 174 (a) Claude Edelman/Photo Researchers, (b) Petit Format-Nestle/Photo Researchers, (c) Petit Format-Nestle/Photo Researchers; p. 178 Photodisc.

Chapter 7   p. 186 Jamie Grill/Getty Images; p. 188 Mary Kate Denny/ PhotoEdit; p. 200 table (top to bottom) Garry Watson/Photo Researchers, Bill Aron/PhotoEdit, Michael Newman/PhotoEdit; p. 200 (bottom) SPL/ Photo Researchers; p. 204 (left) Charles Tatlock; p. 204 (right) AP Photo; p. 209 Luc Beziat/Getty Images; p. 211 Reuters/Corbis.

Chapter 8   p. 216 Leland Bobbe/Getty Images; p. 223 Chuck Savage/ Corbis; p. 225 Mark Peterson/Corbis; p. 226 (top) CNRI/SPL/Photo Researchers, (bottom) Martin M. Rotker/Photo Researchers; p. 233 Rayman/ Digital Vision/Getty Images; p. 235 Science Photo Library/Photo Researchers; p. 236 Oral Health America; p. 237 James Steveson/Photo Researchers.

Chapter 9   p. 250 Corbis; p. 251 Michael Keller/Corbis; p. 270 Peter Nicholson/Getty Images; p. 271 Photolibrary.com/Index Stock Imagery; p. 274 Brian Hagiwara/Foodpix; p. 278 Reg Charity/Corbis.

Chapter 10   p. 287 Comstock Images/Corbis; p. 290 Guang Niu/Corbis; p. 293 Life Measurement, Inc.; p. 300 (left) C Squared Studios/Photodisc, (right) James Noble/Corbis; p. 301 Photodisc/Getty Images; p. 305 (left) Girl Ray/Getty Images, (right) Image Source Pink/Getty Images; p. 312 APF/Liu Jin/Corbis; p. 313 Tammie Arroyo/AP Photo.

Chapter 11   p. 320 Stockbyte/Getty Images; p. 321 Neo Vision/Getty Images; p. 323 Photodisc/Getty Images; p. 324 Burke/Triolo Productions/ Foodpix/Jupiter Images; p. 328 (left to right) Dan Dalton/Getty Images, MIXA/Getty Images, Image Source Pink/Getty Images; p. 332 Nigel Reed/ Alamy; p. 333 Ryan McVay/age fotostock; p. 336 (a–f) Pearson Benjamin Cummings; p. 339 Thomas Northcut/Getty Images; p. 340 Bob Daemmrick/ The Image Works.

Chapter 12   p. 346 Ron Levine/Getty Images; p. 347 Mike Fiala/Corbis; p. 350 (a,b) Visuals Unlimited; p. 357 Chris Fotoman Smith/Alamy Images; p. 361 Donna Day/Stone/Getty Images; p. 373 Anthony Redpath/Corbis; p. 374 (a) James Stevenson/SPL/Photo Researchers, (b,c) P. Marazzi/SPL/ Photo Researchers; p. 377 Joel Saget/AFP Photo/Corbis.

Chapter 13   p. 383 ER Productions/Corbis; p. 390 (a) Gary Gaugler/ Photo Researchers, (b) Linda Stannard, UCT/Photo Researchers, (c) Eye of Science/Photo Researchers, (d) Dennis Kunkel/Phototake USA; p. 402 SPL/ Photo Researchers; p. 403 (a) Steven N. Nussenblatt/Custom Medical Stock Photo, (b) ISM/Phototake; p. 404 P. Marazzi/Science Photo Library/Photo Researchers; p. 406 Steve Hamblin/Alamy; p. 407 Stonehill/zefa/Corbis; p. 409 Nick Ut/AP Photo.

Chapter 14   p. 420 Jim Naughten/Taxi/Getty Images; p. 422 (top, left to right) Fred Prouser/Corbis, Phil McCarten/Reuters/Corbis, Nancy Kaszerman/Corbis; p. 422 (bottom) Image Source/Getty Images; p. 428 John Henley/Corbis; p. 435 Mark Richards/PhotoEdit; p. 436 Chris Harvey/ Getty Images.

Chapter 15   p. 442 Comstock Images/Corbis; p. 446 Richard L'Anson/ Lonely Planet Images/Getty Images; p. 448 Jon Arnold/age fotostock; p. 452 ENERGY STAR; p. 455 Dan Atkin/Alamy.

Chapter 16   p. 463 Stockbyte/Getty Images; p. 464 Jim Sulley/The Image Works; p. 465 Peter Scholey/Getty Images; p. 469 SuperStock; p. 472 Inspirestock/age fotostock; p. 475 A. Ramey/PhotoEdit.

Chapter 17   p. 481 Photodisc/Getty Images; p. 485 Novastock/The Stock Connection; p. 487 Bananastock/Jupiter Images; p. 488 Willie Hill, Jr./The Image Works; p. 489 Plush Studios/Blend Images/Jupiter Images; p. 490 Michael Newman/PhotoEdit; p. 492 Koki Iino/MIXA/Getty Images.

INDEX

Page references followed by *fig* indicate an illustrated figure; followed by *t* indicate a table; followed by *p* indicate a photograph.